Women and Health Series

Women's Health

Complexities and Differences

Edited by

SHERYL BURT RUZEK,

VIRGINIA L. OLESEN,

ADELE E. CLARKE

OHIO STATE UNIVERSITY PRESS

Columbus

Library of Congress Cataloging-in-Publication Data

Women's health : complexities and differences / edited by Sheryl Burt
Ruzek, Virginia L. Olesen, Adele E. Clarke.
    p.   cm. — (Women and health series)
    Includes bibliographical references and index.
    ISBN 0-8142-0704-9 (cloth : alk. paper). — ISBN 0-8142-0705-7
(paper : alk. paper)
    1. Women—Health and hygiene. 2. Women—Medical care. I. Ruzek,
Sheryl Burt. II. Olesen, Virginia L.   III. Clarke, Adele E.
IV. Series: Women & health (Columbus, Ohio)
    RA564.85W66686   1997
613'.04244—dc20   96-34047
                                                               CIP

Text and cover design by Donna Hartwick.
Cover illustration by Jim Griesemer, from photos by Nancy Stoller.
Type set in Goudy by Inari Information Services, Bloomington, Indiana.
Printed by Edwards Brothers, Ann Arbor, Michigan.

9 8 7 6 5 4 3 2 1

We dedicate this book to women who have struggled in the past, in the present, and who will surely do so in the future to improve women's health in diverse communities and in clinical, academic, educational, and policy arenas. We particularly note the women who participated in our Women, Health and Healing Institutes. They taught us and each other much and inspired and encouraged us to complete this book.

Contents

vii

Foreword

HELEN RODRIGUEZ-TRIAS

Reading this landmark book on women's health before its publication was a rare privilege. Exquisitely scholarly, immensely readable, and provocative, this work by women does more than break new ground. Taking us beyond a critique of existing biomedical frameworks of women's health, the authors create totally new territories of consciousness that place women's health solidly in the context of the complexities that define women's diverse lives.

As women sociologists, Ruzek, Olesen, and Clarke have long understood that gender and the great divides of race and class determine our unequal access to health. They propose that to understand how complex, interacting, and overlapping factors affect women and their health, we must first listen to the women themselves.

Starting with the intent of bringing their rich experiences and viewpoints to the ambitious task of collecting source readings in women's health for students and teachers, the editors produced a much larger body of work. What they have accomplished is an outstanding text that is certain to shape future directions for many years. *Women's Health: Complexities and Differences* is a major contribution that for the first time brings together writers who represent and understand the diverse communities of whom they speak. The editors succeeded in gathering distinguished contributors from the ranks of women of color, lesbians, women with disabilities, from rural communities and from aging and other underrepresented and underserved groups. They chose writers whose voices are those of scholars—but scholars who have lived the experiences that they distill into their analyses.

The writers speak with diverse voices, but mostly they share a common connection. Nearly all derive their experiences from participation in the vital, dynamic movement that we recognize as a women's health movement. But, as the editors note in the preface, it took a quarter century of struggles, studies, publications, teaching and learning, organizing, discussion, and disagreement to create and mature a women's health movement that is now beginning to recognize diversities as sources of strength.

Some of my experiences in the women's health movement of the mid-1970s, when the focus was mainly on abortion and other reproductive health issues, illustrate a few of many lessons that the authors of this valuable volume so thoroughly document. In the early years at conferences and other gatherings, it was difficult for black and Latina women to find white women who understood our particular experiences. At that time, in those settings, Native American, Asian, aging, low-income women, and those from rural and other marginated communities were not yet visible, much less vocal. Whereas many white, middle-class women spoke of their individual rights to safe and legal abortions, natural childbirth, and information from their physicians, women of color spoke of their communities' concerns: coercion in sterilization and family planning and their need for jobs, education, and dignity. For many years the struggles for reproductive rights were hampered by disunity and lack of a common agenda. Working through years of painful debates and frequent misunderstandings, white women and women of color were finally able to engage in more productive dialogue. Since then, women of color have created their own advocacy organizations, advancing agendas that respond to the aspirations and priorities of their communities and educating all of us on their issues as well.

The chapters on the dynamics of diversity give us an excellent overview of the leaders and organizations who continue to advance the dialogue among diverse groups of women. We are still learning to provide safe spaces for our discussions and to listen to each other with creativity. We are still learning that to work on commonalities we first have to be clear on the differences. We are still learning, as our sisters living with HIV so poignantly teach us, that only those who live the realities can guide us to their understanding. For solutions to problems that women face, women facing them must define the agenda.

As I continued to read on culture and complexities, I found several authors with whom I have been privileged to work in advocacy and other organizations. I was struck by the hard work women do that they so generously share and how valuable it is to women who are struggling to find their own voices. I recalled an early experience in such sharing that illustrates its immeasurable value. It was how I first learned of Sheryl's work and how much her history of the women's movement (Ruzek 1978) helped me in my own. In 1982, I was a busy pediatrician, running an ambulatory care program, balancing my responsibilities as a single mother, teacher, administrator, and clinician with as much grace as I could rally. Ruth and Victor Sidel, much published writers on health and social issues, were editing a book on the lessons of the struggles to reform medicine, and they asked me to contribute a chapter on the women's health movement (Rodriguez-Trias 1984). Realizing the jam I had gotten into, I called Barbara Seaman, a writer whose groundbreaking books (1969, 1977a, 1977b) had helped launch the women's health movement. Graciously, she lent me her copy of Sheryl's book. I remain eternally grateful to Sheryl for creating a lucid, thoroughly researched analysis that helped frame my contribution. I remain equally grateful to Barbara for her own work and for introducing me to Sheryl's.

Not surprisingly, health care reform is still out of reach in the nineties. The chapters on health care challenge us to become active protagonists in shaping a system that will provide quality care for all. To do so, we need to enter new fields and gain new competencies in health care management and financing, among others. We must also create the institutional norms that will require and welcome participation from women in planning services and assuring accountability.

Out of our political experiences as part of a movement, we are learning to look for systemic solutions to common problems. For instance, we may not yet agree on what the systemic solutions should be to health care reform, but we do agree that small incremental approaches will leave most women out, and that is not acceptable.

I found reading the discussions on power particularly timely as we debate a reduction in public supports that is sure to worsen the lives of countless women and children who are among the least powerful in our society. The authors clearly advance the notion that without social and economic policies to reduce inequities for all marginated groups, we will inevitably widen the gaps in health status among diverse groups of women. Our challenges and choices, as the authors persuasively argue, must hinge on our commitment to struggles for equity.

It is heartening to find that women who navigated the long and difficult trajectory of twenty-five years in the women's health movement have made this great contribution to guide our continuing journey. I know it will inspire readers to continue finding the strengths in our differences and to seek commonalities that will help define our vision for a healthier future. Thank you, dear sisters.

REFERENCES

Rodriguez-Trias, Helen
    1984   "The women's health movement: women take power." Pp. 106–26 in Victor and Ruth Sidel (eds.), Reforming Medicine. New York: Pantheon.
Ruzek, Sheryl Burt
    1978   The Women's Health Movement: Feminist Alternatives to Medical Control. New York: Praeger.
Seaman, Barbara
    1969   The Doctor's Case against the Pill. New York: Avon.
    1977a   Free and Female. New York: Fawcett.
Seaman, Barbara, and Gideon Seaman
    1977b   Women and the Crisis in Sex Hormones. New York: Rawson.

Preface

The day this volume appears will be a most celebrated one by its editors, for in some ways it has been gestating in each of our lives for about twenty-five years. Each of us has studied and taught as sociologists in women's health for about that long. Each of us has yearned for a volume like this for ourselves and our students. And for each of us, bringing it to fruition has been as arduous as it has been fascinating, depressing, worthwhile, and exciting.

Initially we planned this volume to meet a need identified by participants in the three Women, Health, and Healing Summer Institutes that we directed in Berkeley in 1984–86. Those programs, all supported by a grant from the U.S. Fund for the Improvement of Post-Secondary Education (FIPSE), were designed to improve teaching of the social and behavioral aspects of women's health in colleges, universities, and professional schools. A large portion of those sessions focused on the particular experiences and needs of women of color, women who were stigmatized, women who did not fit the "usual white mold."

We discovered that many scholars teach in institutions that have such heavy teaching schedules and limited library resources that assembling course materials largely from current journals and books is just not feasible. In addition, many participants had expertise in one specialized area of women's health, but they were unfamiliar with broader social and cultural issues. What these colleagues sought were books for themselves and their students that addressed key women's health issues within a larger framework of concepts that give coherence to the focus on women's health issues.

Many volumes on women's health that were composed of original research in the social sciences lacked integrating concepts or cohesion, or they were too narrowly specified for our participants' purposes. Textbooks tended to focus primarily on clinical issues for a particular specialty or discipline. "How-to" books were largely informational rather than analyt-ical. Because courses on women's health are being taught in a wide array of college and university settings, what was needed was something beyond what Adele Clarke affectionately calls the "plumbing and politics" of women's health.

In follow-up evaluations, teachers told us that they actually used materials relating to racial, ethnic, and cultural diversities in women's health. We wrote and edited this volume to provide what our colleagues needed for their own classrooms. As we discuss in chapter 3, understand-ing differences in women's health is a critical "next step" in feminist scholarship and in public policy.

Why, one might ask, are three white, middle-class women so com-mitted to this endeavor? And how did we move beyond our particular-istic views of the world to undertake this project? Our individual and collective professional journeys led us to this point together. We agree with the view that members of racial, ethnic, or cultural minority groups should not be expected to take full responsibility for educating majority groups about the needs and perspectives of diverse social and cultural communities. This must be a responsibility shared with many who are willing to make the considerable effort required. Our contributors were specifically urged to address differences among women in each of the chapters, not leaving the health of women of color or other differently situated women to appear only in separate chapters. Persons who belong to subcultures are likely to have insights that outsiders rarely can achieve. So we asked many women to contribute to this volume because of their own lived experiences and special knowledge derived from their involvements in diverse communities.

Our primary work as editors has been to articulate the overall mission of the volume, to sketch out critical issues to consider in consultation with others, and to link diverse perspectives and bodies of information to-gether. Our goal then is to explore, in collaboration with other contribu-tors, complexities and differences *within* as well as *between* groups of women who live in many different Americas. That is, although we focus on the experiences of women in the United States, we see many different lived worlds—worlds that are shaped by differences in ethnicity, race, class, sexualities, disabilities, and regional experiences and opportunities for health. To understand the health situations of women in the United States, many voices need to be heard and understood. We disagree that this "balkanizes" us. Rather, it is the necessary first step we must take together on the long path toward discovering our real commonalities and genuinely appreciating and respecting our differences.

Our personal paths to this point are varied yet bear certain similarities. We share them with you here to give a better sense of how we have come to undertake this work collectively. Virginia Olesen began working in the area of women's health in the late 1960s. She began with a major study in socialization and career issues of student nurses—usually women and usually highly committed to health care. Her work has since expanded to include women clerical workers, estrogen replacement therapy, the tampon alert, issues of women and the body, and health policies.

Sheryl Ruzek's interests in medical sociology, social movements, and social stratification developed in the late 1960s when race and class, but not gender, were considered important dimensions of analysis. Her interest in health movements, particularly the mental hygiene movement of the Progressive Era and alternative health movements in both the late nineteenth and mid-twentieth centuries, gave her conceptual tools with which to understand conflicts and contradictions within the then emerging women's health movement—especially conflicts grounded in race and class divisions. Her work on medical technology assessment, risk communication, and public health policy in maternal and child health have broadened that perspective.

Like many others in the women's health movement, Adele Clarke's interest stems from a personal experience—when she was hospitalized for kidney problems likely induced by the Pill. She first taught a course on historical perspectives on women's health in 1973 and had generated a syllabus so close to one that Sheryl Ruzek had developed that when they met and compared notes in 1980, there was a deep recognition of scholarly and political sisterhood. Adele has gone on to do research on the emergence of American reproductive sciences, contraception, sterilization abuse, RU-486, the Pap smear, and related topics in gender and social studies of science and technology.

Individually, we have spent over a quarter century addressing many of the issues we present here. We have worked together in various ways since the early 1970s. Virginia Olesen taught one of the first university-based courses on women's health in 1973. Sheryl Ruzek, who was studying volunteer health workers, sat in on some of those sessions. When Virginia Olesen convened a conference in 1975, "Women's Health: Research for a New Era," Sheryl Ruzek presented her early research on gynecological self-help, and Adele Clarke was in the audience.

Along with Ellen Lewin, Virginia and Sheryl founded the Women, Health, and Healing Program (WHHP) in 1982 at the University of California at San Francisco. In 1985, Adele Clarke, who had taught women's health and women's studies at Sonoma State University, became a codirector of the WHHP, which offers a specialty in women's health in the doctoral program in sociology.

We have shared many hours laboring to understand what is important and what constitutes health and healing from women's multiple perspectives. Individually and collectively, we have involved ourselves in women's health research, advocacy, and public service and have had the privilege of working closely with many of this book's contributors. This volume represents a culmination of these efforts and our commitments to share with others our evolving understanding.

All books have histories, and the trajectories of edited volumes such as this often are as rich and dense as the volume itself. Part of this wealth is the assistance rendered by almost countless others. We would like to acknowledge a number of people for special assistance of various kinds:

First we acknowledge the participants of the Women Health and Healing Institutes who inspired and encouraged us to create a volume that would reflect their needs. We hope it does. We also thank FIPSE for funding those institutes and giving us a subsequent grant to distribute teaching materials and bibliographical resources on women's health. Our FIPSE program officer, Felicia Lynch, was very helpful. Through the FIPSE project directors' meetings we met Lynn Weber, Bonnie Thornton Dill, and Elizabeth Higginbotham, who have each served as director of the Center for Research on Women at the University of Memphis. They included many materials that we collected in their FIPSE-supported database on "Women of Color and Southern Women." Patricia Anderson and Kristin Hill provided particularly able assistance with the summer institutes and preparation of the curricular materials. Anne Wilson in her consultation on development and fund-raising knowledgeably guided us in an area unknown to us.

Our students in sociology, anthropology, nursing, and public health shaped our thinking and often prompted us to rethink issues in new ways, as did our colleagues who lectured at our summer institutes. Many colleagues read and reread early outlines and drafts and gave us valuable comments for which we are truly grateful. We particularly wish to acknowledge the conceptual contributions of Lynn Weber and Elizabeth Higginbotham, who helped us sketch out what to include in this volume.

Many of our colleagues, friends, and families graciously answered calls for conceptual and editorial advice. Susan Reverby, Jane Zones, Sue Rosser, Anne Kasper, JoAnne Fischer, Diane Depken, Alice Hausman, the late Irving Zola, Andrea Kovach, Mira Katz, Lauren Coodley, and Jennifer Ruzek all read and talked through difficult issues in various parts of the manuscript. Jim Griesemer, who patiently lived through the writing of this book, designed the quilt for the cover and section pages. Nancy Stoller generously provided him with some photographs to incorporate into the images. We have also enjoyed working with each of the contributors, sharing ideas on how to make this volume readable and accessible across a wide range of disciplines.

The Department of Social and Behavioral Sciences, School of Nursing, UCSF, over many years generously provided support for new classes and preparation of the FIPSE grants. This department also provided the academic and intellectual freedom to move into new areas and explore new ideas. Temple University provided Sheryl Ruzek with a research and study leave in the spring of 1994 to work on the project. Patricia Legos, chairperson of the Department of Health Education, deserves particular thanks for her support of this work. Sarah Bauerle Bass ably coordinated preparation of the final manuscript.

We thank Janet Golden and Rima Apple, the Women's Health Series editors, for their enthusiasm and encouragement to complete this book. They, along with Charlotte Dihoff and Ellen Satrom, our editors at Ohio State University Press, provided excellent guidance at every stage of the process. Many people's invisible work turns manuscripts into books. We thank them all, particularly Elaine Durham Otto for careful copyediting and Martin White for preparing the index.

In the end, no volume of this sort is ever "finished." The issues are too broad, too far-ranging, too complex and changing too rapidly to bring closure on the topics we and the contributors address. We can only share with others where we have come on a long journey to understand the complexities and differences of women's health. We hope that we have advanced our collective understandings of women's health and that others will extend them further.

[PART I]

What Is Women's Health?

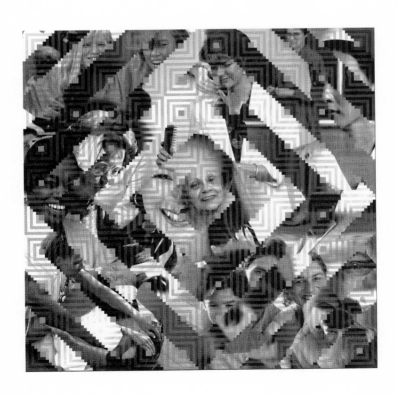

Is women's health the absence of disease, or is it something more? How do we think about our own health and that of other women? Do national agendas for women's health frame the issues in terms of disease prevention, treatment, health promotion, or improvements in living and working conditions? What are the consequences of thinking about women's health in each of these ways?

In this volume we focus on some of the social and behavioral aspects of women's health. In taking this approach, we underscore the importance of understanding the complexities and differences in women's health and life situations, not just the shared characteristics of female organ systems. We attempt to go beyond illnesses and diseases common or particularly important to women. We also seek to go beyond "plumbing and politics," early feminist efforts to teach women how our bodies work and how women's bodies are subject to social control in health and healing systems. While each of these issues is important in its own right, many other aspects of women's health deserve attention. In our view, understanding the diversity of women's health needs, and the complexities of meeting those needs, must be addressed in the social contexts of women's lives.

We are at a critical juncture in understanding and addressing women's health. Over two decades of women's health activism and research in many arenas have "paid off." A record number of women are now in key roles in the health professions, government, and the academy. At the national level, many advocacy organizations provide women with a voice in health matters. The bipartisan congressional Commission on Women's Issues forced the National Institutes of Health (NIH) to address women's health research more adequately. Dr. Bernadine Healy, named to head the NIH in 1991, made a commitment to undertake the Women's Health

3

Initiative the following year. The Women's Health Initiative, the largest study of health interventions and outcomes ever undertaken by NIH, has recruited women from diverse racial/ethnic backgrounds and geographic locations. This and other research efforts, discussed in part 7 of this volume, may provide important information for improving women's health. Overall, women's health research and policy have emerged as national issues.

Along with contributors to this volume, we recognize the importance of clinical advances in women's health. However, we also see a need to broaden awareness of the multiplicity of issues beyond the biomedical domain that too often and too narrowly is taken to constitute women's health studies. A biomedical research agenda is only part of what has been achieved—and needs to be achieved—in women's health research, public policy, and practice. We direct attention here to some of the broader social contexts in which diverse women's health experiences and opportunities must be addressed.

How is women's health conceptualized differently by women in different life circumstances, who occupy different places in society? Scientists, health care providers, insurers, and health advocacy groups all press diverse agendas for improving women's health. But what does "improving women's health" mean? What should such an endeavor include and exclude? These questions are not easy to answer. Taking a historical perspective, we are struck by the complexities and differences in focus and priority that women themselves demonstrate in their daily health practices, their health-seeking behavior, their use of health and healing resources, and their advocacy efforts.

Various models are used to understand health and illness. In biomedical models, analysis focuses on biochemical processes in organ systems, in cells, or increasingly in genes. Social models focus on the values, beliefs, and behaviors of individuals and groups and on psychological processes, social relationships, institutions, and systems of social stratification. Emerging models in mind-body medicine emphasize the role of psychological processes, values, and beliefs in human physiological processes. Epidemiological models can include biomedical, social, psychological, and behavioral variables in studies of the etiology and distribution of disease. Historical approaches to understanding women's health describe and analyze how health beliefs, practices, and social institutions develop in particular times and places—and predictably change over time. Each of these models and analytical approaches is important for understanding one or another dimension of women's health. The burgeoning interest in women's health has brought forth a plethora of scholarship in nursing, medicine, psychology, and related fields that address the clinical and bio-medical aspects of women's health. Historical analysis has documented the malleability—and the fallibility—of both social and scientific views about women's health.

A quick trip to the "women's health section" of any good-sized book-store or a pass through health magazines such as *Prevention* or *Health Quest* reveal a dizzying array of what constitutes "women's health." In academic circles, issues of genetic engineering, infertility treatment, and manipula-tive reproductive technologies evoke heated debate. In the ranks of the National Black Women's Health Project, attention is drawn to gaining access to Medicaid-funded abortions for low-income women, stemming community violence, and adopting positive health practices. "Sandwich generation" women are simultaneously concerned with caregiving facili-ties for their children and for their aging parents, particularly for their mothers who are most likely to live to need supportive services in old age. Some women pursue alternatives to conventional western medicine—in traditional healing practices such as midwifery, herbal therapy, naturopa-thy, homeopathy, chiropractic, or mind-body medicine. Manufacturers of drugs, medical devices, health and fitness equipment, and a dizzying array of products all clamor to show women how using their products will improve their health. Sorting out scientific evidence from snake oil be-comes increasingly difficult as health services become commodities to be bought and sold and to provide stockholders with a good return on their investments.

This layering of exciting and disquieting trends in health and heal-ing reveals a society increasingly anxious and uncertain about how to "produce health," not just for women but for everyone. What has not yet emerged, but is needed, is adequate public dialogue about the social production of health in a society that is divided by race, social class, gender, and growing religious and other forms of intolerance. Women, however, have taken the lead in questioning, organizing, and demanding that the experience of health and illness, of caring, curing, and healing be discussed in new ways. Because women's roles in health and healing are central and affect the lives of their families and communities, what happens in women's health has broad social implications. Health, as a cherished social value, evokes strong sentiments and contributes to cul-tural clashes.

We begin our exploration of what constitutes women's health by considering how social and biomedical models of women's health differ in focus as do traditional healing and emerging mind-body paradigms. Social and cultural beliefs about curing and caring are deeply embedded in these sometimes complementary but often contradictory conceptualizations of health.

The editors and contributors to this volume seek to underscore the importance of conceptualizing health in a broad framework of social relationships and institutions, not simply in terms of diseases or disorders. Many contributors highlight the need to view women's health as embedded in the communities of which women are a part. In our view, women's experiences of health and illness involve mind, body, spirit, social relationships, and working and living conditions. Thus, we argue that it is time to move beyond narrow conceptualizations of health that separate women's health from our roles, responsibilities, and statuses in families, communities, and societies.

Why is women's health so seldom framed this way? Perhaps because biomedical dimensions of women's health are fairly safe and minimally threatening to consider. Who could disagree that cancers, heart diseases, or viruses are "bad" or that women's health would be improved if these could be eliminated or at least substantially reduced? This comfortable but partial view of women's health skirts uncomfortable issues about how health is socially, politically, and economically produced in contemporary society—or how it might be produced differently were we to envision it differently.

In part 1 we explore some of the complexities and differences in women's health that reflect social and cultural as well as biological factors. In chapter 1 we pose questions about how biomedical models differ from social and feminist models of health. Throughout we focus on diversity. Urban, suburban, rural, or reservation residence, country of origin, tribe, social class, language, culture, religion, and length of time in the United States all affect women's health. So do the women's deeply felt parts of self and social identities—religious beliefs, sexual orientations, disabilities, and other identifications.

Many women identify themselves as members of particular racial/ethnic groups; some women see themselves as multiracial.[1] We emphasize here that classification of people into racial/ethnic groups is a social, not a biological, phenomenon. Racial/ethnic identification changes over time. The terminology used to describe racial/ethnic groups generates conflicts and controversies. We note a few of these complexities to illustrate how imprecise, dynamic, and changeable racial designations are at any time.

In official health statistics, Native American women include American Indians and Alaskan Natives (Eskimos and Aleuts), but many women self-identify by specific tribe. The term *Hispanic* refers to Spanish-surnamed or Spanish-speaking residents of the United States and is used in most health statistics.[2] Increasingly national data differentiate "persons of Hispanic origin" by black and white. Terms such as *Latino/Latina*, however, are more often used by people when they describe themselves. Some women refer to themselves as *Chicanas*. Although the term *African American* is commonly used, many women describe themselves as *black*, and many health statistics retain this term. *Asian and Pacific Islanders*, the designation used in official health statistics, refers to both Asian subgroups (e.g., Chinese, Japanese, Filipino, Korean, Vietnamese, Cambodian) and Pacific Islanders (e.g., native Hawaiians, Samoans, Guamanians, Tongans).

We believe that, in daily life, individuals are more likely to see themselves as members of specific racial/ethnic or cultural groups than as members of such broad categories as Asians, Pacific Islanders, or Hispanics. Some women identify (at least at times) with others as women of color, a category that largely separates minorities from dominant group members in the United States. Women who are considered part of the dominant group of whites are least likely to think of themselves in racial/ethnic terms.[3] Few designate themselves as *Euro Americans*, although this terminology is gaining some adherents.

How to characterize mixed racial/ethnic identity grows in social and political importance, as the following story illustrates:

> A few days after Hannah Spangler started the first grade . . . she brought home a school survey form that her mother had difficulty filling out. The form asked parents to check off the race of the child. The choices were (1) white, (2) black, (3) Indian, Eskimo, or Aleut, or (4) Asian or Pacific Islander. The problem? Hannah fits none of these categories. Her father is white. On her mother's side, her grandfather is black and her grandmother is Japanese. "I just checked off all of them," laughs Hannah's mother, Rika Clark, "black, white, and oriental. No one has ever called me up to say, 'Hey, what does *this* mean?'" (Kalish 1995:1)[4]

Because of the complexity of issues involved in the naming of racial/ethnic groups, as editors we have encouraged authors to use terms that seem most appropriate in the context of their own work and perspectives. When citing national health statistics, the terminology used in the original source is generally retained. In chapter 2, Deborah Wingard elaborates on some additional issues in the use of racial/ethnic classifications in national health statistics.

Taken together, the papers in this volume ground our thinking in the specific conditions and experiences of women. They thereby demonstrate how difficult and dangerous it is to generalize about the health or health needs of women without reference to which women and where they are situated in a specific historical period. We deliberately, if reluctantly, limited the scope of this book to women in the United States. We leave global issues in women's health to others expert in these complex arenas. The complexities and differences in women's health in a multicultural society that has not adequately addressed equity in access to medical care, let alone access to working and living conditions that promote health, could alone fill several volumes. We make no claims about being all-inclusive. We emphasize such themes and concepts as intersections of race, class and culture, social control, and women's agency in order to guide readers to a range of issues that affect the health of specific women in particular times and places. We hope that the essays contained here will encourage readers to ask how these women's health issues play out in distinct ways in their own lives and communities.

NOTES

1. There are a growing number of books on racial/ethnic identity. See, for example, Featherstone (1994), Frankenberg (1993), and Zack (1993).

2. Controversies continue about how to classify Hispanic-origin people. See, for example, Zimmerman et al. (1994) for a particularly insightful discussion of the issue of when self-identification is an appropriate inclusionary or exclusionary criterion.

3. Frankenberg raises important questions about the emptiness and meaninglessness of whiteness as a cultural identity. She also points out that "those who are securely housed within its borders usually do not examine it" (1993:228).

4. The question of racial identity is becoming more complex. Between 1978 and 1992, interracial births rose sharply for almost every possible combination and now constitute 3.9 percent of all births. Advocacy groups for multiracial individuals and families are pushing to have the year 2000 Census include a multiracial category. Minority groups could be affected by this in both congressional redistricting and federal program benefits (Kalish 1995).

REFERENCES

Featherstone, Elena
  1994   Skin Deep: Women Writing on Color, Culture, and Identity. Freedom,
          CA: Crossing Press.
Frankenberg, Ruth
  1993   White Women, Race Matters: The Social Construction of Whiteness.
          Minneapolis: University of Minnesota Press.
Kalish, Susan
  1995   "Multiracial births increase as U.S. ponders racial definitions." Popula-
          tion Today 23(4):1-2.
Zack, Naomi
  1993   Race and Mixed Race. Philadelphia: Temple University Press.
Zimmerman, Rick S., William A. Vega, Andres G. Gil, George J. Warheit, Eleni
Apospori, and Frank Biafora
  1994   "Who is Hispanic? definitions and their consequences." American Jour-
          nal of Public Health 84:1985-87.

[1]

Social, Biomedical, and Feminist
Models of Women's Health

SHERYL BURT RUZEK, ADELE E. CLARKE,
AND VIRGINIA L. OLESEN

Integrated models of women's health address the contributions of socially and culturally constructed concepts of caring and curing as well as health practices, medical care, and social investments in the prerequisites for health. These conceptualizations of health differ radically from narrow biomedical models that only acknowledge prevention, detection, and treatment of disease.

What Is Women's Health?

Health activists' quarter century of struggle to place women's health on the national agenda has been partly realized as evidenced by growing attention to women's health issues in many arenas. However, despite the high level of interest, what constitutes this field remains poorly defined. In search of a paradigm, Margaret Chesney and Elizabeth Ozer (1995:4-5) have proposed a framework to organize and "integrate competing approaches to the field of women's health." Their model includes seven content areas: reproductive health, diseases more common in women than men, leading causes of death among women, gender influences on health risk, societal influences on women's health (norms, roles, and poverty), violence against women, and women and health care policy. Although Chesney and Ozer urge attention to the distinct contributions of conceptual models in anthropology, sociology, psychology, and medicine (as well as the variety of research processes and methods used in health research), they do not compare conceptual approaches. We share their desire for new paradigms. "Laundry lists" of health issues are not enough. But where do we start?

In our view, a first step is to recognize how research and public policy have been predominantly biomedical—focusing on a limited range of diseases and conditions taken out of the context of women's daily lives and felt needs. From a biomedical perspective, health is the absence of disease and infirmity. In contrast, the World Health Organization (WHO) has defined health broadly, within a social rather than biomedical frame, for nearly half a century. For WHO, health is a "state of complete physical, mental, and social well-being and not merely the absence of disease or infirmity." However, this broad social model of health has not been used often in the United States to shape research and policy.[1]

We believe that it is useful to contrast some fundamental differences between biomedical and social models of women's health. Feminist models, which spurred national interest in women's health over the past three decades, are themselves inherently social and thus discussed within that framework. We also note the emergence of mind-body models both within and separate from biomedicine. These models emphasize psychological and spiritual dimensions of health that are less often included in discussions of women's health. All conceptualizations of health are dynamic and changing. The breadth and depth of work on women's health that researchers, clinicians, and health advocacy groups have produced over the past three decades have laid the groundwork for new ways of thinking about what actually produces health, not only for women but for families and communities.

As the complexities and differences in women's health take center stage, as they do throughout this book, referring back to underlying conceptual models will help put the various dimensions of health and healing into clearer perspective. Sociologists have long argued that the whole is always more than the sum of its parts. To comprehend the whole of any woman's health or all women's health, it is essential to recognize how partial each of the parts is likely to be. All of us are more than an aggregation of body parts, cells, social actions, or social statuses. No single or singular view of women's health will adequately reflect the complexities of women's lives, although dominant biomedical models are often taken to represent "all" of women's health.

Our critique of biomedical models that dominate thinking about health in the United States is not intended to discount or leave unacknowledged the very real contributions of many individuals who have worked long and hard to change biomedicine to better meet women's needs. What we are suggesting here is that dominant biomedical conceptualizations of health, with their narrow disease-focus, inadequately represent health because they leave out, or only nominally consider, the social forces and contexts that shape women's health and women's lives.

A distinctly social focus is also absent in some, although not all, of the emerging mind-body models. In addition, models that generalize about the needs or nature of disease processes in "all women" ignore the very fundamental differences in what different women need—and how they are likely to respond to medical care.

Within biomedicine, feminist perspectives have spurred recognition of how gender affects the etiology, natural history, and treatment of disease. Results include recent policy changes that ensure inclusion of women in clinical trials and all aspects of biomedical science (discussed in chapter 21). Efforts to incorporate recent research on psychosocial factors in the etiology of disease and gender-related health practices in the use of medical services broaden the biomedical model.[2] But in our view these efforts, no matter how useful, do not adequately represent health. Although these models may recognize social and behavioral dimensions of health, they do so largely within the framework of clinical practice issues. The underlying social dynamics of what actually *produces* health for different groups of women are not integral to biomedical models.[3]

Why Women's Health Needs to Be Reconceptualized

In our view, models of health that reflect the social, not just the biological, dimensions of health and illness must emerge to make space for understanding differences in what women want and need to realize the vision of health set forth by the WHO. These models also need to incorporate psychological and spiritual dimensions of health and healing that have particular significance to women who see these as contributing to their ability to resist and recover from illness.

At the national level, partial and incomplete views of what "needs to be done" to promote women's health are gaining momentum—largely in calls for more biomedical research and wider access to medical services. Although medical care contributes to women's health and well-being, its importance should not be overstated or accepted uncritically. To move beyond a narrow disease-focused model of women's health, we might start by rethinking where health is located.

If we conceptualize women's health as *embedded in communities*, not just in women's individual bodies, we lay a foundation for envisioning very different models of women's health from those that now predominate. Attention to the broader base of what actually *produces* health (as contrasted with managing disease) suggests that social investments in a variety of areas are necessary to promote women's health.[4] When we look closely at the variations in women's health statuses and experiences, the need for doing this becomes clear.

Some Social Features of Health

To conceptualize broader models of health, it is useful to consider what the WHO describes as the prerequisites for health: freedom from the fear of war; equal opportunity for all; satisfaction of basic needs for food, water, and sanitation; education; decent housing; secure work and a useful role in society; and political will and public support.[5]

Each of these prerequisites for health is stated in gender-neutral language, yet access to these prerequisites is shaped by gender as well as social class and many social and cultural factors. For example, the threat of war reduces women's health not only directly through the threat of death, rape, or destruction of working and living conditions but indirectly through emotional stress related to the survival and safety of communities and family members and the disruption of education. Equal opportunity implies elimination of inequalities for women based on gender, race, social class, and other social characteristics such as age, sexual practices, and disabilities that limit the pursuit of health. The quality of housing, education, food, heating, water, and other necessities of life reflect the resources of entire communities and societies.

The importance of political will and support for women's health deserves particular attention. The recent history of women's health movements, especially differences among groups of women, discussed throughout this volume, illustrates how critical these factors are in redefining what is considered important in science and society. Having access to information about the multiplicity of dimensions of women's health is essential to mobilize political support for a broadened vision of what actually contributes to all women's health and well-being.

Too many agendas to promote women's health in the United States seem to take for granted that women *have* the prerequisites for health. This fallacious assumption ensures that the centrality of these prerequisites to health remains submerged, or even repressed, in public policy and in the wider cultural discourse. Moreover, improving the biomedical knowledge base and clinical services for women begs the question of how such improvements will actually benefit women who don't have these basics, even if they manage to gain access to medical care—something that is increasingly problematic in the United States.

Scholars have never fully untangled exactly how improvements in working and living conditions, improvements in medical care, changing economic conditions, and profound changes in patterns of education, employment, marriage, and family life affect patterns of health and illness. Yet we recognize that these dimensions are, in fact, interrelated and consequential. For example, education, which is highly related to socioeconomic status, has clear health effects for women. Data from the National Center for Health Statistics (1995:108) reveal a clear gradient in mortality for white women and for women of all races by educational attainment. In 1992, the death rate was twice as high as for white women and women of all races ages twenty-five to sixty-four who had less than twelve compared with thirteen or more years of education. If national health statistics routinely included information on health status by educational attainment, might the importance of education for women's health be more widely recognized?

Data on health by socioeconomic status is difficult to obtain in national statistics (see chapter 2). When race, but not socioeconomic status, is used in national statistics, the real effects of socioeconomic status are obscured. Health status differences among women within racial/ethnic groups are particularly important to identify because they provide clues to differences between sociocultural and socioeconomic factors that affect health status and thereby suggest different strategies for change. For example, some immigrants have better health and birth outcomes than native-born members of the same racial/ethnic group despite similar poverty levels (Kumanyika and Golden 1991; Scribner and Dwyer 1989).

Because women's health is interdependent, the health of impoverished women affects the health of women in more comfortable circumstances. Examples abound. The spread of HIV, antibiotic-resistant strains of tuberculosis, teen pregnancy, homelessness, and all forms of violence as well as the growing ranks of the uninsured or underinsured affect everyone not only materially but in terms of the kinds of people some Americans are becoming—armed, fearful, and uncaring beyond immediate circles of family and friends. Thus threats to women's health include more than microorganisms, degenerative diseases, bad habits, or failure to map the human genome fast enough to save us from our own bodies! To construct more complete and inclusive models of women's health, models capable of addressing differences and complexities among women, we have to look at some specific limitations of dominant models.

Biomedical Models

Since the U.S. Public Health Service (1991:149, emphasis added) adopted this biomedical conceptualization of women's health, it has been used widely in government and medicine.[6] "Women's health is devoted to the preservation of wellness and prevention of illness in women, and includes *screening, diagnosis and management of conditions* which are unique to women, are more common in women, are more serious in women, [and] have manifestations, risk factors or interventions which are different in women."

The emphasis on the preservation of wellness implies that women have wellness to preserve, but where health comes from, or what is to be done if women do not have health, remains invisible at best or gets glossed over or denied. The biomedical focus on diseases or "conditions" in women is reinforced in the media and in public policy. Cultural metaphors widely used to describe detecting and curing diseases derive from warfare[7] and stir individual and collective action to demand more biomedical interventions. Screening is, in fact, prevention only to the extent that early detection increases the likelihood of early treatment and cure. Americans "race to the cure," declare "war" on cancer, and seek to triumph over the "killer diseases."

The media, in concert with medical experts, promote unrealistic views of miracle cures and prematurely report progress. In contrast, the media pay very little attention to the downside of modern medicine— "cures" that don't actually work and treatments that carry more risk than meets the eye or that contribute little to improved health outcomes. In this cultural context, rational and irrational beliefs about curing support heavy private and public investments in biomedicine.

Efforts to optimize health for individuals through advances in biomedicine consume a growing proportion of what are termed "health expenditures." Conceptualizations of what health *is* reflect this new "market metaphor" of medicine (Annas 1995). The multibillion-dollar annual budgets of the National Institutes for Health, including the commitment to the Human Genome Project, coupled with investment tax credits to the biotechnology industry, are all part of public investments in a narrow range of health resources. Healers, who were transformed into professionals early in the twentieth century, are now being transformed into "providers." Increased expenditures on medical care services inevitably deplete national resources available for critical social investments that promote health such as education, job training, environmental safety, and housing.

Rather than promoting women's health through improvements in these key social areas, national efforts to improve women's health have largely been directed toward making biomedicine more complete and more inclusive of social factors in health. The focus on social factors has been directed to a narrow range of primary prevention activities—largely individual responsibility for personal health practices such as diet, exercise, and avoiding tobacco, which reduce the risk of disease. (Controversies over these approaches to promoting women's health are explored in chapter 5.) Policymakers are eager to promote prevention to reduce costs of medical care. Social and behavioral scientists are increasingly asked to figure out how to do it better, more often, and more cost-effectively. Market concerns drive much of this "outcomes research" designed to rationalize health care service delivery. In medicine, encouraging women to improve health practices is viewed as supporting the "war on disease" while also "saving money."[8]

This is, of course, one of the areas of contradiction in women's health. Greater attention to behavioral factors in health *can* enhance development of risk reduction interventions that meet the needs of distinct populations—smoking cessation designed for low-income pregnant women or for older women. Social and behavioral knowledge can also improve diagnosis and treatment by expanding clinicians' perceptions of sources of women's ill health. Improvements in screening and treatment for battered women have resulted from broader perspectives. For example, Carole Warshaw (1993) and others have called for changes in how women who suffer injuries are treated by emergency personnel. Rather than simply treating a broken nose without considering how it got broken, new clinical protocols help assess how injuries occurred and open opportunities for referring women to supportive community-based shelters and counseling services. These are some of the positive aspects of biomedical approaches to utilizing social and behavioral knowledge. But if we are not careful about how we think, such "improvements" can obscure the likelihood of seeing the social roots of such problems—in gender rules and roles and in social inequities that strain interpersonal relations and undermine human civility.

Mind-Body Models

Emerging mind-body models start with the assumption that the mind and body interact in complex ways.[9] Because these approaches are so varied, characterizing them is problematic. Overall, these models all challenge the dualism of allopathic medicine, which separates mental/emotional states from physical symptoms. Some do this through links with traditional nonwestern healing systems and include spiritual as well as psychological precepts. A few explicitly link these models with social or feminist perspectives. Christiane Northrup, former president of the American Holistic Medical Association, attempts to do this.[10] In her view, "Since Everywoman's problem occurs in part because of the nature of being female in this culture, which programs us to put the needs of others ahead of our own, we need to make radical changes in our minds and lives to get and stay healthy" (Northrup 1994:xxv). Northrup lays out a forceful argument that surgery, drugs, and even good nutrition and health practices are not enough to promote healing. The emotional matters that brought about the physical symptoms must be resolved for real healing to occur.

Mind-body precepts pose a double-edged sword for many women. The assumption of and focus on psychogenesis, the psychological causes of physical disease, have been used in the past against women by physicians. To the extent that women's health problems have been viewed as psychogenic, inaccurately portrayed as "all in the head," most physicians have viewed them as unworthy of scientific investigation or clinical attention.[11] The stigma associated with psychogenic disorders has contributed substantially to women's dissatisfaction with conventional medical treatment. If new research in psychoneuroimmunology and other areas scientifically demonstrates how what happens psychologically and emotionally "gets into the physical body," emerging mind-body paradigms may challenge the biomedical paradigm in critical ways that will benefit women. But paradigms are not easily overturned, and mind-body approaches are likely to meet stiff resistance.

Anthropologist Bonnie Blair O'Connor (1995) points out that there are many nonbiomedical health belief systems in the United States, and they are growing in popularity. These range from folk medicine to newer developments in holistic health and healing.[12] Traditional and alternative healing practices also offer competing paradigms. The popular natural health movements have made an impact on conventional medicine.

Some physicians now offer "complementary medicine," and the National Institutes of Health established an Office of Alternative Health (1994).

Social Models of Women's Health

Neither biomedical nor mind-body models adequately address differences and disparities in women's health within or across social groups. Nor is it clear what direction these models provide for preventing health problems that are rooted in social and cultural factors. The primary prevention model itself, taking action to avoid disease, seems particularly ill-suited for reducing many of the physical and emotional conditions that threaten women's health and well-being. For example, trying to prevent the health consequences of violence (injuries, emergency department visits, mental health problems) does not get to the core social, economic, and cultural factors that cause the violence that "causes" injury! Similarly, focusing only on the medical consequences of unwanted pregnancies, drug addiction, and many other conditions ignores both the causes and consequences of larger social, economic, political, and cultural forces.

Physicians themselves increasingly question medicalizing social problems as medical problems (Schwartz 1995). Social and behavioral scientists have long recognized that women's health problems must be understood as socially, culturally, and economically produced. They are not isolated, individual, biological events that can be explained outside the contexts in which they emerge.

At the same time, demedicalizing health problems carries certain risks. American society is rife with dualistic thinking—medical versus social; responsible versus not responsible; organic versus psychogenic. Raising questions about the nature of health issues raises questions about who will be held responsible for them and who will pay for the medical care that they generate. Tensions over personal responsibility for health are likely to escalate as the social costs of health rise. Living and working conditions, which are changing rapidly (see chapters 6 and 7), will create profound challenges to women's health in the decades to come.

New models must reflect the interconnectedness of working and living conditions, individual health behaviors, and positive biomedical contributions to health and well-being. Such models are needed to develop effective social and public health policy. As a society, we can ill afford to view women's health predominately as the domain of biomedicine and ignore the social forces that actually create—and destroy—health.

More inclusive visions of women's health (that reflected the WHO perspective) have emerged from consumer-oriented and feminist women's health movements in the 1970s. Groups such as the Boston Women's Health Book Collective, the National Black Women's Health Project, and the National Women's Health Network (see chapter 3) envision health, and solutions to health problems, from social perspectives. Feminist conceptualizations of health, like those of many social and behavioral scientists, typically emphasize the ways in which working and living conditions as well as personal health practices create health. The recent scramble for health care reform (more accurately, medical care insurance reform) diverted attention from more fundamental health issues and entrenched biomedical definitions of health even further into public consciousness.

Uniquely, feminist models place women at the center of the analysis, not at the periphery, and emphasize how gender as well as other social roles and rules affect women's health. Feminist models have not, however, always adequately addressed health issues of women whose life circumstances vary by race, class, or a variety of status characteristics, locations, or identities. Tensions and conflicts have erupted over the centrality of particular medical services and social policies for various groups of women (as we discuss in chapter 3). There have also been significant disagreements over what certain biomedical developments, particularly in the areas of manipulative reproductive technologies and genetics, offer or threaten.[13]

Developing more inclusive models of health requires recognizing and dealing with complexities and differences in women's lives. Educational levels, income, culture, ethnicity, race, and a host of other identities and experiences shape women's health. Living and working conditions themselves are shaped by education, economic trends, housing, and other conditions that produce health and prevent illness. Thus health is created in complex, interactive ways that cannot be reduced to any one dimension.

Despite the actual complexities of health, its contours have been described quite well in simple, understandable terms. In the introduction to the popular health book *Our Bodies, Ourselves*, the Boston Women's Health Book Collective describes health this way: "Though medical care sometimes helps us when we are sick, it does not keep us healthy. To a great extent what makes us healthy or unhealthy is how we are able to live our daily lives—how we eat, how we exercise, how much rest we get, how much stress we live with, how much we use alcohol, cigarettes, or drugs, how safe or hazardous our workplaces are, whether we experience the threat or reality of sexual violence" (1992:13).

Feminist conceptualizations of women's health such as this one clearly link the source of health to communities, where food, housing, education, and environmental hazards—the prerequisites to health—are located. Feminist thinking about health also laid important groundwork for expanding the WHO concepts of what produces health. In communities, women not only need to be free from the fear of war but from all forms of violence. American society must come to terms with this prerequisite to health, or all of the breast cancers "caught early," the chronic diseases avoided through positive health practices, and the benefits of new technologies will be undermined and overshadowed. The specter of women being screened annually for a multitude of diseases but remaining fearful of leaving their homes—or perhaps worse yet, fearing to remain in them—raises uncomfortable questions about how narrowly women's health is often defined.

Crafting More Inclusive Models

In carefully crafted inclusive models of women's health, the health of men, children, parents, and life partners would take on particular importance. Extending the analysis of health to include significant others in women's lives in no way dilutes the importance of women's health in its own right. Rather, it underscores the importance of gender in the production and maintenance of women's health. Women from all walks of life emphasize the need to be free from the fear of violence, in all its many sociocultural forms—including violence among men who are women's kin. Addressing violence against women outside the context of male as well as female gender expectations and opportunities is unimaginable. So is the issue of equality of opportunity, a looming challenge for an increasingly divided society. How can the social forces of caring be mobilized—to create health for wider communities, not only for ourselves in personal spheres?

The challenge is to craft inclusive models of health that can mobilize social forces for caring, curing, and concern in new ways to contribute to women's health both as individuals and as members of communities, in their social relations as well as in their bodies. By arguing that women's health resides in communities, we open up new questions about how to balance resources for biomedicine, for promoting individual health practices, and for improving working and living conditions.

As a society, Americans face difficult choices about how to allocate resources to improve women's health. Grafting psychosocial factors onto biomedical models may lead to incremental improvements in primary prevention, screening, and treatment, but these are not adequate substitutes for providing the prerequisites for health. Nor does such grafting even begin to address women's differences and the complexities of meeting their health needs. Women's needs also shift and change as demographic trends in immigration, internal migration, marriage and divorce patterns, and fertility all interact with underlying economic forces.

Troubling social trends make it imperative to develop more inclusive models to guide policymaking, research, clinical practice, and individual behavior. How we think about health shapes cultural beliefs about what women "need" to maintain or improve their health. Currently, biomedical models support excessive investments in medical services without consideration of the underlying social forces that generate health and well-being. As the American economy merges with global economies,[14] excess medical care costs reduce job creation and provide incentives to hire part-time or temporary workers instead of permanent employees who have traditionally received medical benefits from their employers. The stakes are high because jobs are essential for maintaining the prerequisites for health as well as gaining access to medical services. Without creating and maintaining social relationships and institutions that actually produce health, including economically and culturally viable communities in cities as well as suburbs and exurbs, efforts to reduce the burdens of disease and the costs of biomedicine will remain unrealized.

The need for critical thinking about women's health grows daily. Overinvestment in biomedicine, particularly those elements that contribute little to actual improved health outcomes, consumes resources that could be used to extend useful medical care to everyone. Social commitments to education, preserving the environment, spurring economic development, creating safe living and working conditions, and finding new ways to support families and communities are central to an inclusive vision of women's health. Important relational concepts such as caring deserve more recognition. Few research resources are available for studying how caring facilitates health and healing. Caring is not easily measured by checklists of "caring behaviors" or "social supports." These indicators hint at, but miss, the essential experiential aspects of caring or feeling cared for, not only when people are sick but as part of human growth and development. The subjective, experiential dimensions of health and healing, addressed in the qualitative social sciences, in some areas of nursing, and in emerging mind-body paradigms deserve greater attention. So do alternative healing practices and the contributions of a much wider array of healers and helpers than are generally acknowledged under the rubric of "health care workers."

There are no easy recipes or simple formulas for moving beyond narrow biomedical models. A necessary first step is to expand our conceptual and empirical understanding of what actually creates women's health. Collaboration between diverse groups will be needed to enlarge public understanding of how social forces, not just pathogens and biological matter, contribute to women's health. Expanding conceptual and empirical understanding of what actually creates women's health is a daunting task, but if women do not undertake this endeavor, who will?

NOTES

1. This definition first appeared in the 1948 Constitution of the World Health Organization, Geneva. It is reprinted in WHO documents and is widely used throughout the world (see, e.g., Downie, Fyfe, and Tannahill 1990). The WHO is organized into regions, with the United States and Canada falling in the Americas. WHO activities in this region are coordinated under the Pan American Health Organization (PAHO). In practice, PAHO efforts focus heavily on health and development issues in Latin America. The United States and Canada share many health issues with the developed region of Europe and participate in some activities of the WHO Regional Office for Europe. Canada's health policies and medical care systems have developed in the directions set out by the WHO, whereas this has not been the case in the United States. Milio (1989) provides an excellent overview of Canadian health policies. Under the leadership of Ilona Kickbusch, WHO has focused on broad issues in women's health. For a recent example of European perspectives on women's health in WHO, see the "Vienna Statement on Investing in Women's Health in the Countries of Central and Eastern Europe" (1994).

2. Travis (1988) provides an extensive review of biopsychosocial models of women's health.

3. Recent extensive critiques of dominant biomedical models in relation to women include the works of Fee and Krieger (1994), who focus on lack of attention to social class particularly, and Rosser (1994), who focuses on the androcentric bias and denial of diversity in clinical medicine. Rose (1994) takes up the issue of why the sciences have not adequately addressed the needs of women and how that might be changed. Marmor, Barer, and Evans (1994) provide an excellent overview of how U.S. health policy has ignored the centrality of social factors as determinants of health.

4. Our thinking continues to evolve as we struggle with how to present these

issues. Our previous efforts to specify the key elements of feminist perspectives on women's health have appeared in Lewin and Olesen (1985), Ruzek and Hill (1986), and Ruzek (1986, 1993). These ideas have also informed the direction of the courses developed through the Women, Health, and Healing Program.

5. These are described in detail and analyzed by Downie, Fyfe, and Tannahill (1990:62).

6. For example, this definition was adopted 16 September 1994 by the National Academy for Women's Health Medical Education (NAWHME), a joint program of the Medical College of Pennsylvania and the American Medical Women's Association.

7. For a discussion of the metaphors used recently in medicine see Annas (1995).

8. Annas (1995) argues that these mixed metaphors of the medical care world confuse matters and were a factor in the demise of national health reform.

9. The ideas of mind-body medicine are spreading rapidly through the work of clinicians who write for educated lay as well as health professional readers. References to the scientific studies (from widely ranging disciplines) on which their ideas are based are well documented in these works. See also the work on consciousness, spirituality, and medicine by Shealy and Myss (1987). Deepak Chopra (1990, 1994), executive director of the Institute of Mind-Body Medicine and Human Potential, Sharp HealthCare, San Diego, has popularized key mind-body concepts. Proponents of mind-body perspectives also attempt to move the ideas that are particularly well supported by scientific evidence into mainstream medicine. See also the American Holistic Medical Association (1990). Also along these lines, the Society of Behavioral Medicine has launched *Mind/Body Medicine, A Journal of Clinical Behavioral Medicine* under the editorship of Richard Friedman and Herbert Benson and an editorial board of distinguished scholars and clinicians. Western scientific methods may not be fully appropriate for researching some of the central features of these paradigms (i.e., intuitive and spiritual dimensions of health caring and healing).

10. The emerging mind-body paradigms, as they relate to women, are found in the work of Christiane Northrup (1994), who includes an extensive directory of resources ranging from scholarly and popular publications to organizations, products, and practitioners who specifically address women's energy systems and their relationships with psychological issues relating to reproductive organs in particular. Northrup's perspectives build on the feminist psychological perspectives of Anne Wilson Schaef (1992) and proponents of the natural or alternative health and healing practices.

11. Increasingly, physicians recognize that women with breast cancer have better outcomes if they receive support from other women. Efforts to provide group psychological counseling to improve recovery may accelerate given that some research shows that women who perceive themselves as having high-quality emotional support even have an enhanced immune response (Levy et al. 1990). Northrup (1994:288–89) finds considerable evidence of psychological associations between breast cancer and emotional factors in the development of disease. She emphasizes that looking for psychogenic factors in cancer should not be misinterpreted as blaming women for "bringing it on themselves."

12. There is growing interest in African American folk healing: see, for example,

Fontenot (1993) and Snow (1993). Interest in herbal and natural health increased as concerns over conventional medicine increased (Weiss 1984).

13. For discussions of these controversies, see especially Lasker and Borg (1994), Rothenberg and Thomson (1994), Rothman (1989), and Stephens and Wagner (1993).

14. For easily accessible views of the changes that the American economy (and society) are going through, see especially the work of Graef (1992), Harrison (1994), Schwartz and Volgy (1992), Sklar (1995), and Toffler and Toffler (1994).

REFERENCES

American Holistic Medical Association
> 1990   Psychoneuroimmunology: The Scientific Basis for Holism in Medicine. Raleigh, NC: American Holistic Medical Association.

Annas, George J.
> 1995   "Reframing the debate on health care reform by replacing our metaphors." New England Journal of Medicine 332:744–47.

Boston Women's Health Book Collective
> 1992   The New Our Bodies, Ourselves. New York: Simon and Schuster.

Chesney, Margaret A. and Elizabeth M. Ozer
> 1995   "Women and health: in search of a paradigm." Women's Health: Research on Gender, Behavior, and Policy 1:3–26.

Chopra, Deepak
> 1990   Quantum Healing: Exploring the Frontiers of Mind/Body Medicine. New York: Bantam.
> 1994   Creating Health: How to Wake Up the Body's Intelligence. Boston: Houghton Mifflin.

Downie, R. S., C. Fyfe, and A. Tannahill
> 1990   Health Promotion Models and Values. New York: Oxford University Press.

Fee, Elizabeth, and Nancy Krieger, eds.
> 1994   Women's Health, Politics, and Power: Essays on Sex/Gender, Medicine, and Public Health. Amityville, NY: Baywood.

Fontenot, Wonda Lee
> 1993   "Madame Neau: the practice of ethno-psychiatry in rural Louisiana." Pp. 41–52 in Barbara Bair and Susan E. Cayleff (eds.), Wings of Gauze: Women of Color and the Experience of Health and Illness. Detroit: Wayne State University Press.

Graef, Crystal S.
> 1992   In Search of Excess: The Overcompensation of American Executives. New York: Norton.

Harrison, Bennett
> 1994   Lean and Mean: The Changing Landscape of Corporate Power in the Age of Flexibility. New York: Basic Books.

Kumanyika, Shiriki K., and Patricia M. Golden
   1991   "Cross-sectional differences in health status in U.S. racial/ethnic minority groups: potential influence of temporal changes, disease, and lifestyle transitions." Ethnicity and Disease 1:50–59.
Lasker, Judith, and Susan Borg
   1994   In Search of Parenthood: Coping with Infertility and High-Tech Conception, rev. ed. Philadelphia: Temple University Press.
Levy, Sandra, Ronald Herberman, Theresa Whiteside, and Kathy Sanzo
   1990   "Perceived social support and tumor estrogen progesterone receptor status as predictors of natural killer cell activity in breast cancer patients." Psychosomatic Medicine 52:73–85.
Lewin, Ellen, and Virginia Olesen, eds.
   1985   Women, Health, and Healing: Toward a New Perspective. London: Tavistock.
Marmor, Theodore R., Morris L. Barer, and Robert G. Evans
   1994   "The determinants of a population's health: what can be done to improve a democratic nation's health status?" Pp. 217–30 in Marmor, Barer, and Evans (eds.), Why Are Some People Healthy and Others Not? The Determinants of Health of Populations. New York: Aldine de Gruyter.
Milio, Nancy
   1989   Promoting Health through Public Policy. Ottawa: Canadian Public Health Association.
National Center for Health Statistics
   1995   Health, United States, 1994. Hyattsville, MD: Public Health Service.
National Institutes of Health, Office of Alternative Medicine
   1994   Alternative Medicine: Expanding Medical Horizons. A Report to the National Institutes of Health on Alternative Medical Systems and Practices in the United States. NIH Pub. No. 94-066.
Northrup, Christiane
   1994   Women's Bodies, Women's Wisdom: Creating Physical and Emotional Health and Healing. New York: Bantam Books.
O'Connor, Bonnie Blair
   1995   Healing Traditions: Alternative Medicine and the Health Professions. Philadelphia: University of Pennsylvania Press.
Rose, Hillary
   1994   Love, Power and Knowledge: Toward a Feminist Transformation of the Sciences. Bloomington: Indiana University Press.
Rosser, Sue V.
   1994   Women's Health: Missing from U.S. Medicine. Bloomington: Indiana University Press.
Rothenberg, Karen H., and Elizabeth J. Thomson, eds.
   1994   Women and Prenatal Testing: Facing the Challenges of Genetic Technology. Columbus: Ohio State University Press.

Rothman, Barbara Katz
    1989   Recreating Motherhood: Ideology and Technology in a Patriarchal Society. New York: Norton.
Ruzek, Sheryl Burt
    1986   "Feminist visions of health: an international perspective." Pp. 185–207 in Juliet Mitchell and Ann Oakley (eds.), What Is Feminism? London: Basil Blackwell.
    1993   "Towards a more inclusive model of women's health." American Journal of Public Health 83:6–8.
Ruzek, Sheryl Burt, and Jessica Hill
    1986   "Promoting women's health: redefining the knowledge base and strategies for change." Health Promotion 1:301–9.
Schaef, Anne Wilson
    1992   Beyond Therapy, Beyond Science: A New Model for Healing the Whole Person. San Francisco: Harper.
Schwartz, John E., and Thomas J. Volgy
    1992   The Forgotten Americans: Thirty Million Working Poor in the Land of Opportunity. New York: Norton.
Schwartz, Leroy L.
    1995   Special Report. The Medicalization of Social Problems: America's Special Health Care Dilemma. Washington: Public Policy Center for American Healthcare Systems.
Scribner, R., and J. H. Dwyer
    1989   "Acculturation and low birthweight among Latinos in the Hispanic HANES." American Journal of Public Health 79:1263–67.
Shealy, Norman, and Caroline Myss
    1987   The Creation of Health. Walpole, NH: Stillpoint.
Sklar, Holly
    1995   Chaos or Community? Seeking Solutions, Not Scapegoats for Bad Economics. Boston: South End Press.
Snow, Loudell F.
    1993   Walkin' over Medicine. Boulder, CO: Westview Press.
Stephens, Patricia, and Marsden Wagner, eds.
    1993   Tough Choices: In Vitro Fertilization and the Reproductive Technologies. Philadelphia: Temple University Press.
Toffler, Alvin, and Heidi Toffler
    1994   Creating a New Civilization: The Politics of the Third Wave. Atlanta: Turner.
Travis, Cheryl Brown
    1988   Women and Health Psychology: Biomedical Issues. Hillsdale, NJ: Lawrence Erlbaum.
U.S. Public Health Service, Office on Women's Health
    1991   PHS Action Plan for Women's Health. DHHS Pub. No. (PHS) 91-50214. September.

Warshaw, Carole
    1993   "Domestic violence: challenges to medical practice." Journal of Women's
            Health 2:73–80.
Weiss, Kay, ed.
    1984   Women's Health Care: A Guide to Alternatives. Reston, VA: Reston.
World Health Organization
    1994   Women's Health Counts: Vienna Statement on Investing in Women's
            Health in the Countries of Central and Eastern Europe. Copenhagen:
            WHO Regional Office for Europe.

[2]

Patterns and Puzzles:
The Distribution of Health and Illness among Women in the United States

DEBORAH L. WINGARD

Deborah Wingard takes an epidemiological approach to describing health and illness among women in the United States. Here she focuses on variations in mortality, morbidity, fertility, and life expectancy among women from different racial/ethnic groups and age groups. Wingard emphasizes that there is considerable variation in women's health status within as well as between racial/ethnic groups. By studying "patterns and puzzles" in these variations, the complex relationships among social, behavioral, cultural, economic, and biological factors that are associated with women's health and longevity may become better understood.

Women's health is not constant but varies tremendously among socioeconomic and racial/ethnic groups. Women's health also varies by age, geographic area, and time and differs substantially from men's health. To understand this diversity and work toward social equity in health, we must accurately assess these variations and then focus research on reasons for social, racial, and gender differences in health.

Most research to date has focused on white men, reflecting the fact that this research occurred primarily in countries where the most common racial group was Caucasian and where on average men died at a younger age than women. It had also been assumed by most researchers that the process of disease causation and progression was largely the same in men as in women and did not differ by racial/ethnic status. We now know that risk of disease and progression of disease vary by gender and racial status. By studying variations in health by gender and race, we may gain insights into the complex relationships between biological, behavioral, and social factors that influence health and longevity.

In this chapter, I provide an overview of variations in women's health in the United States by racial/ethnic group, age, and time. This epidemiologic overview of the status of women's health focuses on mortality (death rates), morbidity (illness rates), and reproductive health (including fertility, pregnancy complications, death in childbirth, and infant health). The foregoing are widely regarded as good indicators of the health status of particular populations. These data lay the groundwork for subsequent chapters that focus on issues of concern to specific subgroups of women. Taken as a whole, these data underscore the need to guard against overgeneralizing about "women's" health.

It is important to recognize that all commonly recognized racial/ethnic groups are heterogeneous (Manley et al. 1985). African Americans include Haitians, Nigerians, Ethiopians, Ghanians, Jamaicans, and West Indians. Hispanics include Mexican Americans, Puerto Ricans, Cubans, and individuals representing at least sixteen other Spanish-speaking countries. Asians and Pacific Islanders represent at least twenty-five groups: some are recent immigrants, others are established populations. Native Americans include over three hundred tribes and five hundred recognized groups. Each racial/ethnic group has unique genetic, behavioral, and social characteristics that are differentiated by socioeconomic and geographic variations. Many social and cultural dimensions of health in racial/ethnic groups in the United States are discussed throughout this book.

Until recently, few data were available on mortality rates for specific racial/ethnic groups. All racial and ethnic minorities were lumped together into the category "nonwhite," a practice that obscures important differences in health status. In this chapter, I compare the health status of whites and nonwhites only when more specific data are not available. When possible, I also present age-specific and/or age-adjusted[1] data, so that more accurate comparisons between groups can be made. Age adjustment is important. For example, if one ethnic group includes more elderly women than another, its overall death rate will appear "higher" even if individuals in each group actually have the same life expectancy.

Mortality

In 1990 the age-adjusted death rate for nonwhite women was higher than for white women; 510 deaths per 100,000 compared with 370 deaths (National Center for Health Statistics 1994a). This excess of deaths among nonwhite women has persisted throughout the century, although

Figure 2.1 Age-Adjusted Mortality Rates among Women by Race in the United States, 1900–1990

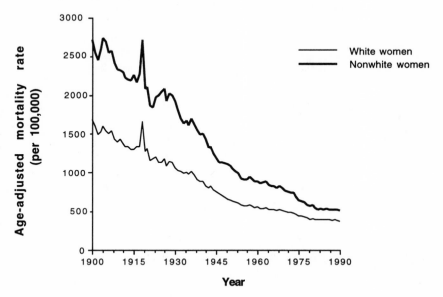

Source: National Center for Health Statistics (1994b).

the magnitude of the difference has decreased from a 60 percent excess in 1900 to a 38 percent excess in 1990 (see figure 2.1).

As shown in table 2.1, mortality rates vary substantially among all women (National Center for Health Statistics 1994a). Note that black women had much higher death rates than white women for all age groups except the very oldest. Mortality rates for black women were two and a half times higher than for white women between the ages of twenty-five and forty-four. However, white women had higher death rates than Hispanic and Asian women in every age group. In fact, Asian women had the lowest mortality rates. Native American women fall in the middle, with death rates as high as black women between the ages of fifteen and twenty-four.

When health statistics are separated into even more specific categories, we see large differences in morbidity and mortality both *within* and *between* different groups and subgroups. For example, table 2.2 presents age- and cause-specific mortality rates among women by racial/ethnic group (National Center for Health Statistics 1994a). For the three leading

TABLE 2.1
Age-Specific and Age-Adjusted Mortality Rates among Women by Race in the United States, 1989-91

Age (years)	White	Black	Hispanic	Asian or Pacific Islander	Native American
1–14	24	40	26	20	29
15–24	47	70	41	28	71
25–44	88	222	74	54	127
45–64	552	994	400	304	548
65–74	1,926	2,880	1,447	1,065	1,677
75–84	4,824	5,768	3,471	2,923	3,338
85+	14,322	13,313	10,183	10,040	7,965
Age-adjusted[a]	370	582	285	222	341

Source: National Center for Health Statistics (1994a).

Note: Mortality rates based on deaths per 100,000 population.

[a]Age-adjusted by the direct method to the 1940 United States population.

causes of death in the United States (heart disease, cancer, and cerebro-vascular disease), black women have the highest mortality rates. Asian women have the lowest rates of heart disease and cancer, and Native American women have the lowest rates of cerebrovascular disease (stroke). Native American women also have the highest rates of death from motor vehicle accidents. Suicide rates vary by age, with Native American women having the highest death rates among women ages fifteen to twenty-four, white women ages twenty-five to sixty-four, and Asian women ages sixty-five and above. Black women are more than twice as likely to be murdered at almost every age, and they have substantially higher rates of mortality from HIV.

Mortality from specific cancers varies substantially by ethnic sub-populations (Horm et al. 1985). For example, between 1973 and 1981 mortality from breast cancer ranged from a low of 8.0 per 100,000 Filipino women to a high of 33.3 in Hawaiian women and 26 in both black and white women. Mortality rates from lung cancer showed a similar pattern: low in Filipino women, high in Hawaiian, black, and white women. How-ever, mortality rates for cervical cancer demonstrated an inconsistent

TABLE 2.2
Age- and Cause-Specific Mortality Rates among Women
by Race in the United States, 1989-91

Cause and Age	White	Black	Hispanic	Asian or Pacific Islander	Native American
Heart disease[a]					
45+	376	597	271	205	274
Cancer[a]					
45+	380	457	238	215	239
Cerebrovascular[a]					
45+	84	158	69	81	63
Motor vehicle					
All ages[a]	11	9	10	8	19
1–14	5	5	6	4	8
15–24	20	10	13	10	30
25–44	10	11	10	7	23
45–64	10	10	11	10	19
Suicide					
15–24	4	2	3	4	8
25–44	7	4	3	4	5
45–64	8	3	4	5	2
65+	7	2	3	9	3
Homicide					
15–24	4	19	7	3	8
25–44	4	21	6	4	9
45–64	2	8	3	3	5
HIV					
25–44	2	24	9	1	2
45–64	1	8	4	1	0

Source: National Center for Health Statistics (1994a).

Note: Mortality rates based on deaths per 100,000 population.

[a]Age-adjusted by direct method to the 1940 United States population.

pattern. White women had high mortality rates for breast and lung cancer and low rates for cervical cancer, whereas Native American women had low mortality rates for breast and lung cancer and high rates for cervical cancer. The experience of disease also varies even within racial/ethnic

TABLE 2.3
Age-Adjusted Incidence and Survival Rates of Cancer by Site among Black and White Women in the United States, 1983-90

Cancer Site	Incidence per 100,000[a] 1990		Five-Year Relative Survival (%) 1983-90	
	White	Black	White	Black
Breast	113.6	95.0	82	66
Respiratory system	42.8	49.0	16	12
Colon	28.2	37.2	60	50
Rectum	9.8	8.3	59	51
Uterus	22.0	14.2	85	55
Cervix	7.5	12.9	70	56
Ovary	15.7	10.0	42	38

Source: National Center for Health Statistics (1994a).

Note: Data are based on the Surveillance, Epidemiology, and End Results Program's population-based registries in Atlanta, Detroit, Seattle–Puget Sound, San Francisco-Oakland, Connecticut, Iowa, New Mexico, Utah, and Hawaii.

[a]Number of new cases per 100,000 age-adjusted by the direct method to the 1970 United States population.

groups. For example, Karen Ito and her colleagues describe how different Asian Americans experience breast cancer (see chapter 12).

Racial/ethnic differences in mortality and survival rates reflect differences in both disease incidence and survival. Table 2.3 compares cancer incidence and survival rates in black and white women by site. In 1990, white women had a higher incidence of breast, uterine, and ovarian cancer, whereas black women had a higher incidence of cervical and colon cancer. However, five-year relative survival rates (1983-90) were higher for white than black women for every site. The extent to which racial/ethnic differences in incidence and survival rates are due to differences in biological/genetic factors, exposure to risk factors, and/or access to medical care is not known.

Studies of migrant populations help separate the effects of genetics from environment and lifestyle. For example, Japanese women who live in Japan have low rates of breast cancer compared with white women in the United States. However, Japanese women who move to Hawaii or to the U.S. mainland have higher rates than Japanese women remaining in Japan. This argues against the difference between Japanese and white women being entirely genetic, and it argues for an environmental or behavioral influence, such as diet. Cancer rates among migrants frequently change to be more similar to the rates among natives of the new country, and migrants who become more acculturated (adopt the behaviors of their new country) demonstrate the greatest change in risk.

For both whites and nonwhites, men have higher mortality rates for virtually all the leading causes of death and higher age-specific and age-adjusted all-cause mortality rates (National Center for Health Statistics 1994b). In 1990, the age-adjusted sex mortality ratio for all causes (male/female) was 1.7; men had a 70 percent higher age-adjusted death rate than women. Even though mortality rates were substantially higher for nonwhites than for whites, the all-cause sex differential was virtually identical: 1.8 and 1.7, respectively. For both whites and nonwhites, the sex differential in mortality has been increasing since the early 1900s, especially for those 15–24 and 55–64 years of age (Wingard 1984). However, since 1970 that trend has slowed.

There is a corresponding race and sex differential in life expectancy. In 1992 (National Center for Health Statistics 1995), life expectancy at birth was 6.6 years longer for white women than for white men (79.8 versus 73.2 years) and 8.0 years longer for nonwhite women than for nonwhite men (75.7 versus 67.7). Note that both white and nonwhite women have a greater life expectancy than either white or nonwhite men. These data underscore the view that what is problematic about women's health is not how long they live but their experience of health, illness, and healing over the life cycle.

Morbidity

Morbidity has been defined in many ways: for example, generalized "poor health," a specific illness, or the sum of a number of illnesses. Each of these in turn has been studied based on self-reported occurrence, restricted activity, doctors' visits, hospitalizations, and (occasionally) screening examinations. No matter how it is defined, morbidity varies by racial/ethnic group.

Between 1985 and 1987, 17 percent of black women in the United States reported fair or poor health on a national survey, compared with 10 percent of white women (National Center for Health Statistics 1990b). Black women also reported slightly more activity limitation resulting from chronic conditions and restricted activity days resulting from

TABLE 2.4
Self-Reported Morbidity among Women by Race
and Family Income Level in the United States, 1985–87

Family Income and Race	Fair or Poor Health[a]	Activity Limitation[b]	Acute Conditions[c]	Restricted-Activity Days[d]
All income levels				
White	10.2	14.4	204	16.5
Black	17.1	15.3	146	19.0
Other	9.1	8.7	184	10.7
<$20,000				
White	17.1	21.8	208	22.8
Black	20.7	18.7	158	22.1
Other	12.3	11.7	192	11.8
≥$20,000				
White	5.4	9.5	210	12.7
Black	8.4	7.5	136	12.6
Other	6.4	6.3	174	9.7

Source: The National Health Interview Survey (weekly probability sample of U.S. households) including interviews with approximately 200,000 white and 28,000 black persons, National Center for Health Statistics (1990a).

[a]Percentage of persons with fair or poor health.

[b]Percentage of persons with limitation of activity because of chronic conditions.

[c]Number of acute conditions per 100 persons per year.

[d]Restricted-activity days per person per year because of acute or chronic conditions.

acute or chronic conditions but fewer acute conditions than did white women (table 2.4). Socioeconomic factors must be considered to interpret these findings (Blendon et al. 1989). Note that within high- and low-income groups, white women report more activity limitation than black women. However, activity limitation is more common in the lower income group. Since more black than white women have low incomes, a larger proportion of all black women report activity limitation.

Morbidity also varies between racial/ethnic subpopulations. For example, in a survey between 1978 and 1980 that identified Hispanic subgroups, the highest rates of bed-disability days, work-loss days, and restriction of major activity as a result of chronic conditions were reported by black, Hispanic, and Puerto Rican women. Puerto Rican women also reported the highest age-adjusted number of acute conditions per year. In almost every category, Mexican women reported the least morbidity (National Center for Health Statistics 1984). There are also important differences in the incidence and prevalence of particular diseases in different groups. For example, black, Hispanic, and Native American women have more diabetes, hypertension, and obesity than white women (Manley et al. 1985). Black women also have more lupus erythematosus than other racial groups, whereas whites have more osteoporosis. Thus far, scientific work has not adequately examined these variations among women.

Although physical and emotional violence affects women of all races and classes (as discussed in chapter 19), homicide and fear of homicide and other forms of violence are acute for African American women. In addition, the consequences of homicide and other forms of violence go far beyond the direct loss of life or physical and emotional injuries, as Nikki Franke points out in chapter 14.

Whether there are racial differentials for violence after controlling for economic status remains hotly debated. Reliable data are difficult to obtain about the actual incidence of domestic violence and sexual assault in any racial/ethnic group. Cultural values and social conditions may lead to different levels of reporting in subpopulations, making comparisons between groups especially problematic. For example, as Jang, Lee, and Morello-Frosch (1990) point out, domestic violence is largely ignored for immigrant and refugee women in the United States. Until recently, there was little interest in identifying the actual incidence of violence in the United States for any subgroup.

Interpreting the racial/ethnic differences in both morbidity and mortality is fraught with methodological and interpretive difficulties (Kumanyika and Golden 1991). In addition to possible (but not scientifically substantiated) biological differences, racial/ethnic groups differ in access to health care and culturally determined aspects of their lifestyles. Socioeconomic and cultural factors also change over time, as newer immigrant groups become acculturated or as existing groups refocus on traditional values and behaviors. Differences may also reflect methodological errors in how racial/ethnic groups are sampled or classified. It is especially problematic when racial groups are combined into whites and nonwhites, as can be seen from the great variability of morbidity and mortality already presented. Even combining ethnic subpopulations, such as specific Hispanic or Asian groups, can camouflage true differences in health status.

TABLE 2.5
Fertility Rates by Race of Mother
in the United States, 1991

Race	Fertility Rate
White, non-Hispanic	60.0
Black, non-Hispanic	86.8
Hispanic[a]	108.1
Mexican	121.6
Puerto Rican	80.9
Cuban	49.1
Other Hispanic	99.3
Asian or Pacific Islander	67.6
Native American	75.1

Source: National Center for Health Statistics (1993).

Note: Fertility rates based on number of live births
per 1,000 women aged 15–44 years.

[a]Hispanic rates based on 47 reporting states.

Reproductive Health

A major component of health for many women includes reproductive
experiences: fertility, pregnancy complications, maternal morbidity and
mortality, and the health of their newborns. Infant mortality rates are
included as part of women's reproductive health status not only because
of the close relationship between a woman's own physical and emotional
health and that of her infant but because these rates are especially useful
for assessing a racial/ethnic group's health status. Infants are particularly
vulnerable to social and environmental conditions as well as genetic/bio-
logical factors (McBarnette 1988). In the United States, reproductive
health status varies tremendously by racial/ethnic group.

In the United States in 1991, fertility rates (number of live births per
1,000 women ages fifteen to forty-four) ranged from a low of 60.0 and 67.6
among white and Asian women to a high of 108.1 among Hispanic
women (National Center for Health Statistics 1993). Even among Hispanic subgroups there was substantial variation in fertility rates, from a low

of 49.1 among Cuban women to a high of 121.6 among Mexican Americans. These differences represent wanted as well as unwanted pregnancies, infertility as well as access to family planning services (see table 2.5).

As can be seen in table 2.6, racial/ethnic groups with low fertility rates (i.e., Asians, Cubans, and whites) have few teenage and unmarried mothers, whereas groups with higher fertility rates (i.e., blacks, Mexican Americans, Puerto Ricans, and Native Americans) have high proportions of teenage and unmarried mothers. For both whites and nonwhites, the proportion of births to teenage mothers increased between 1950 and the early 1970s and has declined since then (Hughes et al. 1988.) The widely cited "epidemic of teen pregnancy" is in fact largely an epidemic of births to *unmarried* teens.

Racial/ethnic differences in fertility rates are influenced by cultural norms as well as socioeconomic access to health services. Groups differ in the value placed on being pregnant, being a mother, or having a large family. They also differ in how they view unwed or teenage mothers; in some cultures or subcultures it is an accepted condition, whereas in others it is a source of shame. Cultures also differ in the importance placed on family support during pregnancy and the acceptability of outside support from the medical establishment. For example, new immigrants are frequently apprehensive about using the health care system, even if they have financial access.

To understand women's reproductive health experiences, it is useful to look at two closely related measures of maternal and infant morbidity—premature delivery and low birthweight—which are presented in table 2.6. Racial/ethnic groups with high fertility rates and the highest proportions of unmarried mothers (i.e., blacks and Puerto Ricans) had the highest proportion of unhealthy outcomes. Groups with low fertility rates and low proportions of unmarried mothers (i.e., whites and Cubans) had the lowest rates of unhealthy outcomes. Asian mothers, especially the Chinese (who had intermediate fertility rates but the lowest rate of unmarried mothers), had fewer low birthweight babies and premature deliveries than any other group. For both whites and nonwhites, the proportion of births at low birthweight has declined since the mid-1960s (Hughes et al. 1988). Some of these differences in infant morbidity may reflect differences in prenatal care. For example, 9 to 12 percent of black, Mexican American, Puerto Rican, and Native American births were to women with little or no prenatal care, while only 2 to 3 percent of births to white or Cuban women fell into this category. Use of prenatal care

TABLE 2.6
Percentage of Births with Selected Characteristics by Race of Mother in the United States, 1991

Race	Teenage Mother[a]	Unmarried Mother	Late or No Prenatal Care[b]	Low Birthweight[c]	Premature Delivery[d]
White, non-Hispanic	3.1	18.0	3.2	5.7	8.7
Black, non-Hispanic	10.3	68.2	10.7	13.6	19.0
Hispanic	6.9	38.5	11.0	6.1	11.0
Mexican	7.2	35.3	12.2	5.6	10.6
Puerto Rican	9.5	57.5	9.1	9.4	13.5
Cuban	2.6	19.5	2.4	5.6	9.7
Central & South American	3.5	43.1	9.5	5.9	10.9
Other Hispanic	8.3	37.9	8.2	7.2	11.1
Asian or Pacific Islander	2.1	13.9	5.7	6.5	—
Chinese	0.3	5.5	3.4	5.1	7.4
Japanese	1.0	9.8	2.5	5.9	7.5
Hawaiian	—	45.0	7.5	6.7	11.2
Filipino	2.0	16.8	5.0	7.3	10.9
Other Asian or Pacific Islander	2.7	13.5	6.8	6.7	10.8
Native American	7.9	55.3	12.2	6.2	11.9

Source: National Center for Health Statistics (1993).

Note: Data based on 49 reporting states and District of Columbia; New Hampshire does not report Hispanic origin of mother on birth certificate.

[a]Teenage mother = younger than 18 years old.

[b]Late or no prenatal care = beginning in third trimester or not at all.

[c]Low birthweight = less than 2,500 grams (5 lbs. 8 oz).

[d]Premature delivery = less than 37 weeks gestation.

reflects socioeconomic access as well as cultural acceptance of prenatal care. A recent study demonstrated that substance use and a relationship with the baby's father were associated with timing of prenatal care, each of which varied by ethnic status (Zambrana, Dunkel-Schetter, and Scrimshaw 1991).

TABLE 2.7
Infant, Neonatal, and Postneonatal Mortality Rates by Specified
Race or National Origin in the United States, 1990

Race	Infant[a]	Neonatal[b]	Postneonatal[c]
White, non-Hispanic	7.4	4.7	2.8
Black, non-Hispanic	17.9	11.4	6.4
Hispanic[d]	7.8	5.0	2.8
Mexican	7.7	4.9	2.8
Puerto Rican	10.2	7.0	3.2
Cuban	7.6	5.6	2.0
Other Hispanic	7.2	4.5	2.6
Asian or Pacific Islander	—	—	—
Chinese	5.5	2.9	2.5
Japanese	4.8	3.1	—
Hawaiian	10.5	5.4	5.1
Filipino	3.1	1.9	1.2
Other Asian or Pacific Islander	5.6	3.3	2.2
Native American	10.7	5.3	5.4

Source: National Center for Health Statistics (1994b).

Note: Mortality rates based on deaths per 1,000 live births.

[a]Infant = younger than one year.

[b]Neonatal = younger than 28 days

[c]Postneonatal = 28 days to 11 months.

[d]Hispanic rates based on 23 reporting states and the District of Columbia.

Some of the racial/ethnic differences in birthweight may not necessarily lead to differences in health. For example, although extreme low birthweight is associated with high morbidity and mortality in all racial/ethnic groups, it has been argued that black infants who are only slightly underweight are at no increased risk (Wilcox and Russell 1990). The appropriate cut point to use for classifying low birthweight babies may be different for different ethnic groups. However, for any cut point, a greater proportion of black babies are underweight, and overall the mortality rate for blacks is higher than for any other racial/ethnic group.

Figure 2.2 Maternal Mortality Rates by Race in the United States, 1940-90

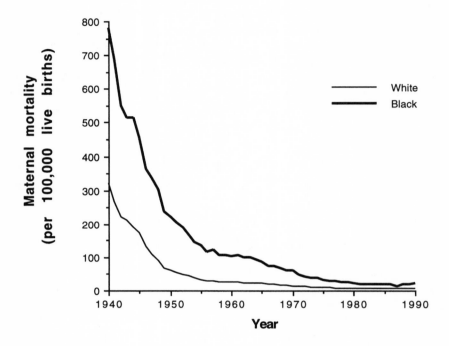

Source: National Center for Health Statistics (1990b, 1994a).

Table 2.7 presents widely varying infant, neonatal, and postneonatal mortality rates in the United States in 1990 (National Center for Health Statistics 1994b). Blacks had more than twice the mortality rates of whites, Hispanics, and Asians. Filipino mothers had among the lowest rates, whereas Native Americans and Hawaiians had comparatively high infant and postneonatal mortality rates (among infants twenty-eight days to eleven months). Although infant mortality has been declining throughout this century, improvement has been faster for whites than blacks, which may reflect their better socioeconomic status.

Black and Native American women also experience higher rates of maternal mortality (18.3 and 12.0 deaths per 100,000 live births in 1983) than white women (5.9 deaths) (National Center for Health Statistics

1990b). Both white and black maternal mortality have declined significantly since 1940, as shown in figure 2.2, but black rates have remained two to three times higher than white rates (Hughes et al. 1988). The leading causes of maternal mortality were the same for blacks and whites: eclampsia and ectopic pregnancy.

Understanding reasons for racial/ethnic differences in reproductive health may help identify effective strategies for reducing social inequities. Those attributable to behavioral or social factors that can be changed easily, or biological differences that are treatable, are more likely to be considered socially and politically acceptable (Ruzek 1993).

Summary and Conclusion

In the United States women's health varies by racial/ethnic group, socioeconomic status, age, and time. Nonwhite women have higher rates of reproductive problems, higher rates of morbidity, and higher rates of mortality from most causes and in virtually every age group. By studying variations in health by gender, race/ethnicity, and age, we may gain insights into the complex relationships between biological, behavioral, and social factors that influence health and longevity. This understanding may in turn help us reduce social inequity in health to the extent that we can modify behavioral and social factors or treat biological differences. But as the essays in this volume show, women in different life circumstances have widely varying values and beliefs, cultural practices, and economic resources. These and other sociocultural factors make reducing inequities in health challenging. The focus on sex and gender issues in health is moving rapidly beyond simplistic comparisons between women and men to complex issues of the social and cultural context of the health of women.

NOTE

1. Age is one of the main determinants of mortality. To compare two populations (e.g., Native American women and Filipino women), it is important to determine whether they have the same age distribution. If they do not, it is necessary to statistically adjust for any age differences or to compare only age-specific data. Age adjustment is a mathematical method used to summarize the mortality rates in different populations while taking into account differences in the age distribution of each population.

REFERENCES

Blendon, Robert J., Linda H. Aiken, Howard E. Freeman, and Christopher R. Corey
   1989   "Access to medical care for black and white Americans: A matter of continuing concern." Journal of the American Medical Association 261:278-81.
Horm, John W., Ardyce J. Asire, John L. Young Jr., and Earl S. Pollack
   1985   "SEER program: cancer incidence and mortality in the United States, 1973-81." DHHS Publication Number (PHS) 85-1837. Bethesda: Public Health Service.
Hughes, Dana, Kay Johnson, Sara Rosenbaum, Elizabeth Butler, and Janet Simons
   1988   The Health of America's Children: Maternal and Child Health Data Book. Washington: Children's Defense Fund.
Kumanyika, Shiriki, and Patricia M. Golden
   1991   "Cross-sectional differences in health status in U.S. racial/ethnic minority groups: potential influence of temporal changes, disease, and lifestyle transitions." Ethnicity and Disease 1:50-59.
Jang, Deeana, Debbie Lee, and Rachel Morello-Frosch
   1990   "Domestic violence in immigrant and refugee communities: responding to the rights and needs of immigrant women." Response 13(4):2-6.
Manley, Audrey, Jane S. Lin-Fu, Magdalene Miranda, Allan Noonan, and Tanya Parker
   1985   "Special health concerns of ethnic minority women." Vol. 2, pp. 37-57 in Women's Health: Report of the Public Health Service Task Force on Women's Health Issues. DHHS Publication Number (PHS) 85-50206. Washington: Public Health Service.
McBarnette, Lorna
   1988   "Women and poverty: the effects on reproductive status." Women and Health 12:55-81.
National Center for Health Statistics; Esther Hing, Mary Grace Kovar, and Dorothy P. Rice
   1983   "Sex differences in health and use of medical care." Vital and Health Statistics, ser. 3, no. 24. DHHS Publication No. (PHS) 83-1408. Public Health Service. Hyattsville, MD: Government Printing Office.
National Center for Health Statistics; Fernando M. Trevino and Abigail J. Moss
   1984   "Health indicators for Hispanic, black and white Americans." Vital and Health Statistics, ser. 10, no. 148. DHHS Publication Number (PHS) 84-1576. Public Health Service. Washington: Government Printing Office.
National Center for Health Statistics; P. Reis
   1990a "Americans assess their health: United States, 1987." Vital and Health Statistics, ser. 10, No. 174. DHHS Publication Number (PHS) 90-1502. Public Health Service. Washington: Government Printing Office.
   1990b "Health of black and white Americans, 1985-87." Vital and Health

Statistics, ser. 10, no. 171. DHHS Publication Number (PHS) 90-1599. Public Health Service. Washington: Government Printing Office.

National Center for Health Statistics

1990c   Vital Statistics of the United States, 1988. Volume 2, Mortality, Part A. DHHS Publication Number (PHS) 91-1101. Public Health Service. Washington: Government Printing Office.

1993   "Advance report of final natality statistics, 1991." Monthly Vital Statistics Report. Volume 42, Number 3, Supplement. Hyattsville, MD: Public Health Service.

1994a   "Health, United States, 1993." Hyattsville, MD: Public Health Service.

1994b   Vital Statistics of the United States, 1990. Volume 2, Mortality, Part A. DHHS Publication Number (PHS) 95-1101. Public Health Service. Washington: Government Printing Office.

National Center for Health Statistics; K. D. Kochanek and B. L. Hudson

1995   "Advance report of final mortality statistics, 1992." Monthly Vital Statistics Report 43(6) suppl. Hyattsville, MD: Public Health Service.

Ruzek, Sheryl B.

1993   "Towards a more inclusive model of women's health." American Journal of Public Health 83:6-8.

U.S. Department of Health and Human Services

1985   Health Status of Minorities and Low-Income Groups. DHHS Publication Number (HRSA) HRS-P-DV85-1. Public Health Service. Washington: Government Printing Office.

1986   Health Status of the Disadvantaged: Chartbook 1986. DHHS Publication Number (HRSA) HRS-P-DV86-2. Public Health Service. Washington: Government Printing Office.

Verbrugge, Lois M.

1985   "Gender and health: an update on hypotheses and evidence." Journal of Health and Social Behavior 26:156-82.

Waldron, Ingrid

1986   "What do we know about causes of sex differences in mortality? A review of the literature." Population Bulletin of the United Nations 18:59-76.

Wilcox, Alan, and I. Russell

1990   "Why small black infants have a lower mortality rate than small white infants: the case for population-specific standards for birthweight." Journal of Pediatrics 116(1):7-10.

Wingard, Deborah L.

1984   "The sex differential in morbidity, mortality, and lifestyle." Annual Review of Public Health 5:433-58.

Zambrana, Ruth E., Christine Dunkel-Schetter, and Susan Scrimshaw

1991   "Factors which influence use of prenatal care in low-income and racial-ethnic women of Los Angeles County." Journal of Community Health 16(5):283-95.

[PART II]

What We Share and How We Differ

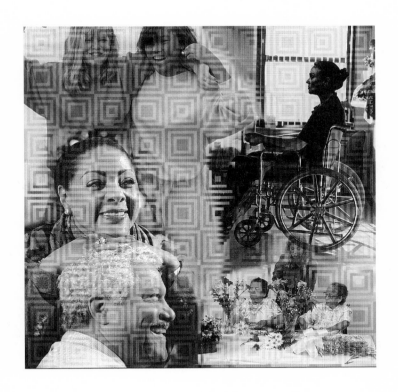

Women's actual biological characteristics, health needs, and priorities for health and healing are complex and highly differentiated. Our own experience and research over the past quarter century makes us wary both of overstating commonalities and of ignoring their importance. In chapter 3, we describe how early feminist assertions about the commonality of women's health experiences in such areas as childbearing and reproductive rights were problematic and obscured important differences in the health perceptions and priorities of white women and women of color. Recognition of differences has directed attention to the particular or special needs of women who have been forgotten and ignored.

But is a "special needs" approach appropriate? Taking a different perspective on what women share and how we differ, Carol Gill argues in chapter 4 that for some women who have been ignored, commonalities with other women, not just special needs, need to be affirmed. As a psychologist and disability rights activist, Gill reveals how women with disabilities want health providers to see them as capable of fulfilling traditional female roles as sexual beings and as mothers, regardless of their disabilities. If their special needs as women with disabilities overshadow their commonalities with other women, they are rendered invisible and placed outside the sisterhood of women.

These contrasting views on what we share as women and how we differ highlight tensions over how to conceptualize women's health in terms of commonalities, differences, and/or special needs. Each perspective adds weight to the argument that truly inclusive views of women's health will emerge only out of the involvement and insights of women from widely diverse social and cultural communities. In terms of health services, the move toward standardization rather than individualization of caring and curing seems particularly at odds with women's complex and different needs. The chapters in this section sound a warning to policy-makers who believe that they can design "one-size-fits-all" medical services. They also make clear why it is so difficult to generalize about "what women want."

[3]

What Are the Dynamics of Differences?

SHERYL BURT RUZEK, ADELE E. CLARKE,
AND VIRGINIA L. OLESEN

Over the past quarter century, feminist health activists
have opened up consciousness of women's health issues in
many arenas. Activist groups that represent the particular
needs of women who share a wide array of social and
political identities have broadened the scope of women's
health agendas and revealed important intersections of
race, class, and gender with life cycle stages, sexual orientations, disabilities, and other life circumstances.

It is not our differences which separate women, but our reluctance to rec-
ognize those differences and to deal effectively with the distortions which
have resulted from the ignoring and misnaming of those differences.
—*Audre Lorde, 1984*

Learning to See Differences

Dealing with differences poses both practical and conceptual problems.
Any journey to understand differences inevitably passes through unfamiliar terrain. Here the traveler will encounter misunderstandings, discover how failing to grasp some particular realities may offend someone
or lead to conflicts. Yet these are the risks that we all need to take to
enable us to take meaningful action in health and health endeavors beyond the narrow confines of our own personal lived experience. This is
how we lift social and cultural blinders and open ourselves to new ways
of seeing, understanding, and being in a world that includes others different from ourselves.

Learning to deal with differences is a shared endeavor. It involves a
commitment to understanding the perspectives of others, particularly
when others challenge one's deeply cherished beliefs about shared
definitions of situations. It also requires affirming that different individuals
and different groups, grounded in their particular life circumstances, will
likely see the world through different lenses than one's own. To hear

51

others as they speak in their own voices requires suspending judgment to facilitate understanding how the world looks from other vantage points.

In this chapter, we place recognition of the importance of multiple perspectives on women's health needs into a historical context. It is critical to recognize that many contemporary women's health issues were initially framed by white, middle-class feminists whose ideologies and social actions reflected their own life experiences and circumstances. Many others—feminists and activists involved in related social movements—broadened awareness of how particular statuses, characteristics, and cultural commitments embedded in race, class, age, sexual orientation, disability, rural life, and religious beliefs all shape distinct perceptions of the salience of particular health issues. To understand different and sometimes competing agendas and priorities for social action, diverse women's underlying perspectives must be understood. Thus we sketch out some of the conflicts and contradictions that taught, and continue to teach, women how partial our own views about women's health are likely to be—and how different the world looks when seen through the eyes of others. To do this we first explore how one women's health movement began around assumed commonalities and then, through confronting many difficult issues, has come to see complexities and differences more clearly.

From Commonalities to Complexities and Differences

Although contemporary feminism has emphasized the primacy of gender in all dimensions of life, differences between groups of women may well be as salient as gender status itself in both the production and experience of health and healing. This is important conceptually, because in the past quarter century of feminist health activism, intense efforts have gone into defining women as a group with special "shared" needs. How, why, and by whom are women viewed as a group? Why do we ourselves, who participated in the construction of women's health as an area of scholarly and political action, see this concept as problematic and in need of revision?

In terms of women's bodies and health issues, women have long been viewed as sharing many characteristics beyond reproductive capabilities. Over two thousand years ago Aristotle described us as colder, weaker, smaller-brained, and generally inferior to men (Tuana 1989). Over the past two centuries physicians, biologists, and other life scientists have played particularly important roles in defining women as members of a group.[1] With the wave of feminism that began in the late 1960s, women themselves have challenged many medical and scientific theories about women and have sought to redefine women's health out of the relatively exclusive domain of medical experts. Not surprisingly, this shift initially reflected the interests, needs, and concerns of the women who were then most involved in feminist health activism—predominately white, middle-class women, with liberal to radical political views. The women's health movement, initially comprised largely, although not exclusively, of middle-class white women, emerged out of several related social movements— the general feminist, childbirth education, and consumer health movements.

A prevailing ideology during the early years of the women's health movement was that health concerns were so fundamental to women that they cut across race and class lines. Thus health was seen as a powerful link that could serve to unite women, all women, into a strong, unified social movement. Whereas many social institutions might divide women, feminism would unite them around health issues because of perceived commonalities surrounding health and health care. However appealing on the surface, this ideology overlooked the critical importance of race and class as sources of different and varied health problems and as sources of different dissatisfactions with health and health care in American society. Moreover, this ideology glossed over the wide array of many women's own perceived priorities for social action that were grounded in very different objective and subjective life experiences.[2]

The serious differences between what some women and other women wanted or needed was lost in global generalizations. For example, as Margaret Nelson (1983) astutely observed, many feminist pronouncements of "what women want" in childbirth glossed over social class differences. Nelson's research clearly showed that the birth preferences of working-class and middle-class women differed in terms of what was considered desirable or undesirable in a hospital setting. Middle-class women wanted fewer drugs and interventions than physicians saw as desirable; working-class women wanted more.

One unintended consequence of assumed commonality was to alienate many women of color. Audre Lorde (1984:497) was one of the first to point out that "there is a pretense to a homogeneity of experience covered by the word *sisterhood* that does not in fact exist." Unlike middle-class white feminists, women of color clearly recognized that the dynamics of race and class as well as gender affected every aspect of their lives, and they were not convinced that gender was as salient as race or class.[3]

From the perspectives of women of color, feminist ideologies of commonalities seemed not only naive and incomplete[4] but—especially in the area of health—dangerously so. For example, although some affluent white women struggled for the right to give birth at home with attendants of their own choosing, many low-income women desperately sought access to hospitals, doctors, and the technologies and interventions that their more affluent sisters struggled to avoid. Why? The "home births" that educated women could have were worlds apart from the "out-of-hospital births" poor women found themselves having not out of choice but out of necessity. Similarly, access to birth control remained problematic for poor women even as middle-class women were critical of its safety. Choosing "good doctors" who communicated well seemed a nearly unimaginable luxury to rural women, who felt fortunate to have any medical care at all.

Critiques of the monolithic view of gender and health in feminism are important to address. African American scholar bell hooks (1981, 1984), one of the first to argue about the importance of both sexism and racism, cogently highlights dilemmas inherent in feminism for women of color. White feminism was predicated on a perception of shared victimization by men in the family, in the workplace, and in health care. For African American women, race and class oppression were far more salient in daily life, and identifying with white women as "victims" strained credulity. Ironically, the women who were most eager to be seen as victims, who overwhelmingly stressed the role of victim, were more privileged and powerful than the vast majority of women in our society (hooks 1984:45).

Although many middle-class white women did see themselves as disadvantaged in relation to men (in their social class) and found support in feminist networks, women of color saw their situations differently—and they found support within their own communities. Esther Ngan-Ling Chow (1987), for example, emphasizes that Asian American women's relative lack of participation in mainstream feminist activities cannot be understood through white women's eyes; it must be understood in terms of Asian American women's own race, class, and cultural experiences. Whereas African American women may derive strength to survive difficult working and living conditions from extended community networks, Asian American women's support and strength comes from the family (Chow 1994). Women of Hispanic origins also had these commitments to family roles (Zavella 1989).

Adding to the blindness of early feminism, in the academy and in the small amount of federally sponsored research on women's health that was funded, even when women of color were nominally included, the diversity of women's experiences and life situations were largely ignored (Zambrana 1987). Given the limited involvement of women of color in mainstream feminism and the patterned ways in which dominant groups generalize their own experience to others *unless directly challenged,* it was predictable that a generalized white, middle-class concept of women's health would emerge.[5]

Much early feminist health research focused on sex differences in health and health-seeking behavior,[6] a focus that did not resonate well with many women of color. Differences between women were rendered invisible as researchers focused on differences between women and men. Research that directly addressed race and class largely focused on institutional stratification, particularly in health occupations.[7] Although increased interest in women's health opened up new areas of inquiry, it did not initially further understanding of women's diverse experiences of health and illness that were grounded in differential experiences such as sexual orientation, disabilities, and geographic location. Nor did feminist analyses (with a few exceptions) address variations in the treatment of women in health and healing systems.

In public policy arenas, the needs and health goals of all women, not just some women, must be addressed. To realize this aim, we argue that understanding women's health must be based on the following premises: Women's health is personally and socially important and warrants serious scholarly attention. It is socially constructed out of specific historical conditions in which one's socioeconomic and social-psychological living and working conditions and culture are as consequential as one's biological makeup. Thus we focus attention on the dynamics of race, class, and gender stratification and cultural factors because women's health status, health behaviors, and health experiences are grounded in these interlocking frameworks of social relations. Understanding the dynamics of multiple differences is challenging and requires suspending assumptions about "all" women and women's experiences. This is the next stage of woman-oriented scholarship, moving beyond the concept that initially opened new areas of women's health scholarship and integrating what has been learned. Ultimately, understanding both the general and the specific, that is, both women's commonalities and differences, is needed to generate health policies, services, and treatments that adequately address the real needs of most, if not all, women.

Some Dynamics of Race, Class, and Gender

Race, class, and gender are interlocking frameworks of social differentiation that are likely to lead to diverse priorities and outright conflicts of interest. In situations that erupt into open conflict, it is easy to see patterns that reveal just how deeply embedded race and class differences are both in "objective" aspects of health status and access to health care and in women's subjective perceptions of what is in their best interest given their overall life circumstances.

To understand women's differences of experience, we next review how concepts of differences emerged historically out of conflict over unexamined assumptions about our commonalities. During the 1970s and 1980s, a period in which health activism coalesced around women's issues, many largely white feminist groups were aware that few women of color joined health movements. Some groups anguished over the lack of women of color in their organizations, and they made efforts to reach out and encourage their participation. It was difficult for many groups to come to terms with the fact that for most women of color, who were actively involved in organizations within their own communities, joining a largely white feminist group was not likely to be a priority.

As Patricia Hill Collins (1990) points out, African Americans are deeply committed to working in their own communities, and this work brings an array of personal rewards and satisfactions. Nonetheless, many feminist health organizations actively attempted to recruit individual women of color into largely white feminist organizations, usually with minimal success. The intentions of feminist groups notwithstanding, we can still ask why would many women of color choose to join groups in which they were likely to feel like "tokens," or "used," when they could be part of a civil rights or church or community group that worked directly for the empowerment of their own communities?

The situation was even more tenuous because women of color who did align themselves with feminist groups sometimes feared that their participation could alienate them from their own communities. Feminism was seen largely as a privileged white women's movement, unlikely to benefit and possibly even harmful to communities of color. Additionally, the individualistic orientation of feminism, and the negativity that was widely expressed toward men and children, conflicted directly with the family and community orientation that many women of color valued.

Some feminist actions also had unintended and unanticipated negative consequences for women of color. These mishaps and misunderstandings heightened tensions around race and class issues. As women of color themselves organized around health and reproductive rights issues during the 1980s, coalition and partnership building between specific women of color organizations and feminist groups became possible. Working relationships between women of color organizations and established groups require dealing with long-standing tensions. Recent conflicts erupted between the National Organization for Women (NOW) and the Women of Color Coalition for Reproductive Health (WCCRH) around the April 1992 Washington March for Reproductive Rights. Members of the WCCRH felt that they had not been adequately included in planning and organizing the event and were not given appropriate prominence in the speaking schedule. The WCCRH's statement highlights tensions that periodically recur over "the uneven power relationship between the long established reproductive rights organizations and the newly established women-of-color reproductive rights organizations." Julia Scott, director of public education and policy for the National Black Women's Health Project in Washington, D.C., commenting on the controversy, suggests that white feminist groups "have to learn to operate differently with us. . . . It's about doing things differently. Realizing that maybe your way isn't the best way. Right now, when faced with diversity, they resist changing" (Martinez 1992:1).

At the same time, many members of established and more powerful groups continue to believe that they have changed and accommodated and that change is not adequately recognized. The painful processes through which others have gone hold clues to understanding what the requisites of cooperation and collaboration are likely to be. They may also reveal likely limits of joint action, limits that are important to understand to facilitate coalition building around issues that are shared to the degree that collaborative efforts are feasible.

Conflicts and Contradictions in Social Change

The specific conflicts that we next present describe how white, middle-class feminists involved in health activism were challenged to rethink some of their basic assumptions about what all women want and need.

Reviewing such conflicts is not intended to discount the enormous contributions to women's health made by these groups, nor is it to suggest
that most feminist health activists knowingly or maliciously disregarded
the needs of women who were not like themselves. The issues in which
these conflicts were grounded go far deeper than mere "lack of sensitivity"
to others by white middle-class feminists. Rather, they derive from underlying structures of inequality (great income disparities, substantial differences in access to opportunities for education, decent paying work,
housing, and other resources and racial discrimination). These are not
simply differences, as some would like to view them. They are fundamental inequities that we, as social scientists, argue inevitably give rise to
conflicts.[8]

Examining conflicts provides an opportunity to look critically at some
of the fundamental assumptions of feminism that are rooted in liberal
western thought. As Cynthia Nelson and Virginia Olesen (1977:13)
noted, "While feminists have conflicting views about *how* equality will be
achieved, the assumption is that it is possible." In questioning key aspects
of this assumption, Nelson and Olesen raised the question of whether
persistent adherence to the view that a "sisterhood of absolute equality"
is indeed possible diverts attention from confronting the inequalities in
all aspects of social life. Here, this perspective is used to explore how and
why many types of conflicts erupt.

Ignoring differences not only distorts "what is" and feeds conflict. It
also obscures some of the larger social forces that shape the "choices"
individuals perceive themselves as making. Such larger social forces include political and economic systems, bureaucracies, and entrenched interest groups. Because "choice" is such a central theme in American
culture and ideologies, including feminist ideologies, it is critical to note
how social actions often fail to address how "choice" is always shaped by
the options that exist within one's specific life circumstances. Women's
"choices" are often rhetorical rather than real.

Learning to recognize differences and diverse interests has come
slowly and painfully.[9] These conflicts have involved issues related to access
to health services and quality control, concepts that are imbued with a
multiplicity of meanings grounded in the socioeconomic and cultural contexts of real women's lives. In complex ways, the social inequalities in
women's life circumstances as they actually are, rather than as anyone
would like them to be, intertwine with social control issues: Who defines
what the acceptable risks and benefits are in a given situation? Whose

interests are served by laws, regulations, and social actions that control access to medical services?

Studying conflict is an important way to deepen understanding of how people or groups define their situations. Conflict requires reexamining what one *thought* was understood about shared definitions of situations. Out of such rethinking may come more complex and complete understanding about what such terms as *access to service* and *quality* mean. And understanding what these things mean to different women is essential for moving beyond simplistic formulations of what women need in health and healing.

Tensions between access and quality or safety erupt in many arenas. In the early twentieth century when the states outlawed American midwives, ostensibly to "improve quality," low-income women who had long depended on ethnic midwives in their communities experienced poorer birth outcomes (Kobrin 1966; Wertz and Wertz 1991). The Flexner Report of 1910, which "cleaned up" the abysmal standard of training in American medical schools, also effectively drove out historically black and women's medical colleges because they could not afford to upgrade and were not given foundation grants to do so as were elite medical schools (Brown 1979). Such tensions and contradictions have riddled women's health activism for three decades.

Access versus Quality Control. One particularly tragic incident that clearly revealed the interplay between race, class, and feminist perspectives precipitated a major early schism within the women's health movement. In this conflict over who should control abortion and who should determine when a woman can give "informed consent" to participate in "medical experiments," sharp differences in interpretation and meaning that emerged were grounded in life circumstances. The incident also laid bare illusions that sisterhood could easily conquer class and race differences.

On Mother's Day 1972, when abortion was still mostly illegal, twenty poor women—most black—were bused from Chicago to Philadelphia for second-trimester abortions after police closed the underground women's clinic where they were scheduled to have abortions.[10] When the Chicago abortionists were arrested, feminists there, in an effort to help, arranged for the women to be bused to Philadelphia. There a local physician agreed to provide abortions assisted by a physician who flew in from California with Harvey Karmen, a well-known underground abortionist and inventor of the Karmen Cannula used widely in vacuum aspiration abortions.[11]

When the Chicago women got to Philadelphia, the abortionists did not use the usual second-trimester "saline" technique (in which salt water is injected into the uterus to trigger an abortion). Instead, they used "super-coils," plastic devices that are inserted into the uterus and left to slowly unwind to cause an abortion (usually within twenty-four hours). It is essential to note that before 1976, medical devices and related procedures were not regulated by the Food and Drug Administration. Experimentation with obstetrical and gynecological devices was common. There was also enormous interest in developing new second-trimester abortion techniques. In this incident, as in others, poor women of color became the subjects of medical experimentation.

The experimental "super-coil" procedure had been tried just previously in Bangladesh where thousands of women were raped in a civil war. For Bangladeshi women, bearing a child under these conditions would have made them social outcasts in their own culture. There the experimental procedure was justified as offering benefits that outweighed the substantial risks. In Philadelphia, the women's situation was also defined by some as an emergency situation. No one except the experimenters had come forward to help the Chicago women terminate their pregnancies.

Half an hour before the Chicago women arrived for the abortions, local feminist groups learned of the experimental procedure. They decided to picket on the clinic steps while the abortions were performed. For the feminist protestors, a critical issue was whether or not the women had been informed that the procedure they were receiving was an "experiment." In the tense situation at the clinic, with the women already in poor health, poor outcomes were not unlikely; one woman required immediate hospitalization. The hospital staff reported the incident to the Department of Public Health, which in turn called the federal Centers for Disease Control (CDC).

In the ensuing investigation, CDC staff documented that 60 percent of the women had complications—three major. Tense conditions during the abortions were noted in the CDC report as contributory factors in the poor outcomes (Copsey 1973). Karmen was arrested, convicted on two counts of practicing medicine without a license, and fined five hundred dollars. The women who had abortions were angry at the feminists who in their view interfered. They were also insulted by a feminist position paper that made them out to be ignorant victims. Two testified for the defense in Karmen's trial, and eight prepared depositions to be included in a libel and slander suit against the feminist groups. Incensed that

Karmen who had helped them was being brought to trial, some felt that it was the feminist picketing, not the procedure, that had caused their problems (Chapman 1973; Women's Health Consumers Union 1973).

Analyzing this situation, it is clear how *safety*, *quality*, and *informed consent* all have relative and situational rather than absolute meanings. The feminist groups that sought to help the Chicago women obtain abortions found themselves at odds with other feminists who operated from the perspective that all women must be afforded protection against experimentation without their explicit consent. The poor women who wanted the abortions saw the situation differently from the Philadelphia women, who had more economic resources and thus more "choices." The lessons learned here transcend simple notions of right and wrong action; they underscore underlying structured inequalities in American women's lives, inequities that shape perceptions of priorities and strategies for change.

Differential Access: Continuing Issues. Access to abortion remains problematic for all women, but it affects poor women and women of color most severely. Historically, unwanted pregnancies have had very different consequences for black compared with white women (Solinger 1992). In the years before abortion was decriminalized in New York, most of the women who died from illegal abortions were black and Puerto Rican. Today, more than twenty years after the *Roe* v. *Wade* decision of 1973, a small number of providers perform most of the abortion services that are concentrated in certain metropolitan areas (Hunt and Joffe 1994). In 1992, 84 percent of all counties had no abortion providers (Henshaw and Van Vort 1992).

Legal abortion remains available largely on the basis of ability to pay and ability to travel long distances. Should the Supreme Court return complete control over all abortion services to the states, the geographic inaccessibility of abortion would further widen socioeconomic differentials of access. And it would likely increase illegal or quasi-legal efforts to retain access (Chalker and Downer 1992).

The Hyde Amendment, first enacted in 1977, which restricted use of federal funds for abortion services, essentially eliminated abortions for poor women under the Medical Assistance (Medicaid) program. According to the Center for Reproductive Law and Policy (1994), only fourteen states authorize abortions for women even for health reasons, and of those, eight do so only under court order. The National Black Women's Health Project regards repeal of the Hyde Amendment as a priority action because it disproportionately affects African American women. (Scott

1994). The project leadership also believes that many feminist groups failed to act vigorously on this issue (Villarosa 1994:196). Staggenborg (1991:144-45), who has studied the pro-choice movement extensively, is not certain that lasting cooperation on a multi-issue pro-choice agenda focusing on the needs of minority and poor women can be achieved because of significant obstacles that emerged in the post-Hyde period.

Contraceptives and Social Control. During the 1960s and 1970s, while largely middle-class, white feminists sought more contraceptive options, including access to sterilization, women of color struggled with the genocidal implications of contraception being imposed on them. One of the key issues here was sterilization abuse, especially of poor women of color. There were clear, well-documented cases of sterilization abuse of black women and girls in the South, Puerto Rican women in New York, Mexican American women in Los Angeles, and Native American women in the Indian Health Service. With the leadership of Dr. Helen Rodriguez-Trias, a Puerto Rican pediatrician in New York City, the Committee to End Sterilization Abuse (CESA) was founded in 1976. CESA and a coalition of other reproductive rights groups pressured New York City to regulate sterilization to prevent its imposition without informed consent or as a condition of receiving medical care, assistance in childbirth, abortion, or welfare. CESA, along with the Committee for Abortion Rights and Against Sterilization Abuse (CARASA), also worked toward federal regulation of Medicaid-funded sterilizations to require a waiting period to obtain voluntary sterilization and to require careful informed consent procedures in a woman's own language and with witnesses to prevent coercive and uninformed sterilizations.[12]

It can be argued that feminist reaction to sterilization abuse was slow in coming largely because it did not affect white middle-class women. People of color were outraged at these abuses because to them what was at issue was genocide of poor people and people of color. In the South, for example, the term *Mississippi appendectomy* was used for sterilization because it was so common, typically done in conjunction with childbirth. In Hartford, Connecticut, in the Puerto Rican community the phrase *estoy operada*, which means "I had an operation," came to mean sterilization because that operation was so common (Gonzalez et al. 1982).

Ultimately, the struggle to end blatant sterilization abuse required coalition building between groups led by women of color and progressive organizations and feminist groups. But coalitions among groups who see the world differently are often forged only after undergoing considerable conflict. In this instance, the National Organization for Women (NOW), at the time the largest feminist group in the United States, testified against sterilization regulations in New York, Washington, and California. NOW's stance was based on the view that there should be no state interference with a woman's right to obtain medical services, a perspective that was central to the campaign for abortion rights. In the case of both abortion and sterilization reform, the ideology reflected the real-life circumstances of NOW's primary constituency: middle- and upper-class white women. For these women, *access* to sterilization, *not protection from it,* was at stake.

To grasp white feminists' stance, it is essential to understand that at the time, white women were largely denied access to contraceptive sterilization because of the "120 rule," the formula that doctors used to determine eligibility. A woman could be voluntarily sterilized only if her age multiplied by the number of her children equaled 120. Thus a woman of thirty would have to have had four or more children to be eligible. The practice of forced or coerced sterilization was virtually unknown to white women, although they were certainly familiar with lack of access to contraception and sterilization. In professional circles, concerns centered largely on the issue of sterilizing mental patients and mentally retarded women (Roth and Lerner 1974). Race and class differentials in access to sterilization were simply not part of most feminists' worldviews.

Following bitter confrontations, coalitions were formed between largely minority health activist groups and white middle-class organizations. From the perspective of women of color, the protection of vulnerable women had to take precedence over other concerns in health policies that affect all women. This view was hard for some feminists to embrace because of their focus on how the state can, and has, used authority to prevent women from exercising the right to control their reproduction in any way they see appropriate.[13]

Contraceptive "Choices." Current controversies over the use of Norplant, a long-term implanted contraceptive device, center around both long-term risks and social control of poor women and women of color. Injectable Depo-Provera, another highly effective but contested method, raises similar concerns[14] (both of which Cheri Pies addresses in chapter 20). Debates over whether Medicaid women are being subtly or not so subtly coerced into use, or if non-Medicaid women with low incomes are being denied access, underscore the diversity of views that surround contraception. In addition, some prominent women of color in medicine take the view that there is a place for Depo-Provera, and banning it would deny some women a useful contraceptive choice.[15] For women who must practice contraception covertly or not at all because of partner disapproval, Depo-Provera is the least likely to be detected.

The historical and contemporary exclusion of women from participation in deciding what kinds of contraception should and will be developed resonate in many arenas.[16] In a diverse society such as the United States, as well as in other countries, how can the advantages and benefits of a particular method for some women be weighed against the costs and dangers it poses for other women, given the differences in their reproductive and health situations broadly defined? In the late 1980s and even more the 1990s internationally, women's health groups increasingly argue that no one group of women should make such decisions for other women. These groups argue for many forms of contraception along with education to allow women themselves to choose what they want, need, or feel is best for them given many considerations including personal access to health care.

The complex issue of "choice" raises the problem of how to approach lived constraints and limits—on access to primary health care, on access to an array of contraceptives, on access to basic health information about reproduction and other issues. The issue of "choice" also raises the problem of the exclusion of women as consumers of contraceptives from participation in designing their means of distribution as well. Increasingly, feminists and others in social studies of science and technology have come to appreciate that the means of distribution and access are integral parts of any technology itself. With whom—what kinds of individuals, agencies, bureaucracies—must you interact to "use" a particular technology? On whom are you dependent if you "choose" to use it? How safe or in danger does the network of distribution make users of different technologies? What kinds of knowledge do you need to be an empowered user? Does the network of distribution easily give you access to that knowledge (Mintzes 1992)?

Another Case of Access and Quality. In October 1991, Med-Tech, a small New York medical device manufacturer, went before the FDA Obstetrics and Gynecology Devices Panel to gain approval for MY-PAP, a tamponlike plastic device that women could use to obtain samples to send to a laboratory for cervical cancer screening. The proposed prescription device was presented by the manufacturer as a mass screening tool for women who did not receive regular medical care. Although it was envisioned as being "prescribed," the prescription was not intended to require a face-to-face encounter with a physician. Although it was unclear how it would actually be distributed given that it was not designed to be sold over the counter, most of the controversy centered around the accuracy of the device. The National Women's Health Network (NWHN) testified before the FDA panel, suggesting that MY-PAP would offer improved access to screening to women of color, who have the lowest rates of cervical cancer screening. The NWHN reflected the perspectives of the board of directors, which now includes a substantial proportion of women who represent women of color health groups. The position taken by the board to support MY-PAP focused on the issue of access, not efficacy.

In the FDA hearing where the request to market the device was rejected, debate centered on the acceptability of a device that was, in the view of FDA staff, consultants, and panel members, substantially less accurate than the conventional Pap test. In contrast, the argument was made by MY-PAP supporters that "some detection was better than none." Although panel members expressed concern over women's lack of access to Pap testing, that problem was defined as a problem of the health care delivery system. Approving an inferior screening device was not a solution to that larger issue. Because MY-PAP produced a high proportion of false negative results (reports of no abnormality when there was one), panel members expressed concern that women who should be followed would not be identified and would instead be lulled into thinking that they did not need medical attention when they did. Concerns were also raised that if marketed, the MY-PAP would be used by women who could have the more accurate Pap test and might have cervical cancer left undetected at an early stage when it could be treated most effectively. Also troubling was the manufacturer's designation of MY-PAP as a prescription device, not to be sold over the counter. How would such a device actually reach underserved populations?

Was this simply a rejection of an ineffective screening device, or was it another instance where some women were denied access to a less effective screening tool to ensure that other women, who have access to care, would not use it? This dilemma goes beyond the feasibility of mediating the needs of one group versus another or determining the best lobbying strategy for groups representing "women's interests." It highlights a dilemma in the regulatory process that is intended to ensure the safety and effectiveness of medical devices for women. Could a regulatory agency have two separate standards of quality for a device—one for women with access to care and another for the underserved? To do so would formally institutionalize race and class inequities. Yet here, "maintaining standards" in the view of the NWHN meant that underserved women continued to go without access to cervical cancer screening of any kind.

What Can Be Learned from These Conflicts?

These events demonstrate how race, class, and gender intersect and affect the experiences and health chances of differently situated American women. These and other confrontations were painful as well as productive for the participants. Conflicts between women of color, poor women, women with disabilities, lesbians, and middle-class white women created opportunities for learning. Some, such as the super-coil controversy and the sterilization abuse campaign, became moments of reconsideration and revision of old understandings of the situations of women, opening the way for participants and wider audiences to grasp that such situations are likely to arise in the future.

Moreover, these events reveal how any women's health movement worthy of the name must address the full diversity of women's situations and on the terms framed by women themselves. To do less would result in health activism becoming only "some women's health movement"— something that early health activists Ehrenreich and English (1973:86–87) cautioned against decades ago. But transforming movements to take knowledge of women's diverse health and life circumstances into account does not come easily, and there is much work yet to be done. We believe that this process of rethinking and revision must be replicated in both scholarship and national policies on women's health. Unless concerted efforts are made to define women's health issues and priorities broadly, making space for the agendas and priorities of diverse groups, the current national attention directed toward women's health may replicate the errors of overgeneralization that have plagued women's health advocacy in the past.

Dimensions of Differences

Women's health activists were not alone in discovering the complexities and differences in women's situations in terms of race, class, and ethnicity. Much of the discovery and learning emerged from "identity movements" composed of women of color, lesbians/gays, older women, and women with disabilities. For women in these movements, health and illness concerns became central to their broader agendas for action.[17]

Given the many dimensions of difference that intersect, what "women want and need" for their health is complex and varied. Thus "what women need" must be reframed to take into account what particular groups of women want and need given their specific life circumstances. How to do this remains problematic. Early efforts to address different women's needs lumped women with particularly visible status characteristics into "special needs" groups—by race/ethnicity, sexual orientation, disability status. This approach, taken, for example, by the U.S. Public Health Service Task Force on Women's Health Issues (1985), ignored differences within these broad groups or categories.[18] The "special needs" approach probably is not well suited for addressing how *overlapping* statuses and situations create multiplicities of needs.

The combinations and permutations of women's needs and perspectives are conceptually overwhelming. Efforts to reduce these needs to more manageable matrices of needs are likely to omit some of the most critical issues for understanding women's health: the meaning of these overlapping characteristics and life circumstances. What does it mean to be a Native American woman on a rural reservation served by the Bureau of Indian Affairs or in a city? Is a lesbian with disabilities "primarily" a lesbian or a disabled woman? How is her identity and health further affected by her racial/ethnic identity, which in itself may be straightforward, complex, or ambiguous? What kinds of health policies will increase the likelihood that all women's health will be addressed most adequately? How will these policies inform health care reform strategies for the next century?

Early thinking about multiplicities of identity tended to be additive—based on a naive and taken-for-granted notion of "combine the elements and stir." This approach has been criticized as inadequate and erroneous, particularly by scholars working in the areas of race, class, and gender issues and in disability studies.[19] To move beyond an additive model of women's experience calls for more interactive and situational models to characterize and understand the experience of women who have multiple statuses that put them outside the mainstream. King (1988) and others suggest an interactive model of "multiple jeopardy" that leads to an understanding of complexities that shape specific practical, ideological, and political choices. For example, there are growing questions about preventive health screening guidelines (see chapter 8). How will mixed-race women be screened for diseases such as breast or cervical cancer if racial/ethnic group–specific guidelines are developed for groups at higher than average risk? Will her "official" racial/ethnic status make her eligible or ineligible for insurance coverage? This is already an issue for Native American women, as Metcalf points out in chapter 11.

The multiplicities of identity are not merely interwoven or inter-leaved or layered in any predictably ordered way (as social scientists might hope to find them!). Instead, various elements of identity can transform each other or "take turns" as the dominant or most pressing identity or set of priorities. Thus multiple statuses are inextricable and emergent in relation to one another in each woman in the very specificities of her situation. At one time one status may override others; at others this same status may be socially irrelevant. For example, lack of money may be the most obvious pressing issue many women face when seeking medical care. But once access to care is achieved, the quality of care provided will be sifted through the lens of what a particular woman needs and how health providers treat her given her other social statuses and their own personal and clinical skills and biases. Some providers, for example, are unfamiliar with how to communicate with patients with hearing impairments. They may fail to make lesbians comfortable or to encourage the degree of individual decision making that many educated women prefer. These same health caregivers may provide excellent care to other women.

Women of color and women with disabilities have been particularly vocal, pointing out how some women's assertions of women's homogeneity denies other women the right to their own voices. Those denied their voices are usually women with the least power in society as a whole. Women's health activists who seek to improve the health of all women are struggling to learn how to move beyond narrow interests to facilitate the development of health policy, clinical services, and research that reflect the real differences in women's needs.[20] How will this take place at the local, state, and national levels? What are some critical elements of this endeavor?

The National Black Women's Health Project included the following in a 1993 position statement:

> Black women are the only appropriate and best qualified indi-
> viduals to define the nature of their health issues and the
> research, programs and services necessary to address them. We
> therefore expect individuals and organizations committed to
> improving the health of women generally, and black women
> specifically, to be sensitive to and encouraging of support for

black women's definition of their health issues, programs and agenda for themselves, and with themselves; to understand that said self-definition and self-governance is the first step toward black women's health, wellness and recovery and to comprehend that indeed, black women are the best able to insure that said agenda/programs are carried forth from the perspective of black women.

Women with disabilities make similar claims. For example, Gill (1992:37) explains:

> Our growing consciousness and willingness to join forces promise to increase our political strength. We must also push for greater self-determination in making health decisions that affect our lives. For too long we have been forced to play the role of passive recipients, while our families and professionals made decisions about our needs. Now we are experiencing that heady realization, familiar to other minority communities, that we are the authentic experts about our own needs. We are demanding, therefore, more input and decision-making authority in the programs that serve us. We are also beginning to expect acknowledgment and compensation for our skills and efforts, and as a result we are pursuing paying jobs and positions of leadership on policy boards in, among others, the organizations that provide our services.

Hearing these voices, we (as scholars and activists) underscore the importance of dismantling a unitary concept of "women's health." Fracturing a unitary view and opening up new questions about what constitutes women's health is crucial. Not all health actions or approaches will work equally well for all women—because not all women share exactly the same problems, concerns, or identities, nor do they have equal resources for creating and managing their health.

At the same time, although different groups of women may have different priorities or prefer to pursue different paths to improving women's health, the need for coalitions and collective action must be recognized. Realistically, this means that all involved will have to learn new ways to compromise, to locate what we describe in chapter 23 as the "contours of women's commonalities," to act jointly on short- and long-term projects.

In working together to write and edit this book, we have struggled to foresee the results of understanding differences—and how they can be addressed. We have contemplated the major contradiction that we will confront—the likelihood that all efforts to improve women's health, no matter how well crafted or intended, will generate some degrees of dissatisfaction for some women. No perfect health care system or set of research priorities can be crafted to meet all of the multiplicity of women's needs and wants. No individual clinician is likely to understand the subtleties and nuances of the experience of health and health caring across all groups of women. Linguistic and communication barriers are likely to continue to exist, and patients and providers will surely make errors of judgment in the course of health and healing activities. Dominant systems of social stratification are likely to continue to produce inequities in both health and health care.

Nonetheless, diminishing "degrees of dissatisfaction" are surely possible. Although the specific needs of many individuals may differ from others with whom they share certain characteristics, in many instances, organizations representing the interests of specific groups can accurately present the needs, priorities, and concerns of identifiable constituencies. It is instructive to listen closely to what their voices are saying. It will be equally critical to insist that they be at the table when national priorities for women's health are established.

Voices from Identity Movements

Different priorities for advocacy, legislative efforts, clinical services, public policies, and research come through in the collective voices of women of color, women with disabilities, lesbians, rural women, and older women. All of these groups make efforts to clearly and directly represent the needs of their constituencies. Their efforts to voice their own health concerns, priorities, and agendas, described briefly here and elaborated elsewhere in this volume, make clear why moving beyond a falsely unitary view of women's health is an essential task for the future.

How Do Women of Color Define Health Issues?

Women of color define women's health issues both from the perspective of their specific racial/ethnic groups and also increasingly as members of women of color coalitions that share some common interests and causes. Thus women of color define their own health issues both through organizations founded specifically to address the needs of particular racial/ethnic groups and through coalitions focusing on the needs of women of color. People of color who work within government agencies are playing active roles in setting federal health agendas for women of color.

Qualitative researchers have generated a considerable body of literature that underscores the importance of understanding the values and beliefs of women about the causes of ill health and strategies for maintaining and improving their health. We review that work in chapter 22. What is important to note is how health beliefs among women of color are not only varied but differ significantly from those held by members of the dominant culture. Typically, health professionals are socialized to take these dominant beliefs as shared when, in fact, this is not accurate (Galanti 1991; O'Connor 1995). Increasingly, professionals' lack of knowledge of the diversity of health beliefs is recognized as contributing to the poorer health status of women of color (Lavizzo-Mourey and Grisso 1994).

The full diversity and range of health issues that women of color define as priorities remains to be mapped.[21] The efforts of some of the most visible national groups are noted in this chapter and throughout this book. Here, some examples of the directions women of color are taking to improve their own health are highlighted.

Many women of color invest themselves heavily in their own community organizations, so the voices of women who are involved in organizations that focus on a broader array of issues that affect communities of color are particularly important to note. African American women's commitments to the health of their communities have been critical for survival (Gilkes 1994; Smith 1995). A survey of national women of color organizations sponsored by the Ford Foundation (Hernandez 1991) provides an overview of the range and breadth of health issues that women of color define as important to address through their own voluntary associations. Many of these organizations are also linked into networks of services for maternal and child health.[22] In the following sections, some of the findings from that survey are noted.

Voices of African American Women. African American women have a long tradition of community health activism. Black club women's public health crusades during the Progressive Era, the work of rural southern midwives, and the Alpha Kappa Alpha sorority health projects during the New Deal era constitute an unbroken line of black women's health activism (Smith 1995). In recent years, the National Black Women's

Health Project (NBWHP) provided leadership for setting priorities and health agendas and community-based services for African American women. Founded by Byllye Avery in 1983, the NBWHP has established 150 self-help groups in twenty-five states that address race- and gender-specific aspects of infant mortality, teen pregnancy, AIDS, substance abuse, cardiovascular disease, cancer, and stress. The organization provides personal health information and policy material on request and is widely credited with pioneering in health and wellness issues for black women. The NBWHP Education Committee's *Body and Soul: The Black Women's Guide to Physical Health and Emotional Well-Being* (Villarosa 1994) includes a discussion of the healing power of spirituality and alternative healing as well as violence, topics that are rarely addressed in mainstream women's health books.

Avery (1994) points out that for black women, violence, particularly battering and sexual abuse, is the number one health issue. It affects black women's mental health and also teen pregnancy, because much teen pregnancy results from incest. Avery's views are reflected in the responses of African American women's organizations to the Ford Foundation survey (Hernandez 1991). All except one of the fourteen African American organizations (in addition to the NBWHP) reported current programs that address one or more health issues. Because these organizations are close to the communities they serve, their programs are likely to reflect felt needs and priorities. Among the organizations that reported current health programs, all but one mentioned teen pregnancy; half reported programs related to some form of violence—domestic violence, sexual harassment, or rape. Ten cited health programs without noting the specific content; three reported reproductive rights, two drug prevention, and one AIDS awareness activities.

Voices of Native American Women. The cultural practices and priorities of Native American women vary considerably by tribe (e.g., Sioux, Navaho, Apache) and by their location—on reservations or in urban areas. Native American groups such as WARN (Women of All Red Nations) have long sought to communicate the ways in which Native women's health perspectives and needs stand in sharp contrast to those of dominant groups (Cook 1980). Some offer services and education. For example, the Native American Women's Health Education Resource Center in Lake Andes, South Dakota, started as a regional community-based health project offering programs on fetal alcohol syndrome, diabetes, and related health issues. It now reaches out to Native American women in the United States and Canada with information on a wide array of issues ranging from toxic waste to racism.[23] In 1990, the Native Women's Reproductive Rights Coalition, comprised of women from over eleven Northern Plains nations, issued an agenda for reproductive rights for Native American women (Astoyer). The Indigenous Women's Health Network, the only Native American women's organization in the Ford Foundation survey (Hernandez 1991), reported program areas in health, teen pregnancy, reproductive rights, and domestic violence.

Drevdahl (1993) points out that Native American women view health holistically and diversely and are interested in health promotion practices, not just illness-care. Above all, they want and need opportunities to blend both traditional Indian and western medicine. In addition to seeking services, Native American women in many areas struggle with maintaining their culture, regretting the loss of their traditions. Joe and Miller (1994), for example, describe how Tohono O'odham and Yaqui women in Tucson, Arizona, struggle with bicultural and even tricultural identities, turning to traditional medicine people and family and friends on the reservation as well as in the city to help them deal with the social and psychological pressures of their lives.

Voices of Latinas. In the Ford Foundation survey, three Latina women's groups reported health-related programs in the areas of teen pregnancy, reproductive rights, general health, and domestic violence (Hernandez 1991). At the local or regional level, Latina health organizing and advocacy reflect various issues. The National Latina Health Organization (NLHO) based in Oakland, California, was founded to raise Latina consciousness about health issues and problems to enable Latinas to take control over their own health and lives. The organization is committed to bilingual access to quality health care and self-empowerment through educational programs, outreach, and research. The NLHO distributes information nationally on reproductive health and locally offers prenatal and other health education classes in Spanish. In 1994, the organization took a stand against a state ballot measure that would establish a single-payer health system on grounds that the plan would exclude illegal immigrants, most of whom are from Latin America.

Health activism for Latinas is often embedded in organizations that serve the entire Latino community. For example, in the Philadelphia area, the Latino Health Issues Forum addresses issues that are specific to particular age groups (infants, children, adolescents, senior citizens). Task forces also work on issues for Latinos with particular characteristics—disabled

persons, sexual minorities, women, and men. The diversity of health activities viewed as important are reflected in *Latinas: Partners for Health
Partnership Directory* (1994). Within Latino/Latina communities, the differences that are significant factors in health are recognized as warranting
direct attention.

In a group as diverse as Hispanic origin women, it is particularly
important to recognize differences in priorities by region and country of
origin. As Zambrana (1994) notes, Puerto Rican women in the United
States are part of a large diaspora in which nearly a third of all Puerto
Ricans live at least part of the year in the United States. Complex migration patterns between the United States and Puerto Rico generate unique
health needs (Lamberty and Coll 1994).

Voices of Asian and Pacific Islander Women. Asian women are an exceedingly diverse group, as Ito and her colleagues show in chapter 12.
Overall, women in this group have excellent health status—better than
that of whites. However, newer immigrant groups do not uniformly share
such favorable health status, nor do they find health services compatible
with their traditional values and belief systems (Kulig 1990). The sheer
diversity of these groups makes generalizing inappropriate.

Asian/Pacific Islanders are well represented in the health professions,
so in large urban areas, culturally appropriate providers may be available
for certain populations. In San Francisco, where there are large, well
established Asian American as well as immigrant populations, there are
numerous clinical services that specifically serve Asian and Pacific Islanders. Both language and culture are important issues, particularly because
of continuing immigration and the diversity of ethnic groups. Beliefs
about the causes of illness among Asian and Pacific Islander women reveal
great diversity. For example, Vietnamese women in the Midwest weight
the causes of illness differently than do most Americans. One study found
that weather or temperature and bad food or water were what women most
frequently saw as the "causes" of disease. Far less often Vietnamese immigrant women cited fatigue, germs, the supernatural, mental state, not
recovering one's health, and personal actions (in that order) as major
sources of illness (Bell and Whiteford 1987). Another study showed that
45 percent of Korean women believe that faith in God is a force in
maintaining health. They also strongly believe in the qualities of hot and
cold food (Park and Peterson 1991).

In Los Angeles, the Asian Health Project provides multilingual
health information and publications to Asian and Pacific communities.

Despite stereotypical views of Asians as "model citizens," domestic violence is an often overlooked health issue. The San Francisco Asian Women's Shelter for battered immigrant women and their children, cofounded by Debbie Lee, provides critical direct services. Lee and others are also active in developing national policy and training on domestic violence for health providers who work with immigrant and refugee communities.[24]

Women of Color Coalitions and Partnerships

Nationally, the Women of Color Partnership formed out of the Religious Coalition for Reproductive Rights (RCRR), an umbrella organization that emphasizes education and advocacy to make reproductive health choices more widely available.[25] Member organizations include Catholic, Protestant, Jewish, and humanist organizations. The Campaign for Abortion and Reproductive Equity (CARE) coordinated by the National Black Women's Health Project and the Campaign for Women's Health, sponsored by the Older Women's League, involve broad-based coalition actions that demonstrate the commitment of women of color organizations to work with others who share common goals. The National Institute for Women of Color reported programs to the Ford Foundation in the areas of teen pregnancy, reproductive rights, and domestic violence. Refugee Women in Development serves primarily low-income Asian, Hispanic, and Caucasian refugee women and reported programs in health, mental health, and domestic violence (Hernandez 1991).

Women of color emphasize that the health of women of color cannot be separated from the health of families and communities of color where race, class, and gender inequities are closely interwoven (Bea 1991). The health of men is seen as central to the health and well-being of women and children's health and is a high priority. For example, African American and Latina women are concerned over the level of all forms of violence in their communities, including homicide, the leading cause of death for young men, which touches virtually every aspect of community life. If feminist health advocates are to work effectively with women of color groups, they will have to respect this stance, not try to change it.

Because women of color emphasize that people of color must define their own issues and set their own priorities and agendas, it is particularly important to note how the themes that recur in women of color health organizations differ most profoundly from the concerns and actions that predominately white feminist organizations have emphasized. These views suggest that national priorities for women's health must be grounded in the felt needs of these groups. In addition to violence, recurring themes include (1) access to conventional medical service for medical problems beyond reproduction; (2) production of culturally sensitive educational materials in languages and language styles other than standard English; (3) reducing the causes and consequences of racial oppression and poverty; and (4) reducing both behavioral and environmental risk factors for the leading causes of death and disability in communities of color.

Women of color view gender differences in health very differently compared with white feminists. Disparities in health status between both women and men of color (compared with whites) are what African American, Hispanic, and Native American women see most clearly. For Asian American women, whose overall health status is more favorable than that of all other women, including white women, culture and language remain priority health issues along with services for new immigrant groups.

The different situations of women are reflected in different perceptions of "what's important." For example, for many African American and Latina women, street drugs are a concern for themselves, their unborn babies, and communities. This contrasts sharply with the focus of white feminists on excessive prescribing of psychotropic drugs to "keep women in their place." Similarly, women of color view male unemployment, not just depressed female wages, as what deprives women of color of access to the economic base needed to maintain healthful living conditions. Environmental concerns of people of color are also different. The United Church of Christ Commission for Racial Justice (1987) has made efforts to address environmental racism—the systematic placement of toxic waste sites in low-income communities of color. When women are fighting the location of solid-waste incinerators and lead poisoning in their communities, they view environmental organizations that are "saving whales and seals" as out of touch with the needs of communities of color (Villarosa 1994:558–65). In short, women of color are likely to see poverty, racism, and their social, political, economic, and behavioral manifestations, not sexism, as "the problem."

How Do Women with Disabilities Define Health Issues?

Ironically, the disabilities rights movement and the women's movement both emerged in the 1970s, but it was almost a decade before the women's health movement embraced concerns about disabled women's health issues. In 1981, some feminist health organizations, such as the Coalition for the Medical Rights of Women (Sprague 1981), took note of disabilities issues. Activists with disabilities enlarged feminist health agendas in several ways. In 1984 the Women and Disability Awareness Project in New York City produced a book, *Building Community*, which attempted to introduce women with disabilities to feminism and to introduce a feminist perspective into disability rights activism. The Project on Women and Disability (PWD) grew out of the Boston Women's Health Book Collective in 1988.

Women with disabilities suffer the costly effects of sexism in employment, but the effects are often amplified by their disabilities. They typically earn less, have less education, are underemployed, and are poorer than their able-bodied peers, all of which have consequences for health and for access to insurance, medical care, and quality of services.

Women with disabilities express concerns about several health issues that do not emerge for able-bodied women and that most feminist health perspectives do not address. These concerns, voiced by scholars and activists[26] and elaborated by Carol Gill in chapter 4, include the following:

1. Health care contexts where access to the site is difficult for persons with physical disabilities or blind people or once in the site, where there are limited facilities for people with hearing impairments or other particular needs.

2. Some providers' assumptions that because a woman is disabled, she is essentially unhealthy or that whatever illness or ailment she currently has is related to her disability.

3. The view that women with disabilities are asexual leads to inadequate counseling as well as limited concern over reproductive health and functioning and inadequate access to contraception.

4. A generally negative attitude about pregnancy for women with disabilities including inattention to the health needs of pregnant disabled women and their capacity to bear and care for children. Access to infertility treatment is rare, and involuntary sterilization is a particular concern.

5. A failure of scholars to address the issues of violence against disabled women, mental health issues, or the extent to which health insurance policies make women with disabilities dependent and keep them from marrying or having children.

Finally, although some women with disabilities have organized around activities that embrace parts of feminist agendas, many are critical or seek to modify such agendas or establish different priorities. Tensions are especially high around abortion of "defective fetuses" (Asch and Fine 1988). Here the feminist and disability rights' movements struggle to accommodate some women's concerns over the difficulties of raising seriously disabled children while simultaneously recognizing that women with disabilities fear that the "search for the perfect child" invalidates their very existence.

How Do Lesbian and Bisexual Women Define Health Issues?

Sexual orientation also shapes perceptions of health needs and experiences in obtaining health care. If lesbians are 10–20 percent of American women, there are 12 to 23 million very diverse lesbians in the United States today. Lesbians come from all social groups, and about one in three is a mother. Many if not most lesbians have long been aware of their lack of access to adequate routine health care because of finances (women earn much less than men—straight or lesbian) or discomfort going to straight providers when they need or desire to stay closeted. Use of gynecological care is reduced by the fact that most women get much of their routine care through birth control/family planning visits, which lesbians do not make. In addition, most gynecological providers routinely assume heterosexuality and do not know enough about lesbian sexuality to be helpful with common concerns and problems (Peteros and Miller 1982; Smith, Johnson, and Guenther 1985).

Other health care issues commonly noted by lesbians and bisexuals include lack of access to health care because of lack of "family" health insurance and resources; lack of access to reproductive rights—including the ability to have joint custody with a co-mother, artificial insemination by donor, or abortions. For bisexuals, these difficulties are often exacerbated by the need to stay closeted because bisexuality is unacceptable not only to straight people but to some gays and lesbians as well (Hutchins and Kaahumanu 1991). Although bisexual women may more comfortably "pass" as straight in seeking gynecological care, it is more difficult to do so in seeking mental health services. Here both lesbian and bisexual women face an array of issues ranging from the need for affordable and positive lesbian/gay/bisexual psychotherapeutic services to services for alcohol and other substance abuse, domestic violence, and child abuse. In chapter 18, Nancy Stoller addresses how stigma and marginality have particularly negative effects on lesbians.[27]

How Do Rural Women Define Health Issues?

The romantic image of rural life as peaceful and free from the dangers and pressures of urban living obscures many conditions that put rural women's health at risk and limit their opportunities for care. As Perry describes in chapter 9, many rural women do not have access to medical care that most urban women take for granted. Rural women often speak of isolation from limited health care facilities, which makes getting help even in crisis situations very difficult. Those who do heavy farm or ranch work also comment on working with heavy machinery or large animals and the threats of being exposed to pesticides, a particular risk for migrant women laborers, most of whom are women of color (Jasso and Mazorra 1984).

Rural economic decline threatens many rural women's health. Women whose family farms or ranches or whose farm jobs are threatened by the economic crisis in American agriculture also experience tension over possible loss of their way of life. Small towns and larger communities have been hard hit by economic difficulties. Environmental disasters such as flooding also threaten to wipe out entire communities. One rural feminist health activist has noted that the economic strains in American agriculture have taken their toll both on rural life and on women organizing around these issues (Bigbee 1985).

In the late 1970s, rural feminists joined with local community organizers to establish rural health care centers in such places as Fayetteville, Arkansas, Santa Fe, New Mexico, and Rutland, Vermont. Rural midwifery took on new importance (Gaskin 1975). In 1981 the Rural Health Issues Committee of the National Women's Health Network, in connection with rural health projects, set out twelve recommendations to frame and guide a focus on rural women's health. Among these were an expanded view of women's health beyond the traditional context of childbearing, distribution of public assistance to rural residents, access for all rural women to full health services, and upgrading health services for older rural women (Rural Health Issues Committee of the National Women's Health Network 1981). This agenda has largely been unrealized because of economic constraints related to both local economies and federal policies. The concerns of rural women continue to focus on economic uncertainties, lack of available medical services, inadequate transportation, and isolation (Gesler and Ricketts 1992; Richardson 1987).

To understand rural women's health, it is important to note that rural values tend to be conservative, most women observe traditional sex roles, and they tend to be socialized to keep their problems to themselves (Bushy 1990). Others (Hansen and Resick 1990; Richardson 1987; Wilson-Ford 1992) emphasize the ways in which self-reliance, religious principles, and subcultural values and beliefs shape rural women's health practices and perceptions. The lack of scholarship on rural women may reflect the degree to which rural women differ significantly from feminist scholars who more often hold liberal political orientations, are career-oriented, individualistic, and favor egalitarian gender roles. A more inclusive understanding of women's health makes space for the situated experiences of rural women who come from many racial/ethnic, socioeconomic, and cultural groups.

How Do Older Women Define Health Issues?

Two organizations emerged to address the needs of older women. The Gray Panthers, founded in 1970 by Maggie Kuhn, addresses a wide array of social and health issues for older women. The Older Women's League (OWL), the largest national grassroots organization for midlife and older women, grew out of the displaced homemakers' movement in the mid-1970s. The organization was formed in 1980 during the White House Conference on Aging and has local chapters throughout the country. OWL president Tish Sommers had previously headed the NOW's Task Force on Older Women. Kuhn and Sommers were concerned that women were "lost" in the two larger movements for the rights of women and for the elderly. Sommers argued (1974:3-4) that "the compounding effects of sexism and ageism have not been sufficiently recognized [because] . . . bureaucracies and disciplines tend to see their field, the elderly, as separate and distinct. They view their constituency as an undifferentiated category especially in regard to sex, so that the specifics are blurred. Older women tend to become invisible in statistics, theories, and social programs in the aging field." In 1980, Sommers and Laurie Shields (founder of the Displaced Homemakers Movement) issued a "gray paper" on "Older Women and Health Care: Strategy for Survival," pointing out that the Boston

Women's Health Book Collective's *Our Bodies, Ourselves* "does not go beyond menopause, as though we cease to exist as women when our reproductive life is over." More recent editions have corrected these omissions.[28]

From the outset, both OWL and the Gray Panthers focused on midlife and older women's economic status and need for access to medical care. Sommers and Shields' agenda—ranging from improved access to medical care to increased biomedical research—became a blueprint for improving older women's health. An early strategy was to seek legislation to relieve the plight of divorced and widowed women who lost medical benefits and had no place to turn until they became eligible for Medicare. Today, insurers cannot simply cut such women off but must allow them to purchase plans for an extended period (if they can afford to do so). Other successful lobbying efforts have included ensuring that the 1993 federal Family and Medical Leave Act included time off to care for an elderly parent, not just a spouse or child.[29]

Sociohistorical Contexts of Women's Lives

As this brief overview of identity movements reveals, the multiplicity of women's concerns defies easy characterization. We underscore that perceptions of "what's important" reflect complex and differential systems of stratification as well as culture. Within patterned group differences, individual women also have complex social and psychological identifications and commitments, each of which adds layers of complexity to defining "what women want." Many of the concerns of women of color may also have particular salience for white women who are at the bottom of the economic ladder. Women of all races, in all regions, who struggle to support families on inadequate incomes must be considered in national discussions of women's health.

Major social and economic shifts in American society are sharpening the need for health perspectives that recognize the complexities and differences in women's life circumstances:

— The growing numbers of single-parent families of all races, mostly headed by women, alter views about woman's traditional place and the role of men and the state in ensuring women's and children's economic survival.

— Increases in homelessness and overcrowding of deteriorating housing leaves families without the security of place that is critical for finding and retaining employment, allowing children to remain in school, and maintaining mental as well as physical health.

— Growing unemployment in cities and states where the cost of doing business is higher than in other regions threatens both single- and dual-worker families who face relocation or loss of work that divides families and strains communities and social support networks.

— Frighteningly rapid technological developments around human, chiefly female, reproductive processes, unregulated and unaccompanied by social customs attuned to such developments, call into question the very definitions and roles of women as mothers.

— Threats to reproductive rights, including terrorism and murder of abortion providers by the Radical Right, and coercion regarding contraceptive technologies create a hostile environment for women, especially younger women learning to be sexual beings.

— The emergence of large numbers of the aged in the American population, the majority of whom are female, raises the specter of a gendered caste seen as pariahs in a youth-oriented, cost-conscious society or alternatively as a power block set on garnering resources for themselves by restricting resources available to young families and children.

— The deterioration of both inner cities and economically depressed rural regions creates the threat of obdurate impoverished substrata with little opportunity to move out of poverty. This increases the likelihood of a growing proportion of children being raised in severe poverty in areas with inadequate education, housing, and health services, all of which have negative health consequences.

— Rising costs of health care and technology development coupled with a growing proportion of the population without medical coverage, or with inadequate coverage, or in fear of losing coverage without hope of ever regaining it further stratifies health care systems.

— Migration patterns highlight cultural differences in health status and care for women, particularly among immigrants—from Southeast Asia, the Caribbean, Central and South America, and the Soviet Union.

These social trends, taken together with the perspectives of various identity movements, make it clear that there is no single, common life experience shared by all women. Identification with one group or another is fluid and changing. The diversity of living and working conditions implied by these social realities demands attention to the differences in women's experience in all aspects of health research, public policy, and clinical practice.

As scholars and health activists, we are aware that assertions of separate and distinct social realities can be misused as rationales for ignoring how others view the world altogether. We share the view of Bannerji and her colleagues (1992:9) that "perceiving the issue as just a matter of who can speak for whom can also offer a way out of dealing with the complexity of women's experience and women's oppression. It permits white women to forget about nonwhite women since 'we have no right to speak for anyone but ourselves.' This reading of the political and theoretical critiques of white feminism can be used to justify ignoring the majority of women in the world altogether."

Our intent in this chapter was to highlight differences in women's health with the expectation that understanding can unite, not divide, women. The challenges of the future will require finding new ways to work together to grow beyond our differences but not evade or ignore them.

NOTES

Lynn Weber and Jane Zones made particularly helpful comments on several early drafts of this chapter. We also wish to acknowledge the research assistance of Leah Greene in preparing this chapter, and we thank the College of HPERD, Temple University, for providing support for her.

1. There is considerable feminist scholarship on this issue. See especially the work of Bleier (1984), Hubbard (1990), and Rosser (1994).

2. For a detailed analysis of the roots of the women's health movement and conflicts and contradictions in this ideology, see Ruzek (1978).

3. For recent perspectives of women of color on the importance of race, class, and gender inequalities and intersections, see especially Cyrus (1993), Baca Zinn and Dill (1994), and Bea (1991). Jean Belkhir, founder and editor of *Race, Gender & Class and Gender, An Interdisciplinary & Multicultural Journal* (Towson, MD: Towson State University) promotes analysis of these intersections.

4. For accounts of the views of women of color on this aspect of feminism, see especially

Baca Zinn (1991), Baca Zinn and Dill (1994), Collins (1990), Cordova et al. (1990), Davis (1981), Dill (1983), hooks (1981), King (1988), and Terrelonge (1989).

5. For a review of the ways in which the experiences of women of color have challenged feminist scholars to rethink the relationship between race and gender, see especially Baca Zinn and Dill (1994) and Collins (1990). In women's health studies there has been less attention to theoretical and conceptual issues and more attention to the health status and medical service needs of various groups.

6. The extensive literature on sex differences in health has been reviewed extensively by Charlotte Muller (1990). In much of this literature, race and class (when included) tended to be "adjusted for" or study groups were made homogeneous to allow for analysis of the variable of interest—differences between men and women (see, e.g., Verbrugge 1985).

7. For the most complete analysis of social class as a critical factor in women's health, see Fee and Krieger (1994).

8. Consciousness-raising, which as a key strategy of feminism in the 1960s and 1970s facilitated new awareness of gender, did not adequately address structural inequities in ways that resulted in effective social action. Consciousness-raising itself largely took place among women who were already similar in terms of socioeconomic status as well as other characteristics.

9. For a more detailed discussion of the roots of these conflicts in the women's health movement during the 1970s, see Ruzek (1978).

10. For the most complete account of this underground abortion service, see Kaplan (1996).

11. The incident described below is analyzed in Ruzek (1978) based on accounts provided by both feminist and medical journalists. See especially BenDor (1973, 1974), Chapman (1973), Copsey (1973), and Dejanikus (1973).

12. For detailed discussion of both blatant and subtle sterilization abuse and efforts to reduce or eliminate it, see especially Clarke (1984), Gonzalez et al. (1982), Rodriguez-Trias (1982, 1984), and Shapiro (1985).

13. This type of controversy has parallels in England. There the campaign against the injectable contraceptive Depo-Provera, used largely on immigrant women of color, involved similar issues about social control and lack of informed consent as well as concerns about safety. At the same time, some feminist critics of Depo-Provera cautiously wondered if, for some women in developing countries who had few options for controlling their fertility and faced multiple health risks, the benefits of this contraceptive might justify the risks (Rakusen 1981).

14. The National Latina Health Organization has raised concerns about lack of informed consent and difficulty in getting Norplant removed (Martinez 1992). Some Native American women view it as an effective addition to contraceptive options and seek better access as well as controls on use (Lewry and Asetoyer 1992). The National Black Women's Health Project has taken the position of supporting new technologies, including Norplant, if they are safe and improve choice. But it also cautions about issues of social control and the failure of adults to "engage young people in thoughtful, honest, realistic discussions about their sexuality and sexual behavior" (Scott 1993:31).

15. For example, Doris E. Tirado (1994), medical director of Planned Parenthood

of Maryland, argues that Depo-Provera is the contraceptive of choice for women with sickle-cell disease because it reduces the severity of episodes.

16. When Margaret Sanger and her colleagues turned the reins of research on contraception over to physicians (Reed 1983) and to reproductive scientists (Clarke 1996) in the 1920s and 1930s, they allowed the contraceptive research agenda to be preempted by nonfeminists and even antifeminists in ways that remain vividly consequential today. See also Gordon (1990).

17. Most women's rights and identity movements emerged in urban centers; rural organizing for economic opportunities and political recognition focused largely on regional needs, not gender. As Judy Perry points out in chapter 9, rural women's health issues are just beginning to be recognized even in regional associations organized to address issues of rural life.

18. For further discussion of the special-needs approach, see also Lin-Fu (1987).

19. An extensive literature now critiques this approach. See particularly critiques that focus on women of color in Anderson and Collins (1992), Baca Zinn (1991, 1994), Baca Zinn and Dill (1994), Collins (1990), Dill and Baca Zinn (1990), DuBois and Ruiz (1990), Garcia (1989), and Lorde (1984). For critical appraisals from disability studies scholars, see especially Browne, Connors, and Sterne (1990), Fine and Asch (1988), Gill (1992), and Saxton and Howe (1987).

20. For elaboration on these points, see especially Bannerji et al. (1992), Blackwell-Stratton et al. (1988), Collins (1990), Gill (1992), hooks (1989), and Nsiah-Jefferson (1990).

21. Diane L. Adams (1995) and Marcia Bayne-Smith (1996) have each edited a volume on health issues for women of color. Neither book was available when this book was completed.

22. For addresses and contact persons in minority health organizations that address maternal and child health issues, see Pickett, Clark, and Kavanagh (1994:6-9). This publication is available at no cost from the National Maternal and Child Health Clearinghouse, 8201 Greensboro Drive, Suite 600, McLean, VA 22102.

23. For Native American women, social and health issues intertwine, as Metcalf points out in chapter 11. See also Abbott (1988), Campbell (1989), and Jaimes (1992).

24. Lee is director of the Family Violence Prevention Fund's National Health Initiative on Domestic Violence, which has been designated as a U.S. Department of Health and Human Services Special Issues Resource Center for Domestic Violence and Health Care Access (Health Watch 1994:15).

25. The RCRR was initially called the Religious Coalition for Abortion Rights (RCAR). Publications are cited by the name used at the time of publication.

26. See various perspectives in Browne, Connors, and Sterne (1990), Deegan and Brooks (1985), Fine and Asch (1988), Finger (1990), Gill (1992), and Hillyer (1992).

27. For reviews of recent scholarship on lesbian health, see especially Rosser (1993), Stern (1993), Stevens (1992), and Stevens and Hall (1991).

28. For more extended discussion of these issues, see especially Doress-Worters and Siegal (1987).

29. Current agendas include (1) universal access to medical care for all Americans,

(2) providing older women with legal knowledge they need to take control of the final years of life, including death, and (3) educating women on how to understand and use Medicare and Medicaid benefits and mobilizing women to fight against supplementary medical care premiums.

REFERENCES

Abbott, Devon L.
   1988   "Medicine for the rosebuds: health care at the Cherokee Female Seminary." American Indian Culture and Research Journal 12(9):59–71.
Adams, Diane L., ed.
   1995   Health Issues for Women of Color: A Cultural Diversity Perspective. Thousand Oaks, CA: Sage.
Anderson, Margaret L. and Patricia Hill Collins, eds.
   1992   Race, Class, and Gender: An Anthology. Belmont, CA: Wadsworth.
Asch, Adrienne, and Michelle Fine
   1988   "Shared dreams: a left perspective on disability rights and reproductive rights." Pp. 297–305 in Michelle Fine and Adrienne Asch (eds.), Women with Disabilities: Essays in Psychology, Policy, and Politics. Philadelphia: Temple University Press.
Avery, Byllye Y.
   1994   "Breathing life into ourselves: the evolution of the National Black Women's Health Project." Pp. 4–10 in Evelyn C. White (ed.), The Black Women's Health Book, rev. ed. Seattle: Seal Press.
Baca Zinn, Maxine
   1991   "Race and the reconstruction of gender." Research Paper 14, Center for Research on Women. Memphis, TN: Memphis State University.
   1994   "Feminist rethinking from racial-ethnic families." Pp. 303–26 in Maxine Baca Zinn and Bonnie Thornton Dill (eds.), Women of Color in U.S. Society. Philadelphia: Temple University Press.
Baca Zinn, Maxine, and Bonnie Thornton Dill
   1994   "Difference and domination." Pp. 3–12 in Maxine Baca Zinn and Bonnie Thornton Dill (eds.), Women of Color in U.S. Society. Philadelphia: Temple University Press.
Bair, Barbara, and Susan E. Cayleff, eds.
   1993   Wings of Gauze: Women of Color and the Experience of Health and Illness. Detroit: Wayne State University Press.
Bannerji, Himani, Linda Carty, Kari Dehli, Susan Health, and Kate McKenna
   1992   Unsettling Relations: The University as a Site of Feminist Struggles. Boston: South End Press.
Bayne-Smith, Marcia, ed.
   1996   Race, Gender, and Health. Thousand Oaks, CA: Sage.

Bea, Irene I.
    1991   La Chicana and the Intersection of Race, Class, and Gender. New York: Praeger.

Bell, S. E., and M. B. Whiteford
    1987   "Tai Dam health care practices: Asian refugee women in Iowa." Social Science and Medicine 24:317-25.

BenDor, Jan
    1973   "Harvey Karman: another vacuum cleaner salesman?" Her-Self 2 (Nov.):9, 21.
    1974   "Super-coil abortion, Karman part 4." Her-Self 2 (Jan.): 8.

Bigbee, Jeri Lynn
    1985   "Rural-urban differences in hardiness, stress, and illness among women." Ph.D. diss., University of Texas at Austin.

Blackwell-Stratton, Marian, Mary Lou Breslin, Arlene Brynne Mayerson, and Susan Bailey
    1988   "Smashing icons: disabled women and the disability and women's movement." Pp. 306-32 in Michelle Fine and Adrienne Asch (eds.), Women with Disabilities: Essays in Psychology, Policy, and Politics. Philadelphia: Temple University Press.

Bleier, Ruth
    1984   Science and Gender: A Critique of Biology and Its Theories on Women. New York: Elsevier Science.

Boston Women's Health Book Collective
    1992   The New Our Bodies, Ourselves. New York: Simon and Schuster.

Brown, E. Richard
    1979   Rockefeller Medicine Men: Capitalism and Medical Care in America. Berkeley: University of California Press.

Browne, Susan E., Debra Connors, and Nanci Sterne, eds.
    1985   With the Power of Each Breath: A Disabled Women's Anthology. Pittsburgh: Cleis Press. Tape version, Womyn's Braille Press.

Bushy, Angeline
    1990   "Rural U.S. women: traditions and transitions affecting health care." Health Care for Women International 11:503-13.

Campbell, Gregory
    1989   "The changing dimension of Native American health: a critical understanding of contemporary Native American health issues." American Indian Culture and Research Journal 13(3-4):1-20.

Center for Reproductive Law and Policy
    1994   Reproductive Freedom in the Courts. Portrait of Injustice. Abortion Coverage under the Medicaid Program. New York: Center for Reproductive Law and Policy, 12 April.

Chalker, Rebecca, and Carol Downer
    1992   A Woman's Book of Choices: Abortion, Menstrual Extraction, RU-486. New York: Four Walls Eight Windows.

Chapman, Frances
    1973   "Supercoil recoil: Karman case comes to trial." Off Our Backs 3 (Nov.):2, 6.
Chow, Esther Ngan-Ling
    1987   "The development of feminist consciousness among Asian American women." Gender and Society 1:284–99.
    1994   "Asian American women at work." Pp. 203–28 in Maxine Baca Zinn and Bonnie Thornton Dill (eds.), Women of Color in U.S. Society. Philadelphia: Temple University Press.
Clarke, Adele E.
    1984   "Subtle forms of sterilization abuse: a reproductive rights analysis." Pp. 188–212 in Rita Arditti, Renate Duelli Klein, and Shelley Minden (eds.), Test-Tube Women: What Future for Motherhood? London: Pandora Press.
    1996   Disciplining Reproduction: Modernity, American Life Sciences, and "the Problem of Sex." Berkeley: University of California Press.
Collins, Patricia Hill
    1990   Black Feminist Thought: Knowledge, Consciousness, and the Politics of Empowerment. Boston: Unwin Hyman.
Cook, Katsi
    1980   "Social control of childbirth: a Native American response." Pp. 251–58 in Helen B. Holmes, Betty B. Hoskins, and Michael Gross (eds.), Birth Control and Controlling Birth: Women-Centered Perspectives. Clifton, NJ: Humana Press.
Copsey, Diana
    1973   "Busing of 15 women to Philadelphia for 'super coil' abortions provokes wide furor." Obstetrics and Gynecology News 34 (1 April):1, 34–37.
Cordova, Teresa, Norma Cantu, Gilberto Cardenas, Juan Garcia, and Christine M. Sierra, eds.
    1990   Chicana Voices: Intersections of Class, Race, and Gender. Albuquerque: University of New Mexico Press.
Cyrus, Virginia, ed.
    1993   Sex, Class, and Race Intersections: Visions of Women of Color. Mountain View, CA: Mayfield.
Davis, Angela
    1981   Women, Race, and Class. New York: Random House.
Deegan, Mary Jo, and Nancy Brooks, eds.
    1985   Women and Disability: The Double Handicap. New Brunswick, NJ: Transaction Press.
Dejanikus, Tacie
    1973   "Super-coil controversy." Off Our Backs 3 (May):2–3, 11.
Dill, Bonnie Thornton
    1983   "Race, class, and gender: prospects for an all-inclusive sisterhood." Feminist Studies 9:131–50.

Dill, Bonnie Thornton, and Maxine Baca Zinn
    1990   Race and Gender: Revisioning Social Relations. Research Paper #11. Center for Research on Women. Memphis, TN: Memphis State University.

Doress-Worters, Paula B., and Diana Laskin Siegal
    1987   Ourselves Growing Older: Women Aging with Knowledge and Power. 1992. New York: Simon and Schuster.

Drevdahl, Denise
    1993   "Images of health: perceptions of urban American-Indian women." Pp. 122–29 in Barbara Bair and Susan E. Cayleff (eds.), Wings of Gauze. Detroit: Wayne State University Press.

DuBois, Ellen C., and Vicki L. Ruiz
    1990   Unequal Sisters: A Multicultural Reader in U.S. Women's History. New York: Routledge.

Ehrenreich, Barbara, and Deirdre English
    1973   Complaints and Disorders: The Sexual Politics of Sickness. Glass Mountain Pamphlet No. 2. Old Westbury, NY: Feminist Press.

Fee, Elizabeth, and Nancy Krieger, eds.
    1994   Women's Health, Politics, and Power: Essays on Sex/Gender, Medicine, and Public Health. Amityville, NY: Baywood.

Fine, Michelle, and Adrienne Asch, eds.
    1988   Women with Disabilities: Essays in Psychology, Culture, and Politics. Philadelphia: Temple University Press.

Finger, Anne
    1990   Past Due: A Story of Disability, Pregnancy, and Birth. Seattle: Seal Press.

Galanti, Geri Ann
    1991   Caring for Patients from Different Cultures: Case Studies from American Hospitals. Philadelphia: University of Pennsylvania Press.

Garcia, Alma M.
    1989   "The development of Chicana feminist discourse, 1970–1980." Gender and Society 3:217–38.

Gaskin, Ina Mae
    1975   Spiritual Midwifery. Summertown, TN: Book.

Gesler, Wilbert M., and Thomas C. Ricketts, eds.
    1992   Health in Rural North America: The Geography of Health Care Services and Delivery. New Brunswick, NJ: Rutgers University Press.

Gilkes, Cheryl Townsend
    1994   "'If it wasn't for the women . . .': African American women, community work, and social change." Pp. 229–46 in Maxine Baca Zinn and Bonnie Thornton Dill (eds.), Women of Color in U.S. Society. Philadelphia: Temple University Press.

Gill, Carol
    1992   "Cultivating common ground: women with disabilities." Health/PAC Bulletin (Winter):32–37.

Gonzalez, Maria L., Victoria Barrera, Peter Guarnaccia, and Stephen L. Schensul
    1982   "'La operacion': an analysis of sterilization in a Puerto Rican community in Connecticut." Pp. 47-61 in Ruth E. Zambrana (ed.), Work, Family, and Health: Latina Women in Transition. Monograph No. 7. Bronx, NY: Fordham University Hispanic Research Center.

Gordon, Linda
    1990   Woman's Body, Woman's Right: Birth Control in America. New York: Viking Penguin.

Hansen, Marie M., and Lenore K. Resick
    1990   "Health beliefs, health care and rural Appalachian subcultures from an ethnographic perspective." Family and Community Health 13:1-10.

Health Watch Information and Promotion Service
    1994   Beating the Odds: Challenges to the Health of Women of Color. A Health Watch National Symposium, New York Academy of Medicine (27-28 April), New York.

Henshaw, Stanley K., and Jennifer Van Vort
    1992   Abortion Factbook: Readings, Trends and State and Local Data to 1988. New York: Guttmacher Institute.

Hernandez, Aileen C.
    1991   National Women of Color Organizations: A Report to the Ford Foundation. New York: Ford Foundation.

Hillyer, Barbara
    1992   "Women and disabilities." NWSA Journal 4(1):106-14.

hooks, bell
    1981   Ain't I a Woman? Black Women and Feminism. Boston: South End Press.
    1984   Feminist Theory: From Margin to Center. Boston: South End Press.
    1989   Talking Back: Thinking Feminist, Thinking Black. Boston: South End Press.

Hubbard, Ruth
    1990   The Politics of Women's Biology. New Brunswick, NJ: Rutgers University Press.

Hunt, Jean, and Carole Joffe
    1994   "Problems and prospects of contemporary abortion provision." Pp. 163-74 in Alice J. Dan (ed.), Reframing Women's Health: Multidisciplinary Research and Practice. Thousand Oaks, CA: Sage.

Hutchins, Loraine, and Lani Kaahumanu, eds.
    1991   Bi Any Other Name: Bisexual People Speak Out. Boston: Alyson.

Jaimes, M. Annette, ed.
    1992   The State of Native America: Genocide, Colonization, and Resistance. Boston: South End Press.

Jasso, Sonia, and Maria Mazorra
    1984   "Following the harvest: the health hazards of migrant and season farmworking women." Pp. 86-99 in Wendy Chavkin (ed.), Double Ex-

posure: Women's Health Hazards on the Job and at Home. New York: Monthly Review Press.

Joe, Jennie, and Dorothy Lonewolf Miller
1994   "Cultural survival and contemporary American Indian women in the city." Pp. 185–202 in Maxine Baca Zinn and Bonnie Thornton Dill (eds.), Women of Color in U.S. Society. Philadelphia: Temple University Press.

Kaplan, Laura
1996   The Story of Jane: The Legendary Underground Feminist Abortion Service. New York: Pantheon Books.

King, Deborah K.
1988   "Multiple jeopardy, multiple consciousness: the context of a black feminist ideology." Signs 14:42–72.

Kobrin, Francis
1966   "The American midwife controversy: a crisis of professionalization." Bulletin of the History of Medicine 40:350–63.

Kulig, Judith C.
1990   "A review of the health status of Southeast Asian refugee women." Health Care for Women International 11(1):49–64.

Lamberty, Gontran, and Cynthia Garcia Coll
1994   Puerto Rican Women and Children: Issues in Health, Growth, and Development. New York: Plenum Press.

Latinas: Partners for Health Partnership Directory
1994   HDI Projects, National Hispanic Education and Communications Project, 1000 16th Street NW, Suite 603, Washington, DC 20036.

Lavizzo-Mourey, Risa J., and Jeane Ann Grisso
1994   "Health, health care, and women of color." Pp. 47–63 in Emily Friedman (ed.), An Unfinished Revolution: Women and Health Care in America. New York: United Hospital Fund.

Lewry, Natasha, and Charon Asetoyer
1992   The Impact of Norplant in the Native American Community. Lake Andes, SD: Native American Women's Health Education Resource Center.

Lin-Fu, Jane S.
1987   Women's Health: A Course of Action. Special Concerns of Ethnic Minority Women. Public Health Reports (supplement to July–August issue):12–16.

Lorde, Audre
1984   "Age, race, class, and sex: women redefining difference." Pp. 114–23 in Sister Outsider. Freedom, CA: Crossing Press. Reprinted, pp. 495–502 in Margaret L. Anderson and Patricia Hill Collins (eds.), Race, Class, and Gender: An Anthology. Belmont, CA: Wadsworth, 1992.

Martinez, Elizabeth
1992   "Caramba, our anglo sisters just didn't get it." Z Magazine (July–Aug.):1–2.

Mintzes, Barbara, ed.
>   1992   A Question of Control: Women's Perspectives on the Development and
>   Use of Contraceptive Technologies. Report of an international seminar
>   held in Woudschoten, the Netherlands, April 1991. Amsterdam:
>   WEMOS, Women and Pharmaceuticals Project.

Muller, Charlotte F.
>   1990   Health Care and Gender. New York: Russell Sage Foundation.

National Black Women's Health Project
>   1993   "Members only! NBWHP membership position statement." Vital Signs 1
>   (Jan.-Mar.):1.

National Women's Health Network
>   1991   "MY-PAP." Testimony before the FDA Obstetrics and Gynecology De-
>   vices Panel (21 October).
>   1992   "Use of Depo-Provera for contraception." Testimony before the FDA
>   Fertility and Maternal Health Drugs Advisory Committee (19 June).

Nelson, Cynthia, and Virginia Olesen
>   1977   "Veil of illusion: a critique of the concept of equality in western thought."
>   Catalyst 10-11:8-36.

Nelson, Margaret
>   1983   "Working-class women, middle-class women, and models of childbirth."
>   Social Problems 30:284-97.

Nsiah-Jefferson, Laurie
>   1990   "Reproductive technology: perspectives and implications for low-income
>   women and women of color." Pp. 93-118 in Kathryn Strother Ratcliff et
>   al. (eds.), Healing Technology: Feminist Perspectives. Ann Arbor: Uni-
>   versity of Michigan Press.

O'Connor, Bonnie Blair
>   1995   Healing Traditions: Alternative Medicine and the Health Professions.
>   Philadelphia: University of Pennsylvania Press.

Park, K.-J. Y., and L. M. Peterson
>   1991   "Beliefs, practices, and experiences of Korean women in relation to child-
>   birth." Health Care for Women International 12:261-69.

Peteros, Karen, and Fran Miller
>   1982   "Lesbian health in a straight world." Second Opinion (April):1-6.

Pickett, Olivia K., Eileen M. Clark, and Laura D. Kavanagh, eds.
>   1994   Reaching Out: A Directory of National Organizations Related to Mater-
>   nal and Child Health. Arlington, VA: National Center for Education in
>   Maternal and Child Health.

Rakusen, Jill
>   1981   "Depo-Provera: the extent of the problem. A case study in the politics of
>   birth control." Pp. 75-108 in Helen Roberts (ed.), Women, Health, and
>   Reproduction. London: Routledge and Kegan Paul.

Reed, James
>   1983   The Birth Control Movement and American Society: From Private Vice
>   to Public Virtue. Princeton: Princeton University Press.

Richardson, Hila
    1987   "The health plight of rural women." Women and Health 12 (3-4):41-54.
Rodriguez-Trias, Helen
    1982   "Sterilization abuse." Pp. 147-60 in Ruth Hubbard, Mary Sue Henifin, and Barbara Fried (eds.), Biological Woman: The Convenient Myth. Cambridge, MA: Schenkman.
    1984   "The women's health movement: women take power." Pp. 106-26 in Victor and Ruth Sidel (eds.), Reforming Medicine. New York: Pantheon Books.
Rosser, Sue V.
    1993   "Ignored, overlooked, or subsumed: research on lesbian health and health care." NWSA Journal 5:183-203.
    1994   Women's Health: Missing from U.S. Medicine. Bloomington: Indiana University Press.
Roth, Robert T., and Judith Lerner
    1974   "Sex-based discrimination in the mental institutionalization of women." California Law Review 62 (May):789-815.
Rural Health Issues Committee of the National Women's Health Network
    1981   "Patterns for change, rural women organizing for health." Washington: National Women's Health Network.
Ruzek, Sheryl Burt
    1978   The Women's Health Movement: Feminist Alternatives to Medical Control. New York: Praeger.
Saxton, Marsha, and Florence Howe, eds.
    1987   With Wings: An Anthology of Literature by and about Women with Disabilities. New York: Feminist Press.
Scott, Julia R.
    1993   "A dangerous combination: Norplant and teens." Vital Signs 1 (Jan.-Mar.):30-31.
    1994   "Memorandum to National Black Women's Health Project Members re: Hyde Amendment." Memo mailed to membership, National Black Women's Health Project, Atlanta.
Shapiro, Thomas M.
    1985   Population Control Politics: Women, Sterilization, and Reproductive Choice. Philadelphia: Temple University Press.
Smith, Elaine M., Susan R. Johnson, and Susan M. Guenther
    1985   "Health care attitudes and experiences during gynecologic care among lesbians and bisexuals." American Journal of Public Health 75:1085-87.
Smith, Susan
    1995   Sick and Tired of Being Sick and Tired: Black Women's Health Activism in America, 1890-1950. Philadelphia: University of Pennsylvania Press.
Solinger, Rickie
    1992   "Wake Up, Little Susie": Single Pregnancy and Race before Roe v. Wade. New York: Routledge.

Sommers, Tish
    1974   "The compounding impact of age on sex." Civil Rights Digest (Fall):1-9.
Sommers, Tish, and Laurie Shields
    1980   "Older women and health care: a strategy for survival." Gray Paper No.
           3, Issues for Action. Washington: Older Women's League.
Sprague, Jane B.
    1981   "Disabled women and the health system." Second Opinion (May).
Staggenborg, Suzanne
    1991   The Pro-Choice Movement: Organization and Activism in the Abortion
           Conflict. New York: Oxford University Press.
Stern, Phyllis Noerager, ed.
    1993   Lesbian Health: What Are the Issues? Bristol, PA: Taylor and Francis.
Stevens, Patricia E.
    1992   "Lesbian health care research: a review of the literature from 1970-
           1990." Health Care for Women International 13 (2):91-120.
Stevens, Patricia E., and Joanne Hall
    1991   "A critical historical analysis of the medical construction of lesbianism."
           International Journal of Health Services 21:291-307.
Terrelonge, Pauline
    1989   "Feminist consciousness and black women." Pp. 557-67 in Jo Freeman
           (ed.), Women: A Feminist Perspective, 3d ed. Mountain View, CA:
           Mayfield.
Tirado, Doris E.
    1994   "Norplant, Depo-Provera, and the Condom: Pros and Cons of Use by
           Minority Populations." Presentation, "Beating the Odds: Challenges to
           the Health of Women of Color." A Health Watch National Symposium,
           New York Academy of Medicine, 28 April.
Tuana, Nancy
    1989   Feminism and Science. Bloomington: Indiana University Press.
United Church of Christ Commission for Racial Justice
    1987   Toxic Wastes and Race in the United States: A National Report on the
           Racial and Socio-Economic Characteristics of Communities with Haz-
           ardous Waste Sites. New York: United Church of Christ.
U.S. Public Health Service
    1985   Women's Health: Report of the Public Health Service Task Force on
           Women's Health Issues. DHHS Pub. No. (PHS) 85-50206. May. Wash-
           ington: Government Printing Office.
Verbrugge, Lois M.
    1985   "Gender and health: an update on hypotheses and evidence." Journal of
           Health and Social Behavior 26:156-82.
Villarosa, Linda, ed.
    1994   Body and Soul: The Black Women's Guide to Physical Health and Emo-
           tional Well-Being. New York: Harper Perennial.

Wertz, Richard W., and Dorothy C. Wertz
    1991   Lying-In: A History of Childbirth in America, rev. ed. New York: Free
            Press.
Wilson-Ford, Vanessa
    1992   "Health-protective behaviors of rural black elderly women." Health and
            Social Work 17:28–36.
Women's Health Consumers Union
    1973   Letter duplicated and mailed to feminist health groups. Printed in Ma-
            jority Report 1974:6.
Zambrana, Ruth E.
    1987   "A research agenda on issues affecting poor and minority women: A
            model for understanding their health needs." Women and Health 12
            (3–4):137–60.
    1994   "Puerto Rican families and social well-being." Pp. 133–46 in Maxine
            Baca Zinn and Bonnie Thornton Dill (eds.), Women of Color in U.S.
            Society. Philadelphia: Temple University Press.
Zavella, Patricia
    1989   "The problematic relationship of feminism and Chicana studies."
            Women's Studies 17:25–36.

[4]

The Last Sisters:
Health Issues of Women with Disabilities

CAROL J. GILL

> Women with disabilities may sometimes have complex
> needs, but failure to acknowledge their commonalities and
> similarities with other women marginalizes and isolates
> women who are struggling to see themselves and wish
> others to see them as women, not as genderless beings.
> Carol Gill raises critical questions about how to meet the
> health needs of women whose place in the diversity of
> womankind has often been neglected.

The needs and concerns of women with disabilities are less exotic than
many nondisabled people might imagine. In fact, the health issues that
women with disabilities highlight as critical may sound unexpectedly familiar. They should sound familiar, because they are *women's* health issues.

When the women's movement attracted national notice almost three
decades ago, many of us with disabilities embraced feminist ideology
wholeheartedly. We had experienced not only women's unequal status but
also the "special" unequal treatment society reserved for persons with
disabilities. Our multiminority group membership impressed in every fiber
of our being that destiny was not determined by biology. Shortly after
joining the struggle for "women's liberation," many of us also joined the
newborn struggle for "disability rights." As our consciousness grew from
both involvements, we realized that most of the barriers we faced in life
were not caused by our somatic differences any more than by our sex. The
major problems we experienced were rooted in the way society responded
to us—by the way we were socially devalued, excluded from the playing
field as women, and rendered invisible both in the health service system
and health reform movements.

Criticism of the women's movement regarding its middle-class, white,
college-educated leadership is addressed by Ruzek, Olesen, and Clarke in
chapter 3. Properly, many feminist organizers responded to charges of
elitism and exclusion by reaching out to poor women, undereducated

women, women working in factories and in fields and in their own homes, women of all colors, and women in the third world. Increasingly over the past fifteen years, all have been invited to join the sisterhood. In recent years, however, the movement has encountered a fresh challenge: Women with disabilities have added a new element to the conscience and consciousness of the women's movement. We have pointed out its ableism. We have complained about meetings held in inaccessible locations with no alternative formats for blind and deaf women. We have protested our omission from agendas purporting to cover women's concerns. We have called for a recognition of our sociopolitical issues and perspective. We have been uniting to write and speak to let other women know that we are here, we are women, and we are sisters.

A striking article appeared in Ms. magazine in 1992 written by Bonnie Klein, a Canadian who acquired a disability after establishing a prominent place in the women's movement. As the permanent effects of her stroke became apparent, she found herself treated as an outsider at feminist gatherings—as if she no longer had women's issues. Her article in Ms. described her process of connecting with other disabled women activists and her successful efforts to remain included in feminist circles. Her message to her sisters, used as the title of her article, was "We Are Who You Are."

Paralleling Klein's analysis, the message of this chapter is this: "Our health issues are your health issues." As women, we share many major areas of health concern with other women. In many cases, our health service needs are identical to those of any woman. Problems arise not inherently from our disabilities but from socially constructed barriers— such as stairways and small print—that impede our access to services. As a minority group of women, however, some of our health issues have a different emphasis or intensity. Thus some of our *needs* may be similar, but *services* must be adapted to the complexities of our disabilities. For example, a woman with a cognitive disability may need contraceptive instructions translated into simpler language. A physically disabled woman might need more time for an exam to accommodate her arduous transfers from wheelchair to examination table. Further, like women in other minority or multiminority communities (e.g., lesbians, African Americans), we sometimes experience "unique" health service needs deriving in two ways from our group membership: (1) needs determined by actual physiological and inherently related lifestyle differences, and (2) those determined by the distinct character of our social oppression.

The reluctance and sometimes outright resistance we have encountered from nondisabled feminists in acknowledging us as part of the sisterhood have been painful, but matters are improving. Particularly frustrating, because it remains incompletely resolved, is our lack of recognition as a social minority group. Many in the women's movement believe, when confronted by our presence, that we deserve inclusion as women and girls "with special needs." However, acknowledgment of our issues as sociopolitical and of our community as a positive and viable component of women's diversity has lagged behind. Yet until the social origin of our marginalization is appreciated as readily as it is for other minority women's communities—until the vile impact of ableism is understood on par with all the other "isms"—our issues, including our health issues, will remain muddled and we will remain unequal within the movement for women's equality. We will be viewed as damaged women instead of women who, like others, are unfairly stereotyped, excluded, and restricted on the flimsy pretext of biology.

A clear sense of disability as a sociopolitical status, then, is the crucial foundation to understanding the health issues of women with disabilities. Because the general economic, social, cultural, and political realities of disabled women's lives have already been well covered (for example, in Fine and Asch's invaluable 1988 text, *Women with Disabilities*), they will not be taken up here. Emphasis will be placed, instead, on clarifying the interface between physiology and social/policy factors in disabled women's health needs. The relation of those needs to the health needs of nondisabled women will also be explored.

At times, we have been treated in health service settings as if our disabilities set us apart from other women when they did not. Conversely, we have sometimes been treated as if our needs were not different from average when they were. Both types of error are trouble for us. To be effective and responsive, our health service providers must know more about exactly how our experiences fit into existing knowledge and planned research on women's health.

Any authentic discussion of health issues affecting women with disabilities will reveal two leitmotives that surface repeatedly to link seemingly disparate topics. One theme is *invisibility*. Women with disabilities have been working hard to emerge from decades of neglect in medical services and research, including programs expressly designed to encompass the diversity of all women's health needs. The second theme is *genderlessness*. When we tell each other our stories, we inevitably exchange complaints of feeling treated not as women at all but as some kind of neutral gender or nonsexual being. Feeling invisible and feeling genderless go hand in hand. If society or the medical system or even our own sisters in the women's movement fail to recognize our womanness, we remain invisible when women's health issues are researched—for example, in studies of pregnancy, contraception, menopause, and sexual abuse.

In the 1990s, we launched a health initiative of our own, organizing across the United States and sometimes internationally. To halt our invisibility and degenderization, we have been publishing, presenting at conferences, developing service, resource, and education programs, and researching our health issues at an unprecedented rate. We are taking the reins in defining our needs, guaranteeing our options, in short, making ourselves hard to ignore. The remainder of this chapter summarizes our efforts.

Access

Women with disabilities share with all women a history of exclusion from health services and research that have traditionally been open to men. Moreover, many disabled women belong to additional disenfranchised groups, serving to undermine further their access to health programs that may benefit them.

Gender Inequity

In health care access, women with disabilities encounter all the problems other women do and then some. We experience the "double whammy" of discrimination as women and discrimination as disabled people, and often that discrimination adds up to more than the sum of its parts. If we hold membership in racial/cultural minorities, have a devalued sexual identity, are old, or are experiencing the poverty that often comes with disability, the resulting oppression escalates. We have had much less attention focused on our health needs compared with men within the specialty of rehabilitation medicine. Historically, medical rehabilitation has focused on the needs of men: soldiers returning from war with injuries; workers who have accidents and need therapy to regain their status as breadwinners; athletes who go down in agony while pursuing the thrill of victory. These have been the clients whom rehabilitation was developed to serve.

Until the last decade, most rehabilitation research, medical and psychological, involved only male subjects. Men dominated studies of organ system functioning in the presence of various disabilities, sexuality, vocational and economic outcome, marital adjustment, depression, and even relationships with children. Women with disabilities have a lot of catching up to do. Like nondisabled women, we reject having our medical needs estimated on the basis of data collected exclusively on men. We must achieve parity with disabled men in access to rehabilitation medicine research and services. Concurrently, we must ensure that women with disabilities are not left out of national research studies focusing on the health needs of women in general. Again, we seek visibility as minority women and inclusion as women.

Service Barriers

Like all women, we want equal access to community health services — to preventive services and treatment. Here, many of our issues are similar if not virtually identical to those of other women. Poverty, loss of insurance, lack of health information, and lack of transportation often keep us from getting to health service facilities at all. Two-thirds of persons with disabilities who wish to work are still denied jobs, and disabled women historically earn significantly less than either disabled men or nondisabled women. Women of color with disabilities earn even less money, and aging women with disabilities often experience increasing social isolation and loss of support for meeting their health needs (Fine and Asch 1988). Thus access obstacles may be more intense and demoralizing for us than for most women.

Women with disabilities must contend with an additional array of barriers unique to the experience of disability in this culture. Man-made physical impediments such as stairs and narrow doorways keep us from entering facilities once we find them. Programmatic barriers are a problem, too, such as scheduling that does not permit us the extra time we need to move or communicate or understand, or not having people on staff who can assist us onto examining tables or who know how to adjust equipment such as mammography machines to accommodate our different sizes and postures. The absence of teletypewriters (TTY), sign language interpreters, and information in Braille or in audiotaped form excludes full and equal utilization of services by deaf or blind women. Most structural and programmatic barriers are addressed in the 1990 Americans with Disabilities Act (ADA), which mandates the removal of discriminatory barriers in buildings, the workplace, communication systems, and transportation. Increasingly, women with disabilities are learning to use the ADA to construct fully accessible health service programs and to counter exclusion in existing programs.

How many women with disabilities are stopped from getting routine physical exams and other health services by remediable physical and programmatic barriers, poverty, lack of insurance, lack of transportation, and discriminatory attitudes in the health service system? It is impossible to know because there is virtually no systematic research documenting the health service experiences of women with disabilities. Baseline information is just starting to be collected about what kinds of health services we are getting, what kinds we are not getting, where we are getting our services, and where we would prefer getting them. I am directing such an investigation through the Health Resource Center for Women with Disabilities in Chicago.[1] Much of this basic fact-finding is being led by researchers and program directors who are, themselves, women with disabilities.

Invalidation of Sexuality and Reproductive Health

In the area of sexuality and reproductive health, as is true for our nondisabled sisters, ensuring our reproductive rights and options has been a long struggle. Unlike nondisabled women, who emphasize the right to delay or bypass having children, we are still fighting for the right to become mothers at all. Society generally invalidates disabled women's sexuality. If anything, our reproductive potential is feared. We are presumed either incapable of producing the kind of babies society wants—healthy babies—or incapable of adequately nurturing children.

Women with disabilities share with nondisabled women a tradition of restricted health service options and society's efforts to control our bodies. For most women, such external control is directed toward ensuring the birth of the next generation and satisfying the sexual and domestic needs of men. For disabled women, whose procreative and aesthetic functions are both devalued, the dynamics of social control are somewhat different. By casting us in the stereotypes of the perpetual asexual child or dried up crone, society justifies its invasive custody over women with disabilities and the prevention of our fertility.

We have endured a long history of medical treatment without consent, including involuntary and concealed contraception, sterilization, and abortion. We are routinely denied critical information regarding our bodies and treatment options while being subjected to unexplained procedures and medications approved by family members, judges, and professionals. Women with disabilities who are either very young or very old, who lack social support, who are impoverished, or who have communication or cognitive disabilities are most likely to be treated in this manner. This kind of thinking has been the basis of a long history of forced sterilization for women with disabilities. It has also been one of the reasons we have so little empirical knowledge of disabled women's reproductive health.

In research, our status parallels that of nondisabled women who are past their reproductive years. Stereotyped as nonbreeders, we are not even considered in reproductive research agendas. Although we are the ones who have the babies, there has been more research on the fertility and sexuality of disabled men than disabled women!

Right now, we know enough about our reproductive health issues to know that we need to know more. We need more scientific information about hormone system functioning in the presence of different disabilities, fertility and contraception, and parenting. We know, for example, that women with some mobility disabilities are likely to have more bone loss at an earlier age than nondisabled women. But how do treatments for osteoporosis affect us? Is calcium supplementation safe for our kidneys if our fluid intake and elimination patterns are affected by disability? Is estrogen replacement safe for women of limited mobility with compromised circulation in the legs? How do specific disabilities interact with contraceptives and with pregnancy? There is anecdotal evidence that pregnancy can be good for certain disabilities, such as arthritis. On the other hand, we know that traditional birthing methods can put some women with disabilities at high risk unnecessarily. For example, some women with spinal cord injuries have died needlessly because their physicians failed to realize that labor contractions can provoke dysreflexia, spiking their blood pressure to levels causing strokes (Verduyn 1994).

Some promising studies are emerging regarding sexuality and reproductive health issues of women with disabilities. Beverly Whipple and her colleagues are studying the sexual response cycle in women with spinal cord injuries (Whipple and Komisaruk 1993). At the Rehabilitation Institute of Chicago, several physicians are examining the interaction between disability and treatment for osteoporosis in menopausal and postmenopausal physically disabled women.

There are also some studies planned on contraception. Women with disabilities need much more information on how available contraceptives affect us. We also want better methods developed—ones that leave us more in control and less reliant on physicians than the injectable and implanted contraceptives commonly administered to women with disabilities. A recent study of high school girls with disabilities revealed an unexpected and alarmingly high rate of unplanned pregnancies in learning disabled teenagers (Wagner et al. 1992). Such results underscore the need for more research on how disabled girls learn about sex and conception as well as how we can provide them with better information. For too long it has been assumed that disabled women cannot manage contraception. It is imperative that we learn *how* to manage the most effective contraception for us, if that is what we want, and how best to have children, if that is what we want.

Women with disabilities are, in fact, losing custody of their children because they are presumed to be incapable parents. Only one organization, Through the Looking Glass in Berkeley, California, has actually formulated and implemented substantial research on the relationship between disabled persons and their children (Kirshbaum 1988). What they found over the past decade refutes all the stereotypes. Not only can disabled women mother in a variety of creative ways, but research shows that our children accept and cooperate with our parenting styles in ways that may, in fact, enhance the mother-child relationship and the development of the child. For example, babies may benefit when mothers who move slowly spend extra time on child-care tasks. Such children learn to coordinate in a matter-of-fact manner with parents who function differently, encouraging their later acceptance of human differences.

Abuse

Perhaps the most striking and dangerous example of disabled women's invisibility is in the area of abuse prevention, intervention, and research.

Like nondisabled women, many of us are victims of assault by partners, relatives, dates, casual acquaintances, service providers, and strangers. Yet we are rarely included in research and service programs that deal with sexual, physical, or emotional abuse of women. I have encountered a shocking level of naïveté on this matter in day-to-day interactions with both women's protection advocates and disability service providers. As one incredulous rehabilitation specialist asked when told of an assault against a woman wheelchair user, "Does this kind of thing really happen?"

We need much more research on violence as a factor in disabled women's lives, including attention to the interaction of disability type, race, and age in mediating risk. From what women with disabilities report, we are at high risk at all ages. In fact, the limited research and anecdotal evidence that address abuse in women with disabilities suggest that our chances of being assaulted may be twice those of nondisabled women. The perpetrators are often the persons we rely on for daily assistance in living, including family members, spouses, and hired personal assistants. According to Margaret Nosek (1995), many disabled women report being abused by professionals in medical settings. The sexual assault of disabled women in residential or educational institutions, including nursing homes and group homes for persons with cognitive or emotional disabilities, is more the rule than the exception. Some studies have indicated that more than 90 percent of all women with disabilities will experience abuse in the course of their lives (Pelka 1993). In Canada, Dick Sobsey (1994) and the DisAbled Women's Network[2] have been collecting important data on assault, but we need more.

In the meantime, the facts are strong enough to demand greater attention to women with disabilities in services and programs for violated women. We must be more widely acknowledged as a defined minority when assault reports are filed. Our statements about the abuse we have experienced must be respected and believed. When we are unable to report our experiences because of fear or disability-related communication difficulties, the possibility that we have been victimized must be considered by health service providers. Women with disabilities who advocate for peers who have been assaulted, such as Veronica Robinson of Access Living,[3] say that most shelters are still inaccessible and unaccommodating to women with mobility, sensory, and cognitive disabilities. The sad truth is that many women with disabilities are forced to stay in dangerous situations because they have been excluded from the safe places other women have provided for each other.

Privacy

Safeguarding our privacy against both offhanded and deliberate violation requires continual vigilance and assertiveness. Most women with disabilities can recount disturbing experiences of medical exams performed with doors or curtains left ajar, information about our private lives carelessly discussed in public places, or authorities monitoring and reporting our sexual behavior. Another form of violation so pervasive and traumatic to us that we have labeled it and categorized it as abuse is "public stripping": the practice of being forced to disrobe and display our different-looking bodies in medical educational settings (Blumberg 1990), often before mixed audiences of professionals and nonprofessionals or photographers. For example, in a 1993 telecast of a popular prime-time "news magazine" show, *NBC Now*, a physician pulled up the T-shirt of a twelve-year-old girl with cerebral palsy and, without even speaking to her, displayed her scoliotic back to a national television audience.

In writing and speaking openly about these violations, women with disabilities have been giving each other validation of our outrage and the courage to oppose further disrespect. Many of us have committed our efforts to educating health professionals and family members of women and girls with disabilities about our rights to privacy, information, and choice in medical settings.

Medical Negligence

All women have long been victims of systemic medical negligence, in that our needs have remained poorly researched and our access to adequate services has been inconsistent. Like other women, women with disabilities often feel that, compared with men, their complaints and questions are taken less seriously by physicians. Devalued populations are also vulnerable to additional forms of medical negligence. For example, physicians' tendency to view disabled women as asexual can result in failure to investigate signs of serious conditions, including cancer, pelvic disorders, sexual dysfunction, and sexually transmitted diseases. Women with disabilities also commonly express the conviction that they are dehumanized or objectified in medical settings—viewed exclusively in terms of their disabilities, not as total persons or women.

I know physicians who have openly admitted their discomfort in responding to disabled women's complaints, particularly those involving the reproductive system, because they felt overwhelmed by the disability and saw the other possible health problems as secondary in importance or as unwelcome complications. Such professionals seemed disturbed by the idea that reproductive health or sexuality would be "significant" to their disabled patients. They prejudged childbearing to be beyond consideration for women with extensive disabilities.

Disabled women commonly complain that their health service providers evade questions about sexuality or body image. They report that their questions about subjects such as orgasm, pain during sex, the advisability of getting pregnant, childbirth, breast size, cosmetic flaws, and weight gain are often brushed off. This can be devastating to women who are already conditioned by society to feel unattractive and invalid as women.

Mental Health

The mental health needs of women with disabilities have received little research attention. There is no reason to believe, however, that having a disability would in any way immunize a woman against depression or other mental illness. In fact, if stress, social isolation, devaluation, and being deprived of meaningful roles contribute to emotional problems in women, as many experts believe, women with disabilities should be considered a group at particular risk.

Stress

According to those who experience it, being female and disabled is one of the most stressful statuses to which you can aspire. Being a woman of color or being a lesbian with a disability may compound the stress. A huge proportion of disabled women are poor and dealing with life without a partner. Each day, such women must deal with access issues, transportation problems, unmet health needs, negative messages about their attractiveness and validity as women, job discrimination, and unfair welfare policies that threaten to reduce even further their paltry resources.

Depression and Suicide

Depression shows up in women in the general population about twice as often as in men. A recent study completed by DAWN in Canada revealed that almost two-thirds of their sample of 391 women with disabilities had considered suicide, and almost one-third of those had attempted it (Masuda 1994). Some observers relate disabled women's despair to social devaluation, our high incidence of abuse, and the fact that society largely prevents us from stepping into the desired roles of mother, partner, and worker. Yet we are often hard pressed to locate accessible, affordable mental health services or professionals who understand our issues.

We may not even receive suicide prevention services. Society seems increasingly willing to sanction the deaths of some disabled women who despair. For example, Jack Kevorkian's first eight "clients" were all middle-aged and elderly women with chronic disabilities or illnesses. Some feminists with disabilities are concerned that women with chronic conditions are becoming easier to discard just as the cost of health care coverage for "incurables" is being debated nationally. The National Organization for Women in several states has endorsed physician-assisted suicide measures. Such endorsements, spearheaded by women who view assistance in dying as a personal choice issue, do not reflect the views of disabled feminists who fear such measures will further oppress and endanger women whom society already views as defective and expendable.

It is imperative that women with disabilities and incurable conditions are included in research on depression, suicide, and other emotional problems. We also must be guaranteed adequate intervention and support when we despair. To be singled out as a group deserving of a hastened exit from life before our needs are adequately understood and our life choices are guaranteed may be the ultimate act of violence against women.

Policy

The new wave of health activism among disabled women includes opposition to public policies that reinforce our invisibility and degenderization. Many of us serve on committees or join disability rights demonstrations to fight for employment equity, accessible transportation, and universal design in the built environment. Unless discrimination is defeated in these areas, many of us will remain segregated—literally invisible in the mainstream—and powerless to achieve self-determination in other aspects of life.

Because a significant proportion of women with disabilities are unmarried and unemployed, many support the idea of universal single-payer insurance that would not be based on employment status and would not exclude "preexisting conditions" or deny expensive disability-related equipment. We generally oppose any plan that would permit capitation or rationing of coverage based on "quality of life" measures or the "irreversibility" of medical conditions, as these criteria too easily can be used to justify withholding benefits from persons with disabilities.

Disabled women activists also publicly denounce policies that undermine or directly oppose our entitlement as women to have children and form families of our own choosing. For example, we fought for the right of Sharon Kowalski, a lesbian disabled in an accident, to live with and have her health services monitored by her chosen lover (Thompson and Andrzejewski 1988). We oppose state policies that wrest custody of babies from impoverished mothers with disabilities, such as Tiffany Callo, who cannot afford private child-care assistance (Mathews 1992).

For many women with disabilities, the availability of a part-time or full-time personal assistant is the deciding factor in whether or not we are able to live in our own homes, raise families, or go to work. The availability of such assistance is capricious, depending on the "in-home care" policy in that person's place of residence, because each state is allowed to set its own rules for the use of federal funds. In many states, in-home assistance is given low priority and citizens with disabilities must have extraordinary information and stamina to fight the bureaucracy to qualify. Consequently, thousands of men, women, and children with disabilities who could live in their own homes with reasonable assistance are incarcerated as "patients" in nursing homes for which the government pays many times what in-home personal assistance would cost. Disability activists across the country are demanding a national personal assistance policy that would divert funds now supporting the profitable nursing home industry into consumer-managed assistance programs that promote independence and dignity.

In some states, even if a woman qualifies for personal assistance funding, she may be penalized by policies that exclude child-rearing as an "activity of daily living" for people with disabilities. Many states pay someone to assist a disabled person with bathing, dressing, driving, food preparation, house cleaning, and even gardening, but strictly forbid the paid assistant from warming a baby's bottle or helping the mother position her infant for breast-feeding. Disabled women across the country have denounced such policies as punitive and disrespectful of our right to parent as well as invasive of the private working relationship between personal assistants and the disabled persons who hire them. Such policies have caused women with disabilities who are impoverished by job discrimination and lack of spousal support to lose custody of their children.

Federal funding policies exact an impossible price from women with disabilities who wish to have full lives and health coverage, too. Barbara Faye Waxman, a colleague who has developed an ingenious program to enable disabled women to gain access to federally funded family planning services,[4] now faces a profound violation of her own right to form a family. She is engaged and wants to marry. Disabled since birth, she uses a power wheelchair and ventilator as well as a full-time personal assistant, all expensive goods and services in our current health system. If she remains single, Social Security disability payments will cover her disability-related expenses. If she marries, however, her husband's income will be considered hers, negating her eligibility for government assistance. Without this assistance, her husband's entire salary will be swallowed by her disability-related expenses, and their new marriage will be subjected to the torture test of instant poverty. As she put it, "I searched until I was 39 years old for both a job that would utilize my worldview and the right man to love me. Now Social Security policies are forcing me to give up one of them if I want to move and breathe!"

We need more research on the way women with disabilities are affected by public policies. We also need more support for programs that are attempting to apply nondiscrimination laws, such as the Americans with Disabilities Act, to secure our rights to accessible health services, protection from abuse, mental health support, family planning, and dignified personal assistance in our own homes.

Gaining Visibility as Women's Health Activists

Our recent efforts to organize around health issues have helped women with disabilities become more visible to each other. This energizing process has revitalized our determination to be included in the women's movement and women's health agenda. We want research and services that acknowledge the complexity of our lives—that acknowledge the sociopolitical reality of disability in our culture rather than merely viewing us through a disease model—but that affirm our membership in the community of all women. We expect to continue exploring and addressing the needs of our minority community in our mentoring programs, health advocacy and resource projects, professional training, and research. This will not, however, impede our intention to take our rightful place in the community of all women as we collectively work for the quality and inclusiveness of health services we deserve.

Increasingly, we realize and want others in the women's movement to realize that by asserting our health needs as a minority community, we are adding to a store of information that benefits all women. Here, diversity is at its paradoxical best. The experience of women with disabilities is set off as "different" when we focus on the particular constellation of variables that determine our health needs. But while the constellation itself may be our signature, the variables composing it—physiological, social, psychological, cultural, political, economic—link us inevitably and inextricably to other women. The experience of women with disabilities, when added to the experiences of other women, then, bring all of us an increment closer to understanding how these forces affect our health and our lives. The added benefit of our inclusion is that together we are all the more powerful in pushing forward our agenda for better and more inclusive policies and services for all women.

NOTES

1. For more information on this research contact Carol J. Gill, Ph.D., Chicago Institute of Disability Research, 7223 S. Kingery #225, Willowbrook, IL 60521.

2. DAWN CANADA: DisAbled Women's Network Canada is an organization of and for women with disabilities that carries out advocacy, research, education, and related services. They can be contacted at 776 East Georgia Street, Vancouver, BC V6A 2A3 CANADA.

3. Veronica Robinson is the deaf services coordinator for the domestic violence program at Access Living, 310 S. Peoria, Suite 201, Chicago, IL 60607.

4. Barbara Faye Waxman is the creator and director of the Americans with Disabilities Act and Reproductive Health Project through the Family Planning Council in California.

REFERENCES

Blumberg, Lisa
    1990   "Public stripping." Disability Rag 11:18–20.
Fine, Michelle, and Adrienne Asch, eds.
    1988   Women with Disabilities: Essays in Psychology, Culture, and Politics. Philadelphia: Temple University Press.

Kirshbaum, Megan
    1988   "Parents with physical disabilities and their babies." Zero to Three 8:8-15.
Klein, Bonnie S.
    1992   "We are who you are: feminism and disability." Ms., March, 70-74.
Masuda, Shirley
    1994   Personal communication.
Mathews, Jay
    1992   A Mother's Touch: The Tiffany Callo Story. New York: Holt, Rinehart and Winston.
NBC Television
    1993   "Do Not Resuscitate." NBC Now, televised 1 December.
Nosek, Margaret A.
    1995   "Sexual abuse of women with physical disabilities." Pp. 487-502 in Trilok N. Monga (ed.), Sexuality and Disability. Philadelphia: Hanley Belfus.
Pelka, F.
    1993   "Rape." Mainstream 18:24-33.
Sobsey, Dick
    1994   Violence and Abuse in the Lives of People with Disabilities: The End of Silent Acceptance? Baltimore: Brookes.
Thompson, Karen, and Julie Andrzejewski
    1988   Why Can't Sharon Kowalski Come Home? San Francisco: Spinsters/ Aunt Lute.
Verduyn, Walter H.
    1994   "A deadly combination: induction of labor with Oxytocin/Pitocin in spinal cord-injured women, T6 and above." Unpublished manuscript. Presented at the Conference on the Health of Women with Disabilities, National Institutes of Health, Bethesda, May.
Wagner, Mary, Ronald D'Amico, Camille Marder, Lynn Newman, and Jose Blackorby
    1992   "What happens next? Trends in postschool outcomes of youth with disabilities. The second comprehensive report from the national longitudinal transition study of special education students." Office of Special Education Programs, U.S. Department of Education.
Whipple, Beverly, and Barry R. Komisaruk
    1993   "Current research trends in spinal cord injuries." Pp. 197-207 in Florence P. Haseltine, Sandra S. Cole, and David B. Gray (eds.), Reproductive Issues for Persons with Physical Disabilities. Baltimore: Brookes.

PART III

Creating Women's Health:
Health Practices, Working and Living Conditions, and Medical Care

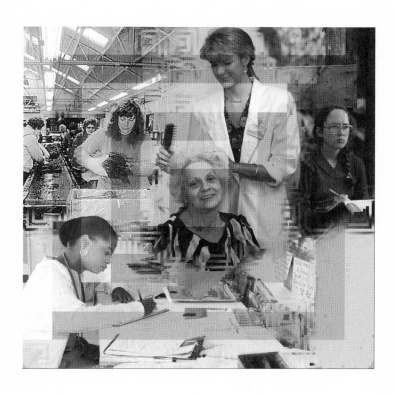

Women's health is shaped by physical, social, and psychological environments. At home and at work, in paid or unpaid labor, living and working
conditions intersect with personal health practices and access to medical
care. Social scientists debate the relative importance of individual compared with social structural factors, such as working conditions, for producing health and illness. The social class gradient in health status,
described earlier, lends weight to the argument that social forces powerfully affect individual health status. But does this invalidate the view that
what individuals do for themselves is secondary? Does positing personal
responsibility for health practices imply "blaming the victim," as some
critics charge? Why are some positive behaviors promoted and others
ignored—by policymakers, employers, and women themselves?

In chapter 5, Sheryl Burt Ruzek explores some of the social and
philosophical issues in promoting women's health through positive health
practices. She argues that health promotion ideologies and intervention
strategies can afford women the ability to act positively in their own
interest. For some women, individual health practices may be one of the
few areas in which they actually have control over their lives.

Recognizing the importance of individual actions that promote health
in no way implies that working and living conditions are unimportant.
On the contrary, social and physical environments present numerous
challenges to our health, including air pollution, improper disposal of
chemical and nuclear wastes, contaminated water, and inadequate transportation systems. In short, a whole array of environmental conditions
must be considered to construct a truly inclusive view of women's health.

Workplaces provide environmental challenges. One is ergonomics—
fitting physical working conditions to workers. Although this is a critical

issue as women enter fields "designed for men," little has been written about this as a "women's health issue." Another challenge is organizing work in ways that increase or decrease the risks and hazards of the workplace. Here we draw attention to the fact that many hazards women face stem not just from "physical things" that are risky but from the way the work is organized and paced. In chapter 6, Julia Faucett addresses the ergonomics of women's work, a largely "invisible" dimension of women's environmental conditions. She also draws attention to efforts to make jobs fit workers better and reduce health risks.

In chapter 7, Virginia Olesen describes some hazards women experience as production workers. Although she focuses on environmental hazards in some emerging areas of manufacturing, agriculture, and electronics assembly, these are intended as examples of what women workers face. Looking at specific working situations makes it easier to see the interrelatedness of women's production efforts and the need for the goods and services that women produce. How does seeing these connections affect one's valuation of products or influence what we believe they are "worth" or what the workers who make them should earn? What are the policy implications of workplace health and safety standards? What kinds of protections may women need to seek to minimize health risks? How can women improve not only their personal health practices but also their working conditions?

In our view, medical care is one of many factors that affect women's health. Medical care can never fully ameliorate or "repair" the damage done by unfavorable living and working conditions or health-damaging behaviors; nonetheless, it is critical to women's health and well-being. Medical care remains, however, unequally available to American women. Unlike other social democracies that provide a "floor of equity" to all citizens or residents, the United States treats medical services as commodities to be bought and sold in the marketplace.

Rapid transformations in the labor force and in the health industry have generated concerns about many features of medical care. In chapter 8, Sheryl Burt Ruzek explores how women fare in the crisis-oriented medical care system, drawing attention to gaps in insurance coverage. She raises questions about where we are headed in the next century as we struggle to juggle access, cost containment, and quality of care. In chapter 9, Judy Perry expands our understanding of "gaps in access" as she explores some sociocultural as well as financial and geographical barriers to medical care in Appalachia, one of America's chronically underserved rural regions.

In sum, the articles in part 3 show why we argue so strongly for conceptualizing health more broadly than "absence from disease." They also illustrate the complexities that must be addressed to understand what actually produces women's health. The multiplicity of factors suggest that improving women's health requires efforts at many levels.

[5]

Women, Personal Health Behavior, and Health Promotion

SHERYL BURT RUZEK

> Debates about the role of individual behavior versus struc-
> tural factors as the "causes" of poor health oversimplify
> complex relationships between individuals and society.
> Productive discussion of these issues is hampered by as-
> sumptions about the political stance of proponents and
> critics of health promotion. More attention needs to be
> paid to the practices that are promoted—as well as ig-
> nored—by all interested parties.

Over the past two decades, scientists confirmed the value of what many of
our mothers and grandmothers exhorted us to do: eat properly, sleep
enough, exercise, think positively, take responsibility for our actions, and
avoid smoking and excessive drinking. Transforming conventional wisdom and maternal advice into scientific knowledge, the experts redefined
bad habits as risk factors for the leading causes of death and disability:
heart disease, cancer, stroke, and injuries. A substantial body of epidemiological research shows that people who follow positive health practices
live longer, healthier lives than those who do not take good care of
themselves.[1] My purpose here is not to assess that body of knowledge but
rather to examine continuing controversies surrounding individual health
promotion and behavioral change for women in diverse life circumstances.

In the United States, politicians and policymakers are increasingly
concerned over how to reduce medical care costs—issues discussed in
chapter 8. Keeping people healthy and out of the hospital or doctor's office
makes good sense, for both individuals and society. One particularly attractive approach to keeping people healthy is promoting healthy lifestyles, encouraging people to take actions in their daily lives that preserve
their health. The individual health promotion paradigm is attractive because it would seem to require little investment in resources, and it puts
the responsibility for health squarely on the individual, the most immedi-

ate beneficiary of good health. The "healthy habits" approach also gives people the sense that what they do for themselves matters, that staying well is a social good to which they contribute and from which they benefit.

Psychologists tend to view individual actions directed to one's own well-being as private matters. Sociologists and political scientists more often see individual actions in terms of the ways they shape and are shaped by larger structural arrangements. A woman's social relationships, family responsibilities, and other living and working conditions all affect her behavior. Larger social structural factors such as poverty, employment opportunities, and environmental conditions also shape how individual women protect or compromise their own health.

As the scientific evidence grows that what we do as individuals affects our health status, staying healthy has become more than a matter of individual preference. But just how responsible should individuals be expected to be for protecting their own health? This question has major social ramifications. Staying healthy not only saves on medical care expenses and contributes to personal enjoyment but may be viewed as a social responsibility or civic duty. Employees, for example, are encouraged to participate in workplace health promotion programs to save on medical care costs as well as to improve morale and increase productivity. Health maintenance organizations pay for programs that help their subscribers learn to stay well.[2] The emerging ethos is that what is good for the individual is good for the group—but does this overlook some critical issues?

Organized health promotion efforts assume that with the right motivation and with opportunities to pursue healthful activities, people will want to do so. This approach to preventing disease and promoting health has been denounced by some as coercive and as a strategy that distracts women from changing the fundamental sources of their ill health—jobs that pay poorly, poor housing, and dangerous environments. Liberal-radical critics argue that society, not individuals, should be viewed as responsible for creating the social conditions that produce the health-damaging behaviors that health promoters purportedly see only as characteristics of individuals. Which risks are considered desirable to reduce or to ignore are social and political issues.

Ever since the "healthy lifestyles" paradigm emerged over two decades ago, academics have been bitterly divided over the implications of health promotion policies that focus so exclusively on the behavior of individuals.

If social conditions account for health-damaging behavior, why are most interventions directed toward individuals rather than toward communities or groups? More often than not, the debate becomes polarized, with one side placing responsibility for poor personal health on individuals and the other on society. Health promotion theorist Lawrence Green (1986) and others rail at what they view as an artificial distinction between individuals and social institutions. Political scientist and public health policy analyst Sylvia Tesh warns that this kind of dualistic thinking about health promotion policies impedes understanding. In her view, "progressive policy analysts who favor shifting responsibility for disease prevention from the individual to the society misunderstand the dialectical relationship between people and their social world. In that relationship each element creates the other, and a disease prevention policy that ignores this reality risks depriving men and women of an opportunity to participate as full citizens in their society" (Tesh 1988:5).

In this chapter, I take the view that neither a purely structural nor an individual paradigm adequately addresses real women's health needs. By rethinking the argument, by envisioning individual and structural approaches as complementary, rather than as oppositional, we open up more opportunities for women to actually improve their personal health. In looking for opportunities to promote women's health, it is striking how some positive behaviors are promoted, whereas others are ignored, but do not have to be—by policymakers, employers, entrepreneurs, and women themselves. By looking at what does and does not get promoted to improve women's personal health practices, we may find strategies that could be used to reshape or fine-tune the contours and contents of both structural and individual health promotion paradigms. Multiple strategies may be particularly important to adopt to meet the complex needs of women in different life circumstances. The "either/or" debates do not serve us well.

Philosophical and Political Perspectives on Personal Practices

Within the self-help and health promotion movements, the concept of "personal responsibility" for health remains fraught with practical and political conflicts, contradictions, and complexities. Contemporary health promotion is not easily categorized, detractors' efforts notwithstanding.[3] Goldstein (1992:141) points out that many progressive and countercultural social forces propelled a highly individualistic health consciousness to the forefront of American life. Conservatives may laud the moral and cost-saving features of self-help and health promotion whereas entrepreneurs may embrace it because it is profitable (Freimuth, Hammond, and Stein 1988; Milio 1988). Although health promotion can be framed in structural terms to include improvements in social institutions that affect living and working conditions (e.g., air quality, work hazards, and public safety), these midrange structural matters do not address fundamental social inequities that some theorists see as the root causes of poor health practices.

Taylor (1989) argues that the prevailing ideology of prevention emerged from a political struggle between advocates of social and individual approaches. In her view, the individual approach to prevention that predominates involves social control and moral judgments about social and individual action. In the United States, most health promotion efforts focus on a narrow range of behaviors: smoking, drinking, sexual practices, diet, and exercise. Thus broader views of health promotion, such as those supported by the World Health Organization,[4] are overshadowed by a narrow focus on what individuals can do to protect their own health.

The focus of health promotion is changing, particularly as it gains momentum in the workplace. Although most workplace programs initially were directed at the individual, specialists in the field increasingly emphasize group and organizational changes to support employee health, including "family-focused" interventions ranging from on-site day care to support for local school and community health projects.[5] Thus it is not entirely accurate to argue that health promotion is practiced only at an individual behavioral level.

Within the individual paradigm, a philosophical and pragmatic issue is the extent to which people make voluntary choices to protect or damage their health in the context of social, economic, and cultural conditions, conditions that may need to be changed. How one envisions the interplay of individuals and social institutions frames larger social questions that continually arise, particularly over the issue of individual responsibility.

— How much responsibility should individuals be expected, or required, to take for their health-damaging actions? For example, should smokers pay higher medical care premiums?
— What are the rights and responsibilities of society for dealing with the health-damaging behavior of

individuals who affect the health and safety of others? For example, should drunk drivers be swiftly removed from the road?
— What rights should individuals have to ignore healthy practices? For example, is remaining sedentary or ignoring medical advice one's right? Is addiction to tobacco or other substances a right?

Questions about how responsible one should be held for one's actions have roots in classical philosophical debates about the extent to which behavior is socially determined or is largely a matter of free will. They also suggest diversity of views around the relative rights and responsibilities of both individuals and society for ensuring public health, safety, and welfare.

What Determines Health Behavior?

In the United States, the ideology of individualism and the myth of the "classless society" obscures complex relationships between social class and personal responsibility for health behavior.[6] The pervasiveness of racial disparities in health and in socioeconomic status, in the face of overt as well as subtle forms of racism, add layers of tension. If resources and opportunities for achieving health were more equitably distributed throughout society, discussion about personal responsibility for health might be different.

Both health status and health-damaging behaviors vary by social class, with those in the lower classes having, on average, poorer health practices and poorer health status. The "uneven distribution of lifestyle risk factors means that the disadvantages that redound to people labeled as high risk tend to fall more heavily on people who are already disadvantaged by being poor or black, or both" (Stone 1990:93). There is considerable disagreement over how personal behaviors contribute to the continuation of disparities in health. Although broader social conditions such as poverty shape individual health practices, do individuals have some control over their health-damaging behaviors?

Economic resources clearly limit many positive actions. Goldstein (1992:133) argues that the health promotion movement, with its emphasis on personal responsibility, is out of reach for many lower-income people:

The possibility of performing the behaviors advanced by the movement (eating a balanced diet, regular exercise, and the like) and maintaining the values the movement espouses (such as deferred gratification, positive outlook) will all be powerfully influenced by class position. For those at the lowest part of the social-class hierarchy, those most vulnerable and most in need of improved health, the movement will appear most remote and unappealing. Their lack of participation is almost pre-ordained. . . . But lack of material resources is not the only reason that the lower social classes find the health movement relatively unappealing. Cultural aspects of lower-class life contribute to this as well.

Bioethicist Robert Veatch (1991) takes a different stance. He rejects the claim that the social environment alone determines personal behavior, because there is great variation in health-damaging and health-promoting behavior *within* all social classes. From this perspective, if social class does not determine lifestyle (in an absolute way), then health behavior is at least partly in the domain of free will and thus the responsibility of the individual.

Although Veatch raises important points about the complexities of human behavior, the disproportionate clustering of health-damaging behavior in economically disadvantaged populations should raise questions about why this is so. Similarly, Goldstein's assertion that positive health practices are culturally unappealing if not incompatible with lower-class life should stimulate investigation into why.

Politics and Polarities

"Liberals," who typically argue that structural factors are what account for health, largely ignore the phenomenon of agency—the capacity of individuals to act on their own behalf in ways that meet their own needs. "Conservatives," who argue that individual actions alone are what create health, largely ignore how difficult living and working conditions make taking positive actions exceedingly difficult. Critics of individual health promotion argue that people should not be blamed for their ill health but should be seen as the "victims" of social conditions that cause their poor health.

Others disagree, arguing that attributing health to social conditions "lets people off the hook" for their own health-damaging behavior. Liberal critics denounce this as "victim blaming"—identifying the individual who suffers from the condition as the one who "brought on" the problem. In their view, focusing on individual behavior not only "blames the victim" but diverts attention from more fundamental social inequities that cause poor health status.[7]

Health promotion proponents who support individual behavioral change reject a purely structural perspective for a variety of reasons.[8] One is that the overly deterministic structural perspective underestimates human agency, the ability of people to take control of their own lives even under seemingly overwhelming conditions. For women, this debate raises personal political issues. To the extent that women see themselves only as "victims" of distant social forces, they remain powerless—incapable of directing their own lives even in personal domains. If women are unable to shape even their own personal health actions, how will they take larger action to bring about structural changes—better medical care, safer working conditions, or cleaner environments?[9]

Individual action must also be understood in terms of the concept of women acting on their own behalf in their own "spheres of influence." This concept bears some resemblance to the feminist stance that the personal is political, a central organizing principle of feminist social action during the 1960s and 1970s. Popular feminist writer Naomi Wolf (1993) argues that somewhere along the way women came to view themselves as "powerless victims." In the realm of personal health practices, are women really powerless? If we believe in our own agency, to what degree do we shape our own destinies?

What individuals can actually do within their own personal spheres of influence to improve their health and well-being warrants closer attention. Understanding the "spheres of influence" concept is central to healthy lifestyles paradigms. Focusing energy on things that we cannot change or influence effectively leads to frustration, not to fruitful results.[10] Thus matters that are outside women's spheres of influence (i.e., only in our spheres of "concern") can be brought into our spheres of influence as we gain greater control over ourselves. Self-mastery, gaining control over personal health, may be a necessary first step to empowering women to bring about wider social change. To the extent that society is created out of social relationships, change even at low levels is important.

From a narrow structural perspective, forces outside one's immediate environment should be seen as the causes of health-damaging behaviors. Smoking, excessive drinking, or failure to exercise are symptoms of problems in women's lives that need resolution. Women need to direct attention to the conditions that cause poor health behavior, not the behavior itself. From an abstract, theoretical perspective this may be true. But how well does this work in daily life for women who are struggling to meet sometimes overwhelming demands of work and family responsibilities?

Women who juggle a shift at work and another at home[11] may not relish the idea of also putting in a "political action" shift. When given a choice between relaxation, meditation, or political action, women will not all want to pursue the same paths. For many women, taking actions that help improve their daily lives may be as far as time and energy can stretch—or should be expected to stretch. Tesh also points out that the broad structural view lacks guidelines for individuals. Personal health policies are different from public ones. We often do need to know what actions we can take. "As long as unhealthy behavior is socially rewarded or difficult to avoid—then it would verge on the suicidal to advocate only prevention policies that require someone else to take action" (1988:81).

Thus although changes in the availability of nutritious food, cigarettes, and exercise would have a wider impact than individual action, individuals can certainly protect themselves through personal actions. The need for taking control of one's behavior is clear in the area of violence prevention. In the long term, improving women's social and economic status will help reduce rape or sexual harassment, but this does not help the woman who has to walk down dark streets at night nor the woman who goes home to a violent man. What she needs is "a *personal* rape prevention policy" (Tesh 1988:81–82).

Victimization versus Empowerment

We must, indeed, develop our own personal prevention policies. The Boston Women's Health Book Collective (1992) has long taken this stance, as have numerous other community-based organizations. The National Black Women's Health Network and other organizations adamantly reject the view that women of color are powerless victims.[12] Women's personal prevention policies embrace a plethora of personal health actions, including efforts to improve workplaces and social environments. The first step, however, is attending to one's own personal health.

Whereas critics of health promotion argue that individual action distracts people from broader issues, many women disagree. Describing the National Black Women's Health Project "walk for wellness" program, Dixon (1993) emphasizes that "we should remember the broader possibilities of our journey. We walk down many paths of destruction like drugs, alcohol, stress, weight, bad diet, stagnation, physical and emotional neglect, and isolation. Women with HIV can no longer afford to walk those paths. Their walk for wellness begins with a journey from within" (1993:12). Although Dixon argues that behavior "plays the largest role" in African American women's risk of HIV, which she relates to self-esteem and inability to make healthy choices, she urges women to view personal change within a framework of understanding that racism, sexism, and classism are real. An Afrocentric definition of personal health behavior, then, does not necessarily distract women from addressing social conditions—as narrow structuralists often argue it does.

In western cultures, false dichotomies between individual and societal responsibility for health behavior divert energy and resources from generating productive solutions to complex problems as do false dichotomies between mind and body. Diverse health movements now challenge dichotomous reasoning, insisting on viewing mind, body, and sometimes spirit as inseparable.[13] Evelyn White, editor of the *Black Women's Health Book*, underscores that black women have a "fierce desire to have healthy bodies, minds, and hearts. Read what you will about the misery and mayhem in our lives but here's what I want you to know: *Sisters want and intend to be well*" (1994:xvii). Positive health actions can be a helpful contrast to many of the overwhelming conditions facing communities of color. The fact that women can modify behavior to reduce heart disease, cancer, diabetes, and violence means that women can exert some control over their own lives.[14]

Women from many walks of life emphasize that they feel better when they exercise, eat well, and maintain a positive attitude.[15] These benefits are real in real women's lives. At the same time, women's personal health behavior remains ensnared in some larger social issues.

From Private to Public Prevention Policies

The popularity of health promotion has been most visible among educated, middle-class women, the very segment of the population that already enjoys the most favorable morbidity and mortality experience (see chapter 2). Such women have access to high-quality health information, and many have chosen to use it. As more is known about personal behavioral risk factors for disease, dominant values reinforce the idea that individuals should choose healthy practices to spare themselves—and society—the personal and financial costs of ill health. Some observers decry this as a creeping health moralism that undermines other social values. Becker (1986:20), for example, argues that health promotion "fosters a dehumanizing self-concern which substitutes personal health goals for more important, human, societal goals." Personal health habits and practices are easy to discount—if you are in a position to "choose" them easily.

Abstract critiques do not square with the voices of women who want to improve their health through their own actions. Even recognizing structural barriers, Angela Davis and June Jordan, for example, eloquently argue for eliminating "the narrow definitions of health imposed on us by people who don't care about us—who don't know how we live or how we die" (Villarosa 1994:xi). In this spirit, the National Black Women's Health Project has launched personal wellness efforts (Avery 1993).

Health promotion in voluntary spheres, in the hands of lay health groups and their professional allies, demonstrates how some women choose to improve their own health. But professionalized health promotion and health paradigm beliefs have entered the formal medical and legal systems where new issues arise. Medicine has long played a social control function in secular society (Zola 1972), and health promotion increasingly does, too. Whether one sees social control largely as oppressive or essential to creating and maintaining social order, social control involves social values.

All groups exert social control over their members to some degree.[16] When there is consensus about the value of personal health behavior, social control remains largely unquestioned and invisible. Most people, for example, accept the idea of immunization as a social good, despite the fact that some people suffer negative health effects from immunization. Children must be immunized to enter school to protect everyone from the spread of disease. Even religious exemptions may be challenged during epidemics.

Objections are sometimes raised that public health policies are paternalistic and controlling. Some feminist critiques center around "overregulation" of women's bodies (Lupton 1995). Beauchamp (1988) argues that many public health measures are misunderstood as intrusive paternalism when in fact such actions are essential for protecting the health and welfare of the larger community.[17] Regulating private life, including personal health behaviors, is problematic, however, because much of it falls within what is generally regarded as a protected private sphere. The regulation of female sexuality, in particular, continues to be a morally and socially contested arena (Nathanson 1991).

Alcohol and tobacco control are also contested, but subject to many social controls—in the forms of sobriety checkpoints, limitations on sales to minors, controls over advertising, and restrictions on use in public places.[18] Medical monitoring of personal health practices (smoking, drug and alcohol use) can have social consequences. Smokers are not hired in smokeless workplaces, and illicit drug users are not hired in critical roles in transit agencies—on the grounds that protecting the public safety warrants routine drug testing.

Controversies over social control of personal behaviors raise questions about the role of the state in health protection and punishment. One example is the situation of pregnant women who take illegal drugs. In some states, women have been charged with child abuse and jailed unless they agreed to accept treatment (Gest 1989). The criminal justice system, already strained beyond capacity, is surely ill-equipped to handle violations of health behavior. The situation is complicated by the fact that testing for drug use targets low-income and minority women. The fact that some judges give pregnant women the *choice* between treatment or jail shows how central individual agency is to dominant groups' cultural beliefs and values.

Here the intersections of individual, societal, and institutional factors become more visible. Women's choices of treatment clearly are constrained—that is, outside of free will—to the degree that facilities that accept pregnant women are scarce and waiting lists are long. Recent estimates show that in some states, drug treatment spaces are available for only one out of every seven women identified as drug dependent (Slutsker et al. 1993). Availability is least adequate for women with few financial resources, those most likely to need help.[19]

Addictions generate other controversies. When hospitals and clinics impose punitive measures such as mandatory drug testing, women avoid prenatal care. Child and women's health advocates struggle over how to balance the needs of all interested parties—neither blaming women for their predicaments nor disregarding child welfare.[20] Even medical personnel who develop positive policies in their own spheres of influence do not typically see themselves as having the power to affect larger structural changes. How, in fact, can society or individuals prevent so many mothers from getting into these painful and health-damaging situations? Do structural critics of conventional perspectives provide useful directions?

Tesh (1988:76–77) argues that many such critics speak in clichés, with "words and phrases so encumbered with stale political thinking" that others refuse to reflect on their interpretations. They are simply dismissed by most of the people who have the power to put their suggestions into practice, and "the critics are left talking only to one another."[21] Clichés do not solve real women's problems.

Morals, Morality, and the Politics of Prevention

The past quarter century has been marked by increasing concerns over morality and moralism. In homogeneous social groups health values can be imposed without much controversy. For example, Seventh Day Adventists, Mennonites, and the Amish all impose strict dietary, social, and religious practices on their members without concerns about violating civil liberties or limiting people's right to choose health-damaging behaviors.[22] People can choose to leave the religion or violate its norms, but ostracism from the group remains a powerful form of social control. These cohesive religious groups enjoy particularly favorable physical and mental health status by contemporary standards of assessment.[23]

In the wider society, moral judgments and social controls that are exerted by closed religious communities are not accepted. Some liberals' fears of imposing some groups' values and standards of behavior on others contrast starkly with some conservatives' efforts to impose their own morality even into domains of life that are protected as private spheres—the family and sexuality.[24] In this highly charged atmosphere, professionals may suspend moral judgments publicly but privately acknowledge discomfort and even anger with patients who remain in addictive lifestyles, fail to use contraceptives, or continue to smoke.[25]

The dilemmas of social control loom ever larger. If a woman smokes, drinks excessively, fails to exercise, or eats inappropriately, should society or other health plan subscribers, for example, bear the cost of her medical care? In a society that values individualism and individual effort, the degree to which people should be held accountable for their health choices and accept responsibility for the consequences of their behavior poses particular challenges.

Social Values in Health Promotion

Public health and health movements, like science and medicine, are not value-free, despite protestations to the contrary. Americans are profoundly ambivalent about values and moral judgments, and they lack consensus about whether, when, and where imposing them on others is appropriate, inappropriate, oppressive, not oppressive enough, or in some other way flawed. In a diverse society, such ambivalence may well be inevitable. In secular social groups, professional values partly shape what is culturally accepted. But as Whatley (1988) points out, questions about interests must be raised because the individual behavioral focus fits so well with conservative political ideologies.

With spiraling health care costs and the need for cost containment, moral values are explicitly justified on economic grounds. For example, Louis Sullivan, former U.S. secretary of health and human services, argued that prevention was essential to reduce the "ever-increasing portion of our resources that we spend to treat preventable illness and functional impairment" (U.S. Department of Health and Human Services 1991:v). Citing the annual costs of smoking as $65 billion, AIDS $4.3 to $13 billion, and alcohol and drugs $10 billion, Sullivan framed solutions entirely in terms of the individual.

> Medical care, alone, will not eliminate the devastating impact of chronic disease on the disadvantaged, nor will it reduce, as much as we would like, the rate of infant mortality or the burden of homicide and violence or any of the other "health" problems that are borne by the poor in our society. If we are to extend the benefits of good health to all our people, it is crucial that we build in our most vulnerable populations what I have called a "culture of character," which is to say a culture, or a way of thinking and being, that actively promote responsible behavior and the adoption of lifestyles that are maximally conducive to good health. This is "prevention" in the broadest sense. (ibid.)

The tension over the "right" amount of attention to behavioral change reflects where people find themselves in the social structure. Addressing a conference on minority health research, Nickens (1993:508) notes that an insidious aspect of American individualism is "national ambivalence" about whether personal health practices are personal choices or fit objects of public policy. This ambivalence has led to "half-hearted research policies and programs."[26] Thus although affluent people (who already enjoy favorable health status) may worry about excessive normative health promotion expectations, those who have the poorest health chide public health officials for failing to find effective intervention strategies to support behavioral change.

The Politics of Prevention

Despite his interest in prevention, Sullivan canceled the previously approved NIH-funded research on adolescent sexual practices that was expected to provide information needed to design more effective pregnancy prevention programs. To the extent that federal efforts to understand adolescent sexuality were thwarted and access to reproductive health services are severely limited, especially for adolescents with low income, federal commitment to assisting "our most vulnerable populations" through primary prevention may be more rhetorical ideology than operative policy.[27]

Conservatives are not the only purveyors of contradictory words and actions. Liberal critics who have long decried the disproportionate attention paid to medical treatment over prevention find themselves in the awkward position of opposing primary prevention when they reject the behavioral change paradigm. This seemingly contradictory position stems from liberal-radical disdain of actions that fall short of altering the root causes of poor health—socioeconomic inequalities. Palliatives *prevent* more fundamental changes by distracting people from the root causes of problems.

Public health practitioners see prevention efforts differently. Primary prevention does not require eliminating the "most fundamental cause" of disease; it only requires altering something to stop the development of disease. For example, immunization interrupts the disease cycle and protects people without necessarily eradicating the pathogens involved. Similarly, food supplements prevent low-income families from developing nutritional deficiency disorders without eliminating the family's poverty. Banning smoking in public places and offering smoking cessation programs can reduce cancer and heart disease without eliminating the reasons that people offer for taking up smoking. People who avoid infectious disease, nutritional deficiencies, cardiovascular disease, and cancer as the result of such interventions are likely to share public health perspectives. This is not to say, however, that greater attention to underlying structural factors that generate ill health are unnecessary. The issue is where they fit in relation to immediate solutions.

How Living and Working Conditions Shape Health Behavior

Women in all social classes engage in many health-damaging behaviors— smoking, overeating, abusing drugs and alcohol, leading sedentary lives— as they cope with loneliness, stress, anxiety, and depression and try to fit in with peer groups. Efforts to encourage women to improve their health practices are likely to widen the gaps in health status between women in different life circumstances. For affluent women, health promotion may include a $400 gym membership, a $300 weight management program, and inpatient alcohol or drug treatment (covered at least partly by health insurance). More affluent women may also have access to more positive outlets for dealing with stress. The sound advice to exercise, talk to friends, eat well, and get adequate rest may sound strangely out of reach to women who raise children alone on limited incomes and who face unemployment and the loss of welfare benefits, housing, or sources of food and heat. That access to these goods is not equally available does not diminish their value. It should raise important questions, however, about why some women do not have adequate opportunities to maintain or improve their health.

Poverty and Health Practices

Women in lower-income groups have, on average, poorer eating, drinking, smoking, and exercise habits than more affluent women. Poverty affects health in many ways, including making it difficult to follow good health practices. Certainly the stresses of daily life are greater for women whose incomes do not meet basic needs for housing, food, clothing, and medical care. Graham (1990) poignantly shows how difficult it is for women living in poverty to eat a healthful diet even if they know how to do so.

Many women lack basic health information—something that many professionals fail to grasp until they have worked with economically disadvantaged groups. Much health information remains out of reach for women who have limited literacy. In the United States, an estimated 23 million adults are functionally illiterate; they read at or below the fifth-grade level, the level needed to understand most everyday information. In one study, patient education material in a Public Health Service hospital on average was written at the tenth-grade reading level. The patients, who were mostly high school graduates, on average actually read only at the seventh-grade level. Reading is not the only issue: people with low literacy also find health workers' verbal communication hard to understand (Doak, Doak, and Root 1985).

The gap between the actual reading level of the population and health educational materials makes food labels, pamphlets, and health handbooks far less accessible than people who take reading for granted might realize. Information at the appropriate reading level is clearly needed, yet improving education, a structural issue, must also be a public health commitment. Because education is highly associated with health status,[28] improving education may be the most far-reaching action that could be taken to improve women's health. Why do we not see this as a national, state, or local "health promotion" policy?

Where Are Health Habits Learned?

Mothers are generally expected to teach their children the basic positive health habits. Yet national survey data show that low-income children of color do not learn adequate health habits in the areas of nutrition, sleeping, and exercise (Cornelius 1991). Where caretakers are addicted to alcohol or drugs or have poor interpersonal communication or conflict resolution skills, who will teach the children? If children do not learn positive physical and mental health practices at home, neither do they at school. One survey of kindergarten through fifth-grade teachers in an inner-city school district revealed that most teachers had never been trained to teach health, and many readily admitted omitting health education entirely or teaching only a few safe subjects such as tooth brushing or food groups. When the local chapter of the American Red Cross was asked to train school staff in basic aid, only one person was willing to go to the schools because they were located in neighborhoods seen as dangerous (Ruzek and Hausman 1993). Thus in some communities, home, school, and voluntary health agencies all fail to provide tools for healthy living.

As social conditions worsen, positive health behavior may be seen as a lower priority in many families than meeting immediate needs for food, housing, or emergency medical care. But the perception that low-income women cannot afford, nor be interested in, prevention should not be overstated. This view can too easily become a rationale for not providing culturally appropriate and accessible services for those who can and will use them.

Health Promotion in Commerce and Communities

Although Tesh views a public health policy that "consists mainly of exhorting individuals to change their behavior" as shortsighted or protective of institutions that do not want to change, she sees the issue as complicated— as do others (Milio 1986; O'Rourke and O'Rourke 1989). Like medical care and education, health promotion activities are increasingly commodities to be bought and sold, and the individual health promotion paradigm is by no means value-free.

Women's health promotion "needs" are the result of highly organized efforts to generate them (Alpern 1987; Whatley and Worcester 1989). This is not actually a new phenomenon. Historically, women have been the targets of an amazing array of health treatments and practices.[29] To some extent health and fitness promotion counters alcohol and cigarette advertising that promotes damaging behavior. Marketing concerns have also generated more services exclusively for women—stress management, eating disorders, smoking, alcohol and drug treatment, and exercise programs—further medicalizing women's lives. Some programs offered exclusively to women at a particular time and place are only superficially different from standard services. Other behavioral interventions are, however, better tailored to meet women's needs. For example, some drug and alcohol treatment programs (slow to adapt gender-appropriate treatment strategies) teach women how to avoid or resist gender-linked situations including negotiating with partners.

Which Risks Get Reduced?

Although professional health educators may recognize social forces that pose significant barriers to behavioral change (e.g., pervasive advertising by the alcohol, tobacco, and processed food industries), these factors are largely ignored. Interventions are designed to teach individuals how to gain control over things that are in their personal realms of influence and control—to use individual agency to counteract opposing health-damaging "pulls." This is not surprising in a society dominated by individualist thinking where efforts to impose "passive controls"—such as regulation of gun purchases, restrictions on advertising, and automatic license suspensions for drunk drivers are widely denounced as infringements on individual liberty and freedom.[30]

Formal behavioral health risk reduction programs reflect what medical personnel are prepared to treat or prevent rather than what might be changed for the improvement of all. This is critical to note because action is not taken in any consistent way to reduce actual threats to health and well-being, even within a behavioral framework, without the political will to do so. As I have argued elsewhere, "In a biomedical model, things are called risk factors when we expect to do something about them" (Ruzek 1993:7). Things that we do not expect to do anything about are called control variables or "nonmodifiable" risks, or they are simply ignored.[31]

What is curious is how many behaviors that *are* modifiable and could improve women's health are ignored. Promoting assertiveness and self-defense skills, for example, would likely improve the quality of women's health. Why do we put such emphasis, then, on motivating women to comply with screening rather than on educating women to protect themselves in positive ways? Where is the individual behavioral paradigm when we need it? Lack of assertive behavior is a risk factor for sexual harassment, economic exploitation, rape, and domestic abuse—all of which compromise health and well-being. Surely self-defense and assertive behavior are within the sphere of individual influence, yet these behavioral skills are rarely offered in health promotion programs. Depken (1992) suggests that part of the problem of defining the parameters of health promotion stems from the fact that most "experts" are men; instructors and users are largely women.

Workplace Health Risk Reduction Priorities

Behavioral factors in workplace health promotion illustrate the complexity and interrelatedness of individual behavior and institutional policies. Some companies have made considerable efforts to improve workers' health through institutional means. On-site child care, flexible work hours, and allowance for "personal days off" that some companies now offer are particularly critical for many women's health and well-being. As with other "benefits," however, women who need them most are least likely to have them. Rural women, women of color, and women of all races with limited education are least likely to be employed in larger firms where health promotion activities and supportive workplace policies are most commonly provided.

The physical and social environment—workstation design, equipment, production schedules, and levels of hazardous chemicals or other toxins—shape health and safety (see chapters 6 and 7). But women also bring personal habits and practices to the workplace, and these interact with working conditions in ways that affect rates of disease and injury. The growth of alcohol and drug treatment programs in industry reflects the severity of addictions throughout society.[32]

A growing health risk in the workplace is sleep deprivation, a complex problem linked to increases in family responsibilities, inadequate social support, changes in transportation and residence patterns, the accessibility of electronic media at all hours, and the growth of shift work and expectations of overtime work. Sleepiness is a well-documented cause of accidents among nurses who work rotating shifts—illustrating the interrelatedness between personal habits and how work is organized (Gold et al. 1992).

In many industries, wearing seat belts and lifting correctly are both under the control of individuals.[33] Although employers may fail to protect workers adequately, workers themselves are not always aware of safe practices, and they may even resist using protective gear and taking precautions.[34] This is not limited to poorly educated employees. Workers in university research laboratories, for example, sometimes disregard safe handling practices even when they know the hazards of chemicals.

The ways in which women's health can be positively affected both by structural and individual change are illustrated in workplace smoking policies. Because chemical exposures interact with tobacco, workers who smoke and are also exposed to chemicals are at particularly high risk of developing cancers and respiratory disorders. Limiting toxic exposure is important, but so is eliminating smoking to lower the overall risk of disease. Creating smoke-free workplaces reduces this risk and also protects others from exposure to secondhand smoke, a known cause of cancer. Prohibiting smoking also creates a culture that helps smokers to quit.

Critics of workplace health promotion programs fear that focusing on individual health behaviors creates an illusion of concern for worker health without addressing more fundamental worker health and safety issues. Such concerns have validity in that workplace health promotion efforts typically offer a catalog of programs such as stress and weight management, exercise, and smoking cessation.[35]

Although these activities may be beneficial, stress management programs teach individuals to alter their responses to "stressors" rather than change the stressors themselves. To the extent that everyone faces situations that they cannot change, some coping strategies are useful, such as regular exercise, time management, stress reduction techniques (e.g., deep breathing, meditation), and learning to say no to nonessential activities.[36]

Organizations bring in stress management trainers more readily than they hire consultants to change the physical plant, improve workstations, or reorganize work and modes of interaction—even though these might actually be much more effective for reducing stress and increasing morale, which in turn improves productivity. Here it is clearest how the individual health promotion paradigm limits how problems and solutions are seen—a fact that is recognized by specialists in the field (DeJoy and Wilson 1995).

Here "victim blaming" can indeed take over. Viewing reactions to situations, not situations themselves, as what "causes" stress can encourage women to view themselves as the cause of their own distress. Failure to "cope effectively" with intolerable conditions can lead to tacit acceptance of unacceptable working conditions. The displaced homemakers' adage "Organize, don't agonize" might be a productive response, although for many women threatened by job loss, this may not be feasible. At some point, health promotion is not enough; government and industry must share a commitment to health protection.[37]

Smoking—A Touchy Issue for Women and Minorities

Employers and government are not alone in seeing disease prevention and health promotion through their own values and perceived interests. Risks are perceived selectively by subcultures as well. Prevention policies around smoking illustrate some tensions between economic interests, personal liberties, and health as a social value.

Tobacco is a major industry in some states, providing both employment and tax revenues. The federal government supports national objectives to reduce smoking while providing the tobacco industry with subsidies. The tobacco industry has promoted ties with communities of color and with women's organizations, clearly with the expectation of influencing these potential markets. By funding social and political activities, the industry has succeeded in preventing women and minority organizations from making tobacco control a health priority (Alexander and LaRosa 1994:130–31). The recent success of a coalition against Uptown, a cigarette aimed at urban African Americans, suggests that communities can fight back—even when they fear immediate economic consequences.

But inattention to smoking and other health-damaging behavior reflects more than just economic interests. For young women, who outnumber young men as new smokers, the ideology of personal choice tacitly includes the right to make negative choices. Many women who elevate choice to a near-ultimate value have equated smoking with independence and liberation. Given this value orientation, it is not surprising that feminists were slow to address the health risks of smoking.

Elizabeth Whelen of the American Council on Science and Health has raised important questions about how a product as deleterious as the cigarette can exist in a country that is so ostensibly health conscious. A primary cause of preventable deaths in the United States, smoking has been a touchy issue for many women. Whelen, who conducted research on the tobacco industry and efforts to overcome it in the mid-1980s, found "a virtual silence on the subject of women's smoking in feminist circles" (1984:206).[38] Even award-winning health writer Barbara Seaman (1969, 1977, 1995), who spearheaded national efforts to warn women about the hazards of oral contraceptives, largely ignored the issue of smoking until recently.[39] The issue is critical, because women who use oral contraceptives and smoke cigarettes are 30–40 percent more likely to develop coronary artery disease, the leading cause of death in women over fifty (Legato and Colman 1991:103). If the choice paradigm were in fact value-free, full information would be publicized about *all* known risks.

Tobacco companies have worked hard to avoid this by sponsoring activities and advertising (Williams 1991). There is a large body of research on the content of advertising in women's magazines. Magazines that run more cigarette and alcohol advertisements publish fewer articles on the dangers of drugs and alcohol than those with fewer cigarette ads.[40] Even *Ms.*, a mainstream feminist magazine that did not accept advertising considered "offensive to women," accepted cigarette ads.[41]

Silencing magazines aimed at women and people of color undermines health because American women get much of their health information from them. Women simply do not learn that heavy smokers in their twenties who continue can expect to die on average eight years sooner than nonsmokers (Thompson 1985:769). Twenty percent of all deaths in the United States are attributable to smoking, and the direct costs of medical care attributable to smoking are estimated at $42.2 billion (Alexander and LaRosa 1994:130).

Some Troubling Questions

Health promotion efforts raise other troubling questions about societal commitments to improving women's health practices—either as individuals or through efforts to alter social conditions to support health-damaging behavior. Some are briefly described below.

1. *Who Has Access to Behavioral Assistance?* Behavioral health interventions may help women, but as discussed in chapter 8, preventive services remain a significant gap in coverage for most women. Those most likely to gain access to behavioral assistance through third-party reimbursement are members of health maintenance organizations. Low-income pregnant women in some states are eligible for behavioral services recommended by the National Academy of Sciences to reduce low birthweight, the major cause of infant mortality and morbidity. These include smoking cessation, dietary counseling, and addiction treatment (Brown 1989).

2. *Whose Health Gets Promoted?* Interest in health promotion for pregnant women raises questions about why women are not valued in their own right but only as mothers. Campaigns to urge women not to drink or to use recreational drugs focus on pregnancy, emphasizing the health of the fetus rather than that of the mother. Critics see growing concerns over substance use as another form of social control over women (Pollit 1990). Reports of women being charged with abuse, neglect, and manslaughter because they drank and/or used drugs while pregnant raise concerns over threats to individual liberties. According to *U.S. News and World Report*, the "pregnancy police" are turning public health issues such as addictive behavior into criminal justice problems—both in inner cities ravaged by illegal drugs and in communities where the search for the perfect child is turning into an obligation (Gest 1989).

Although alcohol, drugs, and nicotine surely are not good for a developing fetus, neither are many of the other factors to which women and fetuses are exposed: violence (including the beating of pregnant women), malnutrition, environmental toxins, inadequate prenatal care, racism, and homelessness. Punitive treatment of pregnant women for personal health practices seems unfair when such major hazards to the fetus are largely ignored.

3. How Adequate Is the Research Base? Although positive health practices are certainly in women's interest, the actual contribution of some health behaviors to health status needs to be examined critically. Some health promotion activities have not been shown to be effective in terms of health benefits (Becker 1993). However, in contrast to clinical research (see chapter 21), epidemiological research on behavioral risk factors for many diseases have included women as subjects.[42] One of the rationales for the Women's Health Initiative is in fact to determine the effects of dietary modifications, vitamin and calcium supplementation, exercise, smoking cessation, and hormone replacement therapies in women (Palca 1991) as well as to collect adequate data on women of color. Russell (1986), however, raises important questions about the soundness of trying to prevent things that might in fact be more easily or cheaply "cured."

4. Do Health Promotion Norms Hurt Women? Health expectations themselves, some argue, cause stress. How does stress related to being overweight diminish health in addition to the physiological aspects of being overweight, particularly in cardiovascular diseases and in diabetes? How do excessive role demands leave inadequate time for healthy meal preparation, time for relaxation and exercise (commonly recommended to reduce stress), and maintaining supportive social relationships with family, friends, and communities? Are single mothers and women with limited incomes oppressed by rising "health norms"?[43]

5. What Does Health Promotion Mean for Stigmatized Women? Alcohol use, adolescent pregnancy, sexual transmission of disease, and illicit drug use affect women in all social groups but are of particular concern to women of color who bear the disproportionate burden of their effects (see chapters 14 and 18). The National Institute on Drug Abuse estimated that in 1989, over 5 million women of childbearing age used an illegal drug; 1 million used cocaine, and 3.8 million used marijuana (Roberts 1991:3).[44] Motherhood remains important to many seriously addicted women, so drugs that undermine their ability to raise their children are profoundly harmful (Regan et al. 1987). Providing drug-addicted women with "parenting skills" may help some women care for their children, yet preventing addiction itself requires helping women get jobs that move them out of poverty and into more healthful social environments.

6. Has Health Promotion Gone Too Far? Some critics believe that Americans are overly concerned with health—seeing all activities as promoting or damaging health rather than viewing them as pleasures or tribulations (Becker 1993; Goldstein 1992; Lupton 1995). Defining "living well" as reducing risk factors reinforces a medicalized view of life that misses some of the essential features of human existence. The fact that there is more to life than risk reduction, or that some women overbuy the health and fitness message, does not invalidate the contribution of personal health practices to health and well-being, but it does raise questions about the values and priorities placed on reducing risk factors narrowly while ignoring education, housing, recreation, and other living conditions that women value.

Beyond Dualistic Theorizing

Health behavior is key to women's health—both for individuals and for social policy. Critics who disdain personal responsibility and deny individual agency leave women at the mercy of distant forces, not only in their everyday lives but too often at a policy level as well. Abstract theorizing about structural factors that cause women to engage in health-damaging behavior may be accurate, but it offers little direction to women whose day-to-day lives are already crammed with at least a "double shift."

At policy levels, attention might be directed toward identifying practical ways in which women's health behaviors could be enhanced to reflect personal goals and priorities that also enhance social conditions. The structure of work should allow families to care for children and others in their lives. Ways should be found to share work to ensure that more people are employed and have access to incomes so that they can maintain their health.

We need to find practical ways to reshape working and living conditions along with practical health promotion policies—the things we all do to preserve our personal health.

NOTES

Diane Depken and Kathy Scafidi both assisted with preparation of this chapter with support from the College of HPERD, Temple University.

1. Reviewing the scientific literature on health behaviors and their contributions to overall mortality and morbidity is beyond the scope of this chapter. Although

experts disagree about the validity and interpretation of studies on various behaviors, the epidemiological basis for the effects of behavior on health is well established. See, for example, Belloc and Breslow (1972), Berkman and Breslow (1983), Breslow and Enstrom (1980), and Winett, King, and Altman (1989). For reviews of behavioral risk factors across various health conditions, see especially U.S. Department of Health and Human Services, Public Health Service (1991).

2. Some HMOs, for example, pay annual health club fees or weight reduction program fees if members document that they used the services and/or maintained their weight.

3. Various schema are used to categorize health promotion efforts from the regulatory level to the individual behavioral level. See especially Bandura (1986), Downie, Fyfe, and Tannahill (1990), Glanz, Lew, and Rimer (1990), Winett, King, and Altman (1989), and Tesh (1988).

4. The WHO views healthy lifestyles broadly and includes health environments such as working and living conditions. See Kickbusch (1981) for one of the earliest explications of this approach. The broad social structural perspective is largely absent in the United States, where the individual behavioral perspective dominates. Coreil and Levin (1985) critique the lifestyle approach. It should be noted, however, that some broad forms of health promotion are addressed in the United States under the rubric of "health protection" objectives. See U.S. Department of Health and Human Services (1991).

5. The field of workplace health promotion has grown dramatically in the past decade. For good summaries of the range of activities included see DeJoy and Wilson (1995) and the Office of Disease Prevention and Health Promotion (1993).

6. In the United Kingdom, where social class is openly recognized as existing and social scientists use standardized measures of social class, such questions are investigated more fully. Indeed, the relative contributions of individual health actions compared with material conditions have been addressed directly and explicitly in regard to women. See, for example, Blaxter (1990), Graham (1990), Hart (1986), and Pill and Stott (1986).

7. This position was popularized by Crawford, who argued that the ideology of individual responsibility promoted a concept of "wise living" that viewed the individual as "independent of his or her surroundings, unconstrained by social events and pressures" (Crawford 1977:677). For discussions of the long-standing controversy over "victim blaming," see DeJoy and Wilson (1995:55–57), Winett, King, and Altman (1989:299–302), and Tesh (1988). Critics of "victim blaming" include Allegrante and Green (1981), Crawford (1978), Minkler (1989), and Wikler (1987).

8. Katz and Levin, nationally recognized proponents of self-care, feel that the argument that individual health action distracts people from more basic issues "oversimplifies to the point of obfuscation" because real life is not so simple. In their view, popular self-help and self-care movements have flourished "exactly because their protagonists are aware of social events and pressures" as threats to health, and that in their view "wise living" requires combating and overcoming these pressures (1980:332–33).

9. Levin (1980:333) has forcefully argued there is no evidence that workers who wear protective equipment are less likely to engage in efforts to change structural

causes of poor health. Rather, "people alert to personal hazards and active in their own self-protection are the people most likely to be concerned with economic and political etiologies."

10. Covey (1989) emphasizes the concept of operating in one's spheres of influence. Mastery over one's self leads to widening spheres of influence.

11. Hochschild (1989) popularized the term *second shift* to characterize the dual burdens that working parents face.

12. For example, bell hooks (1984:45) underscores the need for self-definition and self-determination to bring about social change, arguing that feminism's overwhelming stress on women as powerless "victims" makes identification with feminism problematic. In a more recent work, hooks (1993) focuses on recovery. Similar themes emerge in the work of Collins (1990), who underscores the centrality of concepts of self-reliance and independence in the empowerment of African American women.

13. Goldstein (1992) points out how strong this thesis has been in mid- to late-twentieth-century health movements. Specifically in regard to women, see Northrup (1994) and Villarosa (1994).

14. This theme was repeated throughout "Beating the Odds: Challenges to the Health of Women of Color," a Health Watch national symposium, New York Academy of Medicine (27–28 April), New York City. Nickens (1993) makes a similar point about minorities not having adequate opportunities to learn how to change health-related behaviors.

15. If there are experiences that cut across race and class lines, they are likely the experience of taking control of personal health. African American women describe how changing their health practices and lifestyles has benefited them physically, mentally, and spiritually. See, for example, Arnold (1990), Battle (1994), Harrison (1993), hooks (1993), McDonald (1993), Phillips (1993), Villarosa (1994), and Windham (1993). Similarly, members of the Boston Women's Health Book Collective (1992) describe how positive health practices enhance their sense of well-being. Self-help health books continue to be best-sellers, suggesting that people who buy them find something of value in pursuing positive health. Because behavioral change programs try to teach women how to take control of situations that are potentially within their sphere of control, they hold out the possibility for women to assume greater control in other areas of their lives.

16. Overturning social control is not always as positive as some libertarians hope it will be. Duhl (1994) recollects that civil libertarians who pressed to free mental patients from state institutions and "demedicalize" mental illness transformed it into homelessness.

17. During the FDA hearings on silicone gel-filled breast implants, public testimony involved divergent views on paternalism. Some women (who had implants that had not caused them difficulties) argued that it was paternalistic to regulate what women had a right to have as a matter of choice. Women who had experienced problems wanted the FDA to be, as one woman put it, "paternalistic or maternalistic," trusting the FDA to be in a better position to interpret the scientific evidence than either the public or self-interested manufacturers and doctors.

18. "Passive public health measures" often are resisted by libertarians and others who fear racial and socioeconomic disparities in enforcement.

19. The PACE program in New York reports significant reductions in low birthweight among participants in a program for pregnant women who abused drugs. The cost of treatment, $7,700, may be lower than the cost of neonatal intensive care (LaFrance et al. 1994).

20. For an insightful assessment that does not blame the victim, see Harrison (1991).

21. Tesh also argues that these arguments are flawed by assigning responsibility for social ills to capitalism. This ignores the presence of disease in precapitalist and socialist countries. The dire health conditions that have come to light in eastern Europe since Tesh completed her analysis lend further weight to her argument.

22. The health of these groups receives relatively little attention, although the health status of Seventh Day Adventists has been well researched. For a discussion of these groups, see Simons-Morton, Greene, and Gottlieb (1995).

23. The favorable health of such groups is widely known but seldom discussed publicly by public health professionals. The silence may be grounded in fear of being seen as supportive of conservative ideologies, particularly in the area of sexuality, which many liberals may view as repressive.

24. These strains are well described by Beauchamp (1988), Bellah et al. (1985), and Etzionni (1993).

25. These tensions have been described by Harding (1986), Herzlich and Pierret (1987), Manning et al. (1989), and others. In the realm of sexuality, the problematic efforts of maintaining a "value-neutral stance" are particularly notable (Irvine 1994; Joffe 1986; Nathanson 1991).

26. He goes on to argue that the greatest research challenges to changing minority health status are in learning how race, class, ethnicity, and disease interact and in learning how to change our health-related behavior.

27. As a political appointee, Sullivan may have been carrying out the directives of the Bush administration.

28. The relationship between education and health status for women is well documented. See especially table 36, National Center for Health Statistics (1995:108).

29. Many nineteenth-century women were drawn to popular health movements that emphasized the healthful effects of good nutrition, proper exercise, and treatments ranging from water cures to medicinal potions (Cayleff 1987; Ehrenreich and English 1978; Leavitt 1984). But certainly the women who treated themselves to snake oils, tonics, rest cures, and water cures perceived some need or benefit, no matter how such needs were socially constructed.

30. Health psychologists, who design programs to improve health practices, emphasize group teaching to change knowledge, attitudes, and behaviors that foster healthier practices. Some strategies to reducing barriers to healthy practices include providing information (such as nutritional content of foods) at points of purchase.

31. DeJoy and Wilson (1995) emphasize that workplace health promotion always has to limit actions to modifying conditions that the employers or unions who engage them are willing to support.

32. These issues are widely discussed by occupational medicine specialists. Employee-assistance programs that provide drug and alcohol counseling reflect efforts to address these issues. See especially DeJoy and Wilson (1995).

33. Automobile crashes are the leading cause of death and days of work lost in all U.S. industries, yet only a small proportion of workers regularly use seat belts. See the risk reduction objectives for Occupational Safety and Health in U.S. Department of Health and Human Services (1991:295–312).

34. For examples of efforts to educate women as to what they can do both as individuals and collectively to improve working conditions see Kenen (1993) and Nelson, Kenen, and Klitzman (1990).

35. According to the Office of Disease Prevention and Health Promotion (1993), the increases in workplace fitness, nutrition, weight control, high blood pressure, and stress management activities increased significantly between 1985 and 1992. Gains have also been made in restricting or prohibiting smoking.

36. Barnett, Biener, and Baruch (1987) address many complex aspects of stress and stress reduction for women.

37. Many national objectives for health protection and regulation are often overlooked by those who claim that public health policy ignores institutional issues. See U.S. Department of Health and Human Services (1991). These objectives do not, however, address the fundamental sources of social inequities.

38. Whelen notes that at that time *Our Bodies, Ourselves* made only passing reference to the subject of smoking. The National Organization for Women had not commented on smoking and did not include a single reference to it in its forty-page submission to the 1979 Kennedy hearings on women's health. The National Women's Health Network had "no formal position on smoking," and the San Francisco Women's Health Collective, an organization that devoted its efforts to health education, did not address smoking on the grounds that it was "not a priority."

39. As early as the 1970s, it was known that smoking increased the risk of death even more than oral contraceptives alone. Ms. Seaman has recounted in a personal communication that these risks were not taken seriously at the time; only later did health activists come to see the contradiction of ignoring tobacco risks.

40. For studies of the relationship between advertising and health articles see Ernster (1985, 1986), Kessler (1989), Krupka, Vener, and Richmond (1990), Minkler, Wallack, and Madden (1987), and Warner (1985).

41. Whelen notes that during the years it accepted advertising, Ms. never carried an article on smoking and health (1984:206).

42. Both the Framingham Heart Study and the Alameda County Human Population Laboratory Study, from which much of the evidence has come on the importance of everyday health behaviors, did include both women and men. These early observational studies yielded important information about the role of behavior in morbidity and mortality (see especially Belloc and Breslow 1972).

43. Bair and Cayleff (1993:378) point out that few studies focus on how members of "minority" groups stay well or maintain "physical and mental harmony." It would be useful to have research, not just assertions, about the effects of health norms on different groups.

44. The immediate effects of drug use include premature birth and low birth-weight (Chasnoff, Landress, and Barrett 1990).

REFERENCES

Alexander, Linda Lewis, and Judith H. LaRosa
1994   New Dimensions in Women's Health. Boston: Jones and Bartlett.
Allegrante, John P., and L. W. Green
1981   "Sounding board: when health policy becomes victim blaming." New England Journal of Medicine 305:1528-29.
Alpern, Barbara Bellman
1987   Reaching Women: The Way to Go in Marketing Healthcare Services. Chicago: Pluribus Press.
Arnold, Georgiana
1990   "Coming home: one black woman's journey to health and fitness." Pp. 269-79 in Evelyn C. White (ed.), The Black Women's Health Book. Seattle: Seal Press.
Avery, Byllye Y.
1993   "Launching a dream, walking for wellness." Vital Signs 1 (Jan.-Mar.):5.
Bair, Barbara, and Susan E. Cayleff
1993   Wings of Gauze: Women of Color and the Experience of Health and Illness. Detroit: Wayne State University Press.
Bandura, Albert
1986   Social Foundations of Thought and Action: A Social Cognitive Theory. Englewood Cliffs, NJ: Prentice-Hall.
Barnett, Rosalind C., Lois Biener, and Grace K. Baruch, eds.
1987   Gender and Stress. New York: Free Press.
Battle, Sheila
1994   "Moving targets: alcohol, crack, and black women." Pp. 251-56 in Evelyn C. White (ed.), The Black Women's Health Book, rev. ed. Seattle: Seal Press.
Beauchamp, Dan E.
1988   The Health of the Republic: Epidemics, Medicine, and Moralism as Challenges to Democracy. Philadelphia: Temple University Press.
Becker, Marshall H.
1986   "The tyranny of health promotion." Public Health Reviews 14:15-25.
1993   "A medical sociologist looks at health promotion." Journal of Health and Social Behavior 34:1-6.
Bellah, Robert N., Richard Madsen, William M. Sullivan, Ann Swidler, and Steven Tipton
1985   Habits of the Heart: Individualism and Commitment in American Life. New York: Harper and Row.

Belloc, N. B., and Lester Breslow
    1972   "Relationship of physical health status and health practices." Preventive
            Medicine 1:409–21.
Berkman, Lisa, and Lester Breslow
    1983   Health and Ways of Living: The Alameda County Study. New York:
            Oxford University Press.
Blaxter, Mildred
    1990   Health and Lifestyles. London and New York: Tavistock/Routledge.
Boston Women's Health Book Collective
    1992   The New Our Bodies, Ourselves. New York: Simon and Schuster.
Breslow, Lester, and J. E. Enstrom
    1980   "Persistence of health habits and their relationship to mortality." Preven-
            tive Medicine 9:469–83.
Brown, Sarah S., ed., Institute of Medicine
    1989   Prenatal Care: Reaching Mothers, Reaching Infants. Washington: Na-
            tional Academy Press.
Cayleff, Susan E.
    1987   Wash and Be Healed: The Water-Cure Movement and Women's Health.
            Philadelphia: Temple University Press.
Chasnoff, I. J., H. J. Landress, and M. E. Barrett
    1990   "The prevalence of illicit-drug or alcohol use during pregnancy and dis-
            crepancies in mandatory reporting in Pinellas County, Florida." New
            England Journal of Medicine, 322:1202–6.
Collins, Patricia Hill
    1990   Black Feminist Thought: Knowledge, Consciousness, and the Politics of
            Empowerment. Boston: Unwin Hyman.
Coreil, Jeannine, and Jeffrey S. Levin
    1985   "A critique of the life-style concept in public health education." Interna-
            tional Quarterly of Community Health Education 5:103–14.
Cornelius, Llewellyn J.
    1991   "Health habits of school-age children." Journal of Health Care for the
            Poor and Underserved 2(3):374–95.
Covey, Stephen R.
    1989   The Seven Habits of Highly Effective People: Restoring the Character
            Ethic. New York: Simon and Schuster.
Crawford, Robert
    1977   "You are dangerous to your health: the ideology and politics of victim
            blaming." International Journal of Health Services 7(4):663–80.
    1978   "Sickness as sin." Health/PAC Bulletin 80:10–16.
DeJoy, David M., and Mark G. Wilson
    1995   Critical Issues in Worksite Health Promotion. Boston: Allyn and Bacon.
Depken, Diane
    1992   "Women and wellness." Unpublished paper. Department of Health and
            Physical Education, SUNY College at Buffalo.

Dixon, Dazon
    1993   "Sisterlove: from the AIDS front." Vital Signs 1 (Jan.-Mar.):12.
Doak, Cecilia, Leonard Doak, and Jane Root
    1985   Teaching Patients with Low Literacy Skills. Philadelphia: Lippincott.
Downie, R. S., Carol Fyfe, and Andrew Tannahill
    1990   Health Promotion Models and Values. New York: Oxford University Press.
Duhl, Len
    1994   "Looking backwards: a personal look at community mental health." Journal of Primary Prevention 15:31-43.
Ehrenreich, Barbara, and Deirdre English
    1978   For Her Own Good: 150 Years of the Experts' Advice to Women. Garden City, NY: Anchor.
Ernster, Virginia L.
    1985   "Mixed message for women: a social history of cigarette smoking and advertising." New York State Journal of Medicine 85:335-40.
    1986   "Women, smoking, cigarette advertising, and cancer." Women and Health 11(3-4):217-35.
Etzionni, Amitai
    1993   The Spirit of Community: Rights, Responsibilities, and the Communitarian Agenda. New York: Crown.
Freimuth, Vicki, S. Hammond, and J. Stein
    1988   "Health advertising: prevention for profit." American Journal of Public Health 78:557-61.
Gest, Ted
    1989   "The pregnancy police, on patrol." U.S. News and World Report (6 Feb.):50.
Glanz, Karen, Frances Marcus Lewis, and Barbara K. Rimer, eds.
    1990   Health Behavior and Health Education: Theory, Research, and Practice. San Francisco: Jossey-Bass.
Gold, Diane R., Suzanne Rogacz, Naomi Bock, Tor D. Tosteson, Timothy M. Baum, Frank E. Speizer, and Charles A. Czeisler
    1992   "Rotating shift work, sleep, and accidents related to sleepiness in hospital nurses." American Journal of Public Health 82:1011-17.
Goldstein, Michael S.
    1992   The Health Movement: Promoting Fitness in America. New York: Twayne.
Graham, Hilary
    1990   "Behaving well: women's health behavior in context." Pp. 195-219 in Helen Roberts (ed.), Women's Health Counts. New York: Routledge.
Green, Lawrence W.
    1986   "Individuals vs. systems: an artificial classification that divides and distorts." Health Link 2:29-30.

Harding, Geoffrey
   1986   "Constructing addiction as a moral failing." Sociology of Health and Illness 8:75–85.
Harrison, Michelle
   1991   "Drug addiction in pregnancy: the interface of science, emotion, and social policy." Journal of Substance Abuse Treatment 8:261–68.
Harrison, Tiana
   1993   "Well woman: understanding of self." Vital Signs 1 (Jan.–Mar.):15.
Hart, Nicki
   1986   "Inequalities in health: the individual versus the environment." Journal of the Royal Statistical Society 149:228–46.
Herzlich, Claudine, and Panine Pierret
   1987   "The duty to be healthy." Pp. 230–35 in Claudine Herzlich and Panine Pierret (eds.), Illness and Self in Society. Baltimore: Johns Hopkins University Press.
Hochschild, Arlie
   1989   The Second Shift: Working Parents and the Revolution at Home. New York: Viking.
hooks, bell
   1984   Feminist Theory: From Margin to Center. Boston: South End Press.
   1993   Sisters of the Yam: Black Women and Self-Recovery. Boston: South End Press.
Irvine, Janice, ed.
   1994   Sexual Cultures: Adolescence, Communities, and the Construction of Identities. Philadelphia: Temple University Press.
Joffe, Carole
   1986   The Regulation of Sexuality: Experiences of Family Planning Workers. Philadelphia: Temple University Press.
Katz, Alfred H., and Lowell Levin
   1980   "Self-care is not a solipsistic trap: a reply to critics." International Journal of Health Services 10(2):329–36.
Kenen, Regina
   1993   Reproductive Hazards in the Workplace: Mending Jobs, Managing Pregnancies. New York: Haworth Press.
Kessler, L.
   1989   "Women's magazines' coverage of smoking-related health hazards." Journalism Quarterly 66:316–23.
Kickbusch, Ilona
   1981   "Involvement in health: a social concept of health education." International Journal of Health Education (suppl.) 24(4):1–15.
Krupka, L., A. Vener, and G. Richmond
   1990   "Tobacco advertising in gender-oriented magazines." Journal of Drug Education 20:15–29.

LaFrance, Shawn V., Janet Mitchell, Karla Damus, Cindy Driver, Gladys Roman, Elizabeth Graham, and Lisa Schwartz
    1994   "Notes from the field: community-based services for pregnant substance-using women." American Journal of Public Health 84:1688-89.
Leavitt, Judith Walzer
    1984   Women and Health in America. Madison: University of Wisconsin Press.
Legato, Marianne J., and Carol Colman
    1991   The Female Heart: The Truth about Women and Coronary Artery Disease. New York: Prentice Hall.
Levin, Lowell S.
    1980   "Individual vs. social responsibility for disease." Paper presented at the American Public Health Association annual meeting, Washington, November 1977. Cited on p. 333 in Alfred H. Katz and Lowell S. Levin, "Self-care is not a solipsistic trap: a reply to critics." International Journal of Health Services 10(2):329-36.
Lupton, Deborah
    1995   The Imperative of Health: Public Health and the Regulated Body. Thousand Oaks, CA: Sage.
Manning, W. G., E. B. Keeler, J. F. Newhouse, E. M. Sloss, and J. Wasserman
    1989   "The taxes of sin: do smokers and drinkers pay their way?" Journal of the American Medical Association 261:1604-9.
McDonald, Cornelia
    1993   "Well woman. It's not what I was eating, but what was eating me." Vital Signs 1 (Jan.-Mar.):14.
Milio, Nancy
    1986   Promoting Health through Public Policy. Ottawa: Canadian Public Health Association.
    1988   "The profitization of health promotion." International Journal of Health Services 18:573-85.
Minkler, Meredith
    1989   "Health education, health promotion, and the open society: an historical perspective." Health Education Quarterly 16:17-30.
Minkler, Meredith, Lawrence Wallack, and Patricia Madden
    1987   "Alcohol and cigarette advertising in Ms. magazine." Journal of Public Health Policy (Summer):164-78.
Nathanson, Constance
    1991   Dangerous Passage: The Social Control of Sexuality in Women's Adolescence. Philadelphia: Temple University Press.
National Center for Health Statistics
    1995   Health, United States, 1994. Hyattsville, MD: Public Health Service.
Nelson, Lin, Regina Kenen, and Susan Klitzman
    1990   Turning Things Around: A Woman's Occupational and Environmental Health Resource Guide. Washington: National Women's Health Network.

Northrup, Christiane
    1994   Women's Bodies, Women's Wisdom: Creating Physical and Emotional Health and Healing. New York: Bantam Books.

Nickens, Herbert W.
    1993   "Minority health research issues." Science, Technology, and Human Values 18:506–10.

Office of Disease Prevention and Health Promotion
    1993   Health Promotion Goes to Work: Programs with an Impact. Washington: Department of Health and Human Services.

O'Rourke, T. W., and D. M. O'Rourke
    1989   "Beyond victim blaming: examining the micro-macro issue in health promotion." Wellness Perspectives: Research, Theory, and Practice 6(1):7–17.

Palca, Joseph
    1991   "Healy gets off to a fast start." Science 252:1242–44.

Phillips, Seaman
    1993   "Avoiding self-destruction: how to confront alcoholism in yourself or loved ones." Health Quest 1(1):8–11.

Pill, R., and N. C. H. Stott
    1986   "Looking after themselves: health protective behavior among British working-class women." Health Education Research 1:111–19.

Pollit, Katha
    1990   "A new assault on feminism." Nation, 26 March, 409–17.

Regan, Dianne O., Saundra M. Ehrlich, and Loretta P. Finnegan
    1987   "Infants of drug addicts: at risk for child abuse, neglect, and placement in foster care." Neurotoxicology and Teratology 9:315–19.

Roberts, Dorothy
    1991   Women, Pregnancy, and Substance Abuse. Washington: Center for Women Policy Studies.

Russell, Louise B.
    1986   Is Prevention Better than Cure? Washington: Brookings Institution.

Ruzek, Sheryl Burt
    1993   "Towards a more inclusive model of women's health." American Journal of Public Health 83:6–8.

Ruzek, Sheryl, and Alice Hausman
    1993   Final Evaluation Report on Partners for Health: A Comprehensive School Health Education Project. School District of Philadelphia and Department of Health Education, Temple University, Philadelphia.

Seaman, Barbara
    1969   The Doctors' Case against the Pill. New York: Avon.

Seaman, Barbara, and Gideon Seaman
    1977   Women and the Crisis in Sex Hormones. New York: Rawson Associates.
    1995   Women and the Crisis in Sex Hormones, 25th anniversary ed. New York: Hunter House.

Simons-Morton, Bruce G., Walter H. Greene, and Nell H. Gottlieb
 1995   Introduction to Health Education and Health Promotion, 2d ed. Prospect
        Heights, IL: Waveland Press.
Slutsker, Lawrence, Richard Smith, Grant Higginson, and David Fleming
 1993   "Recognizing illicit drug use by pregnant women: reports from Oregon
        birth attendants." American Journal of Public Health 83(1):61-64.
Stone, D.
 1990   "Preventing chronic disease: the dark side of a bright idea." Pp. 83-103
        in Institute of Medicine, Chronic Disease and Disability: Beyond the
        Acute Medical Model. Washington: Institute of Medicine.
Taylor, Rosemary
 1989   "The politics of prevention." Pp. 367-88 in Phil Brown (ed.), Perspec-
        tives in Medical Sociology. Belmont, CA: Wadsworth.
Tesh, Sylvia Noble
 1988   Hidden Arguments: Political Ideology and Disease Prevention Policy.
        New Brunswick, NJ: Rutgers University Press.
Thompson, Douglass S., ed.
 1985   Everywoman's Health: The Complete Guide to Body and Mind by Fif-
        teen Women Doctors, 4th ed. New York: Prentice Hall.
U.S. Department of Health and Human Services
 1985   The Health Consequences of Smoking for Women. A Report to the
        Surgeon General.
 1991   Healthy People 2000: National Health Promotion and Disease Preven-
        tion Guidelines. DHHS Pub. No. (PHS) 91-50212. Washington: Gov-
        ernment Printing Office.
Veatch, Robert M.
 1991   "Voluntary risks to health: the ethical issues." Pp. 196-210 in The Pa-
        tient-Physician Relation. The Patient as Partner, part 2. Bloomington:
        Indiana University Press.
Villarosa, Linda, ed.
 1994   Body and Soul: The Black Women's Guide to Physical Health and Emo-
        tional Well-Being. New York: Harper Perennial.
Warner, K. E.
 1985   "Cigarette advertising and media coverage of smoking and health." New
        England Journal of Medicine 312:384-88.
Whatley, Mariamne H.
 1988   "Beyond compliance: towards a feminist health education." Pp. 131-46
        in Sue V. Rosser (ed.), Feminism within the Science and Health Care
        Professions: Overcoming Resistance. New York: Pergamon Press.
Whatley, Mariamne H., and Nancy Worcester
 1989   "The role of technology in the co-optation of the women's health move-
        ment: the cases of osteoporosis and breast cancer screening." Pp. 199-220
        in Kathryn Strother Ratcliff et al. (eds.), Healing Technology: Feminist
        Perspectives. Ann Arbor: University of Michigan Press.

Whelen, Elizabeth
    1984   A Smoking Gun: How the Tobacco Industry Gets Away with Murder.
            Philadelphia: George F. Stickley.
White, Evelyn C., ed.
    1994   The Black Women's Health Book: Speaking for Ourselves. Seattle: Seal
            Press.
Wikler, D.
    1987   "Who should be blamed for being sick?" Health Education Quarterly
            14(1):11-25.
Williams, Marjorie
    1991   "Tobacco's hold on women's groups." Washington Post, 14 November,
            A1, A16.
Windham, Yulande Z.
    1993   "Well woman. Do you know how far we had to walk?" Vital Signs 1
            (Jan.-Mar.):15.
Winett, Richard A., Abby C. King, and David G. Altman
    1989   Health Psychology and Public Health: An Integrative Approach. New
            York: Pergamon Press.
Wolf, Naomi
    1993   Fire with Fire: The New Female Power and How to Use It. New York:
            Fawcett Columbine.
Zola, Irving Kenneth
    1972   "Medicine as an institution of social control." Sociological Review
            20:487-504.

[6]

The Ergonomics of Women's Work

JULIA FAUCETT

Women are at greater risk than are men for developing
work-related musculoskeletal disorders of the upper extremities. Many such injuries occur in jobs most often
held by women, such as small parts assembly, office work,
garment manufacture, nursing, food processing, and grocery checking. A nurse researcher explains how ergonomics—the science of fitting the job to the worker—can be
used to reduce risks to women's health.

*Imagine that your job is to travel from farm to farm inoculating turkeys.
You work in a van equipped with cable on a conveyor belt. The two men
who work with you bind the turkeys' legs and hang them upside down on
the conveyor belt cable. Your task is to reach up and grasp the turkeys with
your left hand, pinch a fold of skin, and inject them in the fold using a syringe in your right hand. The helpers are paid by the piece, whereas you
are salaried. You inject over five thousand turkeys a day. Over time, you
develop numbness and tingling in both hands and pain in your right thumb
from pushing the plunger on the syringe. You are told you have bilateral
carpal tunnel syndrome and tendinitis and will be unable to continue working. You can no longer brush your hair or do household tasks, and you are
told not to lift your children.*

Women and Workforce Participation

Occupational illnesses or injuries affect over 735,000 women a year in the
United States. For women, the risk of developing work-related musculoskeletal disorders of the upper extremities is greater than it is for men. In
1993, for example, women sustained 64 percent of occupational disorders
caused by repetitive motion (U.S. Bureau of Labor Statistics 1995). It is
not known whether their increased risk results from genetic predisposi-
tion, the types of jobs that women tend to perform, or both. Over the last
decade, work-related disorders from cumulative or repetitive trauma, primarily musculoskeletal disorders, more than tripled to account for over 60

percent of all occupational illnesses. Many of these injuries occur in jobs held mostly by women, such as small parts assembly and office work.

Between 1987 and 1993, the incidence of cumulative trauma disorders rose from 100 to 347 per 100,000 full-time workers. Carpal tunnel syndrome alone accounted for more than six thousand cases in 1993 in California (California Division of Labor Statistics and Research 1994). Disorders caused by repetitive motion also resulted in the longest absences from work, with a median work loss of twenty days per case (U.S. Bureau of Labor Statistics 1995). Increases in awareness and subsequent reporting of these disorders may account for the growing incidence. Whatever the reason, prevention of occupational musculoskeletal disorders has become a major public health goal (U.S. Public Health Service 1991; National Institute for Occupational Safety and Health 1986).

Ergonomics, the science of fitting the job to the person, investigates the causes of occupational musculoskeletal disorders and their prevention. This chapter considers ergonomic hazards,[1] particularly for women, and will focus on the categories and causes of musculoskeletal disorders that arise as a result of job and work task ergonomics and the use of injury prevention techniques in the work setting.

Ergonomics

The science of ergonomics is concerned with the interaction between human factors and job factors. *Human factors* include the biomechanical and physiological features of the body, such as its size and strength, and the functioning of tissue and organ systems. Human factors also include psychological functions such as cognition, memory, attention, and coordination. *Job factors* include the physical and mechanical properties of workstations, tasks, and tools as well as the organizational features of jobs such as work pace, production quality standards, the supervision and evaluation of work performance, and task diversity. The mismatch between human and job factors was observed by one sewing machine operator: "During the thirty-minute lunch break I had a chance to see the factory. Its improvised aura was underscored by the metal folding chairs behind the sewing machines. I had been sitting in one of these during the whole morning. . . . They were not designed in accordance to the strenuous requirements of a factory job, especially one needing the complex movements of sewing. It was therefore necessary for the women to bring their own colorful pillows to ameliorate the stress on their buttocks and spines. Later on I was to discover that chronic lumbago was, and is, a frequent condition among factory seamstresses" (Fernandez-Kelly 1983:115).

Women differ from men on human factors like size and upper body strength. However, in nontraditional jobs they may be required to use workstations and tools designed for men. For the woman construction worker or machinist, for example, is the handle circumference on the electric drill, the distance between ladder rungs, or the height of the drill press appropriate for her body measurements (anthropometrics)?

An ergonomic *hazard* is a potentially dangerous situation that an employee may encounter on the job. A *risk* exists if the employee is actually exposed to the ergonomic hazard to the degree, or *dose*, that may cause illness or injury. Eliminating the hazard from the workplace is the best way to reduce risk and to prevent a musculoskeletal disorder. However, the presence of an ergonomic hazard need not pose a serious risk to the employee if there are adequate protections available. Organizational job factors, for example, may increase or decrease the exposure of the worker to hazardous physical or biomechanical operations and thus the risk of contracting a musculoskeletal disorder. For example, the operator of a video display terminal (VDT) or computer may sit at a workstation with improper placement of the keyboard and monitor, but if VDT use is limited to one hour per day, the exposure to these ergonomic hazards is low. Likewise, an electronics assembler whose job requires attaching screws to small appliances may grip a screwdriver repeatedly to turn the screws into place. Steadying and turning the screwdriver requires a forceful pinch grip that if performed repeatedly may stress the soft tissues of the hand and cause tendon or nerve-related disorders. If the screwdriver task is alternated with assembly tasks that require other body movements and hand functions, the risk associated with exposure to the pinch grip is reduced.

What are the ergonomic factors associated with work-related musculoskeletal disorders? The most prominent ergonomic problems are repetition, particularly forceful repetition, and awkward and constrained postures (Rempel, Harrison, and Barnhart 1992).[2] These are commonly found in occupations dominated by women (table 6.1). Directory assistance and telephone operators, emergency dispatchers, data processors, billing clerks, reporters, and editors all perform repetitive keying at a VDT. The work of assembly line workers, sewing machine operators and other garment workers, grocery store clerks, postal workers, food packers, and

TABLE 6.1
Ergonomic Hazards Associated with Various Occupations

Ergonomic Hazards	Examples from Occupations
Repetition	Data processing: Continuous keyboard work Grocery stores: Checking barcoded items with laser scanners Assembly work: Assembling small electronics parts, microscopy
Repetition with force	Building maintenance: Pushing floor waxer Shipping: Stapling boxes and containers Poultry processing: Sectioning chickens
Awkard and constrained posture	Sewing machine operation: Shoulders bent over machine, arms elevated to grasp material Post office handling: Repeatedly raising arms to sort mail (casing) Nursing: Bending over to make beds
Vibration	Assembly work: Powered screwdrivers Construction: Powered hand tools Drivers: Vibration from motor vehicle
Exposure to cold temperatures	Meat packing: Working in cold storage rooms Shipping: Working with dry ice (CO_2)

musicians is also characterized by high rates of repetitive motion. Workers themselves realize how their work leads to problems. Lisa, a Mexican American working in a fruit canning factory, explained, "You're just standing there moving your hands and it hurts your lower back" (Zavella 1987:104). Meat, fish, and poultry workers are at a particularly high risk of injury because, in addition to the forceful, repetitive motions required to butcher meat, they also must work in cold environments that decrease the circulation to their hands and arms. One study, for example, reported an incidence of 44 cases of work-related musculoskeletal disorders per 100 meatpackers (Hales et al. 1989). Likewise, vibration from power tools, such as electric grinders and drills, increases the dangers of the forceful and repetitive activities found in assembly or construction work.

Awkward postures of the shoulders, elbows, or hands characterize many of the jobs just cited. For example, VDT operators work with their arms poised above the keyboard, with the hands deviated outward from the wrists and often with downward pressure on the wrist at the crease. Sewing machine operators elevate their arms to grasp and guide material slowly through the machines. Construction work often entails bending and twisting the upper body to reach confined spaces. Poultry inspectors must reach above their heads to grasp and turn chickens passing, assembly line fashion, on a cable. The processing of large postal envelopes or flats requires grasping and passing the flat along an assembly line with the left hand while resting the right arm on the elbow and keying information about it with the right hand. These postural pressures invite injuries for both blue- and white-collar workers.

Musculoskeletal Disorders and Diagnoses

Occupational musculoskeletal disorders may affect muscles, tendons, joints, nerves, and related soft tissues anywhere in the body. The lower back and upper extremities, including the neck and shoulders, are the most common sites. In fact, in 1993, the national incidence of work-related upper extremity disorders surpassed the incidence of back disorders (U.S. Bureau of Labor Statistics 1994). Because repeated exposure to force of the same muscle, tendon, or region may result in trauma, injury, and inflammation to the affected area, such names as *cumulative trauma disorder, repetitive motion injury, repetition strain injury*, and *occupational overuse syndrome* have been applied to these disorders. The proliferation of nomenclature has generated considerable confusion about diagnosis, treatment, and worker compensation. Thus, in a number of industrialized countries, efforts are being made to apply more specific diagnostic terms. Diagnostic categories for work-related injuries may be extremely important because of rights to workers' compensation.

Diagnoses most commonly associated with cumulative or repetitive trauma include *tendinitis*, or inflammation of a tendon, *tenosynovitis*, or inflammation of the sheath surrounding the tendon, *bursitis*, or inflammation of the sack surrounding a joint, nerve entrapments, such as *carpal tunnel syndrome*, which pinches the median nerve at the wrist, or *cubital tunnel syndrome*, which pinches the ulnar nerve at the elbow, and *myalgia* or muscle pain, which may also be referred to as muscle strain, tension neck, or neck and shoulder syndrome (Rempel, Harrison, and Barnhart

TABLE 6.2
Occupational Musculoskeletal Disorders

Body Parts Affected	Examples of Diagnoses
Back	Chronic low back pain Disc disease
Neck and shoulders	Cervical neck syndrome Cervical root syndrome Neck and shoulder syndrome Bursitis Tendinitis Muscle strain Neck torsion syndrome
Elbow	Tendinitis (epicondylitis) Tenosynovitis Ulnar nerve entrapment Cubital tunnel syndrome
Hand and wrist	Hand tendinitis Trigger finger tendinitis De Quervain's tenosynovitis Wrist tendinitis Carpal tunnel syndrome Hand-arm vibration syndrome Raynaud's syndrome
Knee	Tendinitis Tenosynovitis Osteoarthritis

1992). Table 6.2 lists many of the diagnoses associated with occupational musculoskeletal disorders.

An individual may also have more than one type of disorder at one time. It is not unusual, for example, to have elbow tendinitis (epicondylitis) and pain in the neck and shoulder muscles at the same time or to have wrist tendinitis along with carpal tunnel syndrome. As a group, occupational musculoskeletal disorders are characterized by one or all of the following localized symptoms, depending on the type of disorder: pain, stiffness, numbness, tingling, and sometimes weakness. Patients may also refer to aching, burning, or buzzing and may subjectively experience swelling. Pain may extend from the neck and shoulder region down the arm, into the hand, or up to the head and face.

Occupational Risks for Women

Because of the jobs that women typically perform, they are often subjected to ergonomic hazards such as repetitive motion and awkward or constrained postures (Morse and Hinds 1993). High-risk job categories for women include nursing, small parts assembly, office work, and agriculture.[3] Furthermore, women of color tend to occupy the least desirable jobs in these categories, such as nurse's aide or attendant, licensed practical nurse, typist, data entry keyer, file clerk, sewing machine operator, and postal clerk.[4] One researcher has described her experience working on an assembly line:

> You also suffered from various aches and pains. Sitting in the same position all day was almost unbearable — it made me feel like a stiff slug that couldn't even stretch. Backache and neckache were common, and excruciatingly painful. During the first few weeks screwing down resisters on the Maxi, I was in agony because of the way I had to strain forward to hold the airgun. The others had all been through it themselves when they started. Arlene's backache was so bad, she paid 20 pounds to the doctor for painkilling injections so that she could carry on working. If the chairs had been the right height and the jigs the right distance away, most of this would have been avoided. If we'd had the time to stretch and walk about it wouldn't have been so bad, but the pace made it worse because you had to tense yourself up to work as fast as you could. (Cavendish 1982:119-20)

Evidence that women in these occupations experience significant injuries from ergonomic hazards is found in a study by the California Workers' Compensation Institute (Miller 1995). CWCI, whose insurer members underwrite approximately 88 percent of statewide premiums, studied over one thousand randomly selected worker compensation claims for cumulative trauma and specific injuries filed in California in 1990. Based on that study, the CWCI estimated that 41 percent of cumulative trauma disorders in that state occur to service workers in jobs typically dominated by women (e.g., hairdressers, housekeepers, and dental assistants). Another 21 percent occurred to sales and clerical workers (e.g., cashiers and computer operators), a category also dominated by women. In the CWCI study, 29 percent of the cumulative trauma disorders were to the trunk region (back, chest, and pelvis) with an additional 11 percent to the upper extremities (hands, arms, and shoulders), 8 percent to the neck, and 4 percent to the lower extremities. In-depth studies of several at-risk occupational groups provide a closer look at the issues.

Garment Workers

Sokas, Spiegelman, and Wegman (1989) studied musculoskeletal symptoms among sewing machine operators, matching the operators against respondents to the National Health and Nutrition Survey (HANES I). Women constituted 93 percent of the sample, which was also 63 percent black, 36 percent white, middle-aged (mean age = 54 years), and experienced (mean years spent as operator = 26 years). Sewing machine operators generally guide material by hand through the machine, which is operated by knee pedals. To better observe the work, they frequently bend over the machine. Sewing machine operators were found to report significantly more knee and upper back pain; aching fingers, wrists, and elbows; and finger, shoulder, knee, and foot swelling than the national survey respondents. Another study showed that garment workers have a higher risk of work disability than the general population and one that increases with the number of years on the job (Brisson, Vezina, and Vinet 1992). Furthermore, Brisson and colleagues showed that the risk of severe disability is higher for piece workers than for hourly wage workers, reflecting the pressures of that type of compensation. The method of payment in this case is an example of an important organizational job factor that influences exposure to the physical ergonomics of the machine operator's job.

Nurses and Nurse's Aides

Nurses, aides, and other hospital workers are at high risk for back disorders (Agnew 1987). In an Iowa study, the incidence of worker compensation claims for back injuries in the previous year among nurse's aides (4.66%) was found to be much higher than that for registered nurses (1.42%). Twisting and lifting on the job, prior injury, and obesity were identified as risk factors for injury in that study (Fuortes et al. 1994). Videman and colleagues (1984) found that nurse's aides have nearly twice the lifting, bending, and twisting as nurses. In the Videman study, 85 percent of nurse's aides and 79 percent of nurses reported at least one previous episode of back pain, and in the previous five years, 12 percent of aides and 7 percent of nurses had had back pain severe enough to require bed rest. The risk of disability caused by musculoskeletal problems among the nursing workforce studied increased with age, a probable reflection of time on the job, similar to the previously noted sewing machine operators. In another study, 40 percent of a general sample of nurses and 30 percent of nurse's aides reported back pain during their careers (Cust, Pearson, and Mair 1972). The nurses' back pain occurred earlier in their careers and was more often attributed to occupational causes than back pain among a comparable group of teachers. Nurses specializing in geriatrics were particularly prone to back pain, followed by nurses in medicine and surgery. In a study of twenty-six departments in different hospitals, back pain during the previous twelve months was reported by 47 percent, treated in 29 percent, and the cause of sick leave in 16 percent of female hospital workers (Estryn-Behar et al. 1990). The investigators found that long hours of standing and bending in uncomfortable postures, lifting patients, and manipulating or pushing heavy beds or carts all contributed to the women's risk for injury. Because of the diversity of these risk factors, the investigators suggested that simply teaching safe lifting techniques is an inadequate approach to injury prevention, although patient lifting is the most frequently reported cause of acute low back pain among nurses.

Grocery Store Checkers

Grocery store checkers often have to use multiple awkward postures and high levels of repetitive motion in their work. The use of bar code readers or laser scanners has revolutionized grocery check stands, but this may not have improved conditions for workers. For example, an investigation by the National Institute of Occupational Safety and Health found that laser scanner operators were more likely to report musculoskeletal symptoms and significantly more likely to report shoulder symptoms than checkers operating cash registers (Baron, Milliron, Habes, and Fidler 1991). That study found that checkers reported significantly higher rates of shoulder and hand symptoms than noncheckers in the stores. The NIOSH investigators also found that shorter checkers had a higher risk of developing musculoskeletal disorders, presumably because of the misfit of the standard workstation to their body size and proportions. Hispanic and Asian women, because of their shorter stature, may therefore be at greater risk than other women. Investigators found that customer contact rather than restrictions of the checker's workstation resulted in a number of awkward motions. For example, checkers often tied plastic bags of produce and handed them across the workstation to the customer or reached over and retrieved items from the customers' carts.

Two studies of grocery checkers in southern California found that upper extremity musculoskeletal symptoms in general and symptoms of carpal tunnel syndrome in particular increased with the exposure to the task, that is, more hours worked per day and more years worked on the job (Morgenstern, Kelsh, Kraus, and Margolis 1991; Harber, Pena, Bland, and Beck 1992). A northern California study affirmed the increased risk of carpal tunnel syndrome among checkers (together with meat cutters and cake decorators), suggesting that this high-risk group was over eight times as likely to develop carpal tunnel syndrome as a low-risk group of noncheckers (including stockroom clerks, produce workers, and pricers) and that the risk of greater neuropathy increased the longer they worked on the job (Osorio et al. 1994).[5]

Like the grocery store checkers, women assembly line workers have also been shown to have an increased risk of musculoskeletal symptoms, with the odds of reporting symptoms increasing with the pace of the work on the line (Ohlsson, Attewell, and Skerfving 1989).

VDT Operators

Data processors, telephone operators, billing clerks, secretaries, reporters, and copy editors all operate VDTs on the job. Intensive study has confirmed VDT use as a risk factor for upper extremity problems and pointed to links with other types of work stress. Keyboard operators, for example, have been shown to have three times the risk of developing neck problems as compared with the general population (Hagberg and Wegman 1987). Similarly, accounting machine operators have been found to report significantly more hand and arm symptoms than department store saleswomen (Maeda, Hunting, and Grandjean 1980). Long hours of sitting in a static posture and repetitively keying contribute significantly to the development of musculoskeletal symptoms among VDT operators (Knave et al. 1985; Prezant and Kleinman 1987; Rossignol, Morse, Summers, and

Pagnotto 1987). As one of the clerk typists put it in Barbara Garson's (1995) study of routine work, "You push yourself like a machine. . . . You forget you're not a machine." Studies of workstation posture among data processors have also suggested that symptom reports increase with workstation ergonomics such as elevated keyboard placement and poor back support (Ryan and Bampton 1988; Sauter, Schleifer, and Knutson 1991; Stammerjohn, Smith, and Cohen 1981).

Because tedious jobs, less job autonomy, and electronic performance monitoring have also demonstrated significant associations with symptoms, investigators have suggested that VDT operators' musculoskeletal symptoms increase with work stress (Cohen, Smith, and Stammerjohn 1981; Ryan and Bampton 1988; Smith, Cohen, and Stammerjohn 1981; Smith, Sainfort, Rogers, and LeGrande 1990). Faucett and Rempel (1994), for example, reported that poor workstation ergonomics may be particularly problematic for VDT operators who have little control over job-related decisions, such as copy editors, secretaries, and data processors. Similarly, in a study of the *Los Angeles Times*, employees in the circulation, accounting, and classified advertising departments were more likely to have musculoskeletal disorders than employees in the editorial department, who have more control over their jobs (Bernard et al. 1993).

In summary, many jobs that are typically occupied by women have demonstrated considerable risk for musculoskeletal disorders. Such jobs are frequently associated with high degrees of repetitive, often monotonous, and boring tasks that require intense utilization of the hands, wrists, arms, neck, and shoulders. It has long been recognized that women's jobs requiring heavy lifting have high rates of back injury, yet attempts to prevent these disorders have traditionally rested on retraining the workforce rather than examining physical ergonomic or organizational job factors that place workers at risk (Feldstein et al. 1993). The final section of this chapter will discuss approaches to the analysis of jobs and the development of multiple preventive measures.

Preventing Occupational Musculoskeletal Disorders

The prevention of occupational musculoskeletal disorders is best addressed by a team that includes professionals trained in occupational health and safety, the workers themselves, and their managers and supervisors. To address the multiple sociocultural, biophysical, and psychological dimensions of these disorders, the women who actually do the jobs must be involved in the planning and implementation of prevention interventions. Effective prevention depends on employees and managers who are knowledgeable about ergonomic principles and can actively participate in identifying hazards and proposing solutions.

Prevention begins with team analyses of the job, the hazards to which workers may be exposed, and the risks for the workers who perform the job. Ergonomic analyses should take into account the physical fit between the workers and their workstations and tools and the potential for ergonomic hazards associated with each work task (Keyserling and Chaffin 1986). Ergonomic job analyses should also include organizational factors that influence worker exposure such as the diversity of the work tasks in each job, the cumulative risks associated with all of the tasks of a specific job, work pace, production quality standards, the degree of control a worker has over the way the job is done, supervisory systems for evaluating work performance, and supervisor and coworker social support. Such thorough assessment is required to generate an adequate array of control methods to consider for implementation in a given setting.

Risk Reduction

In occupational health, methods to limit the risk of injury and illness are prioritized at three levels. This hierarchy of controls preferentially ranks engineering controls at the top.

Engineering control focuses on eliminating the hazard from the work operation and setting, if possible, or developing effective barriers to prevent exposure from occurring. Thus engineering control is the most effective form of prevention. Examples are designs for keyboards that better fit the structure of the human hand, grocery store check stands that require less twisting and turning, easily adjustable patient beds and chairs that reduce the nurse's need to bend over, needleless injection devices, and adjustable sit-stand sewing machine workstations.

Administrative control is typically ranked second in the hierarchy. Administrative controls focus on reducing the individual employee's exposure to the hazard. Such risk reduction may be accomplished by rotating employees through the hazardous task, including a diversity of tasks on the employee's job, or expanding the degree of control that the employee has over the job, among other techniques. For example, grocery store checkers' task diversity might be increased by rotating them through the produce or stock sections periodically. Likewise, postal workers who operate automated letter sorters might rotate through package handling and hand sorting mail for neighborhood delivery. The hospital labor-management health and safety committee may establish criteria for the use of a lifting team to handle heavier patients. Effective utilization of such criteria, however, may depend on collaborative efforts by the nursing staff and their supervisors. Clerical workers may alternate typing with filing, sorting mail, or photocopying. In garment manufacture, a team of workers may be organized to complete all stages of production, allowing them increased control over job decisions including task assignment and rotation, quality monitoring, and work pace.

Behavioral control focuses on having individual workers learn to protect themselves from exposures that cannot otherwise be eliminated or reduced (Snook 1988). Protections at this level include learning safer work techniques, including the utilization of personal protective equipment. Although we typically think of hard hats, goggles, or respirators as personal protective equipment, examples may be found among the women's jobs discussed here. For example, nursing staff may learn to use lifting equipment and safer lifting techniques. Grocery store checkers may use a footstool to rest one leg while standing and ask customers to unload their own carts. VDT operators often are trained to adjust their workstations, use document holders, type more efficiently, and take frequent short breaks to stretch their arms and hands.

Regardless of the type of controls that are feasible for the job, decisions about their selection and implementation are best facilitated by a joint labor-management health and safety team who are familiar with the jobs being redesigned, the affected workforce, and the organizational priorities and climate in which the changes are being implemented. Workers, managers, ergonomists, safety engineers, risk analysts, and occupational health nurses and physicians all bring skills to the redesign of jobs. Even if experts are not available, workers and managers can and should work together to reduce job risks. Women who work at high-risk jobs are often aware of the hazards they face and the consequences of those hazards. Frequently, they have devised their own creative and inexpensive solutions such as taping grips and handles on tools, padding workstations and protruding corners of equipment, cushioning chairs, or raising VDT monitors with telephone books. There are multiple ways available to include workers in prevention planning (Occupational Health and Safety Administration 1993).

Regulatory Control

The Occupational Health and Safety Act of 1970 requires employers to provide a safe workplace (Public Law 91-596 1987). Worker compensation law requires employers to carry the costs of workers' medical care and disability compensation while it limits employees' rights to sue employers for work-related injuries and illnesses. These laws, and the regulations and standards that emerge from them, reinforce employer efforts to develop adequate hazard controls and limit company costs related to worker compensation and lost productivity. Voluntary employer programs, often promoted by critics of governmental regulation, are not uniformly applied, even though programs to improve job ergonomics have been shown to enhance production levels and employee morale in addition to protecting the workforce.

Many industrialized countries, including Australia, Japan, and some of the European Community, have successfully established governmental standards to facilitate the control and regulation of ergonomic hazards. However, attempts by the U.S. Occupational Safety and Health Administration to adopt general ergonomic standards have been unsuccessful, despite considerable efforts on the part of occupational health care specialists, labor and business leaders, and government regulators. Furthermore, political efforts to limit governmental regulation overall will continue to delay the implementation of such standards to the detriment of many American workers.

Lawsuits against the manufacturers of tools or workstation equipment, such as IBM or Apple computer keyboards, although legal, may be difficult to pursue (Eagen 1995). Even if the plaintiff's injuries are clearly work related, juries may attribute them to the way equipment is used on the job rather than to equipment design. The risk posed by a sewing machine, hospital bed, or hammer may differ depending on other equipment, work task requirements, and work break provisions, which are the responsibility of the employer, not the manufacturer, and fall under the scope of occupational safety and worker compensation laws. Significant incentives may be required before manufacturers consider altering products to increase user safety. For example, efforts to convince manufacturers to develop needleless injection devices have been unrewarding, even though these devices would notably limit the risk of contracting blood-borne diseases by health care professionals and have been shown to be feasible in terms of economics and engineering (Fisher 1994).

Informed action by a knowledgeable workforce and business leadership will be required to facilitate the development of appropriate standards and equipment for worker protection. The jobs that women hold, particularly women with low literacy or language skills, are often characterized by ergonomic hazards. It is important for women to understand the risks posed by their jobs, learn to limit those risks, and influence and collaborate with employers and others to provide for safe jobs and worksites. Even where employers are reluctant to change production processes, women can help each other to learn about injury prevention in their work settings. Tailoring jobs to fit workers remains the ideal of ergonomics.

NOTES

1. Other types of work-related health hazards include chemical, biological, physical, safety, and psychological hazards.

2. The postures most commonly implicated in upper extremity musculoskeletal disorders are extension, flexion, and ulnar and radial deviations of the wrist; pinching using the whole hand; twisting movements of the wrists and elbows; and shoulder abduction and flexion.

3. Women fill most of these jobs: registered nurses (95.8%), secretaries, stenographers, and typists (98.2%), record processing except financial (82.4%), and financial record processing (89.4%) (U.S. Bureau of the Census 1994).

4. Percentages of blacks in the following occupations are licensed practical nurses (17.7%), health aides (16.5%), nurse's aides, orderlies, and attendants (27.3%), typists (13.8%), nonfinancial record processors (13.9%), postal clerks (26.2%), data entry keyers (18.6%), sewing machine operators (15.5%), and pressing machine operators (27.1%). Hispanics make up 14.5 percent of all sewing machine operators and 14.2 percent of all pressing machine operators (U.S. Bureau of the Census 1994). These figures include both men and women, but it is reasonable to assume, given the large numbers of women in these occupations, that the percentages reflect mostly women.

5. Neuropathy, or nerve damage, can occur with the entrapment of any nerve. Entrapments of the median and ulnar nerves at the wrist, the ulnar nerve at the elbow, and cervical nerves in the neck are among the most common causes of neuropathy in occupational health.

REFERENCES

Agnew, Jacqueline
    1987   "Back pain in hospital workers." Occupational Medicine State of the Art
            Reviews 2:609–16.

Baron, Sherry, Monica Milliron, Daniel Habes, and Anne Fidler
    1991   Health Hazard Evaluation Report HETA 88-344-2092 (Shoprite Super-
            markets). Cincinnati: National Institute for Occupational Safety and
            Health.
Bernard, Bruce, Steve Sauter, Martin Petersen, Lawrence Fine, and Thomas Hales
    1993   Health Hazard Evaluation Report HETA 90-013-2277 (Los Angeles
            Times). Cincinnati: National Institute for Occupational Safety and
            Health.
Brisson, Chantal, Michel Vezina, and Alain Vinet
    1992   "Health problems of women employed in jobs involving psychological
            and ergonomic stressors: the case of garment workers in Quebec."
            Women and Health 18:49-65.
California Division of Labor Statistics and Research
    1994   "Number of nonfatal occupational injuries and illnesses involving days
            away from work by selected characteristics and industry division, 1993."
            Unpublished data from the Occupational Injuries and Illnesses Survey.
            San Francisco: State Division of Industrial Relations.
Carter, J. B., and E. W. Banister
    1994   "Musculoskeletal problems in VDT work: a review." Ergonomics
            37:1623-48.
Cavendish, Ruth
    1982   Women on the Line. London: Routledge and Kegan Paul.
Cohen, B., M. Smith, and L. Stammerjohn
    1981   "Psychosocial factors contributing to job stress of clerical VDT opera-
            tors." Pp. 337-45 in G. Salvendy and M. Smith (eds.), In Machine
            Pacing and Occupational Stress: Proceedings of the International Con-
            ference (Purdue University). London: Taylor and Francis.
Cust, George, J. C. Pearson, and A. Mair
    1972   "The prevalence of low back pain in nurses." International Nursing Re-
            view 19:169-79.
Eagen, John
    1995   "RSI battle is over, but war's just begun" San Francisco Examiner, 12
            March.
Estryn-Behar, M., M. Kaminski, E. Peigne, M. F. Maillard, A. Pelletier, C. Berthier, M.
F. Delaporte, M. C. Paoli, and J. M. Leroux
    1990   "Strenuous working conditions and musculoskeletal disorders among fe-
            male hospital workers." International Archives of Occupational and En-
            vironmental Health 62:47-57.
Faucett, Julia, and David Rempel
    1994   "VDT-related musculoskeletal symptoms: interactions between work pos-
            ture and psychosocial work factors." American Journal of Industrial Med-
            icine 26:597-612.
Feldstein, Adrianne, Barbara Valanis, William Vollmer, Nancy Stevens, and Christo-
pher Overton
    1993   "The back injury prevention project pilot study: assessing the effectiveness

of back attack, an injury prevention program among nurses, aides, and orderlies." Journal of Occupational Medicine 35:114–20.

Fernandez-Kelly, Maria Patricia

1983   For We Are Sold, I and My People: Women and Industry in Mexico's Frontier. Albany: State University of New York Press.

Fisher, June

1994   Strategies for integrating health care workers into the process of design, selection, and use of control technologies. In William Charney and Joseph Schirmer (eds.), Essentials of Modern Hospital Safety. Chelsea, MI: Lewis.

Fuortes, Laurence J., Y. Shi, Mingdon Zhang, Craig Zwerling, and Mario Schootman

1994   "Epidemiology of back injury in university hospital nurses from review of workers' compensation records and a case-control survey." Journal of Occupational Medicine 36:1022–26.

Garson, Barbara

1975   All the Livelong Day: The Meaning and Demeaning of Routine Work. New York: Penguin Books.

Hagberg, Mats, and D. H. Wegman

1987   "Prevalence rates and odds ratios of shoulder-neck diseases in different occupational groups." British Journal of Industrial Medicine 44:602–10.

Hales, T., D. Habes, L. Fine, R. Hornung, and J. Boiano

1989   Health Hazard Evaluation Report HETA 88-180-1958 (John Morell & Co.). Cincinnati: National Institute for Occupational Safety and Health.

Harber, Philip, Laura Peña, Gerard Bland, and John Beck

1992   "Upper extremity symptoms in supermarket workers." American Journal of Industrial Medicine 22:873–84.

Keyserling, W. Monroe, and Don B. Chaffin

1986   "Occupational ergonomics: methods to evaluate physical stress on job." Annual Review of Public Health 7:77–104.

Knave, B., R. Wibom, M. Voss, L. Hedstrom, and O. Berkqvist

1985   "Work with video display terminals among office employees: I. Subjective symptoms and discomfort." Scandinavian Journal of Work, Environment, and Health 11:457–66.

Maeda, Katsuyoshi, Wilhelm Hunting, and Etienne Grandjean

1980   "Localized fatigue in accounting-machine operators." Journal of Occupational Medicine 22:810–16.

Miller, Mark L.

1995   Cumulative Injuries and Specific Injuries in California. San Francisco: California Workers' Compensation Institute.

Morgenstern, Hal, Michael Kelsh, Jess Kraus, and Wendy Margolis

1991   "A cross-sectional study of hand/wrist symptoms in female grocery checkers." American Journal of Industrial Medicine 20:209–18.

Morse, Linda H., and Lynn J. Hinds

1993   "Women and ergonomics." Occupational Medicine State of the Art Reviews 8:721–31.

National Institute for Occupational Safety and Health
  1986   Proposed National Strategies for the Prevention of Leading Work-Related Diseases and Injuries: Musculoskeletal Injuries. Cincinnati: Center for Disease Control.
Occupational Health and Safety Administration, Office of Cooperative Programs
  1993   Managing Worker Safety and Health. Washington: Department of Labor.
Ohlsson, Kerstina, Robyn Attewell, and Staffan Skerfving
  1989   "Self-reported symptoms in neck and upper limbs of female assembly workers." Scandinavian Journal of Work, Environment, and Health 15:75-80.
Osorio, Ana Maria, Richard G. Ames, Jeffrey Jones, Joseph Castorina, David Rempel, William Estrin, and David Thompson
  1994   "Carpal tunnel syndrome among grocery store workers." American Journal of Industrial Medicine 25:229-45.
Prezant, B., and G. Kleinman
  1987   "Environmental stressors and perceived symptoms among office workers." Pp. 26-37 in B. Knave and P. Widebackf (eds.), Work with Display Terminal Units 86. North Holland: Elsevier.
Public Law 91-596
  1987   Occupational Health and Safety Act of 1970. (91st Congress, S2193). Washington: Government Printing Office (181-519/64291).
Rempel, David M., Robert J. Harrison, and Scott Barnhart
  1992   "Work-related cumulative trauma disorders of the upper extremity." Journal of the American Medical Association 267:838-42.
Rossignol, A., E. Morse, V. Summers, and L. Pagnotto
  1987   "Video display terminal use and reported health symptoms among Massachusetts clerical workers." Journal of Occupational Medicine 29:112-18.
Ryan, G., and M. Bampton
  1988   "Comparison of data process operators with and without upper limb symptoms." Community Health Studies 12:63-68.
Sauter, S. L., L. M. Schleifer, and S. J. Knutson
  1991   "Work posture, workstation design, and musculoskeletal discomfort in a VDT data entry task." Human Factors 33:151-67.
Smith, Michael J., B. G. F. Cohen, and L. W. Stammerjohn
  1981   "An investigation of health complaints and job stress in video display operations." Human Factors 23:387-400.
Smith, Michael J., P. Sainfort, K. Rogers, and D. LeGrande
  1990   Electronic performance monitoring and job stress in telecommunications jobs. Madison: University of Wisconsin Department of Industrial Engineering and the Communications Workers of America.
Snook, Stover H.
  1988   "Approaches to the control of back pain in industry: job design, job placement, and education/training." Occupational Medicine State of the Art Reviews 3:45-59.

Sokas, Rosemary K., Donna Spiegelman, and David H. Wegman
    1989   "Self-reported musculoskeletal complaints among garment workers." American Journal of Industrial Medicine 15:197–206.
Stammerjohn, L. W., M. J. Smith, and B. G. F. Cohen
    1981   "Evaluation of work station design factors in VDT operations." Human Factors 23:401–12.
U.S. Bureau of the Census
    1994   Statistical Abstract of the United States. Washington: Department of Commerce.
U.S. Bureau of Labor Statistics
    1995   Occupational Illnesses and Injuries. Washington: Department of Labor.
U.S. Public Health Service
    1991   Healthy People 2000. Washington: Department of Health and Human Services.
Videman, T., T. Nurminen, S. Tola, I. Kuorinka, H. Vanharanta, and J. D. G. Troup
    1984   "Low-back pain in nurses and some loading factors of work." Spine 9:400–404.
Zavella, Patricia
    1987   Women's Work and Chicano Families. Ithaca, NY: Cornell University Press.

[7]

"Less than Animals?":
The Health of Women Workers in Garment Manufacture, Agriculture, and Electronics Assembly

VIRGINIA L. OLESEN

Women's work in garment manufacturing, agriculture, and electronics assembly produces essential and useful products for other women and their families. Such products, however, carry hidden costs: health risks to women who create them. Directing attention to the risks that women face in such work draws attention to the interdependence between women in different social classes and life circumstances.

It was incredible. . . . I would never have believed a situation like this could exist in the United States.
        —*Victoria Bradshaw, California labor commissioner*

Commissioner Bradshaw's astonished comments refer to deplorable working conditions discovered in a raid on a Southern California sweatshop. Seventy Thai immigrants, mostly women, who had been brought illegally into the United States, worked seventeen hours a day. One worker told authorities she was forced to work nineteen hours a day: "The supervisor forces me to work because work is all they think about. If I don't finish a job, they don't let me sleep." The women's pay, 69 cents an hour, was much less than the legal minimum wage of $4.25. Most of the meager salary received went to repay the owners for the costs of the trip to the United States. They worked and lived in a fortified prisonlike complex of tiny, airless fiberboard-and-plywood rabbit warrens where they sewed ready-to-wear garments for sale in retail stores. They were threatened with violence or rape if they attempted to leave or escape (*San Francisco Chronicle*, 4 August 1995, A12).

Garment manufacturing is not the only work where women face health risks. Risks of many types—exposure to chemicals, bodily strain and stress—are found in many women's work contexts: domestic labor at home (Rosenberg 1984), managerial (Amaro, Russo, and Johnson 1987), secretarial (Fleishman 1984), health care (Kenen 1993:99–111), educational (Kenen 1993:140–46), and service (Kenen 1993:116–22). However, garment manufacturing (like agricultural production of food, and the manufacture and assembly of electronics devices) employs many women of color, particularly immigrant women. These women create, harvest, and produce products essential to the lives of other women, often in health-threatening situations. Their products are time-sensitive: women's fashions change rapidly, fruits and vegetables ripen quickly, electronics technology is continually revised. This not only necessitates substantial labor but a rapid pace. These are also industries in which "offshore" competition (manufacture or production outside the continental United States) puts pressure on American firms to produce more cheaply.[1] In these three industries, women's health is clearly linked to the fortunes of American business.

Garment Manufacturing

The hapless Thai women caught in the Los Angeles raid were among 100,000 workers, mostly female, in Los Angeles alone who work in sweat-shops. Such manufacturing is also done in San Francisco, New York, and Texas where, as elsewhere, the *maquilladoras* (Spanish for manufacturing) employ large numbers of women, some of them undocumented immigrants from Asia, Mexico, or Latin America. In California alone there are six thousand garment industry firms registered to operate within the state and an undetermined but presumably large number not registered and operating "underground" as was the target of the Los Angeles raid (U.S. Department of Labor 1994a).

These women encounter both health and economic risks in their work, especially if the employer is unscrupulous in the abuse of the employees. At best, garment manufacturing is health threatening: eyestrain, muscle strain, breathing in fibers, noise, and stress exacerbated if pay is on a piecework basis. A 1994 California and U.S. Department of Labor survey of basic labor law compliance in sixty-nine randomly chosen garment firms from those registered with the state found health and safety violations in 93 percent of the firms. Garment work is also dangerous. Of those sixty-nine firms, 35 percent had "serious" violations that pointed to a high probability of death or serious physical harm, such as blocked fire exits, unsafe sewing equipment, and improper electrical connections (U.S. Department of Labor 1994b).

Economic risks to workers also were uncovered. Sixty-eight percent of the firms surveyed worked employees overtime, which meant additional exposure to these hazards and for which they were not paid properly. Half the firms did not pay workers the minimum wage.[2] The report indicated that such violations were probably even more frequent among unregistered firms.

Access to health care for women in such circumstances is at best limited and more often nonexistent if the firm does not carry a health plan, a most unlikely option in sweatshops. For undocumented workers who may have been pirated into such work, access is even more problematic because of their terror of contact with authorities.[3]

Differences among women also characterize the female workers in the garment industry. Many Asian women are particularly isolated because of language difficulties, cultural traditions, and lack of familiarity with legal justice systems,[4] but these problems were differentially experienced by Chinese, Filipina, Korean, Vietnamese, and Cambodian workers, according to one study done in Southern California (Kim et al. 1992). Another survey found considerable heterogeneity in the resources available to these groups of women, overturning the view that Asian workers constitute a single model minority (Yamanaka and McClelland 1994). Even entry into such work can differ among groups. For example, understandings within Dominican immigrant families about women's work in the New York apparel industry departed significantly from those of native-born white and African American families (Pessar 1994).

Not all sites in the apparel industry represent the risky health conditions found in the California-federal study, but the numbers of violations found in registered firms and the existence of unknown numbers of unregistered firms suggest that the health problems for these women workers are far from resolved.

Agriculture

Although some contemporary agricultural food production in the United States is mechanized, much of the cultivation and harvest of perishable fruits and vegetables is still done by hand. The workers who enable Americans to enjoy the abundance of seasonable fruits are primarily members of minority groups: three-fourths identify themselves as such; two-thirds are foreign-born, primarily in Mexico (Moses et al. 1993:921). Women and children, as often as men, labor in the fields.

Whether the crop is strawberries, artichokes, beans, tomatoes, bell peppers, or squash, this arduous work is backbreaking and risky, backbreaking because of frequent stooping and lifting, risky because pesticides are heavily used to assure a good harvest. "Migrant and seasonal farm workers and their children . . . are the largest single group exposed to pesticides" (Moses et al. 1993:914). Although efforts to establish an accurate reporting system on pesticide poisoning among farm workers have failed because of resistance by agricultural and chemical interests to amendments in the federal pesticide law, the Environmental Protection Agency estimates that 20,000 to 300,000 poisonings occur annually in agricultural workers (Moses et al. 1993:938).[5]

Exposure to these chemicals, which can drift far beyond the point of application, can produce acute physical effects as well as long-term physical and mental consequences, including cancer (Moses et al. 1993:926–31) and reproductive risks.[6] Lack of decent living conditions often means that farmworkers cannot bathe or effectively launder their clothes to remove the pesticides from their skin or clothing, and even if they can, the water they use may contain the very pesticides they wish to remove. A Chicana nurse who worked with farmworkers recalled:

> Pesticides. There's pesticide poisoning, and we know there is.
> . . . And I think physicians sometimes miss it, too. They're not really trained as far as pesticides are concerned. We've had incidents every summer. . . . Somebody will come in all swollen all over, difficult respiration, the whole thing, and says, "It was right after I was out there picking tomatoes for an hour or so."
> . . . And there are no warning signs this field has been sprayed.
> . . . Sometimes the grower doesn't even know the pesticides being used because [the company] is afraid to give away that information. (Hacker 1990:78)

Even where workers have been exposed, they may be afraid to seek medical help, fearing loss of their jobs or their income. If they are undocumented immigrants, they, like the garment workers, may fear contact with authorities. Lack of bilingual health facilities is also a deterrent.[7] Moreover, workers' compensation laws, designed for year-round rather than seasonal employees, often do not cover farmworkers: in only eight states are such workers fully covered (Moses et al. 1993:940). Further, growers are not required to provide health insurance. For these workers, whose annual income may be $7,000, well below national poverty levels, buying health insurance is clearly not possible (Bechtel, Shepherd, and Rogers 1995:19).

For women, the lack of lavatories in the fields and the constant pressure to keep picking means incurring frequent urinary tract infections, dehydration, stress, hypertension, and problems resulting from a lack of prenatal care (Bechtel, Shepherd, and Rogers 1995:20). Working long hours in unsafe circumstances in the fields, they also face the double day of preparing meals for families, caring for children or sick family members, often in far less than adequate living circumstances. The health risks to women who produce food for American tables are daily, continual, and for the most part unresolved.

Electronics Assembly

Contrasted with the confined, stuffy, tension-laden work of cutting and sewing garments and the physically arduous and chemically risky cultivation and harvesting of fruits and vegetables, electronics assembly work appears clean, light, far more apt to be regulated by protective labor laws than sectors of the garment industry or agriculture, and much more prone to regulations ensuring minimum wages, worker compensation, and even health benefits.[8] Yet within the sterile white assembly rooms of the electronics industry, health risks are as severe as those experienced by sweatshop seamstresses and farm harvesters. Gradual recognition of those risks has begun to reverse old images (Baker and Woodrow 1984). It is now recognized that electronics assembly workers, many of them Asian or Hispanic women and single mothers (Grossman 1980), face mental and physical health problems including severe eyestrain and muscle strain (see chapter 6).

The history of some of those problems reflects an issue discussed in chapter 22 of this volume, namely, the lack of serious attention given to women's physical complaints and/or the tendency to ascribe such complaints to female hysteria. In the case of women microelectronics workers, complaints of bodily symptoms were attributed to female hysteria, a ready-to-hand gendered and racist interpretation based probably in part on occurrences of mass illnesses ("hysteria") among third world women electronics assemblers and on the fact that many such workers in the United States are women of color. In one case this interpretation held until a male supervisor exhibited the same symptoms (Baker and Woodrow 1984:28).

A series of studies then questioned whether female hysteria was the issue (Brabant, Mergler, and Messing 1990) and demonstrated a relationship between symptoms reported by women and chemical exposure (Parkinson et al. 1990).[9] Further study psychologically assessed former microelectronics workers at two different times and found persistence of mood personality disturbances among *both* men and women that were not reactive, temporary hysterical neurosis, but consistent with organic solvent toxicity—chemical poisoning (Bowler et al. 1992). Electronics assembly work also contains high stresses emergent from demands for productivity that lead to what one study found were additive adverse effects on the health of working women (Bromet et al. 1992).

Electronics assembly work is likely to increase in importance as the United States struggles to remain preeminent in a rapidly changing industry. The question remains whether the health of the many women of color who provide the critical labor force for that industry will also increase in importance.

Conclusion

Asian and Hispanic garment workers cut and sew fashionable apparel in sometimes shocking working conditions. Hispanic and African American women stoop and bend to pick fruits and vegetables in pesticide-ridden air. Asian, Hispanic, and Caucasian women create electronics products amid solvents. They dramatically represent the varying degrees of such health risks in women's work found in many fields not reviewed here, including labor at home.

Women's occupational health issues create an invisible collectivity whose fluid boundaries encompass worker and consumer, privileged and impoverished women, unknown to one another but highly interdependent. Health problems of women workers, particularly low-income workers of color, are threaded into garments, grown into food, and built into the electronic devices that ease and organize lives and give pleasure. Everyone is implicated in their work, their health, and the efforts or lack thereof to alleviate the conditions that produce those health problems.

NOTES

Barbara Burgel and Julia Faucett, Occupational Health Nursing Program, Department of Mental Health, Community and Administration Nursing, UCSF School of Nursing; Pam Tao Li, UC Berkeley Department of Labor and Occupational Health; Leti Volpp and Elia Gallardo, Equal Rights Advocates, San Francisco; and Jeffrey Bauman, International Ladies Garment Workers' Union, San Francisco, all provided helpful leads for the background of this chapter.

The title comes from a comment by a Texas migrant farmworker: "This summer has been one of the hottest. . . . People complain that migrants don't want to work, but I'd like to put them all in the fields for just a half day in 90-degree heat and see how they like it. I mean even mules get put in the shade in the heat of the day. Are migrants less than animals?" (Jasso and Mazzora 1984:92–93).

1. Health problems for women workers in the garment manufacturing industry represent a particularly worrisome convergence of cultural and economic factors. The women's clothing industry, prey to the rapid changes in fashion (see chapter 10), has been fragmented into networks of contractors and subcontractors who must produce clothing quickly and inexpensively if they are to stay abreast of fashion or, put differently, to survive economically (*New York Times*, Week in Review, 20 August 1995). Cheap labor is one "solution."

2. Although the 50 percent figure is shocking, it was an improvement over findings from a 1992 survey in which 80 percent of the firms inspected committed minimum wage or overtime violations (U.S. Department of Labor 1994b).

3. There is some evidence that organized Asian crime is bringing Asian and other foreign workers into the country illegally to work in the garment industry (*San Francisco Chronicle*, 25 August 1995). Several episodes of "pirate" boats dumping illegal immigrants on American shores have occurred recently.

4. Two San Francisco organizations have been working with garment workers. Asian Immigrant Women Advocates in the San Francisco Bay Area attempts to increase literacy and develop leadership skills among immigrant Asian women in Bay Area garment shops (Louie 1992). Equal Rights Advocates' Garment Worker Project provides education on legal rights, represents workers at hearings, and works with other organizations on legislation regulating labor violations. The International Ladies Garment Workers' Union also has a strong safety and health program, but many sweatshops are not unionized or open to unionizing.

5. Farmworkers participating in the Equal Rights Advocates Farm Women's Leadership program in the Castro Valley, south of San Francisco, have conducted educational programs for farm women and men on both pesticide risks and domestic violence.

6. Spontaneous abortion and stillbirth have been reported in the few studies available on farmworkers exposed to pesticides (Moses et al. 1993:935–36). Protection against reproductive problems caused by pesticides can be a double-edged sword that protects women but also shunts them out of work or into lower status jobs (Jasso and Mazzora 1984:96). The tension between "protection" and workplace rights has long characterized women's occupational health issues. Critics point out the discriminatory

features of this (Duncan 1989), the pitting of maternal against fetal rights (Daniels 1991; Gonen 1993; Kenney 1993), and the necessity of maintaining workplace safety for both men and women while preserving women's workplace rights (Kirp 1991; Kotch, Ossler, and Howze 1984).

7. Under the leadership of Dolores Huerta, the United Farm Workers' Union has worked to establish health centers and to obtain health and safety protection for California farmworkers (Jasso and Mazorra 1984:96).

8. These observations do not apply to "offshore" electronics assembly work where pay rates may be at subsistence levels or below. Many women in Asia work in undesirable health and safety conditions in "free trade zone" settings that give economic advantages to companies while failing to protect workers (Grossman 1980).

9. Microelectronics assembly involves frequent exposure or handling of organic solvents, sometimes without adequate ventilation or respiratory protection. (For detailed discussion of those solvents see Baker and Woodrow 1984:24–28; Bowler et al. 1992:32–33.)

REFERENCES

Amaro, Hortensia, Nancy Felipe Russo, and Julie Johnson
    1987   "Family and work predictors of psychological well-being among Hispanic women professionals." Psychology of Women Quarterly 11:505–21.
Baker, Robin, and Sharon Woodrow
    1984   "The clean, light image of the electronics industry: miracle or mirage?" Pp. 21–36 in Wendy Chavkin (ed.), Double Exposure: Women's Health Hazards on the Job and at Home. New York: Monthly Review Press.
Bechtel, Gregory A., Mary Anne Shepherd, and Phyllis W. Rogers
    1995   "Family, culture and health practices among migrant farmworkers." Journal of Community Health Nursing 12:15–22.
Bowler, Rosemarie M., Donna Mergler, Stephen S. Rauch, and Russell P. Bowler
    1992   "Stability of psychological impairment: two-year follow-up of former microelectronics workers' affective and personal disturbance." Women and Health 18:27–48.
Brabant, Carole, D. Mergler, and Karen Messing
    1990   "Va te faire soigner, ton usine est malade." Santi Mentale au Quebec 15:181–204.
Bromet, Evelyn J., Mary Amanda Dew, David K. Parkinson, Shelly Cohen, and Joseph E. Schwartz
    1992   "Effects of occupational stress on the physical and psychological health of women in a microelectronics plant." Social Science and Medicine 34:1377–83.
Daniels, Cynthia R.
    1991   "Competing gender paradigms: gender difference, fetal rights, and the case of Johnson controls." Policy Studies Review 10:51–68.

Duncan, Margaret Post
    1989   "Fetal protection policies: furthering sex discrimination in the market-place." Journal of Family Law 28:727-51.
Fleishman, Jane
    1984   "The health hazards of office work." Pp. 57-69 in Wendy Chavkin (ed.), Double Exposure: Women's Health Hazards on the Job and at Home. New York: Monthly Review Press.
Gonen, Julianna S.
    1993   "Women's rights vs. 'fetal rights': politics, law, and reproductive hazards in the workplace." Women and Politics 13:175-90.
Grossman, Rachael
    1980   "Women's place in the integrated circuit." Radical America 14:29-49.
Hacker, Sally
    1990   "Farming out the home: women and agribusiness." Pp. 69-88 in Dorothy E. Smith and Susan M. Turner (eds.), "Doing It the Hard Way": Investigations of Gender and Technology. Boston: Unwin Hyman.
Jasso, Sonia, and Maria Mazorra
    1984   "Following the harvest: the health hazards of migrant and season farmworking women." Pp. 86-99 in Wendy Chavkin (ed.), Double Exposure: Women's Health Hazards on the Job and at Home. New York: Monthly Review Press.
Kenen, Regina H.
    1993   Reproductive Hazards in the Work Place, Mending Jobs, Managing Pregnancies. New York: Harrington Park Press.
Kenney, Sally J.
    1993   "Who is protected? what's wrong with exclusionary policies?" Women and Politics 13:153-73.
Kim, Richard, Kane K. Nakamura, Gisele Fong, Ron Cabarloc, Barbara Jung, and Sung Lee
    1992   "A preliminary investigation: Asian immigrant garment workers in Los Angeles." Amerasia Journal 18:69-82.
Kirp, David L.
    1991   "The pitfalls of 'fetal protection.'" Society 28:70-76.
Kotch, Jonathan B., Charlene C. Ossler, and Dorothy C. Howze
    1984   "A policy analysis of the problem of the reproductive health of women in the workplace." Journal of Public Health Policy 5:213-27.
Louie, Miriam Ching
    1992   "Immigrant Asian women in Bay Area garment sweatshops: 'after sewing, laundry, cleaning and cooking, I have no breath left to sing.'" Amerasia Journal 18:1-26.
Moses, Marion, Eric Johnson, W. Kent Anger, Virlyn W. Burse, Sanford W. Horstman, Richard J. Jackson, Robert G. Lewis, Keith T. Maddy, Rob McConnell, William J. Meggs, and Shelia Hoar Zahm
    1993   "Environmental equity and pesticide exposure." Toxicology and Industrial Health 9:913-59.

Parkinson, David K., Evelyn J. Bromet, Shelly Cohen, O. L. Dunn, Mary Amanda
Dew, C. Ryan, and J. E. Schwartz
    1990   "Health effects of long-term solvent exposure among women in blue-collar occupations." American Journal of Industrial Medicine 17:661–75.

Pessar, Patricia R.
    1994   "Sweatshop workers and domestic ideologies: Dominican women in New York's apparel industry." International Journal of Urban and Regional Research 18:127–42.

Rosenberg, Harriet G.
    1984   "The home is the workplace: hazards, stress, and pollutants in the household." Pp. 219–45 in Wendy Chavkin (ed.), Double Exposure: Women's Health Hazards on the Job and at Home. New York: Monthly Review Press.

U.S. Department of Labor
    1994a   Memo on the Results of the California Garment Survey. San Francisco: Office of Information.
    1994b   Federal, State Labor Agencies Release Results of Compliance Survey of Garment Industry. San Francisco: Office of Information.

Yamanaka, Keiko, and Kent McClelland
    1994   "Earning the model minority image: diverse strategies of economic adaptation by Asian American women." Ethnic and Racial Studies 17:79–114.

[8]

Access, Cost, and Quality of Medical Care:
Where Are We Heading?

SHERYL BURT RUZEK

Access to medical care involves many factors including eligibility for health insurance through a public or private plan. But not all women are insurable, nor does having coverage mean that critical services are included. Here the author highlights some dangerous gaps in coverage for many of women's most common conditions and raises disturbing questions about where we are headed as we plan how to provide medical care into the next century.

Women's Growing Concerns

Women want to believe that American medical care is the best in the world, but is it? The United States spends 50 percent more per person on medical care than any other country but fails to provide all women with medical coverage. We now rank in the bottom fourth of twenty-four industrialized countries in life expectancy, and we have the highest percentage of babies born at dangerously low weights (Schieber, Poullier, and Greenwald 1994:108).[1] A recent national study showed that people in all socioeconomic groups who lack health insurance use fewer medical services than the insured and are more likely to die (Franks, Clancy, and Gold 1993).[2] Some women underuse preventive screening, and so they fail to detect disease early when they could be treated effectively. Other women are overscreened with little evidence of health benefit. American medical care fails to provide not only a floor of equity but a vision of health. What are the social and political ramifications of allocating resources as we do? Can we find new ways to balance private wants with public needs?

Is Access Diminishing?

Many women and their families face particular trials and tribulations getting medical care from a system that Clancy and Massion (1992) aptly describe as a "patchwork quilt with gaps." The growing ranks of the uninsured form a grim yardstick against which to assess just how secure we are. We hope that *our* insurance benefits, if we have them, remain in our possession. If we are like most people, we are not actually sure what our medical insurance provides—until we get sick or have to change health plans.[3]

Being underinsured creeps gradually into consciousness as television and newspaper headlines warn that Medicare, the national health plan that we thought would provide for us in old age, lurches and lunges toward insolvency. No one wants to get less, but how will we make our resources go around? Is access to quality medical care slipping beyond more and more women's reach? Are the gains women made in health care in recent decades eroding? Can troubling trends be reversed?

Are We Paying More but Getting Less?

Women's personal stories, surveys, and scientific studies reveal troubling conflicts and contradictions in American health care. Over the past two decades, feminist health activists, including many health and science writers, raised women's consciousness about a wide range of health topics.[4] Mass circulation magazines such as *Good Housekeeping, Vogue, Essence, Redbook,* and *Working Woman* regularly report medical news, encourage women to take active roles in decision making, and recommend "shopping around" for compatible doctors.[5] These messages encourage women to think critically about the quality of their care. Over 40 percent of the 2,500 women who answered the Commonwealth Fund Survey of Women's Health (1993) reported having left their doctors because they were dissatisfied. A quarter felt "talked down to" by doctors. African American and Hispanic women, who were less satisfied than white women with their doctors, were less likely to have changed physicians, probably because they had fewer opportunities to do so.

Overall, Americans see doctors less often than do people in many other countries who pay less directly and indirectly (through tax support) and use more medical services.[6] M. Edith Rasell (1995) of the Economic Policy Institute wonders about the long-term consequences of current strategies designed to cut costs. Rasell points out that in 1990, even before the recent round of cost cutting, Americans made on average 5.5 physicians visits— less than half the number made in Japan and Germany and slightly less than in the United Kingdom where medical care costs are much lower. Americans also used hospitals only two-thirds as often as the French and Canadians and less than half as often as Germans. Yet our total spending per person is higher than in any other industrialized country.[7]

Three decades of health activism underscore that spending alone does not ensure that women will get careful diagnosis, caring, and concern from medical providers. Physician Carolyn DeMarco (1994:59-60) writes: "Over the last sixteen years of medical practice, I have seen many women suffer needlessly because their doctors did not really listen to them, told them that physically based complaints were all in their heads, and treated normal events in a woman's life as if they were diseases. Time and time again I have seen women paying a heavy price for the careless prescription of antibiotics, birth control pills, hormones and tranquilizers. . . . Women are not getting healthier. In fact, we see the opposite trend in our practice."

Who Has Insurance?

Increasingly, women face financial difficulties getting medical care at all. For mainstream Americans, widespread anxiety over access to medical care is a recent phenomenon. Both women and men worry about how corporate downsizing and job losses, especially better-paying unionized industrial and middle-management jobs, leave them without adequate medical benefits to pay for rising medical care costs. Between 1971 and 1991, the real cost of medical services rose rapidly. Full-time employees found themselves replaced with "part-timers" or "contract employees" who could be hired without being paid costly benefits.

Upper-, middle-, and working-class people who have had good medical coverage increasingly fear losing medical benefits. In one study, nearly half of all respondents reported difficulty in or anxiety about being able to pay for insurance or medical services, particularly in the event of a major illness. Less than one-third were confident about being able to pay for long-term care (Jacobs and Shapiro 1994). In another study, conducted by the National Opinion Research Center (NORC), 19 percent of all respondents reported having difficulty in paying medical bills in the past year. Of these, 75 percent *had* health insurance (Blendon et al. 1994a).

Most Americans continue to have private health insurance through employment, although the proportion of American households in which neither spouse is eligible for employer-provided health benefits is increasing (Schur and Taylor 1991). Whites are more likely than blacks or Hispanics to have employer-provided insurance (Seccombe, Clarke, and Coward

1994). Women are less likely than men to have insurance through their own employment, but they are twice as likely as men to have it through a spouse.[8] Women are more likely than men to have insurance, largely because women are more likely than men to be eligible for Medicaid, the public insurance for people with low income and disabilities.[9] In 1993, among women ages 15 to 44, about 67 percent had some form of employer-provided insurance, 6 percent had other group or individual private insurance, and 8 percent had Medicaid coverage. Nearly 15 percent were uninsured part of the year, and 8 percent were continually uninsured (Women's Research and Education Institute 1994:5).

The National Center for Health Statistics reports that in 1993, 40 million people under the age of sixty-five were uninsured.[10] Nearly one-third of young adults ages nineteen to twenty-four go without coverage during their prime reproductive years. Many lose insurance when they leave their parents' policies and are unable to obtain their own. Among rural residents, the poor, and minorities, the rates of uninsurance are especially high (Short, Monheit, and Beauregard 1989). In recent years, the number of uninsured Americans increased at four times the rate of population growth (Short, Cornelius, and Goldstone 1990).

The working poor, who constitute the majority of the uninsured, have experienced significant erosion of benefits.[11] The working poor are only one-third as likely to receive insurance from an employer as the nonpoor, and they are over five times as likely to be without insurance from any source (Seccombe and Amey 1995). Being employed actually *restricts* access to medical care for people who are poor because earnings make them ineligible for public health insurance programs (Berk and Wilensky 1987; Seccombe and Amey 1995). Women who are near or only slightly above the poverty level are rapidly joining the ranks of the uninsured. Their modest to marginal earnings[12] make paying premiums for inadequate medical coverage neither rational nor practical. Herein lies what may be the most overlooked impediment to moving women off welfare and into jobs.

Employer-Provided Insurance

Employers offer many types of medical plans. Most require workers to pay a fixed annual deductible and to pay monthly premiums and other expenses. Employers contribute little in firms with a large proportion of part-time workers and in the service sector where women and minorities are concentrated. Just because a woman is eligible for medical coverage does not mean she can afford medical care.[13] Disparities between medical plans for executives and lower-level workers break along gender lines. For example, in one large financial firm on the West Coast, a former administrative assistant said, "All of the partners who were male and earned over $500,000 a year had medical plans that didn't have any co-payments or deductibles and covered all prescriptions. The 'peons,' the women administrative assistants and secretaries [who earned about $25,000 a year], got HMO coverage with large co-payments on office visits and prescriptions."[14] Even if employees all get the same medical plan, virtually all private plans burden lower-income workers. A woman who earns $20,000 and pays a $200 deductible and $600 copayment for hospitalization pays a far greater proportion of her earnings than does the employee who earns $50,000 (Muller 1990:83). Thus employers provide "safety nets" with the largest holes for those with the greatest needs.

Affordability. As a society, we fail to ensure that people can get medical care for themselves and their families on modest or marginal incomes. Women who head families are particularly vulnerable. In 1993, women ages fifteen to forty-four had on average $2,123 in medical expenses— $1,550 paid by insurance and $573 out-of-pocket. Over 25 percent of women who were poor paid over 10 percent of their income for out-of-pocket medical expenses; under 5 percent of women with high incomes spent this much.[15]

Private insurance costs vary widely. Insurers set rates based on a wide array of individual and community factors.[16] Surveys of large companies show that the average annual cost of medical insurance is $3,600 per employee.[17] In the HMOs reviewed by Consumer's Union in 1990–91, the monthly cost of family premiums ranged from a low of $288 to a high of $610.[18] Purchasing even the *cheapest* plan would take 16.6 percent of white and 18.5 percent of black full-time working women's median annual earnings![19]

Some Intersections of Race, Class, and Gender. Medical care coverage amplifies social inequities. Whites are more likely to have private coverage than blacks or Hispanics; women in households with higher incomes are more likely to have private insurance than women with lower incomes. Since 1989, a smaller proportion of men and women had private insurance whereas a growing proportion of women enrolled in public programs (Horton 1995:134). As the private sector withdraws benefits, the public sector expands to "take up the slack." The growth of public sector spending erodes public confidence in government, especially among people who have too much income to qualify for assistance but too little to be able to provide for themselves. This impoverishment of middle- to low-income workers fuels social divisions and political dilemmas.

Health care workers, who are predominately female, provide a case study of how sex, race, and class stratification in the labor force affect insurance status.[20] Nearly one million health care workers, who constitute nearly 9 percent of the civilian health care labor force, do not have health insurance. In nursing homes, one-fifth of employees are uninsured. The largely female food service staffs and aides, who are also most likely to be members of racial/ethnic minority groups, are least likely to be covered. In doctors' offices, over half of all employees pay for their entire policies, whereas 6 percent have no coverage at all (Himmelstein and Woolhandler 1991).

Insurability. On the open market outside of employer-based group plans, many women cannot get insurance. Histories of hypertension, back problems, obesity, cancer, and a growing array of "health risks" turn women into "uninsurables." Genetic testing, screening for HIV and other diseases, and computerized medical records—information age tools—all help insurers and employers keep medical pariahs out of their carefully guarded pools. Women and their families who have chronic conditions, disabilities, or even genetic markers for diseases that they may or may not actually develop get "risked out." Many employers make direct decisions about reimbursement for costly procedures. Some employers "let workers go" when they develop costly illnesses, fearing that large claims will raise their rates. Or they cap the amount of coverage (e.g., at $100,000) and allow employees with chronic or terminal conditions to face financial disaster. Thus those who most need insurance have the most difficulty getting it.

Other life decisions get pulled into the medical care mess. People hesitate to change jobs because they fear they will lose medical coverage. Some mothers stay on welfare to keep Medicaid benefits; others resort to divorce and welfare to get medical care for their children.[21] In the gap between divorce or widowhood and eligibility for Medicare at age sixty-five, women struggle to pay medical bills (Muller 1990:128–29). How well do these safety nets work, how much do they cost, and who is eligible?

Public Insurance

The United States boasts two major public health insurance programs: Medicare, initially designed for persons sixty-five or over, and Medicaid, the program initially designed for economically disadvantaged mothers and children.[22] Both are expanding rapidly and bringing with that expansion political and fiscal problems. Public insurance is a critical "women's issue" because women ages eighteen and older are twice as likely as men to be poor (13.3% compared with 8.4%) and more likely to be eligible for public insurance programs. Black (31%), Native American (29.1%), and Hispanic origin (26.2) women are more likely to be poor than white (10.8%) or Asian (10.9%) women.[23]

Medicare. Medicare, enacted in 1965, provides insurance for more than 99 percent of the elderly. People who are eligible for Social Security disability benefits or end-stage renal disease benefits are also eligible for Medicare. Private insurers widely market "Medi-Gap" policies to cover deductibles and restrictions. In ignorance and confusion, elderly persons underuse services, fail to get reimbursement, and buy duplicate supplementary policies (Muller 1990:129). Medicare recipients pay on average over 18 percent of their annual income for health insurance premiums, deductibles, copayments, and noncovered services (Challenges in Health Care 1991:82). For elderly low-income women, Medicaid, the "insurer of last resort," is a critical safety net.

Medicaid. Medicaid, enacted as a welfare-type program for low-income Americans, remains largely a "women's program." About three-quarters of all Medicaid beneficiaries are low-income women and their children; 12.5 percent of all children in the United States are covered by Medicaid (Challenges in Health Care 1991:102). State Medicaid programs grew dramatically in the past decade when Congress began expanding coverage to pregnant women, infants and children, and low-income older and disabled people. Women with HIV receive Medicaid coverage as do other disabled persons (Kaiser Commission on the Future of Medicaid 1993).

Despite rapid increases in Medicaid spending, less than half of all persons living in poverty are actually covered by Medicaid. With the rising cost of medical coverage and limitations on benefits, a growing proportion of the population remains uninsured until serious illness reduces them to the lowest levels of poverty. Only then do they become eligible for Medicaid. Currently, the states provide Medicaid clients with wide variations in services. In 1993, average payments per Medicaid insured person varied more than twelvefold.[24] As states take on greater control for administering federal programs, variability between states will widen.

Costs and Conflicts in Public Insurance. In 1993, federal, state, and local government combined paid for 43 percent of all personal health care expenditures, largely through Medicare and Medicaid. Both programs are widely regarded as "out of control." Unless dramatic modifications are made in both systems, neither system will be able to meet the growing need for services into the next century. Medicare already consumes an increasing proportion of the federal budget—8 percent in 1987 (Physician Payment Review Commission 1990) and a projected 10 percent in 1996 (U.S. Office of Management and Budget 1996:9). As the population ages, Medicare faces enormous financial pressures. Already, employed persons are being taxed 1.45 percent of current earnings to cover rising costs.[26]

From 1988 to 1991, the cost of Medicaid services alone grew from $51.6 billion to $88.6 billion, primarily because of increases in enrollment, medical price inflation, and increases in expenditures per beneficiary through expansion of federally mandated coverage. Medicaid is now the single largest item in state budgets, and it has forced states to reduce spending on education and welfare (Kaiser Commission on the Future of Medicaid 1993).[27] The elderly and disabled actually account for two-thirds of all Medicaid spending. Medicaid also pays an estimated 40 percent of all care for persons with AIDS. In 1991, these costs were $2.1 billion, estimated to double to $3.8 billion by 1997 (Kaiser Commission 1993:15).[28] The Kaiser Commission concluded that "efforts to resolve a 'Medicaid crisis,' viewed in isolation, are a mistake. Rather, the real crisis is the growing need for health insurance among the poor and disabled, unrestrained health care costs, and fiscal constraints on state and federal governments. These tensions underscore the need for systemwide control of health care costs and national health care reform. Only by addressing these broader problems, and determining the most effective role of a safety net, can we ensure adequate protection for the nation's poor and vulnerable" (1993:37).

Gaps in the Patchwork Quilt

Having medical insurance does not ensure access—or ensure the quality of what women struggle to pay for. As Collins and her colleagues point out (1994:144), at least 60 million people are *underinsured*. Their private insurance is inadequate in terms of what it covers, they risk losing it if they become ill (because of the carrier's right to discontinue), or their policies have such high out-of-pocket charges (deductibles and copayments) that access to medical care is precarious if not entirely out of reach.

Younger, middle-aged, and older women find different gaps in coverage in different insurance plans. Some of the worst gaps are in primary care. Many younger women have inadequate access to maternity and abortion services.[29] Many middle-aged and older women face limited access to preventive screening. All but the most affluent have difficulty finding and paying for long-term care.[30] Women who have chronic mental disorders find mental health services particularly inaccessible and inadequate. Women who are disabled face gaps in accessible and appropriate services even when they have insurance.[31] Gaps in services for women over the life cycle raise troubling issues about how we provide medical care in an advanced industrial nation.

Inadequate Maternity Care Coverage

The Costly American Way of Birth. Over half of all hospital discharges for women ages eighteen to forty-four are for childbirth (Adams and Benson 1991). Each year about 3.7 million women have babies. Eight out of ten women have at least one child, and most eventually have two or three (Alan Guttmacher Institute 1987:5). There are compelling reasons for societies to figure out how to pay for caring for women who are fulfilling their role in continuing the human species. According to the Health Insurance Association of America (1992), the average cost of maternity care in 1991 was $4,720. Physicians charged on average $1,625 and hospitals charged $3,095 for normal deliveries. The average total charge for cesarean births was $7,826.[32] More complicated births cost even more.

Many expectant parents simply cannot pay the costs of maternity care. Over the past two decades, real earnings declined most dramatically for younger workers—those ages fifteen to twenty-four. Between 1981 and 1991, the median income of married couples in this age group dropped by 8 percent (Costello and Stone 1994:330). For all families in this age group (which includes single parents as well as married couples), 1991 median earnings were only $16,848. It would take 18 percent of such a family's annual income to pay the medical costs of an uncomplicated birth and 47 percent to pay for a cesarean birth! On top of this, resources would be needed to cover other costs of pregnancy and birth—maternity clothing, baby clothing, equipment, and food.

Who Pays for Maternity Care? A decade ago, the Alan Guttmacher Institute reported that an estimated 5 million women of reproductive age had private insurance that did not cover maternity care at all. Half a million women without any public or private insurance coverage gave birth each year, mostly in hospitals. Maternity and newborn care, the biggest single source of uncompensated care, constituted almost half of all unpaid bills of more than $25,000. To protect themselves, hospitals refused to admit patients without evidence of insurance. Although Congress authorized penalties for physicians and institutions that turned away women in active labor, the law did not prevent refusing care to women in early stages of labor—"a nice distinction that is more appropriately made in a textbook than in an emergency room" (Alan Guttmacher Institute 1987:46).[33]

The recent expansion of private and Medicaid coverage to pregnant women came in response to national pressure from scientific, professional, and advocacy organizations concerned with women's and children's health. Private insurers and Congress both took considerable flak over America's poor international standing in infant mortality rates. Hospitals, in particular, supported expansion of coverage that helped pay for the growing cost of unreimbursed care and the extra costs that inadequate prenatal care caused. By 1994, most private health plans covered maternity care (Horton:141).

Congress specifically required the states to provide at least minimal coverage for all pregnant women with family incomes up to 133 percent of the federal poverty level. Using the 1990 federal threshold of $13,359 for a family of four, a hypothetical young family who earned under $17,767 that year would have been eligible for Medicaid maternity coverage under federal requirements. Between 1988 and 1991, an additional 900,000 pregnant women who previously would have been ineligible were enrolled (Kaiser Commission on the Future of Medicaid 1993:9). In 1990, uncompensated deliveries declined to about 8 percent, and by 1991, Medicaid paid for 1.24 million births—32 percent of all births in the United States (Singh, Gold, and Frost 1994). If the states covered maternity care for women up to 185 percent of the poverty level as recommended by the federal government, close to half of all U.S. births would be financed at least in part by Medicaid (Rosenbaum 1992).

Ironically, for three decades scholars and activists railed against medicalizing childbirth and adopting birth technologies that have never been shown scientifically to improve birth outcomes.[34] Doctors and hospitals have now made maternity care so costly that we no longer *believe* that we can afford care for women who give birth!

Complexities and Conflicts in Screening

American medicine is acute care oriented. Actually preventing disease falls outside the biomedical model. DeMarco (1994:66–67), reflecting on her own medical training, notes: "Doctors are taught nothing about true prevention. If you asked your doctor what prevention means to her, chances are that she would say Pap smears, mammograms, annual physicals, screening for hidden blood in the stool, and so forth. This concept of prevention really has nothing to do with prevention and everything to do with looking for something after it is too late to stop the process."

Screening to detect disease early before symptoms are noticed is widely promoted but rarely thought about critically. Louise Russell (1994), a prominent public health policy analyst, points out that physicians and patients have embraced the advice of experts on screening without recognizing complexities and trade-offs, the mixture of solid information and educated guesses, that led to their development. She also warns patients, clinicians, and payers to pay closer attention to screening guidelines that gloss over or ignore such important matters as the social, psychological, and financial costs of excessive screening.

For patients, the question Russell raises is whether a screening test is the best way to spend time, emotional energy, and money to improve personal health. For doctors and their professional associations, the questions center on the most productive way to spend the ten or fifteen minutes allotted to each patient's appointment and, of course, the impact of the answers on their professional lives. For payers, the issues have to do with how best to spend employers' or taxpayers' money to improve health—or even whether the money would be better spent in alternative ways (Russell 1994:3). Even strong supporters of screening recognize the adverse social, psychological, and behavioral consequences including negative labeling and stigma, increased anxiety, work absenteeism, and fatalism (Croyle 1995).

There are also inevitable errors—some disease will be missed and some women who do not have disease will be subjected to costly and sometimes risky diagnostic procedures.[35] Neither scientists nor professionals agree on how frequently women at different ages should be screened.

In an era when many women are adamant that biomedicine has "short-changed women," raising questions about the appropriateness of screening may appear contrary. But "uniform standards" and "practice guidelines" for screening "all women" perpetuate misallocation of funds. High-income women (who are least at risk) and low-income women (who are at the greatest risk) for most diseases may not be well served by screening guidelines that treat all women alike, a point that women need to make more forcefully.[36]

Who Gets Screened? Screening rates vary by race/ethnicity, but Hispanic women appear to be least screened.[37] Black women are being screened more often now. National data for 1990 show that a larger proportion of black than white women received Pap tests (to detect cervical cancer), blood pressure checks, and clinical breast examinations. Rates of screening for cervical cancer and clinical breast examinations now appear to be more related to income and education than to race per se (Piani and Schoenborn 1993).

The effectiveness of recent efforts in a Medicaid HMO to increase women's use of screening through reminder letters and phone calls suggests that "hard-to-reach populations" may respond when encouraged to use services. Screening rates remain low, however, for women who have to take time off from work, underscoring the need for services to be available when women can use them (Lantz et al. 1995). The actual costs and health benefits of bringing all women into line with current screening guidelines need to be examined carefully.[38]

Within racial/ethnic populations, disease incidence as well as screening rates differ. These are particularly striking, for example, among Native American and Alaska Native women. Nutting et al. (1994) make a compelling case for questioning whether national guidelines for screening can be established. Such guidelines fail to take into account important differences in the incidence of disease in particular populations and subpopulations. This concern is consonant with calls to stop overscreening low-risk women and ensure access to regular screening for high-risk women (Russell 1994; Miller 1995).

Whose Interests Are Served by Screening? Too many screening programs are thinly disguised marketing tools for hospitals, means for gaining "name recognition" in competitive markets. In a critique of the overselling of osteoporosis and breast cancer screening, Whatley and Worcester (1989:217) point out how the availability of technologies such as bone mass measurement and mammography can be selling points for clinics and profitable services in and of themselves. In their view, these technologies are marketed not with an honest assessment of their value but with the intent of manipulating women's fear of disease. The emphasis on screening as "prevention" confuses the public over what really keeps people free of disease.[39] If women allow screening to be used primarily as a marketing tool, without regard for its "health payoff," we will squander funds that would be better spent on useful services or on improved living and working conditions. Thus far, no one has calculated the "promotional costs" of screening.

Virginia Soffa, cofounder of the Breast Cancer Action Group, questions much of what women are told about screening. In her view, the lack of improvement in longtime survival of women whose breast cancer was detected early makes it unclear whether "early detection actually promotes survival or merely extends the amount of time a woman lives knowing about her breast cancer." The failure of medicine to aggressively research and publicize possible means for reducing risk and the promotion of myths about screening and survival play into dangerous myths about "our collective attitudes of suppression, denial and displaced reality" (1994:181, 189).

Cervical Cancer Screening. Every year about 13,500 new cases of invasive cancer are diagnosed and 4,400 women die of cervical cancer (American Cancer Society 1992).[40] The Pap test reduces the risk of death from invasive cervical cancer, yet women at greatest risk (older women, poorer women) are least likely to be screened. Many private insurance plans do not cover routine screening, and an estimated 680,000 Medicaid eligible women do not have even partial payment for Pap smears (Boss and Guckes 1992). As with other services, screening practices reflect patients' socioeconomic statuses. Race, education, and access to a regular source of care affect the likelihood of being screened (Bernstein, Thompson, and Harlan 1991; Harlan, Bernstein, and Kessler 1991).[41]

Mammography Screening. Breast cancer has long been regarded as the disease that women fear most. Each year some 46,000 women die of breast cancer, and 180,000 new cases are diagnosed (American Cancer Society 1992). Although black women have lower age-adjusted breast cancer incidence than white women, their higher mortality suggests poorer access to medical care. Regular mammograms are associated with a reduction in breast cancer mortality in women ages fifty and older, but most women do not have mammograms or clinical breast examinations regularly.[42] Low education, low income, and lack of a regular source of health care are also associated with lower rates of mammography use.[43] Language and insurance barriers may be hard to separate. For example, among the Hispanic women in one study, 86.4 percent had never had a mammogram, but only 42.5 percent had health insurance (Stein, Fox, and Murata 1991). Kagawa-Singer (1987) points out that many cultural issues are ignored in cancer prevention efforts.[44]

Research on social and psychological factors in screening must be viewed in the financial context of women's lives. A mammogram costs from $50 to $150 or more plus the cost of follow-up to rule out ambiguous results and make a diagnosis.[45] Screening mammograms are not reimbursed in all private insurance plans. Medicaid-eligible women have coverage in only twenty-three states.[46] Not surprisingly, women worry about the cost of mammograms.[47] Physicians themselves say that cost deters them from recommending mammograms (American Cancer Society 1985).

Why is the cost so high? Starr argues that lack of coordination in medical systems drives up price. If mammography machines were fully utilized, screening mammograms should cost no more than $55. Because they were "overbought" (by hospitals competing with one another), they are used far below capacity and are unaffordable. "Only in America are poor women denied a mammogram because there is too much equipment" (Starr 1994:26).

Some Consequences of Ignoring Scientific Evidence. That we have too many machines is a fact. But "poor coordination" begs the question of why they were purchased and promoted inappropriately. The fact is that, in the absence of evidence that mammography reduced breast cancer deaths in women under fifty, professional organizations widely promoted routine screening beginning at age forty. In 1993, the National Cancer Institute (NCI) finally announced that the evidence did not support routine screening mammography for women before age fifty (Volkers 1994). The NCI position was supported by the National Women's Health Network, but fought and then ignored by the American Cancer Society and many physicians. If science fails to inform practice, why, women might ask, do we continue to pay for it?

Reducing the numbers of women who are screened may, in the short run, increase the per-mammogram cost. Had the American Cancer Society refrained from promoting mammograms for women under fifty in the absence of evidence of effectiveness in reducing mortality, and had hospitals not seen mammography as a marketing tool, we might have avoided the excessive inventory of mammography equipment.[48] Now that we have it, how will interested parties resist "keeping down the per-unit costs"? Equipment is precisely what the health industry invests in and must retain, all too often to the detriment of women's health.

Mental Health Services: Stigmatized and Underfunded

For many women, mental health services for serious mental and emotional conditions remain a problematic gap in medical care. Feminist scholarship on mental illness that emerged in the 1970s emphasized the social control function of psychiatry and the ways in which psychiatric diagnosis and treatment institutionalized sex and gender bias in American society.[49] Feminist scholars decried overprescribing of psychoactive drugs[50] and urged their colleagues to address the social nature of many women's psychological problems. Carol Tavris, a fellow of the American Psychological Association, emphasizes how the way we think about problems shapes our actions: "A woman who thinks she has a chronic disease may be persuaded to enlist in group therapy forever, and a woman who thinks she has a personality disorder may begin a lengthy course of treatment. A woman who thinks she needs a better job may enroll in school. If a woman thinks she is angry at her husband because her hormones are out of kilter, she may consult a doctor; if she decides she is angry because she is doing 99 percent of the housework, she may talk to her husband about it" (Tavris 1994:100).

For women who feel that they do need professional mental health services, options are limited by both financial and social barriers.[51] Insurers restrict mental health services stringently. Plans typically require higher cost sharing than for "physical" conditions and frequently deny coverage on the basis of preexisting conditions. Psychiatric benefits for inpatient care are on a par with medical benefits in only 21 percent of large and medium-sized firms in the private sector. Only 2 percent have comparable outpatient coverage.[52] Medicaid reimburses such low rates for psychiatric services that few patients see private providers. Medicare reimburses slightly better (Glied and Kofman 1995:56–58).

Long-Term Care

For older women, both screening and long-term care remain costly gaps. About the year 2011, when the baby-boom generation starts reaching age sixty-five, the cost of medical care will escalate rapidly. For women, long-term care is critical. Already, women are twice as likely as men to be in nursing homes (Challenges in Health Care 1991:82). (See also chapters 16 and 17.)

As elderly persons "spend down" their assets during long illnesses, Medicare transfers them to Medicaid and turns them into "welfare cases."[53] As more elderly women need to be cared for at home, who will do it? Who will define eligibility for assistance with preparing meals or taking medications? Definitions of need are always open to negotiation.[54] For example, gerontologist Jeanne Bader (1994), who developed an extensive list of products that allow elderly people or people with physical, hearing, or visual limitations to live independently, notes that because these products are considered "nonmedical assists," health insurance does not cover them and people with limited means may be unable to purchase them. How will we shift resources from keeping elderly people alive in hospitals, perhaps too long, to helping elderly people continue to lead healthy lives in communities?

Partial Perspectives and Partial Solutions

Overall, women's access to medical care remains spotty, unequal, and costly. Efforts to contain excessive costs reflect partial solutions that fail to go to the root of why American women pay more and get less than citizens of other nations. Rasell (1995) attributes high costs and lower use of medical services in the United States to high prices and physicians' fees, high administrative costs, less efficient delivery of services (because of duplication and underuse of equipment), and the high rate at which many costly procedures are performed. Maternity care and cancer screening provide good examples of the "systems problems" that need to be resolved.

Maintaining the Status Quo

Too many players simply assume that the current organization of maternity care can be "fixed" without rethinking the way we care for women giving birth. Why, one might ask, are obstetricians considered the most suitable provider of routine maternity care? Why is reducing the *number of days women are cared for following birth*, rather than reducing the *cost* of hospital stays, seen as the solution to the "cost crisis"? Why must most maternity care be provided in hospitals at all?

To reduce costs, major insurers began imposing 24-hour discharge in California in the early 1990s. As this policy moved east, public outcries, accompanied by threats of lawsuits and legislation, led major insurers to reinstate routine approval for two-day stays. Childbirth educators and home birth advocates, who have long favored discharging women from the hospital as soon after birth as possible, recognize that predicting the consequences of discharging women early is uncertain. Women who do not have supportive homes to go to, or who have undetected complications, may suffer from pressure to check out early. Nonetheless, insurers implemented this major change in maternity care *without* carrying out any research to identify possible adverse outcomes.[55]

Insurers seem exceedingly willing to risk "taking chances" with women's and infants' health *outside* the hospital. *Inside* the hospital, insurers continue to pay for costly "just in case" technologies—even when scientific evidence fails to document clear beneficial outcomes. Obstetricians, who tend to prefer higher-technology approaches, fear competition from female midwives. States that have tried to reimburse nurse-midwives at the same rate as physicians to increase the pool of providers have met with stiff resistance from organized medical societies.[56]

Seeking Systems Change

Systems change may or may not result from pressures to reduce costs and still compete on the basis of consumer perceptions of quality and desirability.[57] Many observers argue that we need to shift the emphasis of the entire medical system. DeMarco (1994:67), for example, believes that decreased health care costs will come from education, prevention, self-reliance, and "a return to safer, less expensive, and more sane methods of therapy." DeMarco's insight warrants wide discussion. If Americans need to reduce medical costs, why are some forms of out-of-hospital care—particularly home or freestanding birth center care—so strongly resisted despite clear evidence of safety, cost reduction, and parent preferences?[58] Why have nurse-practitioners and other midlevel practitioners remained undervalued and underutilized? Given what primary care providers actually do in day-to-day practice, why are so many physicians needed in this role (Harrison 1994)?

Similar questions should be asked about the long-standing resistance of organized medicine to alternative or holistic health care treatments.[59] Increasingly managed care plans are exploring these services, particularly where there is growing scientific evidence of effectiveness. For example, Kaiser-Permanente in California now strongly supports midwifery care. Sharp HealthCare in San Diego recently acquired the Birth-Place, a free-standing facility run largely by midwives. Here, deliveries cost on average only $2,639, which is 32–46 percent less expensive than hospital births. They also result in higher birthweight rates, lower infant mortality, and greater family satisfaction (Bergman 1994).[60] Midwives simply must be recognized as primary maternity care providers, or access and affordability will be achieved at the expense of women and their families.[61] Consumer demand is likely to be a critical force in bringing about change. As insurers compete for contracts, public demand for benefits relative to costs should become paramount.

Women's health activists have long questioned the ethics of medicine's attachments to technologies that are hazardous or ineffective. Given the growing view that resources should not be squandered on things that don't work, policymakers should give particular thought to achieving cost containment by weeding out ineffective technologies that scientists scorn and patients protest.[62] Responsible managed care organizations have in fact been lauded for producing lower rates of unnecessary or inappropriate surgery (such as hysterectomies and cesarean sections) compared with fee-for-service practice.[63]

Given that a significant proportion of physician-prescribed medical care is unevaluated or has questionable positive effects, many resources are wasted on services that providers want to provide whether or not they improve patient health (Duncan 1994; Lomas and Contandriopoulos 1994). Despite recent efforts by the Agency for Health Care Policy Research to evaluate medical technologies, or the efforts by professional organizations to promote appropriate use of technologies, physician practices change slowly (Fennell and Warnecke 1988; Foote 1987; Kosecoff et al. 1987). Medical outcomes research, which has burgeoned recently (Wennberg 1990), has not been accompanied by mechanisms for disseminating information effectively to practitioners (Detsky 1989; Duncan 1994) or to patients. Funds allocated to assess the efficacy and cost-effectiveness of medical care are essentially wasted if they do not influence practice decisions. If the proliferation of high-technology resources in medicine do not result in improved outcomes or more efficient use of health care dollars, on what grounds can they continue to be supported (Rublee 1994)? For women who want providers to communicate more and attend more to the social-psychological dimensions of health and healing, fiscal priorities clearly need reordering.

Can We Control Technology?

Resources for caring and healing must come from somewhere. That "somewhere" lies in controlling cost escalation that is rooted in technology diffusion. Theoretically, advances in technology should reduce costs, but in fact technology is a central problem.

Is More Better?

Institute of Medicine president Kenneth I. Shine points out that, although technology may lower the cost of a given procedure, medicine has "a fantastic capacity to make up for decreases in cost by increasing volume. We have an insatiable interest in technology. The easier it is to apply, the more we use it" (qtd. in "How Current Technology" 1995:1). In one large health maintenance organization, for example, the introduction of laparoscopic cholecystectomy reduced the cost of conventional gallbladder surgery by 25 percent. But because the volume rose by 40 percent, the overall cost to the system increased by 11 percent. In addition, the introduction of this procedure in New York led to increased morbidity and mortality because inexperienced physicians were using it. Shine states that technology manufacturers should define the learning curve, and "payers should not reimburse providers who are unable to maintain competency levels." New technologies rarely replace old ones— they are used in addition to what is already being used, and they are used far beyond their intended indications. Although some estimate that only 25 percent of increasing medical care costs are due to technology use, Shine suspects that the figure is closer to 50 percent. Here is the Achilles' heel of cost containment (qtd. in "How Current Technology" 1995:1).

Is the Newest Always the Best?

Many seemingly intractable problems in restraining medical costs are rooted in the myth that the latest and newest treatments and technologies are the best. Increasingly, medical insurance excludes "experimental procedures," or services for which there is no proven efficacy. But what is defined as "experimental" or "effective," and by whom, leaves much room for disagreement. Because medicine is constantly evolving and decisions are often made in the absence of certainty, some disagreements over reimbursement are probably inevitable.[64]

Controversies over access to rapidly developing technologies should raise questions about whether the latest (or the most expensive) is the best, particularly considering the history of medical experimentation on women. As Rothman (1986) points out, it is fortunate that all women were not required to take DES, thalidomide, or high-dosage oral contraceptives or to subject themselves to a number of technologies each of which has been proven to be harmful. Whether the new technology is a contraceptive (e.g., Norplant, Depo-Provera), an abortifacient (e.g., RU-486 or one of several highly toxic cancer drugs used "off-label"), a breast cancer inhibitor (e.g., tamoxifen), or one of many birth technologies, women need reliable, unbiased scientific evidence that documents claims about both efficacy and adverse effects. Ironically, some women's health advocacy groups have sought reimbursement for experimental treatments without fully considering the implications of this expectation in the long run (Ruzek 1995). The situation is reminiscent of the conditions that led to the growth of the women's health movement—a medical environment marked by widespread, harmful experimentation on women.[65] The urgency of accurately assessing the value of medical technologies is heightened by media pressures. Television too often offers only partial and biased views of "high-tech" medicine that inflate public expectations.[66]

How Much Are Women Likely to Benefit from Medical Advances?

With the national focus on women's health, tensions are likely to mount. The surge of interest in breast cancer prevention and treatment, some of it long overdue, brings with it new risks. Fugh-Berman (1994), for example, warns that the NIH prevention trial of tamoxifen, a drug previously used only to treat breast cancer, sets a dangerous precedent. For the first time, a drug with many known severe side effects (e.g., uterine cancer, blood clots, retinal eye problems, depression, vaginitis, and hot flashes) is being given to a healthy population. Women over sixty (who have only a 10 percent lifetime risk of developing breast cancer) are eligible to enter the trial.

Researchers are also looking for ways to prevent breast cancer by reducing women's exposure to "incessant ovulation." Fugh-Berman explains how: "In the name of preventive medicine women's reproductive hormones (estrogen and progesterone) are shut down by monthly injections of gonadotropin-releasing hormones, and then small amounts of estrogen and progesterone are added back into their bodies. This artificial hormone regimen is expected to decrease the number of breast, ovarian, and uterine cancers all of which are connected to estrogen output. However, after tests revealed that study subjects lost two percent of their bone mass per year, an additional male hormone—testosterone—was added to the cocktail in order to minimize osteoporosis in this young, previously healthy population" (1994:84–85).

Such efforts to "restructure" women's physiology surely will have long-term effects on women's health. Already the adverse effects of manipulative reproductive technologies are coming to light (Koch 1993; Rothenberg and Thomson 1994; Stephenson and Wagner 1993). Considering the history of technology development and its consequences for women over the past half century, women's health advocates as well as scientists and proponents of mind-body medicine would seem to be ideal allies of responsible managed care groups in reframing the cost containment debate from excessive reliance on controlling costs by realigning financial incentives to discourage use of medical services into dramatically different terms. Quality along with cost *in relation to effectiveness* must move to the center of debate and action.

Refocusing on Quality—Challenges for the Future

Consumer perceptions of quality and quality standards by which providers are formally judged are not necessarily those that were considered by the architects of failed health reform—access to care, appropriateness of care, health outcomes, health promotion, disease prevention, and satisfaction with care (Mangano 1995). What women say they want is greater responsiveness and attention to their personal felt needs, to the psychological and spiritual, not just to the "hardware" of modern medicine. Many middle-class patients insist on being seen as active participants in decision making, and they expect professionals to take time to listen, communicate, and share information to enhance their emotional as well as physical states. As O'Connor (1995:167) points out, patients constitute an increasingly knowledgeable group who value their own intellects and autonomy. Many have pursued holistic health movements, actively seek and advocate for the widest variety of alternative healing modalities, and most firmly expect— even require—clinicians to be accessible and accountable to them.

Emanuel and Dubler (1995) argue that a central factor in the failure of health reform was inattention to the doctor-patient relationship—the heart of what women want. Although most Americans are satisfied with their regular doctors, many have had to search long and hard to find good doctors and are loathe to give them up.[67] This theme resounds in a Harvard Community Health Plan survey. When asked "What kind of information would be most important to you in choosing your own health plan?" with five items to check (choice of doctor, results of patient satisfaction surveys, ease of access, the overall benefits package, and standardized measures of quality), 48 percent identified choice of physicians as most important. When questioned about the benefit package, respondents viewed preventive care as more important (55%) than prescription drug benefits (37%) or mental health/substance abuse coverage (22%). Over half indicated that the reputation of the plan among their friends, family, and coworkers was more important than satisfaction surveys or standardized quality ratings (Raymond 1995).[68]

These findings highlight two things that cost containers and health planners will have to contend with to succeed: First, in seeking medical care, people grasp the importance of the fit between the patient and doctor. Second, in choosing doctors, people trust family members, friends, and coworkers—members of what social scientists call lay-referral networks—more than impersonal indicators. Thus patients' subjective experience of quality must be addressed. Patient satisfaction surveys, used increasingly in managed care to identify the degree to which patients have experiences that will likely keep them in the system rather than send them shopping elsewhere, may fail to tap what matters most to patients. In most patient satisfaction surveys, quality indicators are defined in terms of waiting time to get appointments, time spent with claim forms, rates of cancer screening, immunization, blood pressure checks, and perceived accessibility of chosen doctors and specialist care.[69] What these surveys fail to tap are patients' subjective experiences of seeking health care. Thus these surveys understate women's deep dissatisfaction with medical care.

Subjective Dimensions of Quality

Health care systems can ill afford to ignore consumers' subjective experience of seeking medical care. The depth of patients' concerns about retaining choice of physicians, even if they choose them out of a telephone book or by word of mouth, indicates that the word *quality* has many meanings to patients. Cultural values and beliefs about science and medicine, the social-psychological experience of being a patient, and interpersonal communication all shape perceptions of quality. Quality of care and quality of life issues in human, subjective terms are difficult to measure objectively, but patients are understandably wary about ignoring these factors. They are at the core of what patients find wrong with medicine.

Biomedicine largely discounts the patient's own experience of physical, social, and psychological disequilibrium—until it can be shown to be "objectively measurable."[70] The subjective aspects of childbirth, for example, are so devalued that hospitals buy costly machines but fail to provide human contact, despite evidence that many of the machines are ineffective or counterproductive whereas simple personal support improves outcomes.[71] To address quality of care we must include women's emotional needs and the social and psychological aspects of illness.[72] As feminist ethicist Caroline Whitbeck (1991) points out, greater attention must be directed to the ethical issues surrounding the effects of medical technologies on relationships, families, and communities.

Despite the obvious importance of women's social, familial, and emotional needs, these are widely ignored by health professionals when treating women for serious, even life-threatening, diseases.[73] Qualitative studies and narrative accounts of women who have lived through serious illnesses or dealt with the iatrogenic effects of medical treatment raise provocative questions about how one can best assess quality.[74] Women's perspectives of living with breast cancer, or the threat of cancer, provide insights into what women who have this disease experience in terms of quality of life and quality of care.[75]

Objective Dimensions of Quality

Despite the limitations of current "quality assurance" efforts, women stand to benefit greatly from the objective performance measures that are emerging. Encouraging patients to use standardized performance measures to make informed choices about medical care plans and providers is likely to enhance patients' real control over medical care (Raymond 1995). Managed care has not yet realized its potential for educating women about the benefits of avoiding inappropriate interventions, something that will be critical in the future. Tensions will likely arise, however, over how to balance indicators of quality of care for the individual and for the population, or subpopulations, as wholes. Bringing women into the discussion of meeting population needs, rather than simply using resources carelessly to support personal preferences, must also be a national priority.

Into the Future: Rethinking Rationing

Even with more efficient organization of health resources, choices will have to be made about what should be paid for universally, what levels of care will be defined as discretionary on the basis of some agreed-upon criteria. All societies ration medical care, although Americans largely deny that we have "come to this yet." More affluent members of society fail to acknowledge that we "came to it" long ago. Many Americans seem uncannily accepting of distributing medical care on the basis of ability to pay, whereas members of other western industrialized societies view the state as responsible for providing at least some basic level of care.[76]

Rationing, or apportioning, medical care on anything other than wealth rests on the notion that some larger social good is served by providing some acceptable level of care to everyone. That level of care must be based in part on the individual's needs, not just ability to pay. The dilemma is how to generate public discussion of the matter without feeding into public fears, fears that are exploited by interests who profit by maintaining the current inequitable, and profitable, system of private insurance and acute care medicine. American medicine is also rapidly shifting financial incentives—from fee-for-service medicine that leads to overtreatment to managed care that puts patients at risk of undertreatment. New balances will have to emerge.

Universal access, which progressive reformers seek, will only be achieved by accepting responsibility for making hard choices about "who gets what." Whether universal access can be achieved through market mechanisms remains to be seen. Leaving a growing proportion of the population uninsured or underinsured suggests the folly of failing to take national action to ensure and even require everyone to have some form of health plan. Women and cost containers continue to inhabit separate intellectual and political spheres, poorly informed about each others' concerns and quandaries. To benefit women, medical care insurance *must be separated from employment*. Because women are particularly disadvantaged in access to employer-provided coverage, this policy direction is critical. Providing at least some choice of health plans is also essential to provide women with diverse needs access to many types of health care.

What the needs of society might be for medical care as a social good, and the extent to which resources should be devoted to that good above all other social goods, has not yet emerged as a dominant moral framework within which access to medical care or resources spent on it are debated. Women who lay claim to promoting social values that support human needs cannot ignore what "we" as a society need and concentrate only on what "we" as individual patients want. From women's perspectives, care should always be tailored to meet individual needs. Balancing the needs of typical, hypothetical patients and real ones poses practical as well as fiscal problems. Insurers need to provide patients and providers more latitude for negotiating how to meet conflicting wants and needs. But we, as consumers, may also have to rethink our own expectations—and reorder our expectations.

Can Access, Cost Containment, and Quality Be Achieved?

National commitment to universal access is segmented, tenuous, and hampered by lack of clarity of just what it might entail. Supporters of universal access appear willing to extend access to others only on the condition that their own benefits do not decline. Although it has been argued that American women view universal access as a priority for government, and women may in fact be willing to pay higher taxes to achieve it (Kasper 1994b), the lack of clarity about what various groups of women "want" makes generalizing highly problematic. Take one issue that is hotly debated and socially divisive: Should universal access be extended to all U.S. residents or only to citizens and legal immigrants? Social consensus about a right to health care has not yet emerged. Nor has there been forthright discussion of what proportion of societal resources should be spent on medical services or what proportion of one's income might be "reasonable" to pay.

Will Cultural Change Occur?

Lack of social consensus on these issues, coupled with unrealistic expectations about the role of medicine in promoting health, makes public policymaking inherently problematic. Most Americans are loathe to give up the notion of "unending medical progress," and recently appeared unwilling to make "trade-offs"—even between broader coverage but longer waits for elective procedures. In the coming decades, Americans will be forced to rethink the view that medical care should be unlimited and the idea that access can be widened without imposing restrictions on reimbursement. Reducing financial incentives to "overtreat" can in fact benefit women if we reduce overuse of costly, ineffective technologies and overpaid, excessively specialized providers for routine medical care. Reversing financial incentives will fail to benefit women if clarity and conscience lose out to vested interests that ignore either scientific evidence of efficacy or "what matters" to women—communication, caring, and continuity of care.

The Gender Divide in Health Reform

Change will not come easily. Economists, whose concerns about costs are well founded, seem ill prepared to address how cost containment strategies will affect quality of care in human terms. Women's health advocacy groups, who grasp the human side of quality, fail to confront hard questions about how to finance services or how to temper "entitlements." We need a new consensus around principles to help a wealthy, industrialized nation provide a "floor of equity" for medical care.

The economics of health care and health care financing have received scant attention in national women's health conferences, publications, or discussions. In these arenas, women focus on gaps and limitations in health services and on "what women want." Questions about how to pay for what we need or want and make hard decisions are too often ignored or even resisted. This is an intellectual and political gender gap that women can ill afford. Outside of a few policy corridors of Washington, too many women readily accept a gendered division of labor: The content and experience of health care continues to be "women's work," whereas health care financing is left to men.

Men need to understand women's perspectives on quality of care, particularly the interpersonal aspects of caring and healing. But women need to grasp the social consequences of controlling—or failing to control—medical care costs. Daily decisions about how to control costs have profound implications for women's health. Women must assert women's perspectives in the realms of health care financing to ensure that women become the architects of the health systems that society sorely needs. Whether women can become drastically different kinds of architects, putting caring and healing back into a central place in medicine, remains to be seen, but we will not have the opportunity of doing so if we hold ourselves aloof from cost considerations.

Is Social Justice Possible?

The profound inequities in the current patchwork of services will not be solved easily or without social conflict. For a society to provide at least some universal care to older citizens, but not to women and children, pits the young and old against one another in a society already deeply divided by social class and race. Failing to provide all citizens primary and preventive care, while supporting costly tertiary care and a massive biomedical research enterprise, institutionalizes inequalities that neither promote women's health nor minimize societal costs for ill health. The specter of further divisions in society based on ability to pay for medical care underscores the urgency of bringing new views and new visions to the table.

Moral and ethical issues are embedded in fiscal matters. How can a society tax the many to support the development of biotechnologies that will benefit only the few who can afford them? How can a society tax low-wage female workers (who are likely to be uninsured or underinsured) to subsidize medical benefits for high-income workers and affluent elderly persons as well as the most vulnerable—the disabled and the most economically disadvantaged? How can a wealthy society leave so many gaps in the medical care crazy quilt for so many?

What Values, What Directions?

The medical care crisis is really one of confusion and disagreement over values, not just how much money can be spent.[77] Health and medical care are complex social and cultural creations that require more than a change of financial incentives to "fix." Entrenched interests continue to find ways to keep medical care coverage focused on costly capital-intensive curative medicine, giving only lip service to the ideology of "managed care" and prevention (Shortell et al. 1993). Preventive and primary care services are inherently labor-intensive and cannot produce profits like capital-intensive medical machinery and drugs do so readily. As the medical care system becomes increasingly privatized and controlled by overtly for-profit corporations whose mission it is to provide a return on capital to investors, women must ask hard questions about how quality and cost will be balanced. Women need to be prepared to ask these questions:

— How "medically necessary," "safe and effective," and "quality" of services will be defined and by whom?
— On what moral and ethical as well as scientific basis will value judgments about "what matters" in medical coverage be made?
— Whose interests do decisions reflect, and how will they be rationalized?
— What arrangements will be made for caring for patients who get sucked into insurance plans that don't "survive" market competition? How can we avoid setting up another "savings-and-loan" bailout scenario that rewards bad decision making?

How we, as a society, transform our health and healing systems will be a legacy for future generations. As we pay more and get less, the urgency of hearing women's voices increases. What women know about gaps not only in services but in caring needs to be heard and used to formulate public policy. Mending the holes in the "patchwork quilt" of medical care requires more than lobbying for expansion of coverage and ensuring universal access to what passes for health care. In the next wave of health reform, the medical care organizations now evolving, with a variety of financing incentives, will be the entrenched interests that control the hard choices about what women will get.[78] Choices are inevitable, so health advocates had best prepare to make them unless we are content to let others make them for us.

NOTES

Andrea Kovach, Anne Kasper, and Jennifer Ruzek each made substantial contributions to the development of this chapter.

1. Morbidity and mortality are affected by far more than health care, but lack of medical care is widely associated with poor health status and excess risk of death.

2. This effect remains even after controlling for sociodemographic differences in insured and uninsured groups.

3. Studies done during the 1993–94 health reform debates showed that most people did not know what their own insurance covered, nor did they know the basic features of different types of insurance coverage (Blendon et al. 1994b).

4. As noted in chapter 5, women's magazines have failed to address smoking as a women's health issue.

5. Health and science writers such as Barbara Seaman (1995:1–7)) played critical roles in bringing investigative reporting to medical care. Seaman herself wrote regularly for *Ladies' Home Journal, Bride,* and *Good Housekeeping,* reaching an audience of 12–15 million women monthly. Her 1969 book, *The Doctors' Case against the Pill* (reissued in 1995), is widely credited as one of the major forces that brought about national recognition of problems in medical care for women. Newsletters of women's health advocacy groups ensure wide and rapid circulation of health information to interested audiences. The popularity of women's health and self-help books, visible in any bookstore, is another indicator of the role that journalists and laypersons, not just medically trained experts, play in public understanding of health and medical care. Mass circulation women's magazines, such as the *Ladies' Home Journal, Family Circle,* and *Woman's Day,* provide a good barometer of women's concerns with American medical care and an indicator of how widely available biomedical information has become.

6. The average American makes six doctor visits each year, whereas Canadians average seven, Australians nine, and Japanese and Germans twelve (Schieber, Poullier, and Greenwald 1994:107).

7. In 1992, per capita health care expenditures (translated into U.S. dollars) were $3,086 in the United States, $1,949 in Canada, $1,775 in Germany, and $1,376 in Japan (National Center for Health Statistics 1995:30).

8. The literature on employment and insurance is growing rapidly. For good overviews see especially Collins et al. (1994) and Horton (1995:133–36). Key data on insurance status come from Short, Monheit, and Beauregard (1989); National Center for Health Statistics (1995); and the Commonwealth Fund's background paper on insurance (Reisinger 1995).

9. Estimates from the Bureau of the Census show that men ages 18–64 are more likely to be uninsured than women at every income level and that insurance status is directly related to income level for both women and men. The differences between women and men are greatest in the lowest income groups and smallest in upper income groups. For a comparison of these rates see Costello and Stone (1994:145). In comparing insurance status of women and men, it is important to remember that a larger proportion of women than men are poor, but that variations in different racial and ethnic groups reflect fundamental economic inequities in access to medical care.

10. Between 1980 and 1993, the age-adjusted percentage of persons under age sixty-five who were uninsured grew from 12.5 to 17.3 percent of the total population (National Center for Health Statistics 1995:35).

11. The working poor are defined as workers with household incomes below the federal poverty line. Poverty level is based on definitions originally developed by the Social Security Administration, which set income thresholds that vary by family size and composition. The thresholds are updated annually by the U.S. Bureau of the Census to reflect changes in the Consumer Price Index. In 1993, the average poverty threshold for a family of four was $14,654. For procedure used, see National Center for Health Statistics 1995:291.

12. In 1991, black women who worked full-time had median annual earnings of $18,720; white women earned $20,794 (Horton 1995:136).

13. Over two-thirds of employees pay the full cost of insurance for family members (Horton 1995:136).

14. This example was provided by Jennifer Ruzek, September 1995.

15. The Women's Research and Education Institute (1994:9) defined women who had incomes at or below the federal poverty level as poor and those with incomes at 400 percent or more of the federal poverty level as high income.

16. Insurance carriers, or managed care companies, negotiate "prices" for coverage with large employers and charge smaller employers higher rates. The cost of coverage is related to a number of factors including the "benefit package" (i.e., what is covered), copayments (what patients are charged over and above what the insurance pays), and deductibles (for both individuals and families).

17. These include the National Health Interview Survey, the National Medical Expenditure Survey, and the Current Population Survey. Data on insurance are summarized in National Center for Health Statistics (1995:35). For reviews of these issues see Horton (1995:133–35) and Costello and Stone (1994:322–26).

18. The costs listed were $288 for the Health Insurance Plan of Greater New York, $288 for Kaiser Foundation Health Plan, $559 for HMO of Pennsylvania, and $610 for CaliforniaCare (Editors of Consumer Reports 1992:94–99).

19. In 1991, the median incomes of female-headed households were $19,547 for whites, $11,414 for blacks, and $12,132 for Hispanics (Costello and Stone 1994:330). A growing proportion of women head households—13.5 percent of all white women, 46.4 of all black women, and 24.4 of all Hispanic origin women headed households in 1991 (U.S. Bureau of the Census 1992). Families headed by a woman are apt to be poor. Statistical data on trends in the economic status of female-headed families, from the Bureau of the Census and Bureau of Labor Statistics, are found in Costello and Stone (1994:327–43).

20. For a particularly good recent analysis of the economic conditions of allied health workers, see Muller (1994). Butter et al. (1994) include a detailed analysis of race, class, and gender stratification in the health care labor force.

21. Efforts to "move women off welfare to work" will only be successful if provision is made for medical insurance that is currently unavailable through low-paying jobs.

22. The Department of Veterans Affairs and the military also provide smaller public insurance programs.

23. Estimates of the poverty status of men and women are based on the 1991 Bureau of the Census Current Population Survey. See Collins et al. (1994:143).

24. Arizona spent the least ($524) and New York the most ($6,402). The states with the highest average payments per recipient were predominately in the Northeast; the lowest were in the South and West (National Center for Health Statistics 1995:44).

25. The cost of Medicare varies by age, sex, race, and region. In 1992, average payments per enrollee were $3,190 for white women and $3,591 for women of all other races (National Center for Health Statistics 1995:244–45).

26. As the large "baby-boom" generation become Medicare eligible, the propor-

tionately smaller "baby-bust" generation will be left to pick up the tab. The next generation of workers (currently entering the labor force) are economically disadvantaged relative to previous birth cohorts (U.S. Bureau of the Census 1992, table B-10). Their contributions will not support rising Medicare costs. Jones and Estes discuss issues in Medicare for women in chapter 17. Current trends are troubling because income disparities make younger, low-wage workers particularly disadvantaged in access to medical care. Regressive taxation of low- and moderate-income families for services that they cannot afford for themselves is socially divisive. In my view, inadequate attention has been directed to the specific ways in which social policies have put medical care and quality education out of reach of working Americans, how the "welfare state" has left out those who are disproportionately taxed to pay for it. Sklar (1995) views hostility toward the poor and minorities largely as scapegoating.

27. In 1993, Medicaid costs averaged $4,160 per enrollee in the ten states with the highest level of benefits and under $3,000 in the states with the lowest level of benefits (National Center for Health Statistics 1995:46). Although recent Medicaid expansion of coverage to pregnant women and children raised the number of enrollees substantially, these programs account for only a small proportion of cost growth (10.8%).

28. The term "persons with AIDS" (PWA) has obscured differences between men and women. The research on the lifetime cost of treating HIV typically fails to differentiate the costs of treating women compared with men or the costs in different subgroups.

29. For an overview of other reproductive medical care needs see Gold and Richards (1994) and Nsiah-Jefferson and Hall (1989).

30. For other medical care needs of older women see chapter 17.

31. Carol Gill addresses many of these issues in chapter 4, so they will not be repeated here.

32. Prices actually vary greatly throughout the United States. Claims data from Metropolitan Life Insurance Company (1994), for example, showed an average of $11,000 for cesarean and $6,430 for uncomplicated vaginal deliveries. The range for uncomplicated cesareans differed by as much as 77 percent between states—from $13,700 in New York to $7,730 in Oklahoma. For vaginal births, the average charge in New York ($8,840) was 2.1 times higher than the charge in Arkansas ($4,190).

33. The most complete analysis of maternity coverage was published in 1987 by the Alan Guttmacher Institute, which found that dependents who were not spouses were excluded from maternity coverage in about 35 percent of typical family policies, leaving 2.7 million unmarried teenagers (who are supposedly insured) without coverage for a common event—birth. Their babies were not insured in over two-thirds of these plans whether or not the teenager herself was covered. Only 7-8 percent of participants in group plans were fully covered for hospital room and board and other charges such as anesthesia. Only 26 percent were fully insured for physician charges, although the proportion was greater in HMOs (92%). Fourteen percent of health plans did not cover injections essential to prevent miscarriage or stillbirth for pregnant women with blood type Rh-negative, 50 percent did not cover routine physician care for newborns in the hospital, and 18 percent limited hospital days for newborns to

three days (Alan Guttmacher Institute 1987:318–19). With the massive changes taking place in medical care, new studies of maternity care coverage are sorely needed.

34. For critiques of the inappropriate use of birth technologies in the United States see especially Brackbill, Rice, and Young (1984), Corea (1985), Guillemin (1981), Guillemin and Holmstrom (1986), Rothman (1982, 1989, 1993), Ruzek (1980, 1993), Wagner (1994, 1995), and Wertz and Wertz (1989).

35. Cases that are missed are referred to as false negatives; cases that are incorrectly identified as disease are referred to as false positives. No mass screening test is ever entirely accurate, and there is always a degree of uncertainty over whether or not a person who tests positive for disease actually has the disease. The actual predictive value of positive tests is related not only to the "accuracy" of the test but to the prevalence of the condition in the screened population. For technical discussions of screening tests, see a standard text such as Sackett et al. (1991). The questions about screening for cancer discussed here apply equally to prenatal and other forms of genetic screening (see Rothenberg and Thomson 1994).

36. Because the predictive value of positive tests is lower in groups that have a lower prevalence of disease, the high-income groups that are screened frequently are particularly at risk of being subjected to costly and psychologically harmful follow-up procedures. Lower-income women, for whom positive tests have a higher predictive value because of the higher prevalence of disease in the group, are less likely to have access to follow-up care. The ethics of screening without making provision for follow-up care must be addressed.

37. For a good overview of the literature on frequency of screening by race and education see especially Horter (1995:143–44). For research on other screening issues relating to women of color, see Jacob, Spieth, and Penn (1993); Saint-Germain and Longman (1993); Leigh (1994); and Kagawa-Singer (1987). For screening by insurance status, see Himmelstein and Woolhandler 1995).

38. The financial cost of finding each case, termed the *cost of case-finding*, is calculated by dividing the total number of cases detected by the total cost of screening in the population. The follow-up costs, however, are not always included in these calculations, and thus the *real* cost may be obscured.

39. They also argue that there is little value in offering bone mass measurement for osteoporosis screening, although the research potential is excellent. The controversies and problems surrounding mammography also warrant attention.

40. See National Center for Health Statistics (1995:151) for information on the incidence and mortality from cervical cancer in different racial and ethnic groups. As Wingard points out in chapter 2, variations are important within as well as between racial/ethnic groups.

41. In this study, black women through age 69 reported being screened at similar or slightly higher rates than white women. Latinas, especially those who speak only or mostly Spanish, were much less likely than black or white women to have Pap smears or to know about them. Women with less than a high school education were three times more likely never to have heard of the Pap test than women with more education. Women frequently reported that health providers had never told them to be screened. Many women did not understand the importance of screening.

42. A recent review by the National Center for Health Statistics found that in 1992, only half of the women ages 50–64 and 39 percent of women ages 65 and older reported a recent mammogram. Among uninsured women ages 50–64, only 19 percent reported having had a mammogram (Makuc, Freid, and Parsons 1994). See Soffa (1994) for a critical lay appraisal of the scientific evidence on the effectiveness of mammography.

43. There are a growing number of studies on screening for breast cancer. For some that address social and cultural factors as well as rates, see Stein, Fox, and Murata (1991), and Saint-Germain and Longman (1993).

44. Research efforts are under way to fill this gap. Dr. Carol D'Onofrio, emerita associate professor of health education, School of Public Health, University of California, Berkeley, and her associates are engaged in a multiethnic study of women and screening practices.

45. The cost of follow-up is high. Physicians tend to prefer to err in the direction of performing further tests and surgical diagnostic procedures on any suspicious finding than chance missing a case of early cancer. The costs are very high for following up on the large proportion of mammogram readings that are suspicious but prove not to be cancer. The social and psychological costs to women who undergo this process are significant (see especially Lerman and Rimer 1995; Marteau 1995).

46. In twelve states, no mammogram coverage is provided for an estimated 570,000 Medicaid-eligible women aged 45 to 84 (Boss and Guckes 1992).

47. In one study nearly half reported that they would not pay $150 each year to be screened (Horton, Romans, and Cruess 1992). For other studies of cost as a barrier to mammography, see Stein, Fox, and Murata 1991; Rimer et al. 1989; Urban, Anderson, and Peacock 1994.

48. There is growing concern that the American Cancer Society is too closely linked to the financial interests of hospitals and doctors who profit from mammography to take an objective stand on this issue.

49. A full discussion of this is beyond the scope of this chapter. See Tennov (1975) and Howell and Bayes (1981) for examples of this perspective.

50. See for example Fidell 1981; Verbrugge 1982.

51. The National Coalition for Women's Mental Health, the National Institute of Mental Health (Russo 1990), and the Commonwealth Fund Commission on Women's Health (Glied and Kofman 1995) all detail serious gaps in mental health services for women. The contributions of socioeconomic factors, race, and ethnicity as well as gender roles to the etiology and treatment of mental and emotional disorders also need to be more fully researched (Amaro and Russo 1987).

52. Over 70 percent of employer-provided insurance limits inpatient coverage to 30–60 days per year (Frank, Goldman, and McGuire 1992). HMOs tend to have the most restrictive policies on psychotherapy.

53. There is growing controversy over how to interpret the increase in the elderly Medicaid population. Some observers argue that the growth in Medicaid spending for the elderly may reflect in part middle-class strategies to pay for long-term care. Ginzberg (1994:41), for example, argues that many upper- and middle-income families find legal or quasi-legal ways to transfer family assets to others to make themselves

eligible for Medicaid reimbursement for long-term care, putting a financial strain on an already overburdened system. Over 50 percent of all nursing home costs are now covered by Medicaid.

54. If the strictest eligibility criteria were used, only 1.5 percent of all elderly would receive home care. Less restrictive definitions would provide 15.5 percent with assistance (Stone and Murtaugh 1990).

55. Doctoral students and I have been unable to locate any published research on this topic as of April 1995.

56. For a recent medical critique of these issues, see especially Wagner (1995).

57. The need to compete for maternity patients brought about some changes in hospital birth practices in the 1970s and 1980s, but hospitals tended to co-opt the idea of "home-style" birth rather than actually support it (Ruzek 1980).

58. Numerous scholars have explored the tensions between midwives and physicians. See especially DeVries 1996; Rothman 1982; and Wertz and Wertz 1989.

59. A growing number of physicians are "breaking away" from this position and openly criticizing conventional American medicine. See, for example, the newsletters published by David G. Williams, M.D., "Alternatives for the Health Conscious Individual" (Mountain Home Publishing, P.O. Box 329, Ingram, Texas 78025); Julian Whitaker, M.D., "Health and Healing," and Christiane Northrup, M.D., "Health Wisdom for Women" (both from Phillips Publishing, 7811 Montrose Road, Potomac, Maryland 20854).

60. Freestanding birth centers are often assumed to have such good outcomes because they only care for low-risk patients. Controlled studies, however, show that their results are favorable compared with hospital births among similar groups of women. Historically, midwives have provided important care for low-income and rural women. See note 34 above.

61. For the short overview of the history of birth practices, see Bogdan (1993). For fuller histories that include controversies over midwives, see especially Eakins (1986), Leavitt (1986), and Wertz and Wertz (1989).

62. Barbara Seaman (1995) is widely acknowledged for playing a catalytic role in raising public awareness of how scientific evidence of the safety and effectiveness of technologies that affect women is ignored and disregarded. For other critiques of how medicine ignores evidence, see, e.g., Corea (1985), Ratcliff et al. (1989), Ruzek (1993, 1995), Scully (1980), Seaman and Seaman (1977).

63. Research has shown that as much as 30 percent of the surgery performed in the United States is unnecessary (Starr 1994). For medical audits and analyses of unnecessary surgery during the second half of the twentieth century, see Bunker (1970), Lembke (1956), Scully (1980), Stafford (1990), and Wennberg, Barnes, and Zubkoff (1982).

64. High-level insurance executives often insist that their companies do not reimburse for "experimental procedures" or for drugs or devices that are not FDA approved. In fact, many do reimburse when pressured. Malpractice attorneys point out that juries rarely grasp scientific distinctions between proven and unproven therapies. When faced with cases that have jury appeal, insurers may "roll over and pay" rather than face litigation.

65. See especially Corea (1985), Grant (1992), Ruzek (1978, 1980), and Seaman (1995).

66. For example, in a widely publicized case, Nelene Fox brought a lawsuit against her insurer, HealthNet, for failing to pay for a $170,000 autologous bone marrow transplant (ABMT) with high-dose chemotherapy (HDC). Her story on ABC television's 20/20 on 15 April 1994 centered around her insurer's denial of payment—without addressing the question of whether the bone marrow transplant could have saved her life. An independent technology assessment concluded that data from clinical trials do not support the view that ABMT with HDC is superior to standard chemotherapy. It is also far more costly and debilitating. This case is discussed in "Technology Assessment: Public Access, Public Trust" (1994) and Ruzek (1995).

67. Emanuel and Dubler (1995:324) assert that despite differences and disagreements over what the ideal might be for individuals, "core understandings that are widely, if not uniformly, shared are embodied in six Cs—choice, competence, communication, compassion, continuity, and (no) conflict of interest." Trust is not an independent element, they argue, but the culmination of all the others. Although many patients drift in and out of being insured or are served in hectic clinics where these six Cs are out of reach, these patients want the same thing that affluent patients are more likely to have.

68. This information was circulated to health care leaders by Bader and Associates, Washington.

69. The importance of measuring patient satisfaction is a growing theme in managed care. See, for example, the ongoing National Research Corporation's "Satisfaction Report Card" survey, NRC 1033 O Street, Lincoln, Nebraska 68508. Group Health Association of America, 1129 20th Street N.W., Suite 600, Washington, D.C. 20036, the primary association for the managed care industry, is actively involved in disseminating quality improvement strategies to its members.

70. Historically, much of women's subjective experience of health has been discounted by medical experts but eventually recognized as valid. For example, pain in labor, menstrual disorders, and other conditions that have been shown to have an organic base have been dismissed as psychogenic disturbances and not treated seriously (Lennane and Lennane 1973). A common complaint of women is that their physical complaints are often ignored unless laboratory tests confirm some objective pathological condition. Too often, the signs and symptoms may not be recognized or taken seriously. For example, women's complaints about side effects of oral contraceptives and IUDs were routinely discounted by many doctors until objective scientific evidence confirmed that there were serious hazards including death (Corea 1985; Seaman 1995; Seaman and Seaman 1977). Women's concerns about silicone gel-filled breast implants used for reconstructive and cosmetic surgery were similarly ignored for years until the evidence became so compelling that the FDA had to act (Zones 1992).

71. The effectiveness of a support person for improving birth outcomes (see, e.g., Sosa et al. 1980) has not had the attention that machines have had, nor have other labor-intensive approaches to birth. The consequences go beyond the birth suite and nursery. Cohen (1993:123) links the frequency and intensity of depression following

birth to "obstetrical attitudes, philosophies, interventions, and methods accepted and practiced in the United States."

72. For the most thorough discussion, see Northrup 1994.

73. For example, surgeons defended radical mastectomy for many years despite evidence that it did not improve survival compared with minimal surgery. Pressure from consumer groups increased awareness of the psychological aspects of treatment; state breast cancer informed consent laws were also enacted to get surgeons to inform women adequately of all treatment options (Montini and Ruzek 1986). Difficulties in access to care may also increase psychological problems. Saint-Germain and Longman (1993) discovered that women who experienced more barriers to access to breast cancer screening expressed more severe levels of turmoil than women with fewer barriers.

74. See studies of the experiences of women with conditions such as lupus (Charmaz 1991; Jones 1994), sickle cell anemia trait (Hill 1994), diabetes (Williams 1994), physical and emotional disabilities (Fine and Asch 1988), and undesired hysterectomies (Behar 1994). Medical personnel could also learn about quality of medical care from accounts of women who have suffered as a result of medical treatments—for example, the stories of women who were exposed to DES (Bell 1989) or who used the Dalkon shield (Hicks 1994; Grant 1992). Similarly, health personnel need exposure to how women of color are particularly vulnerable to toxic work environments (Fox 1992).

75. For patient perspectives, see especially Lorde (1980), Butler and Rosenblum (1991), and Kasper (1994a). These complex works give human meanings to *quality*, *safety*, *risk*, and *satisfaction* that surveys simply cannot provide. Checklists of disembodied "satisfaction levels" or indices of "access" do not provide planners with critical information that they need to create health care systems that meet women's real needs.

76. Norsigian (1994) has been one of the few feminist health advocates who has squarely noted the issue of rationing.

77. The lack of attention to values has been noted by Duncan (1994) and Dubler and Nimmons (1992).

78. For prognostications about difficult issues that will have to be addressed, see especially Callahan (1987), Conrad and Brown (1993), Duncan (1994), Mechanic (1989), and Schroeder (1994).

REFERENCES

Adams, P. F., and V. Benson
1991   "Current estimates from the National Health Interview Survey." National Center for Health Statistics. Vital and Health Statistics 10(181):1–232.

Alan Guttmacher Institute
1987   Blessed Events and the Bottom Line: Financing Maternity Care in the United States. New York: Alan Guttmacher Institute.

Amaro, Hortensia, and Nancy F. Russo, eds.
1987   "Hispanic women and mental health: contemporary issues in research and practice." Psychology of Women Quarterly 11 (special issue).

American Cancer Society
  1985   "Survey of physicians' attitudes and practices in early cancer detection."
         CA-A Cancer Journal for Clinicians 35:197-213.
  1992   Cancer Facts and Figures—1992. Atlanta: American Cancer Society.
Bader, Jeanne E.
  1994   Assistive ('Prosthetic') Devices. Long Beach, CA: Center for Successful
         Aging, California State University at Long Beach.
Behar, Ruth
  1994   "My Mexican friend Marta, who lost her womb on this side of the
         border." Pp. 129-38 in Alice J. Dan (ed.), Reframing Women's Health:
         Multidisciplinary Research and Practice. Thousand Oaks, CA: Sage.
Bell, Susan E.
  1989   "The meaning of risk, choice, and responsibility for a DES daughter." Pp.
         245-62 in Kathryn Strother Ratcliff et al. (eds.), Healing Technology:
         Feminist Perspectives. Ann Arbor: University of Michigan Press.
Bergman, Rhonda
  1994   "Quality watch: the birthplace boom." Hospitals and Health Networks
         (5 Dec.):46-48.
Berk, Marc L., and Gail R. Wilensky
  1987   "Health insurance coverage of the working poor." Social Science and
         Medicine 25:1183-87.
Bernstein, A. B., G. B. Thompson, and L. C. Harlan
  1991   "Differences in rates of cancer screening by usual source of medical care:
         data from the 1987 National Health Interview Survey." Medical Care
         29:196-209.
Blendon, Robert J., K. Donelan, and C. A. Hill et al.
  1994a "Paying medical bills in the United States." Journal of the American
         Medical Association 271:949-51.
Blendon, Robert J., J. Martilla, J. M. Benson, M. C. Shelter, F. J. Connolly, and T.
Kiley
  1994b "The beliefs and values shaping today's health reform debate." Health
         Affairs 13(1):274-84.
Bogdan, Janet Carlisle
  1993   "Childbirth practices in American history." Pp. 69-71 in Barbara Katz
         Rothman (ed.), The Encyclopedia of Childbearing. New York: Henry
         Holt.
Boss, L., and F. Guckes
  1992   "Medicaid coverage of screening tests for breast and cervical cancer."
         American Journal of Public Health 82(2):252-53.
Brackbill, Yvonne, June Rice, and Diony Young
  1984   Birth Trap. The Legal Low-Down on High-Tech Obstetrics. St. Louis: C.
         V. Mosby.
Bunker, John
  1970   "Surgical manpower: a comparison of operations and surgeons in the

United States and in England and Wales." New England Journal of Medicine 282(1):135–44.

Butler, Sandra, and Barbara Rosenblum
    1991   Cancer in Two Voices. San Francisco: Spinsters.

Butter, Irene H., Eugenia S. Carpenter, Bonnie J. Kay, and Ruth S. Simmons
    1994   "Gender hierarchies in the health labor force." Pp. 79–96 in Elizabeth Fee and Nancy Krieger (eds.), Women's Health, Politics, and Power. New York: Baywood.

Callahan, Daniel
    1987   Setting Limits: Medical Goals in an Aging Society. New York: Simon and Schuster.

Challenges in Health Care: A Chartbook Perspective
    1991   Princeton, NJ: Robert Wood Johnson Foundation.

Charmaz, K.
    1991   Good Days, Bad Days: The Self in Chronic Illness and Time. New Brunswick, NJ: Rutgers University Press.

Clancy, Carolyn M., and Charlea T. Massion
    1992   "American women's health care: a patchwork quilt with gaps." Journal of the American Medical Association 268(14):1918–20.

Cohen, Nancy Wainer
    1993   "Emotional recovery following obstetric intervention." Pp. 122–23 in Barbara Katz Rothman (ed.), The Encyclopedia of Childbearing. New York: Henry Holt.

Collins, Karen Scott, Diane Rowland, Alina Salganicoff, and Elizabeth Chait
    1994   "Assessing and improving women's health." Pp. 109–53 in Cynthia Costello and Anne J. Stone (eds.), The American Woman, 1994–95: Where We Stand, Women and Health. New York: W. W. Norton.

Commonwealth Fund
    1993   Commonwealth Fund Survey on the Health of Women. (14 July) New York: Commonwealth Fund.

Conrad, Peter, and Phil Brown
    1993   "On rationing medical care: a sociological reflection." Research in the Sociology of Health Care 10:3–22.

Corea, Gena
    1985   The Hidden Malpractice: How American Medicine Mistreats Women, rev. ed. New York: Harper and Row.

Costello, Cynthia, and Anne J. Stone, eds. for the Women's Research and Education Institute
    1994   The American Woman, 1994–95: Where We Stand, Women and Health. New York: W. W. Norton.

Critical Choices in Health Reform
    1994   League of Women Voters Education Fund and the Henry J. Kaiser Family Foundation.

Croyle, Robert T., ed.
  1995   Psychosocial Effects of Screening for Disease Prevention and Detection.
          New York: Oxford University Press.
DeMarco, Carolyn
  1994   "Medical malepractice." Pp. 59–70 in Karen Hicks (ed.), Misdiagnosis:
          Woman as a Disease. Allentown, PA: People's Medical Society.
Detsky, Allan S.
  1989   "Are clinical trials a cost-effective investment?" Journal of the American
          Medical Association 262(13):1795–1800.
DeVries, Raymond G.
  1996   Making Midwives Legal: Childbirth, Medicine, and the Law. 2d ed. Co-
          lumbus: Ohio State University Press.
Dubler, Nancy, and David Nimmons
  1992   Ethics on Call: A Medical Ethicist Shows How to Take Charge of Life-
          and-Death Choices. New York: Harmony Books.
Duncan, Karen A.
  1994   Health Information and Health Reform: Understanding the Need for a
          National Health Information System. San Francisco: Jossey-Bass.
Duran, A. M.
  1992   "The safety of home birth: the farm study." American Journal of Public
          Health 82:450–53.
Eakins, Pamela, ed.
  1986   The American Way of Birth. Philadelphia: Temple University Press.
Editors of Consumer Reports
  1992   How to Resolve the Health Care Crisis: Affordable Protection for All
          Americans. Yonkers, NY: Consumer Report Books.
Emanuel, Ezekiel J., and Nancy Neveloff Dubler
  1995   "Preserving the physician-patient relationship in the era of managed
          care." Journal of the American Medical Association 273:323–29.
Fennell, Mary L., and Richard B. Warnecke
  1988   The Diffusion of Medical Innovations: An Applied Network Analysis.
          New York: Plenum Press.
Fidell, Linda S.
  1981   "Sex differences in psychotropic drug use." Professional Psychology
          12:156–62.
Fine, Michelle, and Adrienne Asch, eds.
  1988   Women with Disabilities: Essays in Psychology, Culture, and Politics.
          Philadelphia: Temple University Press.
Foote, Susan B.
  1987   "Assessing medical technology assessment: past, present, and future."
          Milbank Quarterly 65:59–80.
Fox, Steven
  1992   Toxic Work: Women Workers at GTE Lenkurt. Philadelphia: Temple
          University Press.

Frank, R. G., H. H. Goldman, and T. G. McGuire
    1992   "A model mental health benefit for private insurance." Health Affairs
            11:98–117.
Franks, Peter, Carolyn M. Clancy, and Martha R. Gold
    1993   "Health insurance and mortality: evidence from a national cohort." Jour-
            nal of the American Medical Association 270:737–41.
Ginzberg, Eli, with Miriam Ostow
    1994   The Road to Reform: The Future of Health Care in America. New York:
            Macmillan.
Fugh-Berman, Adriane
    1994   "The new dangers of medical prevention." Natural Health
            (Mar./Apr.):84–87.
Glied, Sherry, and Sharon Kofman
    1995   Women and Mental Health: Issues for Health Reform. Background paper,
            Commonwealth Fund Commission on Women's Health. New York:
            Commonwealth Fund.
Goad, G. Pierre
    1991   "Canada seems satisfied with a medical system that covers everyone."
            Wall Street Journal (3 Dec.):A10.
Gold, Rachel Benson, and Cory L. Richards
    1994   "Securing American women's reproductive health." Pp. 197–222 in Cyn-
            thia Costello and Anne J. Stone (eds.), The American Woman, 1994–
            95: Where We Stand, Women and Health. New York: W. W. Norton.
Grant, Nicole J.
    1992   The Selling of Contraception: The Dalkon Shield Case, Sexuality, and
            Women's Autonomy. Columbus: Ohio State University Press.
Guillemin, Jeanne H.
    1981   "Babies by cesarean: who chooses, who controls?" Hastings Center Re-
            port 11(3):15–18.
Guillemin, Jeanne H., and Lynda L. Holmstrom
    1986   Mixed Blessings: Intensive Care for Newborns. New York: Oxford Uni-
            versity Press.
Harlan, L. C., A. B. Bernstein, and L. G. Kessler
    1991   "Cervical cancer screening: who is not screened and why?" American
            Journal of Public Health 81(7):885–90.
Harrison, Michelle
    1994   "Women's health: new models for care and a new academic discipline."
            Pp. 79–92 in Alice J. Dan (ed.), Reframing Women's Health: Multidis-
            ciplinary Research and Practice. Thousand Oaks, CA: Sage.
Health Insurance Association of America
    1992   Source Book of Health Insurance Data, 1990. Washington: Health Insur-
            ance Association of America.
Hicks, Karen M.
    1994   Surviving the Dalkon Shield IUD: Women v. the Pharmaceutical Indus-
            try. New York: Teachers College Press.

Hill, Shirley A.
  1994   Managing Sickle Cell Disease in Low-Income Families. Philadelphia:
          Temple University Press.
Himmelstein, David U., and Steffie Woolhandler
  1991   "Who cares for the caregivers? Lack of health insurance among health
          and insurance personnel." Journal of the American Medical Association
          266:399–401.
  1995   "Care denied: U.S. residents who are unable to obtain needed medical
          services." American Journal of Public Health 85:341–44.
Horton, Jacqueline A.
  1995   Women's Health Data Book: A Profile of Women's Health in the United
          States, 2d ed. Washington: Jacobs Institute of Women's Health. Elsevier.
Horton, Jacqueline A., M. C. Romans, and D. F. Cruess
  1992   "Mammography attitudes and usage study, 1992." Women's Health Issues
          2:180–86.
"How current technology practices increase healthcare costs."
  1995   Health Technology Assessment News (July–Aug.):1, 4.
Howell, Elizabeth, and Marjorie Bayes
  1981   Women and Mental Health. New York: Basic Books.
Jacob, Teresa C., Leslie E. Spieth, and Nolan E. Penn
  1993   "Breast cancer, breast self-examination, and African American women."
          Pp. 244–56 in Barbara Bair and Susan E. Cayleff (eds.), Wings of Gauze:
          Women of Color and the Experience of Health and Illness. Detroit:
          Wayne State University Press.
Jacobs, L. R., and R. Y. Shapiro
  1994   "Public opinions tilt against private enterprise." Health Affairs
          13(1):285–98.
Jones, Vida Labrie
  1994   "Lupus and black women: managing a complex chronic disability." Pp.
          160–66 in Evelyn C. White (ed.), The Black Women's Health Book, rev.
          ed. Seattle: Seal Press.
Kagawa-Singer, Marjorie
  1987   "Ethnic perspectives of cancer nursing: Hispanics and Japanese-Ameri-
          cans." Oncology Nursing Forum 14:59–65.
Kaiser Commission on the Future of Medicaid
  1993   The Medicaid Cost Explosion: Causes and Consequences. Baltimore:
          Kaiser Commission on the Future of Medicaid.
Kasper, Anne
  1994a   "A feminist, qualitative methodology: a study of women with breast
          cancer." Qualitative Sociology 17(3):263–81.
  1994b   "The making of women's health policy: health care reform." Paper pre-
          sented at the University of Illinois, Chicago Intensive Summer Institute:
          Reframing Women's Health, July.
Koch, Lene
  1993   "Physiological and psychosocial risks of the new reproductive technologies."

Pp. 122–34 in Patricia Stephenson and Marsden G. Wagner (eds.), Tough Choices: In Vitro Fertilization and the Reproductive Technologies. Philadelphia: Temple University Press.

Kosecoff, Jacquiline, David Kanouse, William Rogers, and Lois McCloskey
1987   "Effects of the National Institutes of Health consensus development program on physician practice." Journal of the American Medical Association 258(19):2708–13.

Lantz, Paula M., Debra Stencil, MaryAnn T. Lippert, et al.
1995   "Breast and cervical cancer screening in a low-income managed care sample: the efficacy of physician letters and phone calls." American Journal of Public Health 85:834–36.

Leavitt, Judith Walzer
1986   Brought to Bed: Childbearing in America, 1750–1950. New York: Oxford University Press.

Leigh, Wilhelmina A.
1994   "The health status of women of color." Pp. 154–96 in Cynthia Costello and Anne J. Stone (eds.), The American Woman, 1994–95: Where We Stand, Women and Health. New York: W. W. Norton.

Lembke, Paul A.
1956   "Medical auditing by scientific methods, illustrated by major female pelvic surgery." Journal of the American Medical Association 162:646–55.

Lennane, K. J., and R. J. Lennane
1973   "Alleged psychogenic disorders in women—a possible manifestation of sexual prejudice." New England Journal of Medicine 288:288–92.

Lerman, Caryn, and Barbara K. Rimer
1995   "Psychosocial impact of cancer screening." Pp. 65–81 in Robert T. Croyle (ed.), Psychosocial Effects of Screening for Disease Prevention and Detection. New York: Oxford University Press.

Lomas, J., and A. P. Contandriopoulos
1994   "Regulating limits to medicine: toward harmony in public- and self-regulation." Pp. 253–83 in Robert G. Evans, Morris L. Barer, and Theodore R. Marmor (eds.), Why Are Some People Healthy and Others Not? The Determinants of Health of Populations. New York: Aldine De Gruyter.

Lorde, Audre
1980   The Cancer Journals. San Francisco: Spinsters/Aunt Lute.

Makuc, Diane M., Virginia M. Freid, and P. Ellen Parsons
1994   "Health insurance and cancer screening among women." Advance Data No. 254 (3 Aug.). National Center for Health Statistics.

Mangano, Joseph
1995   "Report cards come of age." Pp. 1–13 in Karen J. Migdail and Maralee Youngs (eds.), Medical Quality Management Sourcebook: Health Care Information Center. Washington: Faulkner and Gray.

Marteau, Theresa M.
1995   "Toward an understanding of the psychological consequences of screening." Pp. 185–99 in Robert T. Croyle (ed.), Psychosocial Effects of

Screening for Disease Prevention and Detection. New York: Oxford University Press.

Mechanic, David
1989   Painful Choices: Research and Essays on Health Care. New Brunswick, NJ: Transaction.

Metropolitan Life Insurance Company
1994   "Average charges for uncomplicated cesarean and vaginal deliveries, United States, 1993." Statistical Bulletin (Oct./Dec.):27–36.

Miller, Anthony B.
1995   "Editorial: failures of cervical cancer screening." American Journal of Public Health 85:761–62.

Montini, Theresa, and Sheryl Burt Ruzek
1986   "Overturning orthodoxy: the emergence of breast cancer treatment policy." Research in the Sociology of Health Care 8:3–32.

Moon, Marilyn
1994   "Women and long-term care." Pp. 223–50 in Cynthia Costello and Anne J. Stone (eds.), The American Woman, 1994–95: Where We Stand, Women and Health. New York: W. W. Norton.

Muller, Charlotte F.
1990   Health Care and Gender. New York: Russell Sage Foundation.
1994   "Women in allied health professions." Pp. 177–203 in Emily Friedman (ed.), An Unfinished Revolution: Women and Health Care in America. New York: United Hospital Fund of New York.

National Center for Health Statistics
1995   Health United States, 1994. Hyattsville, Maryland: Public Health Service.

Norsigian, Judy
1994   "Women and national health care reform: a progressive feminist agenda." Pp. 111–17 in Alice J. Dan (ed.), Reframing Women's Health: Multidisciplinary Research and Practice. Thousand Oaks, CA: Sage.

Northrup, Christiane
1994   Women's Bodies, Women's Wisdom: Creating Physical and Emotional Health and Healing. New York: Bantam Books.

Nsiah-Jefferson, Laurie, and Elaine J. Hall
1989   "Reproductive technology: perspectives and implications for low-income women and women of color." Pp. 93–117 in Kathryn Strother Ratcliff et al. (eds.), Healing Technology: Feminist Perspectives. Ann Arbor: University of Michigan Press.

Nutting, Paul A., Ned Calonge, Donald C. Iverson, and Larry A. Green
1994   "The danger of applying uniform clinical policies across populations: the case of breast cancer in American Indians." American Journal of Public Health 84(10):1631–36.

O'Connor, Bonnie Blair
1995   Healing Traditions: Alternative Medicine and the Health Professions. Philadelphia: University of Pennsylvania Press.

Physician Payment Review Commission
    1990   Annual Report to Congress. Washington: Physician Payment Review Commission.
Piani, A., and C. Schoenborn
    1993   "Health promotion and disease prevention: United States, 1990." National Center for Health Statistics. Vital and Health Statistics Series 10(185):1–88.
Rasell, M. Edith
    1995   "Cost sharing in health insurance: A reexamination." New England Journal of Medicine 332 (27 Apr.):1164–68.
Ratcliff, Kathryn Strother, Myra Marx Ferree, Gail O. Mellow, Barbara Drygulski Wright, Glenda D. Price, Kim Yanoshik, and Margie S. Freston, eds.
    1989   Healing Technology: Feminist Perspectives. Ann Arbor: University of Michigan Press.
Raymond, Alan G.
    1995   "Giving health care consumers the quality information they need." Quality Letter for Healthcare Leaders 7 (Feb.):15–18.
Reisinger, Anne Lenhard
    1995   Health Insurance and Access to Care: Issues for Women. Background paper, Commonwealth Fund Commission on Women's Health. New York: Commonwealth Fund.
Rimer, Barbara K., M. K. Keintz, H. B. Kessler, P. F. Engstrom, and J. R. Rosan
    1989   "Why women resist screening mammography: patient-related barriers." Radiology 172(1):243–46.
Rosenbaum, Sara
    1992   "Medicaid expansions and access to health care." Cited p. 9 in the Kaiser Commission on the Future of Medicaid, 1993. The Medicaid Cost Explosion: Causes and Consequences. Baltimore: Kaiser Commission on the Future of Medicaid.
Rothenberg, Karen H., and Elizabeth J. Thomson, eds.
    1994   Women and Prenatal Testing: Facing the Challenges of Genetic Technology. Columbus: Ohio State University Press.
Rothman, Barbara Katz
    1982   In Labor: Women and Power in the Birthplace. New York: W. W. Norton.
    1986   "When a pregnant woman endangers her fetus: commentary." Hastings Center Report 16:24–25.
    1989   Recreating Motherhood. Ideology and Technology in a Patriarchal Society. New York: W. W. Norton.
Rothman, Barbara Katz, ed.
    1993   The Encyclopedia of Childbearing. New York: Henry Holt.
Rublee, Dale A.
    1994   "Medical technology in Canada, Germany, and the United States: an update." Health Affairs 13(4):113–17.

Russell, Louise B.
1994   Educated Guesses: Making Policy about Medical Screening Tests. Berkeley: University of California Press.
Russo, Nancy F.
1990   "Overview: forging research priorities for women's mental health." American Psychologist 45:368–73.
Ruzek, Sheryl Burt
1978   The Women's Health Movement: Feminist Alternatives to Medical Control. New York: Praeger.
1980   "Medical response to women's health activities: conflict, accommodation, and cooperation." Research in the Sociology of Health Care 1:335–54.
1993   "Social and cultural constructions of reducible birth risks." Human Nature 4:383–408.
1995   "Technology and perceptions of risks: clinical, scientific, and consumer perspectives in breast cancer treatment." Executive briefing. Health Technology Assessment Information Service, ECRI-WHO Collaborating Center for Technology Transfer, Plymouth Meeting, PA (Jan.):1–6.
Sackett, D. L., R. B. Haynes, G. H. Guyatt, and P. Tugwell
1991   Clinical Epidemiology: A Basic Science for Clinical Medicine, 2d ed. Boston: Little, Brown.
Saint-Germain, Michelle, and Alice Longman
1993   "Resignation and resourcefulness: older Hispanic women's responses to breast cancer." Pp. 257–72 in Barbara Bair and Susan E. Cayleff (eds.), Wings of Gauze: Women of Color and the Experience of Health and Illness. Detroit: Wayne State University Press.
Schieber, George J., Jean-Pierre Poullier, and Leslie M. Greenwald
1994   "Health system performance in OECD countries, 1980–1992." Health Affairs 13:100–112.
Schroeder, Stephen
1994   "Rationing medical care—a comparative perspective." New England Journal of Medicine 331 (20 Oct.):1063–67.
Schur, Claudia L., and Amy K. Taylor
1991   "Choice of health insurance and the two-worker household." Health Affairs 10(1):155–63.
Scully, Diana
1980   Men Who Control Women's Health: The Miseducation of Obstetrician-Gynecologists. Boston: Houghton Mifflin.
Seaman, Barbara
1995   The Doctors' Case against the Pill, 25th anniversary updated ed. Alameda, CA: Hunter House.
Seaman, Barbara, and Gideon Seaman
1977   Women and the Crisis in Sex Hormones. New York: Rawson Associates.
Seccombe, Karen, Leslie L. Clarke, and Raymond T. Coward
1994   "Discrepancies in employer-sponsored health insurance coverage among

Hispanics, blacks and whites: the effects of sociodemographic and employment factors." Inquiry 31:221-29.

Seccombe, Karen, and Cheryl Amey
  1995   "Playing by the rules and losing: health insurance and the working poor." Journal of Health and Social Behavior 36:168-81.

Short, Pamela Farley, Llewellyn J. Cornelius, and Donald E. Goldstone
  1990   "Health insurance of minorities in the United States." Journal of Health Care for the Poor and Underserved 11:9-24.

Short, Pamela Farley, Alan Monheit, and Karen Beauregard
  1989   A Profile of Uninsured Americans. DHHS Publication No. PHS 89-3443.

Shortell, Stephen, Robin R. Gillies, David A. Anderson, John B. Mitchell, and Karen L. Morgan
  1993   "Creating organized delivery systems: the barriers and facilitator." Hospital and Health Services Administration 38(4):447-66.

Singh, S., R. B. Gold, and J. J. Frost
  1994   "Impact of the Medicaid eligibility expansions on the coverage of deliveries." Family Planning Perspectives 26:31-33.

Sklar, Holly
  1995   Chaos or Community? Seeking Solutions, Not Scapegoats for Bad Economics. Boston: South End Press.

Soffa, Virginia
  1994   "The boob trap: debunking myths about breast cancer." Pp. 177-90 in Karen Hicks (ed.), Misdiagnosis: Woman as a Disease. Allentown, PA: People's Medical Society.

Sosa, Roberto, et al.
  1980   "The effect of a supportive companion on perinatal problems, length of labor, and mother-infant interaction." New England Journal of Medicine 303(11):597-600.

Stafford, Randall S.
  1990   "Cesarean section use and source of payment: an analysis of California hospital discharge abstracts." American Journal of Public Health 80(3):313-15.

Starr, Paul
  1994   The Logic of Health Care Reform: Why and How the President's Plan Will Work. Rev. ed. New York: Whittle Books/Penguin Books.

Stein, Judith A., Sarah A. Fox, and Paul J. Murata
  1991   "The influence of ethnicity, socioeconomic status, and psychological barriers on use of mammography." Journal of Health and Social Behavior 32:101-13.

Stephenson, Patricia, and Marsden G. Wagner
  1993   Tough Choices: In Vitro Fertilization and the Reproductive Technologies. Philadelphia: Temple University Press.

Stone, Robyn I., and Christopher M. Murtaugh
    1990   "The elderly population with chronic functional disability: implications for home care eligibility." Gerontologist 30:491–96.

Sullivan, C. B., and T. Rice
    1991   "The health insurance picture in 1990." Health Affairs 10(2):104–15.

Sulmasy, D. P.
    1995   "Managed care and managed death." Archives of Internal Medicine 155:133–36.

Tavris, Carol
    1994   "Why women are 'crazy,' but men have 'problems.'" Pp. 99–102 in Karen Hicks (ed.), Misdiagnosis: Woman as a Disease. Allentown, PA: People's Medical Society.

"Technology assessment: public access, public trust"
    1994   Health Technology Assessment News. May–June:1–3.

Tennov, Dorothy
    1975   Psychotherapy: The Hazardous Cure. New York: Abelard-Schuman.

Urban, N., G. Anderson, and S. Peacock
    1994   "Mammography screening: how important is cost as a barrier to use?" American Journal of Public Health 84:50–55.

U.S. Bureau of the Census
    1992   "Money income of households, families, and persons in the United States: 1991." Table B-10.

U.S. Office of Management and Budget
    1996   A Citizen's Guide to the Federal Budget, FY 1996. Washington: Government Printing Office.

Verbrugge, Lois
    1982   "Sex differences in legal drug use." Journal of Social Issues 38(2): 59–86.

Volkers, N.
    1994   "NCI replaces guidelines with statement of evidence." Journal of the National Cancer Institute 86:14–15.

Wagner, Marsden
    1994   The Birth Machine: The Search for Appropriate Birth Technology. Camperdown, New South Wales: ACE Graphics.
    1995   "A global witchhunt." Lancet 346 (14 Oct.):1020–22.

Wennberg, John E.
    1990   "What is outcomes research?" Pp. 33–46 in A. C. Gelijns (ed.), Medical Innovation at the Crossroads. Vol. 1: Modern Methods of Clinical Investigation. Washington: National Academy Press.

Wennberg, John E., Benjamin A. Barnes, and Michael Zubkoff
    1982   "Professional uncertainty and the problem of supplier-induced demand." Social Science and Medicine 16(7):811–24.

Wertz, Richard W., and Dorothy C. Wertz
    1989   Lying In: A History of Childbirth in America, rev. ed. New Haven, CT: Yale University Press.

Whatley, Mariamne H., and Nancy Worcester
    1989   "The role of technology in the co-optation of the women's health movement: the cases of osteoporosis and breast cancer screening." Pp. 199-220 in Kathryn Strother Ratcliff et al. (eds.), Healing Technology: Feminist Perspectives. Ann Arbor: University of Michigan Press.

Whitbeck, Caroline
    1991   "Ethical issues raised by the new medical technologies." Pp. 49-64 in J. Rodin and A. Collins (eds.), Women and New Reproductive Technologies: Medical, Psychosocial, Legal, and Ethical Dilemmas. Hillsdale, NJ: Lawrence Erlbaum.

Williams, K. Malaika
    1994   "The best foot forward: a black woman deals with diabetes." Pp. 167-71 in Evelyn C. White (ed.), The Black Women's Health Book, rev. ed. Seattle: Seal Press.

Women's Research and Education Institute
    1994   Women's Health Insurance Costs and Experiences. Washington: Women's Research and Education Institute.

Zones, Jane
    1992   "The political and social context of silicone breast implant use in the United States." Journal of Long-Term Effects of Medical Implants 1:225-41.

[9]

A Note from Louise:
Understanding Women's Health in Appalachia

JUDY M. PERRY

Gender expectations and sociocultural factors as well as economic disadvantage and geographical isolation leave Appalachian women with inadequate access to medical care. Here nursing researcher Judy Perry describes how indigenous health workers do more than deliver ancillary services in these disadvantaged rural communities; they teach health professionals how to understand and serve their patients through training approaches that contrast starkly with professional school models.

April 16, 1992
The woman's name is Martha Doe. She is from Hisel, close to Drip Rock. She has lumps in both breasts. One she has had for several years. I called the health department, and they recommended that she get a mammogram right away (she only had to wait three days). The day I took her over to the hospital for the mammogram they said she needed a ultrasound. The nurse told me the health department cannot pay for this ultrasound. Nobody in her family is working, and she doesn't have a medical card or any insurance. Her children have health problems too. I would like her to get some help with this ultrasound and whatever else follows. I have been to see her four times, and I am really concerned about her. She does not have a phone, and I hated so bad to go tell her she couldn't get the ultrasound. She was all cleaned up and ready to go to the hospital with me. She was bad disappointed. I sat and talked with her for a long time. She has no transportation but me.

This note, left on my desk, was signed Message from Louise, Mt. Scout. Louise is a trained indigenous community health worker in a small rural Appalachian county in Kentucky. She embodies the qualities characteristic of indigenous health workers. Louise possesses the social, environmental, and ethnic qualities of Appalachian subculture. She shares Appalachian verbal and nonverbal language, understands community health beliefs and barriers to care, and feels a genuine empathy with and responsibility toward her community and its health service needs.[1] Like many indigenous health workers, Louise provides woman-to-woman care in a medically underserved area.

The Roles of Indigenous Health Workers

Studies have shown the effectiveness of indigenous workers in improving women's health. For example, Vanderbilt University's Maternal and Infant Health Outreach Project has demonstrated that using indigenous home visitors (known as natural helpers) can improve pregnancy outcomes and the quality of the home environment for rural low-income mothers and children (Clinton 1992). Johnson, Howell, and Mooly's (1993) controlled trial of 232 first-time mothers found that after one year of monthly home visits from an indigenous lay worker in addition to traditional clinic services, children of mothers in the intervention group were more likely to receive immunizations, to be read to daily, and to play more cognitive games. Both mothers and children had better nutritional intake than the control group.

The utilization of indigenous health workers in Appalachia follows and expands on international experiences with village health workers. Programs utilizing indigenous health workers have developed in settings throughout the United States, primarily among poor underserved populations (Dunford 1987; Eng 1989; Frate, Whitehead, and Johnson 1983; Service and Salber 1977). However, the published literature seldom reports on such programs. Chapman, Seifel, and Cross (1990) suggest three factors that contribute to this void: (1) programs are begun as service to the community without research design, theoretical frameworks, or evaluation components in place; (2) staff turnover in community-based programs makes long-term evaluation difficult; and (3) when programs appear successful, staff energy goes toward replication and securing continued funding rather than toward rigorous evaluation or analysis and publication. Consequently, there is still much to be understood about why, how, when, where, and under what conditions indigenous lay workers can be used effectively. In Appalachia as elsewhere, soaring health care costs and health problems have brought national attention to the need for cost-effective community-based health promotion and disease prevention strategies.

Need for Indigenous Workers in Kentucky

Louise is an integral part of a community-based program aimed at increasing the utilization of available services for prevention and early detection of breast and cervical cancer. The Mountain Surveillance and Counseling Outreach Program (Mt. Sc-Out), located in rural Kentucky, trained, supervised, and employed local women as community health workers. It is an example of a working partnership between community-based organizations, Appalachian Communities for Children and Whitley County Communities for Children, the Kentucky Cancer Program, and local health departments. The program was initiated in response to studies indicating cervical cancer rates among Appalachian women in southeastern Kentucky were higher than national rates (Hinds, Skaggs, and Hernandez 1985; Pickle, Mason, and Howard 1987). Closer scrutiny revealed that the incidence of invasive cervical cancer among white women2 in thirty-six counties of southeastern Kentucky (14.9 per 100,000) was nearly two times higher than that of white women in other parts of the United States (7.8 per 100,000) and was in fact similar to that of African American women in urban centers (15.3 per 100,000). In addition, breast cancer mortality in Central Appalachia was rising rapidly in comparison with the rest of the United States (Friedell et al. 1992; Friedell and Rubio 1993). This community-based demonstration project emerged from concern that poor women of Appalachia, like other economically disadvantaged groups, experienced higher rates of cancer mortality as a result of late-stage diagnosis attributable to social and economic obstacles to quality health care. The link between higher cancer mortality and poverty has been well established (Couto, Schott, and Boyd 1994; Farley and Flannery 1989; Freeman 1989; Pamies and Woodard 1992; U.S. Department of Health and Human Services 1991).

Breast and cervix cancer are distinctly "women's problems," and thus to be effective, prevention efforts are needed to address women's needs as women and specifically as mountain women who have a distinct culture including gender expectations that influence health beliefs and practices. The project coordinators recognized the significance of crafting culturally specific interventions, and to do this they sought to involve the women whom the program hoped to serve. Focus groups were conducted as part of the initial planning process and again later to guide creation of educational materials.

What Do Appalachian Women Want?

University researchers speculate that mountain women, particularly older women, might be too modest to discuss "female health issues" publicly. However, the focus groups were well attended by low-income women, ages eighteen to eighty-five, who openly shared their experiences and ideas.

Information. The participants consistently expressed a desire for accurate, straightforward information about women's health. For example, when asked about preferences regarding educational videos, the majority of women preferred seeing a woman actually undergo a mammography rather than watching a simulation. One woman explained, "I want to see a real person going through it, not just a doctor or nurse telling you what it is like when they have not experienced it."

Gender Preferences. Most of the women stated they were uncomfortable talking with men about "female problems" and they expressed a preference for female health care providers. Female family members were most commonly identified as the person they would consult first about health concerns. Overall, data collected from the focus groups underscored the significance of sociocultural influences on health beliefs and practices of Appalachian women.

Sociocultural Influences

Cancer Fears. Fear of cancer was a major theme. As expected, reluctance to participate in screening procedures was associated with fear of what might be found. Overall, the women had little confidence in cancer treatment. Many shared stories of family members or friends for whom treatment had failed. For example, one woman described a coworker's experience: "She was working every day until she went for that test. They took her breast off. She got worse and worse and then died. If it's me, I'd rather not know." Surprisingly, some women associated the occurrence of breast cancer with immoral behavior and recalled women they knew who had kept lumps and even open lesions a secret out of embarrassment or shame. In describing her aunt's death, one woman explained, "She never went to the doctor even though she had a knot on her breast. It was an old tale that you were not a good person if you had cancer in the breast. That's why she never went to the doctor even though she had an actual running sore." She went on to say the family might never have known except for a grandchild's hug that caused the drainage to leak through her blouse. This alarmed her daughter, who insisted she go to the hospital, where she died in a few short weeks. Beliefs linking shame and stigma with breast cancer were validated in all the focus groups; however, some women were quick to point out that this is an old myth largely rejected by younger women.

Religion and Health. A number of women identified religious beliefs as having significant influence on health decisions. Some indicated they would consult with their pastors before agreeing to medical treatment. It was explained that those who are of the "Holiness" faith are likely to rely on lay healing within the church and may be reluctant to utilize main-stream medicine. Some thought that the churches would be a good way to reach women to teach about health issues. One woman stated, "You could teach in the church if you have the preacher's permission and the meeting is all female and private. The body is the temple of the Lord, so we can use the church to teach how to take care of it."

Gender Roles and Rules. Male dominance and influence over women's health decisions was a consistent theme in the focus groups and is a concept that warrants further investigation. For example, one young woman stated she did not go for yearly pelvic exams because her husband did not want another man to see or touch her. There was general agree-ment that this was a factor for some women. An older woman explained, "Usually after women start having babies the men get over that non-sense." The focus groups also revealed that males often control use of vehicles and either are not able to miss work or are unwilling to provide transportation to medical appointments. Some women said their husbands would not allow them to drive on the interstate or in unfamiliar areas. In some instances women were quite independent and admonished others for being submissive. One woman said, "Honey, you better get over that. Nobody is going to take care of you but you." With only a few exceptions, a commonly expressed view was that men are not concerned about women's health.

Barriers to Careseeking

Economic barriers to utilizing available services included the anticipated factors of perceived cost, lack of insurance, and fear of inability to pay.

Many women questioned the logic of going for screening procedures. One explained, "If they find something, I can't afford to go to the hospital anyway." As expected, barriers to health care also included problems with transportation, child care, inconvenient clinic hours, and negative past experiences with health care providers.

Rural women are less likely to be insured than are urban women, and they are much less likely to have employer-provided insurance. Whereas rural women are more likely than urban women to be poor, they are less likely to have Medicaid coverage. Kentucky and West Virginia are among the rural states that fail to provide Medicaid coverage to all financially needy women and children. Often rural families are excluded from Medicaid coverage because they own small farms, automobiles, or trucks. Even work tools can put families over eligibility limits (Hughes and Rosenbaum 1989). According to the National Center for Health Statistics (1988), low-income rural women are less likely to obtain adequate maternity care than their urban counterparts, and full-term healthy infants born in rural areas are more likely to die.

Like other underserved populations, Appalachian women have been exposed primarily to individual focused, acute medical care, often imposed upon them with little consideration of social and cultural processes that affect health. Services are not only scarce but those that exist are fragmented and underutilized. Health care professionals become frustrated and are often perplexed by underutilization of services and resistance to prescribed treatment. Health care, especially preventative services, are often a low priority for women struggling to cope with the daily realities of life in poverty.

Different Worlds and Different Meanings

It is essential to consider the profound differences that may exist between health professionals and rural low-income women in regard to the definitions and meanings ascribed to preventive measures. Failure to understand the importance of the assumptions and beliefs individuals bring to a health care encounter can create situations in which both the caregiver and the careseeker leave the interaction feeling diminished and rejected. To explain how events and behavior may be interpreted differently, the following scenario was developed from an actual medical care situation.[3]

The Health Care Provider

The health care provider views prenatal care as a necessity.

The health care provider believes it is essential for a pregnant woman to keep medical appointments in order to have a healthy pregnancy and good birth outcome. The health care provider's belief is that mothers who are concerned about their health and the health of their children will keep appointments and follow their doctor's orders.

The health care provider is helpful and friendly when the woman comes in for her first prenatal visit. Later, when she returns having missed two appointments, the provider is impatient, aloof, and speaks firmly to the woman about the inconvenience caused when appointments are not kept.

The health care provider later questions why he/she continues trying to practice medicine with people "who don't care about their health, won't follow advice, and don't even show up half the time."

Low-Income Woman in Appalachia

She may view prenatal care as a luxury or as a good idea but not as an absolute necessity.

She may feel that going to the doctor when she doesn't feel sick is not critical and may be a waste of time and money. If she has nothing more important to do, it's a good idea to go ahead and go. The woman knows that her own grandmother had eight healthy babies at home without a doctor or any prenatal care, so she is not overly concerned about medical appointments, especially early in the pregnancy.

The woman makes and keeps her first appointment. When her aunt becomes ill and she is called upon to care for her small cousins, she misses her next prenatal appointment. The clinic calls and reschedules, but the woman does not have transportation when the appointment time arrives. Her sister, who has a car, comes over later in the day and drives her to the clinic. She is seen but feels put down by both the receptionist and the provider.

Going to the clinic is a hassle and the people there make her feel bad. She doesn't know whether or not she will go back. If she does go back, she plans to say whatever they want to hear.

In Appalachia, the persistence of poor health status has often been attributed to individual behavior and culture with little attention to the larger

economic, political, and structural components of society that act to encourage, produce, and support poor health. When Appalachian women fail
to keep appointments or follow treatment regimes, they are labeled deviant
and noncompliant. Both the popular media and academic scholars have
portrayed mountain people as fatalistic, flawed, and deficient, thus perpetuating the culture of poverty (or blaming the victim) explanation for the
persistent problems of the region. Many attribute the poor health status of
Appalachian people to geographic isolation, overly close family ties, and
dependency. Some have gone so far as to classify the entire region as a deviant subculture (Finney 1969; Looff 1971; Toynbee 1947; Weller 1965).

Appalachian Myths and Stereotypes

Common stereotypes about Appalachian women include high incidence
of incest and genetic abnormalities linked to intermarriage, lack of restraint regarding fertility, and the belief that mountain women prefer folk
remedies over modern medicine. Furthermore, those seeking to study and
describe the region tend to ignore the presence of African and Native
American populations and the middle and upper classes. This distorted
perception perpetuates the false image of Appalachian women as "poor,
white, barefoot, and pregnant." These myths are not supported by current
studies (Cavender 1992; Hufford 1992; Zahorik 1989).

   Though small in number, new voices are emerging to challenge the
old models of dependency and deficiency. They seek to reexamine regional
health problems from the perspective of how the people of the region see,
define, and create the social and physical worlds in which they live
(Couto, Simpson, and Harris 1994; Keefe 1988).

Expanding Training Models

In the spirit of community-based health promotion and building upon the
successes and lessons of the Mt. Sc-Out project, the 1994 Kentucky
legislature approved funding for lay health worker training in three sites
throughout the state. Now known as the "Kentucky Homeplace" project,[4]
thirty-five indigenous workers, predominantly women, are being trained
and employed as health advisors. The core elements for training of health
advisors are notable in the ways in which they deviate from narrowly
focused biomedical training. Unlike most university-based professional

education, the training is responsive to the perceived needs of the learner and intuitive knowing is affirmed as valid. Teachers must recognize and respect the knowledge the lay worker brings to the training experience because the goal is to connect new learning with what is already known. The training is designed to be nonhierarchical in that all who participate are considered both teachers and learners. Trainers must be flexible and responsive to adult learning styles and cultural influences on the teaching learning process. Avoidance of rigid didactic teaching methods and involvement of the lay workers in development of the training program are essential elements.

Ideally, some components of training will involve both health professionals and lay workers because they have much to teach one another. Experiential learning is the primary methodology. Content focuses on interpersonal skills and role development as learner, teacher, advocate, and friend rather than on accumulation of facts about symptoms and disease. It is family and community centered. Content includes information about community resources and the health care system; however, such knowledge is considered of little use unless combined with the development of skills necessary to assess services in relation to affordability, accessibility, and acceptability to local people.

Identifying Key Roles and Relationships

Some commonly recurring needs of low-income rural families have been identified. Lay health workers must be able to provide information about health services that are affordable, and they must be able to teach others how to seek and request health care when they don't have the means to pay for it. They must know how to arrange for transportation to local clinics and remote medical centers. They must become adept at helping people improve their living conditions through use of available community resources such as local health departments, churches, and other support services. Communication skills are of paramount importance. The lay health worker serves as an interpreter of meaning, a bridge between the health care system and families struggling to avoid and survive poverty. Serving as a role model, she must be able to teach other women how to talk assertively with health professionals when there is a need to convey or request information about health status, medical treatments, or home care. The indigenous health worker has a particularly important role in helping women who feel disenfranchised from the health care system to redefine themselves as health care consumers. This redefinition of self is gradual and continual, so there is a great need for ongoing interaction and relationships.

Measuring Success

Utilizing indigenous lay workers for health promotion is but one strategy for bridging the gap between women in the community and health care systems. It is neither a bottom-up nor a top-down approach but an effort to meet halfway. It appears to be an effective means of promoting utilization of health services when the health care system is receptive to lay involvement. In Kentucky's demonstration project, two of the three counties served by Mt. Sc-Out had 80–100 percent increases in the number of women who received Pap tests and mammography screening in the first year. A third county reported less success. The willingness of health professionals to work collaboratively with lay workers and the flexibility of local health departments were identified as factors accounting for differences in outcome (Friedell and Rubio 1993).

Many questions remain unanswered relating to role development and effective utilization of indigenous health workers for health promotion in Appalachia and elsewhere. Ongoing quality training and program evaluation are greatly needed. A number of excellent training manuals, kits, and guides have been developed around the country and are readily available.[5] However, there is a disturbing absence of systematic evaluation of training effectiveness and little awareness of gender issues. Increased knowledge of sociocultural and gender influences on health in Appalachia is essential for effective planning and implementation of services that will be useful and acceptable to Appalachian women. It is also important that physicians, nurses, and social workers understand that indigenous workers do not merely do what professionals do not have time to do. They are valuable team members who possess knowledge and skills that may not be available to the professional. As Louise's note reveals, what the lay worker brings to health work is not likely to be covered in professional education.

Shaping Our Future

In rural communities throughout Appalachia, community leaders and activists from grassroots organizations, schools, and churches are coming together to address the alarming incidence of new and old public health issues such as teen pregnancy, family violence, medical indigency, AIDS, substance abuse, and cancer. Many innovative programs use lay health workers, mostly women, to provide outreach, peer counseling, and other health promotion activities. However, these programs often have tenuous links or no links at all with traditional health care systems. Successful, lasting programs seem to be those that are able to establish and maintain partnerships with health professionals and existing institutions in the community. Such partnerships are essential in addressing issues related to training, supervision, funding, continuity, and quality of services needed to improve rural women's health.

NOTES

1. In a study of programs utilizing indigenous health workers, Giblin (1989) defined the common traits found in successful programs.

2. Although this study targeted white women in Appalachia, the reader should keep in mind the ethnic and racial diversity of the region.

3. Thanks to Lisa Raymer for contributing to the development of this scenario.

4. Established in 1994 at the University of Kentucky Center for Rural Health, the Kentucky Homeplace demonstration project is ongoing and will seek to evaluate the effectiveness of family-centered lay health advisors in improving health status of Kentucky families. One of the three sites is an urban non-Appalachian, predominantly African American community in southwest Louisville.

5. For information about the *Kentucky Homeplace Training Manual*, contact the University of Kentucky Center for Rural Health, 100 Airport Gardens Road, Suite 10, Hazard, Kentucky 41701. (606) 439-3557.

REFERENCES

Cavendar, A. P.
    1992   "Theoretic orientations and folk medicine research in the Appalachian South." Southern Medical Journal 85(2):170–78.
Chapman, J., E. Seifel, and A. Cross
    1990   "Home visitors and child health: analysis of selected programs." Pediatrics 85(6):1059–68.
Clinton, Barbara
    1992   "Maternal and infant health outreach worker project: Appalachian communities help their own." Pp. 23–45 in M. Larner, R. Halpern, and O. Harkavy (eds.), Fair Start for Children: Lessons Learned from Seven Demonstration Projects. New Haven: Yale University Press.

Couto, Richard, C. S. Schott, and N. R. Boyd
  1994   "Socioeconomic status and cancer." Pp. 122-37 in Richard A. Couto,
          Nancy K. Simpson, and Gale Harris (eds.), Sowing Seeds in the Moun-
          tains. NIH Pub. No. 94-3779. Rockville, MD: National Institutes of
          Health.
Couto, Richard A., Nancy K. Simpson, and Gale Harris, eds.
  1994   Sowing Seeds in the Mountains: Community-Based Coalitions for Can-
          cer Prevention and Control. NIH Pub. No. 94-3779. Rockville, MD:
          National Institutes of Health.
Dunford, Christopher
  1987   Mississippi Applied Nutrition Program. Davis, CA.: Freedom from Hun-
          ger Foundation.
Eng, Eugenia
  1989   PINAH Evaluation Progress Report. Chapel Hill: University of North
          Carolina.
Farley, T. A., and J. T. Flannery
  1989   "Late stage diagnosis of breast cancer in women of lower SES: public
          health implication." American Journal of Public Health 79:1508-12.
Finney, J. C.
  1969   Culture Change, Mental Health, and Poverty. Lexington: University of
          Kentucky Press.
Frate, Dennis, T. L. Whitehead, and S. A. Johnson
  1983   "The selection, training, and utilization of health counselors in the man-
          agement of high blood pressure." Urban Health 12:52-54.
Freeman, H. P.
  1989   "Cancer in the socioeconomically disadvantaged." CA: Cancer Journal
          for Clinicians 39:266-88.
Friedell, G. H., and Angel Rubio
  1993   "Cancer control in Kentucky: lessons in the care of rural poor women."
          Proceedings of the Health Care Needs of Appalachia Conference. Uni-
          versity of Kentucky, Lexington.
Friedell, G. H., T. C. Tucker, E. McMammon, M. Moser, C. Hernandes, and M. Nadel
  1992   "Incidence of dysplasia and carcinoma of the uterine cervix in an Appa-
          lachian population." Journal of the National Cancer Institute
          84(13):1030-32.
Giblin, Paul T.
  1989   "Effective utilization and evaluation of indigenous health care workers."
          Public Health Reports 104(4):361-68.
Hinds, M. W., J. W. Skaggs, and C. Hernandez
  1985   "Cervical cancer mortality trends in Kentucky, 1972." Journal of the
          Kentucky Medical Association 83:186-92.
Hufford, D. J.
  1992   "Folk medicine in contemporary America." Pp. 14-31 in James Kirkland,
          H. F. Mathews, C. W. Sullivan, and K. Baldwin (eds.), Herbal and Magical
          Medicine: Traditional Healing Today. Durham, NC: Duke University Press.

Hughes, Dana, and Sara Rosenbaum
> 1989 "An overview of maternal and infant health services in rural America." Journal of Rural Health 5(4):299–319.

Johnson, Z., F. Howell, and B. Mooly
> 1993 "Community mothers program: randomized controlled trial of non-professional intervention in parenting." British Medical Journal 306:1149–52.

Keefe, Susan, ed.
> 1988 Appalachian Mental Health. Lexington: University Press of Kentucky.

Looff, David H.
> 1971 Appalachia's Children: The Challenge of Mental Health. Lexington: University Press of Kentucky.

National Center for Health Statistics
> 1988 Vital Statistics of the United States: II. Mortality, Part A. Pub. No. (PHS) 87-1102. Washington: Department of Health and Human Services.

Pamies, R. J., and L. J. Woodard
> 1992 "Cancer in socioeconomically disadvantaged populations." Primary Care 19(3):443–50.

Pickle, L. W., T. J. Mason, and N. Howard
> 1987 Atlas of U.S. Cancer Mortality among Whites. DHHS Pub. No. (NIH) 87-2900. Washington: Department of Health and Human Services.

Service, Connie, and Eva J. Salber
> 1977 Community Health Education: The Lay Advisor Approach. Community Health Education Program, Duke University, Durham, NC.

Toynbee, Arnold
> 1947 A Study of History. Vol. 2. New York: Oxford University Press.

U.S. Department of Health and Human Services
> 1991 Healthy People 2000: National Health Promotion and Disease Prevention Objectives. DHHS Pub. No. (PHS) 91-50212. Washington: Government Printing Office.

Weller, Jack E.
> 1965 Yesterday's People: Life in Contemporary Appalachia. Lexington: University Press of Kentucky.

Zahorik, P.
> 1989 "Night comes to the chromosomes." Now and Then 6(1):23–24.

[PART IV]

Culture and Complexities

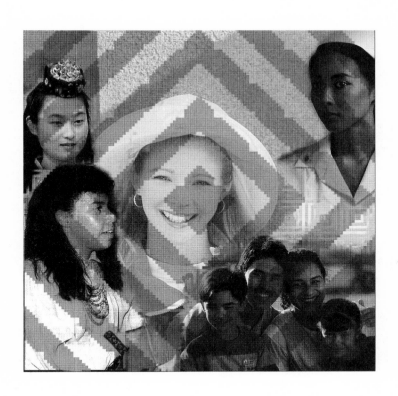

Culture shapes women's health in countless ways. Health beliefs, practices, and illness behavior are cultural productions. Anthropologists, sociologists, and psychologists have long pointed out many of the cultural dimensions of health and illness: how pain is experienced and expressed, what foods to eat or avoid to cope with illnesses, and which healers to seek out. Members of particular cultures or subcultures often share expectations about common health events over women's life cycle: birth, the onset of menstruation, sexual activity, menopause, and death. Not all cultures medicalize these life experiences to the degree that most late-twentieth-century Americans do. Some women who use western medical services do so in tandem with traditional cultural healing practices. As Bonnie Blair O'Connor (1995:161) points out, in the United States "non-biomedical health belief systems are alive and well." In her view, the multiplicity of healing systems used by Americans suggests a health pluralism that is rarely acknowledged in the dominant medical system.

Health and healing relationships and experiences predictably have different meanings to women from different cultures and subcultures. The contributors in part 4 draw attention to cultural complexities in women's health that go beyond stereotypical views that can result from focusing too generally on the health of women who belong to the major racial groups. In chapter 10, Jane Sprague Zones looks at how dominant cultural values and beliefs about beauty affect most American women's health. Cultural expectations about beauty are difficult, if not impossible, to escape, as subcultures develop their own norms and values in relation to the norms and values in the larger culture. Next, Ann Metcalf raises provocative issues about Native American women's health. Her deft analysis of access to medical care through the U.S. Public Health Service reveals a troubling history of cultural conquest—and the importance of providing services that are culturally specific, sensitive, and appropriate.

These themes echo in chapters 12 and 13, each based on qualitative fieldwork. Ito, Chung, and Kagawa-Singer report on the distinct social and cultural health and illness experiences of Japanese American and Southeast Asian women. Scrimshaw, Zambrana, and Dunkel-Schetter analyze birthing experiences of Latinas in the United States. None of these chapters is intended to "cover" the array of distinct health issues of any racial/ethnic or subcultural group.

Attempting to summarize these rapidly growing bodies of scholarship on women of color in the United States would fill a volume in itself. For example, Diane L. Adams (1995) has assembled such a volume, *Health Issues for Women of Color: A Cultural Diversity Perspective.* Barbara Bair and Susan E. Cayleff include an excellent bibliography on the topic in their 1993 volume, *Wings of Gauze: Women of Color and the Experience of Health and Illness.* The Center for Research on Women, University of Memphis, maintains a bibliographic reference service on women of color and southern women that includes decades of research on health and cultural issues. Here, we provide specific examples of how health, healing, and culture intersect and affect women's health.

REFERENCES

Adams, Diane L.
  1995 Health Issues for Women of Color: A Cultural Diversity Perspective. Thousand Oaks, CA: Sage.
Bair, Barbara and Susan E. Cayleff
  1993 Wings of Gauze: Women of Color and the Experience of Health and Illness. Detroit: Wayne State University Press.
O'Connor, Bonnie Blair
  1995 Healing Traditions: Alternative Medicine and the Health Professions. Philadelphia: University of Pennsylvania Press.

[10]

Beauty Myths and Realities and Their Impact on Women's Health

JANE SPRAGUE ZONES

Imbedded in the political economy of the cosmetics and fitness industries, the unrealizable myth of beauty for women in American society serves to suppress diversity. Moreover, the social consequences for some women are depression and lowered self-esteem if they believe they do not meet elusive standards for presenting themselves and their bodies. Sociologist Jane Zones discusses both inter-personal and policy strategies to counter these problems.

Of all the characteristics that distinguish one human being from the next, physical appearance has the most immediate impact. How a person looks shapes the kinds of responses she or he evokes in others. Physical appearance has similar effects on other social statuses. Those considered beautiful or handsome are more likely to accrue benefits such as attributions of goodness and better character, more desirability as friends and partners, and upward social mobility. Those considered unattractive receive less attention as infants, are evaluated more harshly in school, and earn less money as employees. The significance of physical appearance shifts in intensity as it interacts with other statuses, such as gender, race/ethnicity, age, class, and disability. For groups targeted for social mistreatment, such as women and racial or ethnic minorities, physical appearance has profound implications not only for the creation of first impressions but also for enduring influence on social effectiveness. The power of appearance pushes people to assimilate in order to avoid unwanted attention or to attract desired attention. The pushes and pulls to look "conventionally attractive" constitute assaults on diversity.

In this chapter, I describe and evaluate some of the ways that social concerns with women's appearance affect physical and emotional health status and limit the range of perceived and actual possibilities open to individuals and to groups. My particular focus is on how physical appearance is perceived by and affects women of color, those in various social classes, and women who are older or disabled. A review of research and literature that reflect women's personal experiences indicates that cultural preoccupation with how we look militates against the appreciation and expression of women's diversity.

I find two major bodies of research on this topic: the experimental social psychology and the body-image literatures. Much of what we know academically about appearance and its social effects is derived from experimental social psychology, mostly studies of the human face. This body of work generally neglects analyses of social status other than gender distinctions that affect interpersonal (usually romantic) attachment. This research, carried out mainly in university settings with primarily white undergraduate students, is paralleled by a smaller number of studies using other populations that yield comparable results. Global measures of physical attractiveness are employed, in which judges rate "stimulus persons" (either human confederates or photographic images of people with "normal" features) along a continuum ranging from very low to very high physical attractiveness (Patzer 1985). The body-image literature comes primarily from clinical psychology and feminist theory. Body-image scholars (Iazzetto 1988) typically cite historical evidence and open-ended interviews with informants to support their arguments. This school is much more attentive than are the experimentalists to the interaction of social statuses and physical appearance and to social and political contexts generally. Both approaches contribute to understanding the real effects of physical appearance. This chapter interweaves these two strands to show commonalities and differences between women in an attempt to understand the power of appearance in women's lives.

Commonalities in Perception of Beauty

Many women concur that personal beauty, or "looking good," is fostered from a very early age. It is probably true that the ways in which people assess physical beauty are not naturally determined but socially and culturally learned and therefore "in the eye of the beholder." However, we tend to discount the depth of our *common* perception of beauty, mistakenly assuming that individuals largely set their own standards. At any period in history, within a given geographic and cultural territory, there are relatively uniform and widely understood models of how women "should" look. Numerous studies over time reinforce this notion (Iliffe 1960; Patzer 1985; Perrett, May, and Yoshikawa 1994).

Although there have always been beauty ideals for women (Banner 1983), in modern times the proliferation of media portrayals of feminine beauty in magazines, billboards, movies, and television has both hastened and more broadly disseminated the communication of detailed expectations. There are increasingly demanding criteria for female beauty in western culture, and women are strongly pressured to alter their appearance to conform with these standards.

Naomi Wolf, in her book *The Beauty Myth* (1991), contends that the effect of widespread promulgation of womanly ideals of appearance perpetuates the myth that the "quality called 'beauty' objectively and universally exists. Women must want to embody it and men must want to possess women who embody it. This embodiment is an imperative for women and not for men, which situation is necessary and natural because it is biological, sexual, and evolutionary" (12). Wolf declares that this is all falsehood. Instead, beauty is politically and economically determined, and the myth is the "last, best belief system that keeps male dominance intact" (12). She argues that as women have emerged successfully in many new arenas, the focus on and demand for beauty has become more intense, attacking the private sense of self and creating new barriers to accomplishment. In Wolf's view, the increasing obsession with beauty is a backlash to women's liberation.

Beauty's Social Significance for Individuals

Much of the evidence from studies done by experimental social psychologists shows why people assign such importance to their appearance. They have found that people judged to be physically attractive, both male and female, are assumed to possess more socially desirable personality traits and expected to lead happier lives (Dion, Berscheid, and Walster 1972). Social science research shows that "cute babies are cuddled more than homely ones; attractive toddlers are punished less often. Teachers give special attention to better-looking pupils, strangers offer help more readily to attractive people, and jurors show more sympathy to good-looking victims" (Freedman 1986:7–8). This principle holds in virtually every aspect of our lives from birth to death and across racial and ethnic groups (Patzer 1985:232–33). The effects of these myriad positive responses to and assumptions about people who are considered attractive have self-fulfilling aspects as well. The expectations of others strongly shape development, learning, and achievement: people thought to be attractive become more socially competent and accomplished (Goldman and Lewis 1977).

Appearance-based discrimination targets women more than men. Women's self-esteem and happiness are significantly associated with their physical appearance; no such relationship exists for men as a group (Allgood-Merten, Lewinsohn, and Hops 1990; Mathes and Kahn 1975). Women's access to upward mobility is also greatly affected by physical appearance, which is a major determinant of marriage to a higher status man. By contrast, potential partners evaluate men more for intelligence or accomplishment. The significance of beauty in negotiating beneficial marriages is particularly true for white working-class women (Elder 1969; Taylor and Glenn 1976; Udry 1977; Udry and Eckland 1984). Banner (1983), who has traced the shifting models of beauty and fashion over two hundred years of American history, concludes that although standards of beauty may have changed, and women have greatly improved their access to social institutions, many females continue to define themselves by physical appearance and their ability to attract a partner.

The preoccupation with appearance serves to control and contain women's ambitions and motivations to gain power in larger political contexts. To the degree that many females feel they must dedicate time, attention, and resources to maintaining and improving their looks, they neglect activities to improve social conditions for themselves or others. Conversely, as women become increasingly visible as powerful individuals in shaping events, their looks become targeted for irrelevant scrutiny and criticism in ways with which men in similar positions are not forced to contend (Freedman 1986; Wolf 1991). For example, Marcia Clark, the lead prosecutor in the O.J. Simpson trial, was the focus of unremitting media attention for her dress, hairstyle, demeanor, and private life.

The major difference between discrimination based on appearance and mistreatment based on gender, race, or other social attributes is that individuals are legally protected against the latter (Patzer 1985:11). In an eye-opening review of legal cases related to appearance and employment, Wolf documents the inconsistencies that characterize decisions to dismiss women on the basis of their looks. "Legally, women *don't* have a thing to wear" (1991:42). Requirements of looking both businesslike and feminine represent a moving target that invites failure. In *Hopkins v. Price-Waterhouse,* a woman who brought in more clients than any other employee was denied a partnership because, her employers claimed, she did not walk, talk, or dress in an adequately feminine manner nor did she wear makeup. In another court case, it was ruled "inappropriate for a supervisor" of women to dress "like a woman" (Wolf 1991:39). If one appears businesslike, one cannot be adequately feminine; if one appears feminine, one cannot adequately conduct business.

Beauty Myths and the Erosion of Self-Worth

Perhaps the biggest toll the "beauty myth" takes is in terms of women's identity and self-esteem. Like members of other oppressed groups of which we may also be part, women internalize cultural stereotypes and expectations, perpetuating them by enforced acceptance and agreement. For women, this is intensified by the interaction of irrational social responses to physical appearance not only with gender but with other statuses as well—race, class, age, disability, and the like. Continuous questioning of the adequacy of one's looks drains attention from more worthwhile and confidence-building pursuits.

A number of years ago, novelist Alice Walker was invited to speak at her alma mater, Spelman College, the highly regarded historically black women's college in Atlanta. She used the opportunity to describe her experience of feeling as if she had reached the extent of her capacities for accomplishment a few years prior. "I seemed to have reached a ceiling in my brain," Walker recalled. She realized that "in my physical self there remained one last barrier to my spiritual liberation, at least in the present phase. My hair." Walker recognized it was not the hair itself but her relationship with it that was the problem. Months of experimentation with different styles followed. From childhood, her hair had endured domination, suppression, and control at the hands of outsiders. "Eventually I knew *precisely* what hair wanted: . . . to be left alone by anyone, including me, who did not love it as it was" (Walker 1988:52–53). With that realization, the ceiling at the top of Walker's brain lifted, and her mind and spirit could continue to grow. Many African American women have sought just such a liberation from their hair, and others have celebrated its possibilities (Mercer 1990).

Glassner argues that the dramatically increased attention to fitness, diet, and physical well-being in recent years has been accompanied by a plummeting of satisfaction with our bodies (1988:246). There seems to be little relationship between actual physical attractiveness (conformance to culturally valued standards determined by judges) and individual women's satisfaction with their own appearance (Murstein 1972). Both men and women are unrealistic about how others perceive their bodies, but men tend to assume that people think they look better and women tend to assume that they look worse than they actually are perceived (Fallon and Rozin 1985). A recent poll of United States residents (Cimons 1990) found that fewer than a third of adults were happy with their appearance. Women were twice as likely as men to consider themselves to be fat.

Nagging self-doubts about weight emanate from the difference between projected images of women, many of which depict severely undernourished bodies, and our everyday reality. Half of the readers of *Vogue* magazine wear size 14 or larger (Glassner 1988:12), tormenting themselves with images of models with size 6 or smaller figures in every issue. Female models are 9 percent taller and 16 percent thinner than average women. Even the majority of women runners who are in good physical condition and fall within the ranges of weight and body fat considered desirable describe themselves as overweight (Robinson 1983). Research consistently shows that women not only overestimate their own size (Penner, Thompson, and Coovert 1991; Thompson and Dolce 1989) but they expect men to prefer thinner women than is the actual case (Rozin and Fallon 1988).

Internalizing the oppressive messages and images from outside has the effect of making the situation seem intractable. In Alice Walker's case, the distress that she had internalized from the ways in which people (or ads or media impressions) had communicated concern or distaste for her hair distracted her from her work, eroded her confidence, and slowed her progress. Competition between women is a prominent feature of internalized sexism, reflecting women's collusion with beauty expectations that are both limiting and unrealistically demanding. Women become each other's critics, keeping each other anxious and in line, thereby maintaining the status quo. In *Memoirs of an Ex-Prom Queen*, one of the enduring feminist novels of the 1970s, Alix Kates Shulman created a teenage protagonist so obsessed with and insecure about her looks that she realizes she actually is beautiful only after she learns that her closest friends hate her for it.

Internalized oppression causes additional harm by redirecting mistreatment from the dominant culture to other members of one's own group (Lipsky 1987). A transcript of a kitchen table conversation between two black women illustrates how the preferential treatment of lighter-skinned slaves by their masters (who frequently fathered them) during the slavery era has produced continuing conflict among African Americans to the present day (Anderson and Ingram 1994). Tamara, a dark-skinned woman, recounts being ridiculed by family and neighbors as "ugly and black. . . . That's when I stopped liking black kids altogether. They hated me, and they made me hate my best friend [who was darker]. I remember everything about my childhood. It's like a diary. . . . I kept telling myself, 'There's got to be a way to get over this. One day this is going to stop.' But it never did. As I grew older, it just got worse. . . . To this day, I still find myself walking with my head down and trying to cover up my body" (358, 361). The preoccupation with skin color also had hurtful repercussions for Michele, a light-skinned black woman. "Light-skinned blacks resent it when people say we are trying to be or act white. . . . On the other hand, society, both black and white, gives us these messages that we are 'better' than darker-skinned blacks. It's sort of like we're in limbo" (359). The acting out of internalized oppression between members of a group creates additional pressures to assimilate or avoid visibility, and it disrupts the unity essential for social progress.

Quantifying Beauty: Conventionality and Computer Enhancement

The predominant, nearly universal standard for beauty in American society is to be slender, young, upper-class, and white without noticeable physical imperfections or disabilities. To the extent that a woman's racial or ethnic heritage, class background, age, or other social and physical characteristics do not conform to this ideal, assaults on opportunities and esteem increase. Physical appearance is at the core of racism and most other social oppressions, because it is generally what is used to classify individuals.

Although expectations relative to appearance vary in style and interpretation, there are commonalities in their effects on women. Bordo (1993) makes a strong philosophical case for examining the multiplicity of interpretations of the body. She cautions, however, that we must at the same time recognize the significant leveling effect of "the everyday deployment of mass cultural representations. . . . First, the representations *homogenize*. In our culture, this means that they will smooth out all racial, ethnic, and sexual 'differences' that disturb Anglo-Saxon, heterosexual expectations and identifications. . . . Second, these homogenized images *normalize*—that is, they function as models against which the self continually measures, judges, 'disciplines,' and 'corrects' itself" (24–25).

In a number of studies, conventionality has been found to be the most important component of beauty (Webster and Driskell 1983). Judith Langlois and colleagues used a computer to blend likenesses of individuals into composites, mathematically averaging out their features. Undergraduate students judged composites of sixteen or thirty-two faces to be significantly more attractive than individual faces for both male and female images. Composites made from blending thirty-two faces were judged more attractive than those composed of only sixteen (Langlois et al. 1990, 1991). A similar study, using Japanese and Caucasian judges and subjects found that "aesthetic judgements of face shape are similar across different cultural backgrounds" (Perrett, May, and Yoshikawa 1994:239) and that the raters had the highest regard for a computerized caricature that exaggerated the ways that the fifteen most preferred faces differed from the average sixty.

This research is now being applied in the popular media. A computer-generated multiethnic supermodel cover face on a major women's magazine labeled "Who Is the Face of America?" accompanies a story lauding our "radically diversifying demographics" (Gaudoin 1994) when the image projected is one of convergence rather than diversity.

Beauty and the Challenge of Social Diversity

Although significant beauty ideals appear to transcend cultural subgroup boundaries, appearance standards do vary by reference group. Clothing preferred by adolescents, for example, which experiences quick fashion turnover, is considered inappropriate for older people. Body piercing, a current style for young white people in urban areas of the United States, is repellant to most older adults and some ethnic minorities in the same age group. Religious and political ideologies are often identified through appearance. Islamic fundamentalist women wear clothing that covers body and face, an expression of religious sequestering; Amish women wear conservative clothing and distinctive caps; orthodox Jewish women wear wigs or cover their hair; African American women for many years wore natural hairdos to show racial pride; and Native American women may wear tribal jewelry and distinctive clothes that indicate their respect for heritage. In recent years, the disability rights movement has encouraged personal visibility to accompany the tearing down of barriers to access, resulting in a greater variety of appliances (including elegant streamlined wheelchairs) and functional clothing.

Although there are varying and conflicting standards of good looks and appropriate appearance that are held simultaneously by social sub-groups, the dominant ideals prevail and are legitimated most thoroughly in popular culture. Webster and Driskell (1983) contend that physical appearance has effects similar to those of other social statuses such as gender, race, age, class, and so on, conferring superiority or inferiority in the social hierarchy. The implications of physical appearance gain in intensity when they are confounded with other statuses. Wendy Chapkis (1986) presents the perspectives of women from many groups—elderly, fat, black, Asian, lesbian, disabled, and so on—who describe the injuries they have experienced as a result of their combined oppressions. To avoid social harassment and discrimination because of appearance, women frequently alter their looks to appear more conventional, an unwitting attack on diversity. Lisa Diane White, a leader in the Black Women's Health Project's self-help movement, addresses challenges involved in showing diversity. "With the recent upsurge of pride in our African heritage, we like to think that we as black women feel better about ourselves today than our sisters did in the past. . . . But I think a lot of us are striving still for standards of beauty and acceptability that aren't our own, and we're suffering the pain inherent in this kind of quest" (quoted in Pinkney 1994:53).

One major way that dominant social forces have dealt with those who diverge is to remove these expressions from view—through ghettoization, anti-immigration policies, special education programs, retirement policies, and so on. The ultimate social insult is to render the oppressed invisible. Social barriers to visibility are expressed as well in pressures to avoid drawing attention to oneself. Those features that render us "different" are frequently the objects of harassment or unwanted attention. We learn to appear invisible. In the following sections, the gender effects of appearance in combination with other social statuses are described through personal accounts and social research.

Race and Ethnicity. In recent years, there has been a burgeoning of women's literature that provides a rich context for the significance of appearance in women's lives. Analyzing Toni Morrison's *The Bluest Eye,* a novel about a poor black family, Lakoff and Scherr describe how the author shows "ugliness seeping through the skin, becoming conviction." The dominant culture's imposition of white standards of beauty presents an added and impossible burden for women of color. Lakoff and Scherr's interviews with women of color found that as children they grew up feeling ugly and knowing that there was nothing they could do about it. "For these women the American Dream of beauty was a perpetual reminder of what they were not, and could never be" (Lakoff and Scherr 1984:252).

An examination by Patricia Morton (1991) of scholarly portrayals of black women in American history and social science during this century showed persistent "shaping and endorsement of a distinctive and profoundly disempowering, composite image of black womanhood . . . as a natural and permanent slave woman" (ix). The introduction of the black liberation movement with its slogan "Black Is Beautiful" meant to many African American women a welcome contradiction to the assorted ways in which racism had imposed feelings of ugliness. The impossibility of ever achieving the dominant culture's ideal, or even coming close, was deeply daunting. But ethnic pride movements also bring about pressures of their own for their constituents to look a particular way, fulfill a particular ideal (Mercer 1990).

Among white Americans who identify with ethnic minority groups, appearance plays a similar role, sometimes with frightening intensity. A Holocaust survivor continues to dye her hair blonde into old age because it was her light hair color that allowed her to pass as a non-Jew and avoid the Nazi death camps as a young adult. Her current feeling of security, unrelated to actual safety, remains bound up in her ability to pass.

A study of physical features of faces in photographs of "Miss Universe" contestants, half of whom were white, the others black or Asian, found that black and Asian beauty pageant contestants possessed most of the patterns of features associated with attractiveness in the white entrants (Cunningham 1986) Even though contestants were selected by their own nations, and judges for the international contest were from the Japanese contest site, the researcher suggests that both western and nonwestern national representatives were selected because they approximated western standards of beauty.

A comparison of U.S. women with women and girls in nonwestern countries shows that American females have a poorer self-image and diet more (Rothblum 1990). A parallel finding from a study by Aune and Aune (1994) found that white American women and men paid more attention to their appearance than African Americans and that, of the three groups, Asian Americans were the least concerned about personal appearance. Western beauty ideals have permeated the "global village," but their psychological effects appear to be greatest at the source. The pursuit of beauty has provided more and more commodities to offer on the world market, and in this industry, the United States is on the surplus side of the trade balance.

Age. Youthful appearance is a major feature of the beauty standard. In American society, peoples' worries about aging center around economic need, disability, dependency, and death, all very significant and frightening issues. Consequently, visible signs of age on face and body often provoke dread. In *The Coming of Age* (1972:297), Simone de Beauvoir remarks that she has "never come across one single woman, either in life or in books, who has looked upon her own old age cheerfully. In the same way, no one ever speaks of 'a beautiful old woman.'"

Experimental studies corroborate the association of youthful features with attractiveness. Johnson (1985) points out that it is perceived age, not actual age, that is the decisive factor, and he concludes from his research on white women and men that "maintaining or recapturing youthful vigor is an important determinant of judged attractiveness" (160). However, gender differences appear to be related to age. In further studies, female judges found photos of men maintained their level of attractiveness across groups of increasing age, whereas male judges found photos of older women less attractive than those of younger women (Mathes et al. 1985).

Although there are limits to what an individual can do to stave off the physical effects of aging over a lifetime, many products and services claim to prolong youth. Raising fears about aging is a major tool in marketing cosmetics, hair coloring, and cosmetic surgery. Mary Kay Ash, addressing women who sell her cosmetic line, stated that "very young girls with perfect complexions can possibly be naturally beautiful, but at about age 25, things begin to happen. And senility begins at 28" (Rubenstein 1984). Of course, fostering the notion that young adults should begin to consider themselves beset by physical deterioration greatly extends the market for Mary Kay's products.

Wolf (1991:14) argues that aging in women is considered ugly because women become more powerful with age. Stronger attacks are required upon personal worth to undermine the threat posed by accumulation of experience and influence as we grow older.

Disability. Erving Goffman's classic studies of stigma (1963) provided the underpinnings for much of the research on physical appearance. His work focused on the negative social consequences of visible disability and other attributes that are socially devalued. To the extent that individuals have visible physical differences, they are at greater jeopardy of being perceived as and viewing themselves as unattractive.

Alice Walker wrote of being blinded in one eye by a BB pellet at age eight. She changed overnight from being a confident, cute whiz in school to a withdrawn and scared child who did not raise her head. She faced the unwanted curiosity of others because of the noticeable white scar tissue on the eye. At night she pleaded with the eye to clear up. "I tell it I hate and despise it. I do not pray for sight. I pray for beauty" (Walker 1990:284). After the scar tissue's removal at age fourteen, Walker emerged with greater confidence, but the inner scars of self-doubt remained to be battled into adulthood.

A survey of college students with disabilities indicates that they view their visible disabilities as being the primary referent in interactions with others. One student summed it up: "I think the visual impact of a person sitting in a chair with wheels on it is so great as to render all other impressions, such as dress or grooming, virtually insignificant" (Kaiser, Freeman, and Wingate 1984:6). Nevertheless, the authors conclude that people with physical disabilities respond to the labeling process by managing aspects of their appearance over which they can exert some control. Much of the effort goes toward "normalizing" appearance, attempting to make the disability less obvious.

In *Autobiography of a Face,* Lucy Grealy describes the effects of disfiguring cancer surgery that removed much of her jaw at age nine. In adolescence her face constitutes her identity, not unlike other girls her age, but because of the disfigurement, to an even greater extreme: "By equating my face with ugliness, in believing that without it I would never experience the deep, bottomless grief I called ugliness, I separated myself even further from other people, who I thought never experienced grief this deep" (Grealy 1994:180).

Class. Class status has a complex relationship to physical appearance, shaping standards of beauty that may be expensive and dysfunctional and requiring adherence to standards for class membership and identity. Similarly, physical beauty has ramifications for class status: people judged to be physically attractive stay in school longer, get better jobs, and have higher incomes — the three primary components of socioeconomic status.

Devotion of energy to "improvement" of appearance sometimes has dysfunctional results. Sociologist Thorstein Veblen noted a century ago in *The Theory of the Leisure Class* that the major characteristic of envied

clothing is that it is impractical for any kind of work. Little did he antic-
ipate the popularity of Levi's 501 denim jeans for people of all classes in
the 1990s.

To generate continued profits, the fashion industry promotes frequent
and dramatic changes in style that require investment in new clothing
and "looks." These fashions come from many sources: media and sports
stars (expensive high-top shoes, for example), the ghetto (cornrows, baggy
pants, do-rags), as well as Paris fashions (ready-to-wear copies) (Davis
1992). Considerable resources are expended by people of all income levels
to give the appearance of currency and affluence.

One researcher reports that appearance is more significant for African
American women who are better educated than for those with less education (Udry 1977). Michele, a professional, who identifies herself as
light-skinned, describes her repugnance at assumptions she feels black
men often make about her because of her skin color: "They think I'm
attractive, some kind of 'catch.'. . . For instance, I went out with this dude
recently. Mr. Fiction Writer, Would-be Lawyer, whatever. We met at a
cafe. No sooner had we sat down than he puts his arm out and says, 'Umm,
I like that. It's not often I get to go out with a person around the same
shade as I am.' I thought, 'Oh, my God, this man is colorstruck.' All he
could talk about was color, color, color. . . . I was so offended. We are just
obsessed with shade" (Anderson and Ingram 1994:360).

Color is also used to make insidious class distinctions among Latinos.
Richard Rodriguez, a California-raised Chicano, would incur his mother's
wrath when he let himself be darkened by the summer sun as a boy. "You
know how important looks are in this country. With *los gringos* looks are
all that they judge on. But you! Look at you! You're so careless! . . . You
won't be satisfied till you end up looking like *los pobres* who work in the
fields, *los braceros* [physical laborers]" (Rodriguez 1990:265).

The Commercial Imperative in the Quest for Beauty

Standards of beauty are continually evolving and proliferating, and as new
standards develop, "bodies are expected to change as well" (Freedman
1986:6). Unlike race, gender, or age, attractiveness may be considered to
some extent an "achieved" characteristic subject to change through individual intervention (Webster and Driskell 1983). As Wolf puts it, "The
beauty myth is always actually prescribing *behavior* and not appearance"
(1991:14; emphasis added). In her study of black and white Baltimore

women of various ages, both working class and middle class, Emily Martin found a common theme in ways that women discussed their health, which she summarized as "your self is separate from your body" (1989:77). Participants in Martin's study saw the body as something that must be coped with or adjusted to.

To accommodate expectations for physical appearance, women are exhorted to invest large amounts of time, money, and physical and emotional energy into their physical being. "The closer women come to power, the more physical self-consciousness and sacrifice are asked of them. 'Beauty' becomes the condition for a woman to take the next step" (Wolf 1991:28). Geraldine Ferraro, who was the first female candidate for vice president of the United States nominated by a major political party, noted in her autobiography that there were more reports on what she wore than on what she said.

Although there are many compelling theories about how the cultural preoccupation with feminine appearance evolved, it is clear that at present it is held in place by a number of very profitable industries. The average person is exposed to several hundred to several thousand advertisements per day (Moog 1990). To pitch their products, advertisers create messages that cannot immediately be recognized as advertising, selling images in the course of selling products. Two-thirds of the models who appear in magazine ads are teenagers or young adults. Although we are now seeing greater diversity in models, older people, low-income people, and people with disabilities rarely show up in advertisements because they do not project the image that the product is meant to symbolize (Glassner 1988:37). In numerous ways, advertising attacks women's self-esteem so they will purchase products and services in order to hold off bad feelings (Barthel 1988).

Most women's magazines generate much of their revenue from advertisers, who openly manipulate the content of stories. Wolf (1991:81–85) documents incidents in which advertisers canceled accounts because of editorial decisions to print stories unsupportive of their products. Ms. magazine, for example, reportedly lost a major cosmetics account after it featured Soviet women on the cover who were not wearing makeup.

Americans spend an estimated $50 billion a year on diets, cosmetics, plastic surgery, health clubs, and related gadgets (Glassner 1988:13). A review of costs of common beauty treatments itemized in a 1982 newspaper story found that a woman of means could easily rack up the bulk of an annual salary to care for her physical appearance. This entailed frequent visits to the hair salon, exercise classes, regular manicures, a home skincare program with occasional professional facials, a monthly pedicure, professional makeup session and supplies, a trip to a spa, hair removal from various parts of the body, and visits to a psychiatrist to maintain essential self-esteem (Steger 1982). The list did not include the expense of special dietary programs, cosmetic surgery or dentistry, home exercise equipment, or clothing.

As new standards of beauty expectations are created, physical appearance becomes increasingly significant, and as the expression of alternative looks are legitimized, new products are developed and existing enterprises capitalize on the trends. Liposuction, developed relatively recently, has become the most popular of the cosmetic surgery techniques. Synthetic fats have been developed, and there is now a cream claimed to reduce thigh measurements.

Weight Loss. Regardless of the actual size of their bodies, more than half of American females between ages ten and thirty are dieting, and one out of every six college women is struggling with anorexia and bulimia (Iazzetto 1992). The quest to lose weight is not limited to white, middle-class women. Iazzetto cites studies that find this pervasive concern in black women, Native American girls (75 percent trying to lose weight), and high school students (63 percent dieting). However, there may be differences among adolescent women in different groups as to how rigid their concepts of beauty are and how flexible they are regarding body image and dieting (Parker et al. 1995). Studies of primary school girls show more than half of all young girls and close to 80 percent of ten- and eleven-year-olds on diets because they consider themselves "too fat" (Greenwood 1990; Seid 1989). Analyses of the origins, symbolic meanings, and impact of our culture's obsession with thinness (Chernin 1981; Freedman 1989; Iazzetto 1988; Seid 1989) occupy much of the body-image literature.

Concern about weight and routine dieting are so pervasive in the United States that the weight-loss industry grosses more than $33 billion each year. Over 80 percent of those in diet programs are women. These programs keep growing even in the face of 90 to 95 percent failure rates in providing and maintaining significant weight loss. Congressional hearings in the early 1990s presented evidence of fraud and high failure rates in the weight-loss industry, as well as indications of severe health consequences for rapid weight loss (Iazzetto 1992). The Food and Drug Administration (FDA) has reviewed documents submitted by major weight-loss programs and found evidence of safety and efficacy to be insufficient and unscientific. An expert panel urged consumers to consider program effectiveness in choosing a weight-loss method but acknowledged lack of scientific data for making informed decisions (Brody 1992).

Fitness. Whereas in the nineteenth century some physicians recommended a sedentary lifestyle to preserve feminine beauty, in the past two decades of the twentieth century, interest in physical fitness has grown enormously. Nowhere is this change more apparent than in the gross receipts of some of the major fitness industries. In 1987, health clubs grossed $5 billion, exercise equipment $738 million (up from $5 million ten years earlier), diet foods $74 billion, and vitamin products $2.7 billion (Brand 1988). Glassner (1989) identifies several reasons for this surge of interest in fitness, including the aging of the "baby boom" cohort with its attendant desire to allay the effects of aging through exercise and diet, and the institution of "wellness" programs by corporations to reduce insurance, absentee, and inefficiency costs. A patina of health, well-toned but skinny robustness, has been folded into the dominant beauty ideal.

Clothing and Fashion. For most of us, first attempts to accomplish normative attractiveness included choosing clothing that enhanced our self-image. The oppressive effects of corsets, clothing that interfered with movement, tight shoes with high heels, and the like have been well documented (Banner 1983, 1988). Clothing represents the greatest monetary investment that women make in their appearance. Sales for *exercise* clothing alone in 1987 (including leotards, bodysuits, warm-up suits, sweats, and shoes) totaled $2.5 billion (Schefer 1988). To bolster sales, fashion leaders introduce new and different looks at regular intervals, impelling women to invest in what is currently in vogue. Occasionally the designers' new ideas are rejected wholesale, but this is generally a temporary setback. John Molloy's best-selling *Woman's Dress for Success Book* (1977) attempted to resolve this problem for women by prescribing a skirted suit "uniform" that women could wear at work much like the standardized clothing that businessmen wear. He was able to demonstrate its utility in allowing women to project themselves as competent and effective in the workplace. Furthermore, to the extent that women who worked outside the home adopted this outfit, they would not become prey to the vagaries and expense of rapidly shifting fashion. The clothing industry orchestrated a wholesale attack on Molloy's strategy, labeling his uniform unfeminine, and another sensible strategy failed (Wolf 1991:43-45).

Cosmetics. The average person in North America uses more than twenty-five pounds of cosmetics, soaps, and toiletries each year (Decker 1983). The cosmetics industry produces over twenty thousand products containing thousands of chemicals, and it grosses over $20 billion annually (Becker 1991; Wolf 1991). Stock in cosmetics manufacturers has been rising 15 percent a year, in large part because of depressed petroleum prices. The oil derivative ethanol is the base for most products (Wolf 1991:82, 307). Profit margins for products are over 50 percent (McKnight 1989). Widespread false claims for cosmetics were virtually unchallenged for fifty years after the FDA became responsible for cosmetic industry oversight in 1938, and even now, the industry remains largely unregulated (Kaplan 1994). Various manufacturers assert that their goods can "retard aging," "repair the skin," or "restructure the cell." "Graphic evidence" of "visible improvement" when applying a "barrier" against "eroding effects" provides a pastiche of some familiar advertising catchphrases (Wolf 1991:109-10).

The FDA has no authority to require cosmetics firms to register their existence, to release their formulas, to report adverse reactions, or to show evidence of safety and effectiveness before marketing their products (Gilhooley 1978; Kaplan 1994). Authorizing and funding the FDA to regulate the cosmetics industry would allow some means of protecting consumers from the use of dangerous products.

Cosmetic Surgery. In interviews with cosmetic surgeons and users of their services, Dull and West (1991) found that the line between reconstructive plastic surgery (repair of deformities caused congenitally or by injury or disease) and aesthetic surgery has begun to blur. Doctors and their patients are viewing unimpaired features as defective and the desire to "correct" them as intrinsic to women's nature, rather than as a cultural imperative.

Because of an oversupply of plastic surgeons, the profession has made efforts to expand existing markets through advertising and by appeals to women of color. Articles encouraging "enhancement of ethnic beauty" have begun to appear, but they focus on westernizing Asian eyelids and chiseling African American noses. As Bordo (1993:25) points out, this technology serves to promote commonality rather than diversity.

Plastic surgery has been moving strongly in the direction of making appearance a bona fide medical problem. This has been played out dramatically in recent times in the controversy regarding silicone breast implants, which provides plastic surgeons with a substantial amount of income. Used for thirty years in hundreds of thousands of women (80 percent for cosmetic augmentation), the effects of breast implants have only recently begun to be studied to determine their health consequences over long periods (Zones 1992). In a petition to the FDA in 1982 to circumvent regulation requiring proof of safety and effectiveness of the implants, the American Society of Plastic and Reconstructive Surgeons stated, "There is a common misconception that the enlargement of the female breast is not necessary for maintenance of health or treatment of disease. There is a substantial and enlarging body of medical information and opinion, however, to the effect that these *deformities* [small breasts] are really a disease which in most patients result in feelings of inadequacy . . . due to a lack of self-perceived femininity. The enlargement of the underdeveloped female breast is, therefore, often very necessary to insure an improved quality of life for the patient" (Porterfield 1982:4–5; emphasis added).

Cosmetic surgeon James Billie of Arkansas, who claims to have operated on over fifteen thousand beauty contestants in the past ten years, maintains that three-quarters of Miss USA pageant contestants have undergone plastic surgery (Garchik 1992). Cosmetic surgery generates over a third of a billion dollars per year for practitioners, some of whom offer overnight household financing for patients. The hefty interest rates are returned in part to the surgeons by the finance corporation (Krieger 1989). Although cosmetic surgery is the biggest commercial contender in the medical realm, prescription drugs are increasingly lucrative ventures (such as Retin-A to reduce wrinkling skin, and hormones to promote growth in short boys and retard it in tall girls).

Health Risks in Quest of Beauty

Physicians and medical institutions have been quoted as associating beauty with health and ugliness with disease. Dr. Daniel Tostesen of Harvard Medical School, whose research is supported by Shiseido, an expensive cosmetics line, claims that there is a "'subtle and continuous gradation' between health and medical interests on the one hand, and 'beauty and well-being on the other'" (Wolf 1991:227). The imperative to look attractive, while promising benefits in self-esteem, often entails both serious mental and physical health risks.

Mental Health. For most women, not adhering to narrow, standardized appearance expectations causes insecurity and distraction, but for many, concerns about appearance can have serious emotional impact. Up until adolescence, boys and girls experience about the same rates of depression, but at around age twelve, girls' rates of depression begin to increase more rapidly. A study of over eight hundred high school students found that a prime factor in this disparity is girls' preoccupation with appearance. In discussing the study, the authors concluded that "if adolescent girls felt as physically attractive, effective, and generally good about themselves as their male peers did, they would not experience so much depression" (Allgood-Merten, Lewinsohn, and Hops 1990:61). Another study of the impact of body image on onset and persistence of depression in adolescent girls found that whereas a relatively positive body image does not seem to offer substantial protection against the occurrence of depression, it does seem to decrease the likelihood that depression will be persistent (Rierdan and Koff 1991; Rierdan, Koff, and Stubbs 1989).

Physical Health. Perceived or actual variation from society's ideal takes a physical toll, too. High school and college-age females who were judged to be in the bottom half of their group in terms of attractiveness had significantly higher blood pressure than the young women in the top half. The relationship between appearance and blood pressure was not found for males in the same age group (Hansell, Sparacino, and Ronchi 1982).

Low bodyweight has been heavily promoted as a life-prolonging characteristic. There is evidence to support this contention, but the effect of advocating low weight in collusion with the heavy cultural prescription for a very slender look has led people into cycles of weight loss and regained weight that may act as an independent risk factor for cardiovascular disease (Bouchard 1991). A recent review of the medical literature on weight fluctuation concludes that the potential health benefits of moderate weight loss in obese people, however, is greater than the known risks of "yo-yo dieting" (National Task Force 1994). Women constitute 90 percent of people with anorexia, an eating disorder that can cause serious injury or death. The incidence of anorexia has grown dramatically since the mid-1970s, paralleling the social imperative of thinness (Bordo 1986).

There are direct risks related to using commodities to alter appearance. According to the Consumer Products Safety Commission, more than 200,000 people visit emergency rooms each year as a result of cosmetics-related health problems (Becker 1991). Clothing has its perils as well. In recent years, meralgia paresthetica, marked by sciatica, pain in the hip and thigh region, with tingling and itchy skin, has made an appearance among young women in the form of "skin-tight jean syndrome" (Gateless and

Gilroy 1984). In earlier times, the same problems have arisen with the use of girdles, belts, and shoulder bags. The National Safety Council revealed that in 1989 over 100,000 people were injured by their clothing and another 44,000 by their jewelry (Seligson 1992). These figures greatly underestimate actual medical problems.

Approximately 33 to 50 percent of all adult women have used hair coloring agents. Evidence over the past twenty-five years has shown that chemicals used in manufacturing hair dyes cause cancers in animals (Center 1979). Scientists at the National Cancer Institute (NCI) recently reported a significantly greater risk of cancers of the lymph system and of a form of cancer affecting bone marrow, multiple myeloma, in women who use hair coloring (Zahm et al. 1992). In the last twenty years, the incidence of non-Hodgkin's lymphoma in the United States increased by more than 50 percent largely as a result of immune deficiency caused by HIV. However, the NCI researchers conclude that, assuming a causal relationship, hair coloring product use accounts for a larger percentage of non-Hodgkin's lymphoma among women than any other risk factor. These conclusions have been challenged, however, by more recent research (Fackelmann 1994).

Because no cosmetic products require follow-up research for safety and effectiveness, virtually anything can be placed on the market without regard to potential health effects. Even devices implanted in the body, which were not regulated before 1978, can remain on the market for years without appropriate testing. During the decade of controversy over regulating silicone breast implants, the American Society of Plastic and Reconstructive Surgeons vehemently denied any need for controlled studies of the implant in terms of long-term safety. The society spent hundreds of thousands of dollars of its members' money in a public relations effort to avoid the imposition of requirements for such research to the detriment of investing in the expensive scientific follow-up needed (Zones 1992). Although case reports indicate a potential relationship between the implants and connective tissue diseases, recent medical reports discount the association. Definitive research will take more time to assuage women's fears.

Health consequences of beauty products extend beyond their impact on individuals. According to the San Francisco Bay Area Air Quality Management District, aerosols release 25 tons of pollution every day. Almost half of that is from hairsprays. Although aerosols no longer use chlorofluorocarbons (CFCs), which are the greatest cause of depletion of the upper atmosphere ozone layer, aerosol hydrocarbons in hairsprays are a primary contributor to smog and ground pollution.

The Beauty of Diversity

Both personal transformation and policy intervention will be necessary to allow women to present themselves freely. Governmental institutions, including courts and regulatory agencies, need to accord personal and product liability related to appearance products and services the attention they require to ensure public health and safety. The legal system must develop well-defined case law to assist the court in determining inequitable treatment based on appearance discrimination.

Short of complete liberation from limitations imposed by appearance expectations, women will continue to attempt to "improve" appearance to better social relations. Ultimately, however, this is a futile struggle because of the depth and intensity of feelings and assumptions that have become attached to physical appearance. The predominant advice given to women in the body-image literature is to seek therapeutic assistance to transform damaged self-image into a more positive perspective on oneself. Brown (1985) recommends a social context in which such transformation can take place, as does Schwichtenberg (1989), who suggests that, failing women's unified rejection of costly and potentially dangerous beauty products and processes, women should band together into support networks. Lesbian communities have led the way, showing how mutual support can diminish the effects of the dominant society on women. By using supportive relationships as an arena to experiment with physical presence, women create a manageable and enjoyable social situation. The Black Women's Health Project has successfully modeled the formation of local support groups to encourage members to lead healthier lives. Having a small group as referents reduces the power of commercial interests to define beauty standards. Overweight women have created such resources in the form of national alliances (such as the National Association to Advance Fat Acceptance), magazines (such as *Radiance*), and regional support systems (Iazzetto 1992).

The personal solution to individual self-doubt or even self-loathing of our physical being is to continuously make the decision to contradict the innumerable messages we are given that we are anything less than lovely as human beings. Pinkney (1994) suggests several ways to reshape "a raggedy body image" by improving self-perception: respect yourself, search for the source of the distress, strut your strengths, and embrace the aging process. In a passage from *Beloved,* Toni Morrison demonstrates the way: "Love your hands! Love them. Raise them up and kiss them. Touch others with them, pat them together, stroke them on your face 'cause they don't love that either. *You* got to love it, *you!*" (1994:362).

REFERENCES

Allgood-Merten, Betty, Peter M. Lewinsohn, and Hyman Hops
    1990   "Sex differences and adolescent depression." Journal of Abnormal Psychology 99:55-63.

Anderson, Michele, and Tamara Ingram
    1994   "Color, color, color." Pp. 356-61 in Evelyn C. White (ed.), The Black Women's Health Book, rev. ed. Seattle: Seal Press.

Aune, R. Kelly, and Krystyna S. Aune
    1994   "The influence of culture, gender and relational status on appearance management." Journal of Cross-Cultural Psychology 25(2):258-72.

Banner, Lois W.
    1983   American Beauty. Chicago: University of Chicago Press.

Barthel, Diane
    1988   Putting on Appearances: Gender and Advertising. Philadelphia: Temple University Press.

Beauvoir, Simone de
    1972   The Coming of Age. New York: Putnam.

Becker, Hilton
    1991   "Cosmetics: saving face at what price?" Annals of Plastic Surgery 26:171-73.

Bordo, Susan
    1986   "Anorexia nervosa: psychopathology as the crystallization of culture." Philosophical Forum 17:73-104.
    1993   Unbearable Weight: Feminism, Western Culture and the Body. Berkeley: University of California Press.

Bouchard, Claude
    1991   "Is weight fluctuation a risk factor?" New England Journal of Medicine 324:1887-89.

Brand, David
    1988   "A nation of health worrywarts?" Time, 25 July, 66.

Brody, Jane E.
    1992   "Panel criticizes weight-loss programs." New York Times, 2 April, A10.

Brown, Laura S.
    1985   "Women, weight, and power: feminist theoretical and therapeutic issues." Women and Therapy 4:61-71.

Chapkis, Wendy
    1986   Beauty Secrets: Women and the Politics of Appearance. Boston: South End Press.
Chernin, Kim
    1981   The Obsession: Reflections on the Tyranny of Slenderness. New York: Harper Colophon Books.
Cimons, Marlene
    1990   "Most Americans dislike their looks, poll finds." Los Angeles Times, 19 August, A4.
Cunningham, Michael R.
    1986   "Measuring the physical in physical attractiveness: quasi-experiments on the sociobiology of female facial beauty." Journal of Personality and Social Psychology 50:925–35.
Davis, Fred
    1992   Fashion, Culture and Identity. Chicago: University of Chicago Press.
Decker, Ruth
    1983   "The not-so-pretty risks of cosmetics." Medical Self-Care (Summer):25–31.
Dion, Karen, Ellen Berscheid, and Elaine Walster
    1972   "What is beautiful is good." Journal of Personality and Social Psychology 24:285–90.
Dull, Diana, and Candace West
    1991   "Accounting for cosmetic surgery: the accomplishment of gender." Social Problems 38:54–70.
Elder, Glen H., Jr.
    1969   "Appearance and education in marriage mobility." American Sociological Review 34:519–33.
Fackelmann, K. A.
    1994   "Mixed news on hair dyes and cancer risk." Science News 145 (5 Feb.):86.
Fallon, April E., and Paul Rozin
    1985   "Sex differences in perceptions of desirable body shape." Journal of Abnormal Psychology 94:102–5.
Freedman, Rita
    1986   Beauty Bound. Lexington, MA: Lexington Books.
    1989   Bodylove. New York: Harper and Row.
Garchik, Leah
    1992   "Knife tricks come to the rescue." San Francisco Chronicle, 1 September, C5.
Gateless, Doreen, and John Gilroy
    1984   "Tight-jeans meralgia: hot or cold?" Journal of the American Medical Association 252:42–43.
Gaudoin, Tina
    1994   "Is all-American beauty un-American?" Mirabella (Sept.):144–46.

Gilhooley, Margaret
    1978   "Federal regulation of cosmetics: an overview." Food Drug Cosmetic Law
            Journal 33:231-38.
Glassner, Barry
    1988   Bodies: Why We Look the Way We Do (and How We Feel about It).
            New York: Putnam.
    1989   "Fitness and the postmodern self." Journal of Health and Social Behavior
            30:180-91.
Goffman, Erving
    1963   Stigma: Notes on the Management of Spoiled Identity. Englewood Cliffs,
            NJ: Prentice-Hall.
Goldman, William, and Philip Lewis
    1977   "Beautiful is good: evidence that the physically attractive are more so-
            cially skillful." Journal of Experimental and Social Psychology 13:125-30.
Grealy, Lucy
    1994   Autobiography of a Face. Boston: Houghton Mifflin.
Greenwood, M. R. C.
    1990   "The feminine ideal: a new perspective." UC Davis Magazine (July):8-11.
Hansell, Stephen, J. Sparacino, and D. Ronchi
    1982   "Physical attractiveness and blood pressure: sex and age differences."
            Personality and Social Psychology Bulletin 8:113-21.
Iazzetto, Demetria
    1988   "Women and body image: reflections in the fun house mirror." Pp. 34-53
            in Carol J. Leppa and Connie Miller (eds.), Women's Health Perspec-
            tives: An Annual Review. Volcano, CA: Volcano Press.
    1992   "What's happening with women and body image?" National Women's
            Health Network News:1, 6, 7.
Iliffe, A. H.
    1960   "A study of preferences in feminine beauty." British Journal of Psychology
            51:267-73.
Johnson, Douglas F.
    1985   "Appearance and the elderly." Pp. 152-60 in Jean Ann Graham and
            Albert M. Kligman (eds.), The Psychology of Cosmetic Treatments. New
            York: Praeger.
Kaiser, Susan B., Carla Freeman, and Stacy B. Wingate
    1984   "Stigmata and negotiated outcomes: the management of appearance by
            persons with physical disabilities." Annual meeting of the American
            Sociological Association, San Antonio, TX.
Kaplan, Sheila
    1994   "The ugly face of the cosmetics lobby." Ms. (Jan.-Feb.):88-89.
Krieger, Lisa M.
    1989   "Fix your nose now, pay later." San Francisco Examiner, 30 October, 1.
Lakoff, Robin Tolmach, and Raquel L. Scherr
    1984   Face Value: The Politics of Beauty. Boston: Routledge and Kegan Paul.

Langlois, Judith H., Lori A. Roggman, and Loretta A. Rieser-Danner
   1990   "Infants' differential social responses to attractive and unattractive faces."
           Developmental Psychology 26:153–59.
Langlois, Judith H., Jean M. Ritter, Lori A. Roggman, and Lesley S. Vaughn
   1991   "Facial diversity and infant preferences for attractive faces." Developmen-
           tal Psychology 27:79–84.
Lipsky, Suzanne
   1987   Internalized Racism. Seattle: Rational Island.
Martin, Emily
   1989   The Woman in the Body: A Cultural Analysis of Reproduction. Boston:
           Beacon Press.
Mathes, Eugene W., and Arnold Kahn
   1975   "Physical attractiveness, happiness, neuroticism, and self-esteem." Jour-
           nal of Psychology 90:27–30.
Mathes, Eugene W., Susan M. Brennan, Patricia M. Haugen, and Holly B. Rice
   1985   "Ratings of physical attractiveness as a function of age." Journal of Social
           Psychology 125:157–68.
McKnight, Gerald
   1989   The Skin Game: The International Beauty Business Brutally Exposed.
           London: Sidgwick and Jackson.
Mercer, Kobena
   1990   "Black hair/style politics." Pp. 247–64 in Russell Ferguson, Martha Gever,
           Trinh T. Minh-ha, and Cornel West (eds.), Out There: Marginalization
           and Contemporary Cultures. Cambridge: MIT Press.
Molloy, John T.
   1977   The Woman's Dress for Success Book. New York: Warner Books.
Moog, Carol
   1990   Are They Selling Her Lips? Advertising and Identity. New York: William
           Morrow.
Morrison, Toni
   1994   "We flesh." P. 362 in Evelyn C. White (ed.), The Black Women's Health
           Book, rev. ed. Seattle: Seal Press.
Morton, Patricia
   1991   Disfigured Images: The Historical Assault on Afro-American Women.
           New York: Praeger.
Murstein, Bernard I.
   1972   "Physical attractiveness and marital choice." Journal of Personality and
           Social Psychology 22:8–12.
National Task Force on the Prevention and Treatment of Obesity
   1994   "Weight cycling." Journal of the American Medical Association
           272(15):1196–1202.
Parker, Sheila, Mimi Nichter, Mark Nichter, Nancy Vuckovic, Colette Sims, and
Cheryl Ritenbaugh
   1995   "Body image and weight concerns among African American and white

adolescent females: differences that make a difference." Human Organization 54(2):103-13.

Patzer, Gordon L.
1985   The Physical Attractiveness Phenomena. New York: Plenum Press.

Penner, Louis A., J. Kevin Thompson, and Dale L. Coovert
1991   "Size overestimation among anorexics: much ado about very little?" Journal of Abnormal Psychology 100:90-93.

Perrett, D. I., K. A. May, and S. Yoshikawa
1994   "Facial shape and judgments of female attractiveness." Nature 368:239-42.

Pinkney, Deborah Shelton
1994   "Body check." Heart and Soul (Summer):50-55.

Porterfield, H. William
1982   Comments of the American Society of Plastic and Reconstructive Surgeons on the Proposed Classification of Inflatable Breast Prosthesis and Silicone Gel-Filled Breast Prosthesis, submitted to the Food and Drug Administration. Washington, 1 July.

Rierdan, Jill, and Elissa Koff
1991   "Depressive symptomatology among very early maturing girls." Journal of Youth and Adolescence 20:415-515.

Rierdan, Jill, Elissa Koff, and Margaret L. Stubbs
1989   "Timing of menarche, preparation, and initial menstrual experience: replication and further analyses in a prospective study." Journal of Youth and Adolescence 18:413-26.

Robinson, Jennifer
1983   "Body image in women over forty." Melpomene Institute Bulletin 2:12-14.

Rodriguez, Richard
1990   "Complexion." Pp. 265-78 in Russell Ferguson, Martha Gever, Trinh T. Minh-ha, and Cornel West (eds.), Out There: Marginalization and Contemporary Cultures. Cambridge: MIT Press.

Rothblum, Esther
1990   "Women and weight: fad and fiction." Journal of Psychology 124:5-24.

Rozin, Paul, and April E. Fallon
1988   "Body image, attitudes to weight, and misperceptions of figure preferences of the opposite sex: a comparison of men and women in two generations." Journal of Abnormal Psychology 97:342-45.

Rubenstein, Steve
1984   "Cosmetic queen tells her women to think pink." San Francisco Chronicle, 3 February, 5.

Schefer, Dorothy
1988   "Beauty: The real cost of looking good." Vogue (Nov.):157-68.

Schwichtenberg, Cathy
1989   "The 'mother lode' of feminist research: congruent paradigms in the analysis of beauty culture." Pp. 291-306 in Brenda Dervin, Lawrence

Grossberg, Barbara J. O'Keefe, and Ellen Wartella (eds.), Rethinking Communication. Newbury Park, CA: Sage.

Seid, Roberta Pollack
    1989   Never Too Thin: Why Women Are at War with Their Bodies. New York: Prentice Hall.

Seligson, Susan
    1992   "The attack bra and other vicious clothes." San Francisco Chronicle, 13 January, D3-D4.

Shulman, Alix Kates
    1972   Memoirs of an Ex-Prom Queen. New York: Bantam Books.

Steger, Pat
    1982   "The making of a BP: how to diet, polish and pay your way to well-groomed perfection." San Francisco Chronicle, 3 August, 15.

Taylor, Patricia Ann, and Norval D. Glenn
    1976   "The utility of education and attractiveness for females' status attainment through marriage." American Sociological Review 41:484-98.

Thompson, J. Kevin, and Jefferey J. Dolce
    1989   "The discrepancy between emotional vs. rational estimates of body size, actual size, and ideal body ratings: theoretical and clinical implications." Journal of Clinical Psychology 45:473-78.

Udry, J. Richard
    1977   "The importance of being beautiful: a reexamination and racial comparison." American Journal of Sociology 83:154-60.

Udry, J. Richard, and Bruce K. Eckland
    1984   "Benefits of being attractive: Differential payoffs for men and women." Psychological Reports 54:47-56.

Veblen, Thorstein
    [1899] The Theory of the Leisure Class. Boston: Houghton Mifflin.
    1973

Walker, Alice
    1988   "Oppressed hair puts a ceiling on the brain." Ms. 16(6):52-53.
    1990   "Beauty: when the other dancer is the self." Pp. 280-87 in Evelyn C. White (ed.), The Black Women's Health Book. Seattle: Seal Press.

Webster, Murray, Jr., and James E. Driskell Jr.
    1983   "Beauty as status." American Journal of Sociology 89:140-65.

Wolf, Naomi
    1991   The Beauty Myth: How Images of Beauty Are Used against Women. New York: William Morrow.

Zahm, Sheila Hoar, Dennis D. Weisenburger, Paula A. Babbitt, et al.
    1992   "Use of hair coloring products and the risk of lymphoma, multiple myeloma, and chronic lymphocytic leukemia." American Journal of Public Health 82:990-97.

Zones, Jane Sprague
    1992   "The political and social context of silicone breast implant use in the United States." Journal of Long-Term Effects of Medical Implants 1:225-41.

[11]

Old Woes, Old Ways, New Dawn:
Native American Women's Health Issues

ANN METCALF

Anthropologist Ann Metcalf puts the health of Indian women into historical context by tracing the history of colonization, the role of the Bureau of Indian Affairs, and recent migration from reservations to urban areas. She addresses how recent attention to women and alcohol has lead to blaming women for alcohol problems, but she also argues that new ways must be found to help women. Her description of culture matching and culture cultivating treatment modalities illustrate what may be involved in making behavioral interventions more than superficially culturally appropriate.

Statistics detailing the continued economic and social disadvantage of American Indians abound, and in many ways Native American health status differs little from that of other groups caught in cycles of poverty and discrimination. There are, however, some very important characteristics that set Native Americans off from other groups and that set Native American women apart from other members of their communities. In addition, there are important differences in health status among Native American women themselves that are related to their varying patterns of social and cultural characteristics. Here I will outline those differences, comment on their significance, and conclude with implications for the future of Native American women's health.

Old Woes

Review of Indian Policy

It is necessary to begin any discussion of the current status of Native Americans with a review of federal Indian policy.[1] Such a discussion can serve several purposes in understanding health issues affecting Native American women. First, federal policy has had a significant impact on the delivery of health care services to Native Americans; second, the etiology of many health problems, especially those that come under the rubric "mental health," can be directly traced to federal policy; and finally, federal policy has had an important impact on defining and redefining differences within the Native American population, differences which in turn have affected Indian women's health.

Treaty Rights. One of the most important distinctions between Native Americans and other ethnic groups is the special relationship that Indians have had historically with the federal government. This relationship, known as sovereignty, is based on treaty law and gives Indians certain assurances that do not legally extend to other citizens. The federal government must see to it that these assurances are indeed carried out. Most Native Americans interpret this special relationship as including the right to federally provided health care.

Treaty law, sovereignty, and the trust relationship are often difficult for non-Indians to understand and can create confusion among service providers and resentment from other ethnic groups. These principles of Indian policy have roots in the relationships that were established between the various European nations and the Native American groups they encountered during the colonial period. To gain access to Indian lands or to secure individual tribes as allies in their struggles with one another, European nations negotiated treaties with tribes. The treaties were made on the same principles that operated when one European nation dealt with another; that is, Indian groups were identified as sovereign nations with clear rights to their own territories and internal political control. In exchange for Native American "rights" (mostly those to land), Europeans offered other "rights" (usually dealing with trade).

After the American Revolution, the concept of treaty rights for Indians was firmly established and became a part of the United States Constitution. The implications were far-reaching, setting up the federal government as the only entity that had the power to deal with Indians; states could not, municipalities could not, individuals could not without the express approval and/or involvement of Congress. Treaty law can be seen as something of a gigantic real estate deal where, in exchange for being forced to give up a continent, Native Americans were granted certain services in perpetuity, "as long as the grass shall grow and the rivers shall flow." The fact that, almost without exception, the treaties were broken does nothing to invalidate them as legal documents, and Indians recently have been able to win court cases based on these early agreements. Treaty making was officially halted in 1871 and was replaced by congressional statute law. The principle of federal trust responsibility survived, however.

Treaty Rights to Health Care. The first mention of health care as a part of the trust responsibility came in 1836 in a treaty with the Ottawa and Chippewa (Ojibwe) nations. In exchange for giving up land, the Indians were granted annual payments for vaccines, medicines, and services of physicians—provided, of course, that they stayed on their reservations and did not bother the white settlers. Since that time, similar clauses have been included in treaties and statutes until health care has become a clearly established right in the eyes of Native Americans.

Furthermore, Indians have their own federally financed, federally staffed, and federally run health care provider, the U.S. Indian Health Service (IHS). Other U.S. citizens, even those entitled to Medicaid or similar programs, do not go to a federal facility to get care. Instead, the government helps them pay for care at private, state, or community facilities. The only other federally run health service is for the military and its related agencies. Health care for Indians is not linked to employment (as is the case for most private health insurance programs), it is not linked to age or special infirmities (as is the case for Medicare or government-funded disability programs), and it is not linked to past military service (as is the case with the Veterans Administration program). It is simply a right due to Indians.

It should be noted that Indians are eligible, should they meet the criteria, for any and all other forms of health care as well; the elderly are eligible for Medicare, veterans are eligible for VA benefits, employed persons receive their company policy, and so on. This situation has caused confusion and not a little rivalry among the various health care systems. The question of which system to charge for medical services to Indians has had important consequences affecting Indians' access to medical care, a point to which I will return later.

Shifts in Service Delivery. Originally, federal health care services (like all other guaranteed services) were geared toward reservation Indians. The agency responsible for delivering them was the Bureau of Indian Affairs (BIA), which is a part of the Department of the Interior. In the 1950s, that responsibility shifted to the Public Health Service in the (then)

Department of Health, Education, and Welfare for a variety of reasons, not all of them sympathetic to Indian treaty rights.

One reason frequently given for the transfer of Indian Health Service (IHS) from the Bureau into the Public Health Service was the abysmal state of Native American health in the 1950s. For example, infant mortality was 53.7 per 1,000 compared with 27.1 for all Americans. The average age at death was 41.8 compared with 62.3 for the rest of the population. Leading causes of death included intestinal infections (about eight times the national average), accidents, homicide, influenza and pneumonia (all at about three times the national average), and cirrhosis (twice the national average). On the other hand, deaths due to heart disease, stroke, or cancer were only about half the national average (Brophy and Aberle 1966).

These figures present some very disturbing trends. First, the things that Native Americans were dying from either were preventable given good medical care (e.g., antibiotics and good sanitation) or were related to severe sociocultural stress (e.g., accidents, homicide, cirrhosis). Second, Indians were not dying from diseases of old age; they simply were not living long.

These statistics became part of the rationale for shifting Indian health into PHS. Whenever the "plight" of Native Americans is discovered or rediscovered, a certain amount of Bureau bashing seems to be in order; that is, Indians, the general public, and policymakers all put the blame on the BIA for not doing its job. One solution is to put some other agency in charge. In the case of Indian health, the Public Health Service seemed a likely candidate. But there was another and perhaps more important reason—from the policymakers' viewpoint—for making the move. That other reason is known in Indian country as Termination.

Termination Policies. Termination refers to a set of policies enacted after World War II aimed at abrogating or "terminating" Native American treaty rights and the federal trust relationship. The policy was pushed by congressmen from western states who had the most to gain from the defederalization of Indian lands and by conservative budget cutters recoiling from the Roosevelt administration. Besides the severance of federal ties to specific tribes (over one hundred were cut off from their treaty-derived relationship with the federal government), Termination also included policies aimed at decreasing services to Indians. The transfer of Indian Health Service into PHS is an example of the latter because it was thought by the architects of the policy that such action would eventually lead to the termination of health care rights for American Indians.

What in fact happened is considerably more complicated. The Indian Health Service, in its new home in Public Health, did some impressive work. New sanitation programs on reservations decreased the numbers of Indians affected by bacterial infections and tuberculosis; access to newly constructed clinics and hospitals meant that infant mortality and diseases of early childhood were reduced (as well as maternal death rate); and average life span was increased. For example, infant mortality decreased by 69 percent from the 1950s to the 1970s, hospital admissions for tuberculosis declined by 95 percent, and life expectancy rose to sixty-five years (U.S. Indian Health Service 1980:20).

Relocation: From Reservation to City. The Termination-era policy with perhaps the most lasting and serious consequences for Native Americans was Relocation. The premise was simple: get Indians into the city and, as one congressman put it, "get out of the Indian business" (the late Senator Watkins of Utah as quoted in Bryant 1969). Under Relocation, thousands of Indians were moved off reservations and into urban areas in a federally subsidized program. In 1950, before the policy was officially established, only 16.3 percent of Indians lived off reservations in urban areas (Neils 1971:19); by 1980, 54 percent did (Office of Technology Assessment 1986:4).

Relocation cuts at the heart of the sovereignty principle. Do urban Indians have the same rights as reservation Indians? With respect to health care, must the IHS minister to urban Indians? And, in particular, how has this policy affected women's health?

Relocation usually involved a six-month program of job training, subsidized housing, and certain benefits including a medical insurance program. After six months, Indians were on their own as far as the BIA was concerned. If they were employed, they would be covered by their employee benefits. More often than not, however, they were unemployed. If they sought treatment from city or county facilities, the officials there were likely to refer them back to the BIA. The BIA countered that they were no longer covered. What ensued was a ping-pong ball situation resulting in little care for Indians in need.

Because of these situations, in the 1970s urban Indians pressured the IHS to extend services to Indians in the city. Now, most major relocation centers have some form of IHS-supported facilities. Some are connected to nearby rural or reservation programs such as Seattle's Indian Health

Board; some are geared to specific kinds of services such as Oakland's alcoholism treatment center; most receive only partial funding from the IHS and exploit other resources such as Medicaid.

The Issue of Eligibility. Termination as an official policy ended in the early 1970s, and Relocation ended in 1980; however, the legacy remains. Because the federal government has been unsuccessful in phasing out health services to Indians on a programmatic basis, it is attempting to do so on an individual basis. Recent policy changes have focused on tightening eligibility rules.

Initially, Indian Health Service established hospitals on reservations to serve the resident population. All Indians living on the reservation were eligible for service. Budget constrictions, changing demographic trends, and the persistent push toward assimilation have changed that simple equation. Now the concern is "Who is a 'real' Indian?" In other words, who is eligible for services?

Indianness has been officially defined by the Bureau and the IHS as the amount of "blood quantum" an individual possesses. Full-blood means that all four of one's grandparents were Indian, half-blood means at least two grandparents were, and so forth. Most tribes maintain official rolls that list individuals according to their blood quantum. Tribes differ as to how much blood quantum is required for membership, but the use of the concept is an accepted criterion for enrollment in most federally recognized tribes and has become a standard classification used by Indians and non-Indians alike.

It should be noted that blood quantum as officially defined is at best a quasi-definition of Indian; it does not take into consideration differences in cultural behavior or sense of allegiance to the group. For example, an Indian who was adopted into a non-Indian home as an infant may have no sense of ethnic identity as a Native American, although her blood quantum is full-blood; whereas, a quarter-blood who grew up on the reservation, speaks the native language, and participates in tribal ceremonies is sociologically more "Indian." Given these distinctions, who should be eligible for services under IHS guidelines?

Most Indian-run programs, including those that have partial funding from the IHS, define an Indian as one who is recognized as such by the community. The IHS, however, maintains that an Indian eligible for services is one who is enrolled in a federally recognized tribe and is quarter-blood if on the reservation or half-blood if residing off the reservation. Furthermore, IHS has begun to issue plastic identity cards, similar to those used by many health insurance providers. To receive services, an individual must produce a card. What this means is that members of all nonfederally recognized tribes can be classed as ineligible (that includes tribes who were terminated as well as those who were never officially recognized). It also means that Indians in the cities are placed under more stringent requirements than those on the reservation.

Complicating the eligibility issue is the question of whether or not access to medical care is an entitlement for Indians. As pointed out above, the concept of treaty law and trust responsibility would argue that it is. However, IHS regulations stipulate that it is a "residual provider," meaning that all other sources of funding must be exhausted before IHS will pay. What happens is that IHS will treat Indians in its facilities and then try to bill other sources, such as private insurers, Medicaid, and county resources, for the treatment. The problem is that some of those other resources, especially county and state facilities, also consider themselves to be residual providers and try in turn to bill the IHS. Technically, Congress is the only constitutional body with the authority to solve this dilemma, but given the recession-ridden economy in recent years, it is not likely to do so soon. Meanwhile, access to medical care for Native Americans is further hampered.

The shift in eligibility requirements is especially difficult for Indian women in the city and their children. Many tribes only enroll members who are born on the reservation; therefore, urban Indian women must travel to the reservation to have their babies if they want them enrolled. Further, Indian women in the city are much more likely to marry non-Indian men than are their reservation counterparts; therefore, their children are more likely to be less than half-blood. The overall result in the policy shift is that fewer and fewer Indian children, especially those born in the city, are eligible for IHS services. Eligibility requirements can thus be seen as the Termination policy of the 1980s and 1990s.

Current Health Status

To put health statistics in perspective, it is important to take an overall look at the socioeconomic status of Native Americans. As a group, Indians are more likely to be poor, unemployed, and undereducated than other U.S. populations. Table 11.1 gives selected statistics derived from the 1990 census. Median family income is less than half that of the nation as a whole, the percentage of individuals living below the poverty line is

TABLE 11.1

Selected Characteristics of the American Indian Population as Compared with the U.S. Total Population, 1990

Characteristic	American Indian	U.S. Total
Median family income	$14,886	$30,056
% Poverty rate of persons	31.6	13.1
% Unemployed		
Male	16.2	6.4
Female	13.5	6.4
% College graduates	9.0	20.3

Source: U.S. Indian Health Service (USIHS) 1994, 32, table 2.5.

2.4 times the national average, and unemployment is twice as high as for non-Indians. All of these factors, of course, impinge on health status.

Life expectancy for American Indians went from 61.0 in 1972 to 73.2 in 1990. Life expectancy for non-Indians in 1990 was 75.4, yielding a ratio of 0.97 of Indian to non-Indian (USIHS 1994:77, table 4.33). The increase in life expectancy can largely be explained by consistent decreases in maternal death rates and infant mortality rates, especially since the 1970s. Infant mortality decreased by 54 percent, and the maternal death rate fell 65 percent (USIHS 1994:79).

Indians have one of the highest birth rates of any U.S. population (28.1 for Indians versus 16.7 for non-Indians), making them a relatively young and rapidly growing population. In 1990, 34 percent of the Indian population was under fifteen years of age whereas only 6 percent was over sixty-four. Comparable figures for non-Indians were 22 percent and 13 percent, respectively (USIHS 1994:29).

Although the life expectancy figures are encouraging, given the skewed age distribution of the Native American population, data from age-adjusted death rates provide a more detailed look at Indian/non-Indian differences.[2] Of the ten leading causes of death for Indians, six are above the national average. Four of these are related to sociocultural stress factors: accidents (2.6 times the national average), cirrhosis (3.5 times), homicide (1.5 times), and suicide (1.4 times). Diabetes (2.5 times the national average) appears to be related to such environmental factors as diet and nutrition including alcohol abuse, whereas pneumonia and

TABLE 11.2
Age-Adjusted Death Rates for Leading Cause of Death among American Indians Compared with Rates for U.S. Total Population, 1990

American Indian Leading Cause of Death	American Indian Rate	U.S. Total Rate	Ratio of Indian to U.S. Total
1. Heart disease	132.1	152.0	0.9
2. Accidents	86.0	32.5	2.6
3. Malignant neoplasms	94.5	135.0	0.7
4. Diabetes mellitus	29.7	11.7	2.5
5. Liver disease/Cirrhosis	30.3	8.6	3.5
6. Cerebrovascular diseases	25.2	27.7	0.9
7. Pneumonia/Influenza	20.5	14.0	1.5
8. Suicide	16.5	11.5	1.4
9. Homicide	15.3	10.2	1.5
10. Pulmonary diseases	13.8	19.7	0.7

Source: U.S. Indian Health Service (USIHS) 1994, 53, Table 4.9.

Note: Death rates based on number of deaths per 100,000 in population.

influenza (1.5 times the national average) are related to poor sanitation and housing and inadequate access to health care (see table 11.2).

The other four leading causes of death were below the national average: heart disease (0.9 times), cerebrovascular diseases (0.9 times), cancer (0.7 times), and pulmonary diseases (0.7 times). These conditions, often indicating diseases of the aged, remind us that Native Americans still do not live as long, on average, as non-Indians. In 1991, 32 percent of Indian deaths occurred to those younger than forty-five; the comparable figure for the United States as a whole was 11 percent (USIHS 1994:56).

Diabetes has emerged as a major health problem in Native American communities; it is the fourth leading cause of death. Indications are that it is a relatively recent phenomenon and has been increasing significantly in the latter half of the twentieth century (Ghodes 1986). Although exact causal relationships have yet to be defined, changes in diet and increases in obesity have been implicated. Justice (1988) points out, however, that current research is inconclusive. A long-term epidemiological study is under way on a sample of Pima Indians in Arizona that may be able to provide some answers to questions of cause and prevention (OTA 1986:141).

In 1986, the Office of Technology Assessment (OTA)[3] completed a detailed study of Indian health that included comparisons by gender. In that study, overall death rates due to diabetes show little difference when Indian women are compared with Indian men; for women the age-adjusted death rate is 28.8 whereas for Indian men the figure is 26.7. Yet, there is considerable variation by IHS service area, indicating differences by tribe. In six of eleven areas, the diabetes death rates for women are higher than those for men, reaching nearly two times higher in the Billings area (OTA 1986:93, 100).

Indian women are about three times as likely as women in the general population to die of diabetes. The highest rates for women are in the Tucson, Phoenix, Billings, and Aberdeen areas where death rates are over five times higher than for other U.S. women. Alaska is the only area where the rate for Indian and native women is lower than that for women in the general population (OTA 1986:93, 100).

As with many other health issues, women are singled out not only because of their own susceptibility to certain diseases but also because of their position as potential mothers. For example, Justice concludes his paper on diabetes in Native American communities by asserting: "Pregnant, obese, hyperglycemic mothers seem to represent the major biological mechanism that leads to higher diabetic rates in the next generation. . . . Therefore, this group should be singled out to receive modern prenatal medical services with the aim of weight control and blood sugar control, and delivery of a healthy infant" (1988:7).

While not among the leading causes of death, tuberculosis remains a significant health problem among Native Americans. Although the age-adjusted death rate from tuberculosis dropped 74 percent from 1972 to 1990, it still remains 5.4 times higher than the non-Indian rate (2.7 per 100,000 to 0.5 per 100,000) (USIHS 1994:74.).

Pneumonia and influenza represent the seventh leading cause of death among Native Americans. Rates for women vary from over three times the rate for all U.S. women in the Aberdeen, Alaska, Phoenix, and Billings areas to about the same (1.07 times the national rate for women) in the Oklahoma area. When Indian women are compared with Indian men, women's rates never exceed those of men. Pneumonia accounts for most deaths in this category and is related to inadequate access to care. It should be noted that deaths due to pneumonia and influenza have been on the decrease among Indians, dropping from the third leading cause of death in the 1950s (OTA 1986:99–100).

Information on the health status of urban Indians is virtually impossible to find. Even in areas where the Indian Health Service funds urban projects, detailed statistics are not gathered and analyzed. Furthermore, because Native Americans constitute less than 1 percent of most urban populations, they are simply lumped in the "other" category when general health statistics for specific cities are computed. In 1986, OTA was only able to generate crude death rate information from vital statistics on Indians in standard metropolitan statistical areas. These figures were not broken down by sex. It would appear, however, that urban patterns do not differ much from reservation patterns.[4]

In sum, Native Americans' health status continues to lag behind that of other Americans. Most differences can be attributed to sociocultural stress and access to care.

The distribution of resources in the IHS is not immune to the complex maze of federal Indian policy. For example, IHS allocates resources on a "historical" or "program continuity" basis (OTA 1986:27). What that system means is that budgets are based on expenditures from the previous fiscal year plus a percentage increase across the board for cost-of-living adjustments. Demonstration of need is not the major consideration in funding. The system favors tribes and communities with long-standing service delivery programs and, because of them, better health status. In contrast, those areas with fewer facilities, and concomitantly greater need, receive fewer resources. Issues of eligibility and federal recognition further complicate access to care and serve to exacerbate differences in health status among Native Americans.[5]

Alcohol as a Women's Issue

It is virtually impossible to discuss Indian health issues without a detailed look at the significant role that alcohol plays. The statistics referred to above regarding accidents, suicides, homicides, and, of course, cirrhosis are all alcohol related. Accidents are usually automobile accidents where the driver was under the influence; homicides and suicides are usually committed by persons who are inebriated; cirrhosis is usually due to a career of alcohol abuse. Combined, these conditions account for an estimated 35 percent of all Indian deaths (Andre 1979). Such statistics have led Indian leaders themselves to define alcohol abuse and its attendant consequences as the primary health problem of Native Americans for nearly two decades.[6]

The literature on Native Americans and alcohol is enormous, but almost all of it deals with men. (For comprehensive surveys see Leland 1976; Lex 1985.) The few available studies suggest that women are less likely than men to be problem drinkers and that men are more likely than women to succumb to alcohol-related deaths. Thus alcohol abuse has not been widely defined as a "woman's problem."

These gender-related generalizations are supported when the age-adjusted death rates for accidents, cirrhosis, homicide, and suicide are used (with caution) as proxy measures of the relative severity of alcohol abuse in Native American communities. Indian men die in accidents 3.0 times more often than Indian women, they succumb to cirrhosis 1.4 times more often, they are victims of homicide 2.7 times more often, and they commit suicide 6.3 times more often. We get a different perspective when Indian women are compared with white women. Here the significance of alcohol-related deaths for Indian women becomes striking. Indian women are 3.0 times more likely than white women to die in accidents, 7.2 times more likely to succumb to cirrhosis, and 4.0 times more likely to be victims of homicide. The suicide rate is the same for white and Native American women; however, the involvement of alcohol is probably higher for the Indian group. (Statistics are computed from OTA 1986:93, table 4.6.)

As revealing as these figures are, they still do not convey the full significance of alcohol on the lives of Native American women. As with other populations, marital discord and dissolution are related to alcohol abuse in Native American communities, as are spouse abuse and child abuse/neglect (DeBruyn and Lujan 1986). Therefore, even if an Indian woman does not drink, she may find herself and her children at risk if her male partner drinks. Secondly, when Indian women begin heavy drinking, they are likely to suffer severe health consequences more rapidly than are men, a trait known as "telescoping" that they share with women in the larger population (Lex 1985).

Most observers agree that alcohol consumption is increasing among Native American women (Lex 1985:153; Young, n.d.:6). Due to the general lack of research on Indian women, however, it is unclear whether these impressions are caused by an actual increase in alcohol abuse or a recent increase in attention being paid to Indian women and alcohol.

Cultural Variations. There is considerable variation among tribal groups. In the case of cirrhosis, the highest rates are found in the areas with the highest concentrations of Plains Indians: Billings (109.0, 14 times the rate for all women) and Aberdeen (86.3, 11.7 times the rate for all women).

Navajo has one of the lowest rates (20.5, about three times the national rates). These figures (OTA 1986:100) are consistent with the literature on tribal drinking. For example Whittaker (1972) found the highest rate of drinking among Plains Indian women (50–55%), whereas the lowest rates were recorded for the Navajo and Pueblos of the Southwest (13–26%) (Levy and Kunitz 1974). In their studies of fetal alcohol syndrome, May and his associates (1983) also found the highest rates in Plains tribes and lowest in Navajo and Pueblo tribes. They attribute the differences to cultural patterns: "The Plains tribes allow for considerably more individuation of behavior, especially alcohol-abusive behavior. . . . More Plains women are permitted to follow abusive behaviors, while the low incidence rates of the Pueblo and Navajo exemplify tighter control exercised on individuation and alcohol abuse" (383).

The question that usually arises at this point is whether or not there is some genetic basis for the widespread evidence of alcohol abuse among Native Americans. Although some interesting research has been done, the question has not been clearly answered (see, e.g., Mello 1983). Even if a genetic link is found, many questions remain unanswered. For example, how do we explain why Indians begin drinking in the first place? If there are genetic problems (e.g., metabolism problems), how do we explain why people resume drinking after having gone through detoxification and treatment? As Schaefer (1981) points out, the best studies on alcohol sensitivity by "race" show a high sensitivity among Asian populations. Yet Asians do not have high rates of alcohol-related health problems. More to the point, if there are genetic links, how do we explain that alcohol abuse seems least pervasive among the most genetically "pure" tribes (e.g., Navajo) and most pervasive among tribes that have the most genetic mix (e.g., Plains tribes)?

In the voluminous literature on Native Americans and alcohol, most authors rely on some form of sociocultural explanation. There are certainly many possible culprits: a history of oppression, forced acculturation, low educational achievement, to name just a few. Critical analyses are available in Leland (1980) and Lex (1985). Most theories, as pointed out above, are based on studies of Indian men. It is rare to find family life mentioned in such studies. In contrast, the sparse but growing literature on Indian women almost always focuses on their positions as mothers.

Fetal Alcohol Syndrome. It is becoming clear that Indian women who drink have become a major source of concern in the Indian community. The Indian woman who drinks is at great risk for family disruption; if she is suspected of child neglect following alcohol abuse, her children are likely to be removed from her care. Further, once removed, they are not likely to return to the Indian community because they are usually placed in non-Indian foster homes (Blanchard and Barsh 1980; Byler 1977; Center for Social Research and Development 1976). Understanding this risk, many Indian women are reluctant to enter treatment programs (Metcalf 1987).

But it is the specter of *fetal alcohol syndrome* (FAS) which has accelerated the community concern. FAS refers to the permanent damage done to a fetus as a result of maternal drinking, especially damage that produces mental retardation. The term *fetal alcohol effects* refers to the same constellation of symptoms, only to a less severe degree. From the time of the first studies on FAS conducted in this country, Native American women were implicated. One of the first identified cases was an Indian baby described in the landmark University of Washington study (Jones et al. 1973). His picture, shown in medical journals around the world, combined with the dismal statistics on alcohol abuse in Native American communities and culminating with the publication of the poignant and disturbing book, *The Broken Cord*, by Michael Dorris (1989), has led to a near-hysterical concern about FAS in Indian communities.

In *The Broken Cord* Dorris chronicles the story of his adopted son, a Lakota Sioux, who suffers from fetal alcohol effects. Like all other authors concerned with Indian health issues, Dorris ponders the question of why alcohol abuse is so pervasive among Native Americans, and he speculates on what can be done about it. Unlike most other authors, Dorris's focus is on women, especially those Indian women who give birth to FAS babies.

Mothers, Alcohol, and Self-Determination. The publication of *The Broken Cord* heralds an important shift in attitudes and emphasis regarding alcohol and Native Americans. Two decades ago concern about alcohol abuse, especially among women, probably would have been dismissed *within* the community as a racist invention of non-Indian anthropologists, social workers, or medical personnel leading to the negative (and presumed inaccurate) stereotype of the "drunken Indian." Denial of the problem was widespread. When I first began work in the San Francisco Bay Area community twenty years ago, there was a not-so-subtle message that alcohol use was not to be mentioned in any reports or proposals. At the same time, there were no overt sanctions against drinking; beer was widely available at community powwows, for example. Now alcohol and drugs are specifically banned at such events, and the rule is enforced by the community. Today, Indians themselves are the ones who identify alcohol as the primary health problem and who heap praise on writers like Dorris (who is himself Native American). What has accounted for the change in attitude?

I do not think that it is any accident that the willingness of the community to confront alcohol abuse has coincided with the definition of the problem as a women's issue. As long as alcoholism was seen as a problem unique to a few single men, if indeed it was seen as a problem at all, it could be conveniently ignored or downplayed by the community. But when Indian women, specifically Indian *mothers*, were implicated, the community shifted its attitudes. The result has been both a blessing and a burden for women.

I think we can trace the redefinition of the problem in large part to a set of policies known as Self-Determination. These policies emerged in the 1970s when, after centuries of dependence on the federal government, Indians began to regain control over some social programs. The argument is that Indians know best how to deal with their own issues and should run their own service delivery system. Given the responsibility (and some limited resources) to identify and treat social problems, many leaders within the community were thus forced to confront the issue of alcohol abuse. And when they did, women moved to center stage in their role as family caretakers.

One example can be seen in the case of an urban child welfare organization. In 1974, the Urban Indian Child Resource Center (CRC) was established in Oakland, California. Funded under the National Center on Child Abuse and Neglect, the center was charged with helping Indian children in abusive and/or neglectful families. Operating under the assertion that there was no true abuse or neglect in the Indian community, the center concentrated its efforts on educating child protective services personnel on cultural differences between Indian and non-Indian child-rearing practices and on providing emergency services for young families migrating to the city on the Relocation program. The goal was to stop the flow of children into the non-Indian foster care system.

In 1978, I completed an evaluation of the services delivered by the center. What emerged were two client profiles. One involved young parents with young children, unversed in urban survival strategies, living on the brink of unemployment and poverty, isolated in the inner city without a support group. This profile was what the CRC expected, and it responded by providing emergency child care and arranging for various benefits such as food stamps, school registration, and transportation. The second profile typically involved an unmarried teenager with small children. The mother was usually involved in drug abuse (with alcohol being the drug of choice). As a result, her children had been severely neglected and sometimes abused; they were either in foster care or about to be placed when the family arrived at CRC.

Faced with this new clientele, CRC was forced to redefine the problem and change its services. It is now a foster placement agency that identifies and certifies Indian homes. In addition, CRC provides a limited mental health treatment program primarily serving young alcoholic mothers and their abused and neglected children.

A similar shift has occurred in the local alcoholism treatment center. It began about twenty years ago, and like most such programs, it served only men. Later, women were admitted, but the ratio of men to women was about 5:1. At first, the program had the reputation (as did most of the Indian-run programs) of being a place where "hard core" alcoholic men came to dry out when they needed food and shelter. But over the years, Indian Health Service, which is the major funding source, has steadily increased its demands for accountability. More careful reporting systems are now in place because the program needs to justify itself annually in order to receive continued funding. Its services have become more professional and less custodial; counselors are trained in local community colleges, a certification program has been instituted, and outside experts are called in for consultation and staff training. One result has been an increased interest in serving a younger population, in providing preventative services, and in reaching out to women. In other words, the program is seeking to maximize its effectiveness with the realization that early intervention, especially with young mothers, has the greatest probability for success over the long haul.

Blessing or Burden? Self-Determination has issued a challenge to Native Americans: define and solve your own problems. How the problem is defined and which model—individual or community—is chosen to guide the search for solutions will be crucial in the coming years.

An individual model looks to the woman, her family of origin, and her personal and psychological development for the source of the problem. It emphasizes her responsibility for her children and sees any lapse in executing that responsibility as a failure on her part. An individual model, often punitive in its implications, can lead to such intervention policies as locking a pregnant woman in jail until the birth of her child to ensure that she does not deliver an FAS baby.

In contrast, the community model stresses institutional causes for the problem. It traces the etiology of alcoholism to the cultural genocide policies of the federal government, including forced removal of children into boarding schools, aggressive foster placement and adoption programs, and enforced acculturation. The antidote is to rebuild the community and change the institutions that caused the problem in the first place. Individuals under this model deserve treatment, to be sure, but the ultimate goal is to reunify families, strengthen community bonds, and maintain cultural integrity.

I said before that the shift in community attitudes toward alcohol and alcohol abuse signals both a blessing and a burden for Indian women. It is a blessing in that attention is finally being paid to the Indian woman and her needs—new programs, new research. It is a burden in that she is in danger of being blamed for the next generation's woes. Whichever way it goes, it seems to me, will depend on whether an individual or a community model is chosen to guide Indian Self-Determination and the programs designed to serve Indian people.

Old Ways, New Dawn

Articles like this one about Native American women's health issues, or for that matter almost any contemporary issue within Native American communities, usually emphasize the negative. It seems that problems are what interest readers, and they certainly are what interest funding agencies. Therefore, research tends to focus on the downside of Native American life. There *are* positives, and I would like to discuss some of the most important ones. This is not to say that everything is rosy, but if Indians, the tribes, the Bureau, the IHS, and the federal government seek solutions, here are some areas where they are likely to find them.

Beyond Stereotypes. First, it is necessary to emphasize that not every Native American woman is alcoholic, diabetic, prone to accidents, suicidal, or the mother of an FAS child. To say that Indian women are overrepresented in these categories is not the same as saying that all or even the majority of Indians succumb to these conditions. Nonetheless, the very real problems that confront the Indian family and community make it easy to fall into that kind of stereotypical thinking. It seems to me that what is more important in the long run is to ask a set of questions about Indian women and health as opposed to Indian women and ill health. Which health promoting or healing strategies show promise? Where can we look for strength?

As with any population, access to decent health care is key; that was proved for Indians when the IHS took over in the 1950s and greatly improved the health status on reservations. What is important to note now in the 1990s is that more and more of the programs that are designed to serve Native Americans are being run by Native Americans. Both the Bureau of Indian Affairs and the Indian Health Service have a policy of Indian preference in hiring, and their contract services are delivered under the provisions of the "Buy Indian Act." This act specifies that only Indian-run organizations can negotiate to deliver selected services and products.

These policies combined with specially funded scholarship and training programs have meant that clinics, welfare agencies, and schools, whether run by the Bureau and IHS or by tribes and Indian nonprofits, are increasingly being staffed with professionally trained Indians. Although the percentage of Indian physicians and dentists in IHS facilities is low (about 3.3% each), nearly half (49.0%) of the nurses and four-fifths (79.6%) of the administrative staff are Indian. (Figures computed from OTA, table 5.3, p. 163.) Given that women are overrepresented in the last two categories, these figures mean that career opportunities for women in the health care field are on the rise. Such programs as the University of North Dakota's INMED, a program designed to assist Indians going to medical school, are working hard to increase women's representation in the ranks of physicians as well (Steele 1985).

A look at changes in the San Francisco Bay area illustrates the magnitude of changes in Indian control of service programs, including health care. In one of the first studies of urban Indians, Ablon (1964) noted that in 1960 there were twenty-one Indian organizations in the Bay Area, most of which were small tribal social clubs such as athletic teams or dance/powwow groups. There were two Indian centers, both organized and run by non-Indian churches, that primarily offered cultural activities. Only one of the organizations Ablon noted was health or service oriented: the San Jose Indian Alcoholics Anonymous.

In 1970, over forty groups were mentioned in a Human Rights Commission report (Metcalf 1980). They included a miscellany of student organizations at local universities, political action groups, and art, cultural, and athletic organizations. Significant among them, however, were agencies delivering health and social services. A fledgling clinic, a Head Start program, and several information and referral services were opened. Three Indian centers—one each in San Francisco, Oakland, and San Jose—were now run by Indian boards, and all included service delivery as well as cultural activities.

In 1995 there are three full-fledged Indian clinics. Most of the staff members are Indian and include physicians, nurses, dentists, and master-level public health administrators. A licensed foster placement agency is staffed with Indian MSWs. The three residential alcoholism treatment programs employ certified counselors, and each Indian cultural center also provides social work services. There is an employment and training organization, a preschool, and three legal services.

A significant proportion of the clientele in these organizations are women and children; for example, the clinics offer prenatal, perinatal, and pediatric services, the foster placement agency primarily serves young single-mother families, and one of the alcoholism programs is exclusively dedicated to the treatment of women and their children. Furthermore, women are conspicuously well represented on the boards and senior staffs of all these organizations.

Culture Cultivating. Along with the increase in Indian-run programs has come an increased determination to provide culturally relevant services. Using alcoholism as an example, there is growing indication that programs designed to treat non-Indians do not succeed with Indian clients (Levy and Kunitz 1974; Morrisette 1991); most observers call for intervention programs that are culturally relevant (Hall 1985; May 1986; Topper 1985; Weibel-Orlando 1987).

Two major types of culturally relevant programs are emerging as Indians look to the "old ways" to help solve contemporary problems. The first I call "culture matching." In this type, the clientele usually come from a clearly defined tribal orientation; therefore, traditions from that tribal heritage are used to facilitate the healing process. For example, Topper (1985) describes programs to treat Navajos that use Navajo language, traditions, and medicine people.

Under the culture matching model, variations in client culture are seen as variations along a traditional-to-acculturated continuum. None-theless, the assumption is that at base the clients come with a grounding in a specific traditional Native American culture. However, the assumption that client characteristics vary only along a traditional-to-acculturated continuum may not reveal the full heterogeneity of the population. Recent research has suggested that some Native Americans are neither grounded in their own tribal culture nor acculturated to the dominant culture (Metcalf 1982).

In an exploratory study, I found that the clientele in an urban treatment program fell into the last category; that is, they were marginal to both cultures (Metcalf 1987). Many had been removed from family and culture at an early age through foster care placement or boarding school. Often clients came from mixed tribal backgrounds as well as from mixed Indian/non-Indian backgrounds. They had little education, limited facility in English, few job skills, and few connections to institutions in the dominant culture such as churches or clubs. Yet they could not speak a native language, had little knowledge of native traditions, and knew little of the skills common in native communities, including native arts and crafts.

In this situation, an exciting and innovative culturally relevant treatment model is developing that can be called "culture cultivating." Under this model, the treatment program begins with the assumption that the opportunity to learn native culture has been disrupted. Federal Indian policies such as boarding school education, Relocation, and Termination are held responsible for separating the younger generation from their heritage. In order to commence the healing process, clients must be taught or retaught the basics of their culture. The theory is that, once grounded in Indian traditions, a new sense of identity and community can be fostered, which in turn will increase self-esteem and provide the support groups necessary for the client to become and remain sober. It should be pointed out that skills necessary for survival in the dominant culture are not neglected under this model; clients also receive vocational rehabilitation services, literacy training, education for the GED, etc. The ultimate goal is to produce a bicultural orientation.

Whether culture matching or culture cultivating, reliance on the old ways—the healing power of Indian spirituality and native medicine, the strength of traditional kinship bonds and communal orientation—shows promise in the struggle to break the cycle of dependency and despair that has plagued Indian families and communities. Especially as applied to treatment programs for women in their roles as mothers, culturally relevant programs seek to reach the next generation. To borrow a metaphor from the name of one of the first treatment lodges for Indian women, this cultural renaissance may provide a new dawn for Native American women and their communities.

NOTES

I thank Betty Cooper for her wisdom and vision; Felicia Hodge for her professional support and access to data; Robert Anderson for being my colleague and mentor; Sheryl Ruzek for encouragement and editorial acumen. Any mistakes in fact or interpretation are, of course, mine alone.

1. This overview is necessarily brief and very general. For the interested reader who wishes more detailed analyses of the complexity of federal Indian policy, I recommend the following: Brophy and Aberle 1966; American Indian Policy Review Commission 1977; Deloria 1985; Dorris 1981; Office of Technology Assessment 1986, chap. 2; selected articles in the *American Indian Law Review.*

2. Where age-adjusted rates are cited, they refer to rates per 100,000; for stylistic reasons, I have used an abbreviated terminology.

3. The OTA report is based on data from the early 1980s. Although overall rates have changed somewhat since then, the relative status of women compared with men has not. I therefore have relied on the detailed information from the earlier OTA report when doing a comparative analysis.

4. Leading causes of death for 1980–82 were (1) diseases of the heart; (2) accidents and adverse effects, particularly motor vehicle accidents; (3) cancer; (4) liver disease and cirrhosis; (5) diabetes mellitus; (6) cerebrovascular diseases; (7) homicide; (8) suicide; (9) pneumonia and influenza; and (10) conditions arising in the perinatal period (Office of Technology Assessment 1986:104).

5. As this volume goes to press, Indian Health Service policies are being reviewed, and proposals for significant revisions are being put forward. It is not possible to know the final outcome of these proposals at this time, but the reader is cautioned to expect such changes as severe funding cuts, mergers and/or elimination of urban programs, stricter eligibility requirements, and a general shift to a managed-care model of service delivery.

6. For example, in 1977 the American Indian Policy Review Commission stated that alcohol abuse was "the most severe and widespread health problem among Indians today" (27).

REFERENCES

Ablon, Joan
    1964   "Relocated American Indians in the San Francisco Bay area." Human Organization 24:296–304.

American Indian Policy Review Commission
  1977   Final Report. Vols. 1 and 2. Washington: Government Printing Office.
Andre, J. M.
  1979   The Epidemiology of Alcoholism among American Indians and Alaska Natives. Albuquerque, NM: Indian Health Service.
Blanchard, Evelyn, and Russell Barsh
  1980   "What is best for tribal children? a response to Fischler." Social Work 25:350-57.
Brophy, William A., and Sophie D. Aberle
  1966   The Indian: America's Unfinished Business. Report of the Commission on the Rights, Liberties, and Responsibilities of the American Indians. Norman: University of Oklahoma Press.
Bryant, Hilda
  1969   "Loneliness in the white man's city." Seattle Post-Intelligencer, 14 December.
Byler, William
  1977   "Indian Child Welfare Program." Pp. 1-11 in Steven Unger (ed.), The Destruction of American Indian Families. New York: Association on American Indian Affairs (1977).
Center for Social Research and Development (CSRD)
  1976   Indian Child Welfare: A State-of-the-Field Study. Denver Research Institute, University of Denver: CSRD. DHEW Pub. No. 76-30095.
DeBruyn, LeMyra, and Carol C. Lujan
  1987   Family Alcohol Abuse and Child Abuse and Neglect: An Intergenerational Study of the Native American Population Served by the Santa Fe Service Unit, Indian Health Service. Albuquerque: Indian Health Service.
Deloria, Vine, Jr., ed.
  1985   American Indian Policy in the Twentieth Century. Norman: University of Oklahoma Press.
Dorris, Michael A.
  1981   "The grass still grows, the rivers still flow: contemporary Native Americans." Daedalus 110:43-69.
  1989   The Broken Cord. New York: Harper and Row.
Ghodes, D. M.
  1986   "Diabetes in American Indians: a growing problem." Diabetes Care 9:609-13.
Hall, Roberta
  1985   "Distribution of sweat lodge in alcohol treatment programs." Current Anthropology 26(1):134-35.
Jones, K. L., D. W. Smith, C. N. Ulleland, and A. P. Striessguth
  1973   "Pattern of malformation in offspring of chronic alcoholic mothers." Lancet 1:1267-71.
Justice, James W.
  1988   Bio-Social Predictors of Non-Insulin Dependent Diabetes in Populations.

Paper presented to the 46th International Congress of Americanists, Amsterdam, The Netherlands.

Leland, Joy
1976   Firewater Myths. New Brunswick, NJ: Rutgers Center of Alcohol Studies.
1980   "Native American alcohol use: a review of the literature." Pp. 1–56 in P. D. Mail and D. R. MacDonald (eds.), From Tulapi to Tokay: A Bibliography of Alcohol Use and Abuse among Native Americans of North America. New Haven, CT: HRAF Press.

Levy, Jerrold E., and Stephen J. Kunitz
1974   Indian Drinking and Anglo-American Theories. New York: Wiley-Interscience.

Lex, Barbara W.
1985   "Alcohol problems in special populations." Pp. 89–187 in J. H. Mendelson and N. K. Mello (eds.), The Diagnosis and Treatment of Alcoholism. New York: McGraw-Hill.

May, Phillip A.
1986   "Alcohol and drug misuse prevention programs for American Indians: needs and opportunities." Journal of Studies on Alcohol 47:187–95.

May, Phillip A., Karen J. Hymbaugh, Jon M. Aase, and Jonathon M. Samet
1983   "Epidemiology of fetal alcohol syndrome among American Indians of the Southwest." Social Psychology 30:374–87.

Mello, N. K.
1983   "Etiological theories of alcoholism." Pp. 271–312 in N. K. Mello (ed.), vol. 3, Advances in Substance Abuse. Greenwich, CT: JAI Press.

Metcalf, Ann
1980   "The Indians of the San Francisco Bay area." In Urban Indians: Proceedings of the Third Annual Conference on Problems and Issues Concerning American Indians Today. Center for the History of the American Indian. Chicago: Newberry Library.
1982   "Navajo women in the city: lessons from a quarter-century of relocation." American Indian Quarterly 6:71–89.
1987   Native American Women and Alcoholism: Treatment Issues. Paper presented to the Society for Applied Anthropology. Oaxaca, Mexico, April.

Morrisette, Patrick J.
1991   "The therapeutic dilemma with Canadian native youth in residential care." Child and Adolescent Social Work 8(2):89–99.

Neils, Elaine M.
1971   Reservation to City. Research Report No. 131. Chicago: Department of Geography, University of Chicago.

Office of Technology Assessment (OTA)
1986   Indian Health Care. (OTA-H-290, Congress.) Washington: Government Printing Office.

Schaefer, James M.
1981   "Firewater myths revisited." Journal of Studies on Alcoholism (suppl.) 9:99–115.

Steele, Lois
  1985   Medicine Women. Grand Forks, ND: INMED.
Topper, Martin
  1985   "Navajo 'alcoholism': drinking, alcohol abuse, and treatment in a chang-
          ing environment." Pp. 227–51 in L. A. Bennett and G. M. Ames (eds.),
          The American Experience with Alcohol: Contrasting Cultural Perspec-
          tives. New York: Plenum Press.
U.S. Indian Health Service (USIHS)
  1980   The Indian Health Program. DHHS Pub. No. (HSA) 80-1003. Washing-
          ton: Government Printing Office.
  1994   Trends in Indian Health. Department of Health and Human Services.
          Rockville, MD: USIHS.
Weibel-Orlando, Joan
  1987   "Culture-specific treatment modalities: assessing client to treatment fit in
          Indian alcoholism programs." Pp. 261–83 in M. Cox (ed.), Alcoholism
          Treatment and Prevention. New York: Academic Press.
Whittaker, J. O.
  1972   "Alcohol and the Standing Rock Sioux tribe." Quarterly Journal of Stud-
          ies of Alcohol 23:468–79.
Young, Robert
  n.d.   A Review of Treatment Strategies for Native American Alcoholics: The
           Need for the Cultural Perspective. Monograph series. University of Ari-
           zona Native American Research and Training Center.

[12]

Asian/Pacific American Women and Cultural Diversity:
Studies of the Traumas of Cancer and War

KAREN L. ITO, RITA CHI-YING CHUNG,
AND MARJORIE KAGAWA-SINGER

These researchers take an anthropological approach to understanding the complexities of women who are classified in this exceedingly heterogeneous racial/ethnic group. They emphasize the multiplicity of factors that shape women's experiences of health and health care and present qualitative data to illustrate how sociocultural expectations and experiences are central to health behavior. Their case studies of coping with cancer and mental disturbances related to traumatic migration experiences provide vivid examples of the complexities and differences that can be found within one officially designated racial/ ethnic group.

Health and health care for Asian/Pacific American women is complicated by their diversity. They encompass at least seventy-one ethnic, cultural, national, and regional groups, including Bangladeshi, Bhutanese, Burmese, Chamorro (indigenous people of Guam and the Northern Marianas), Chinese, Fijian, native Hawai'ian, Hmong, Indian, Indonesian, Japanese, Cambodian, Korean, Laotian, Malaysian, Nepalese, Okinawan, Pakistani, Palauan, Filipino, Samoan, Singaporean, Sri Lankan, Tahitian, Taiwanese, Tibetan, Tongan, Thai, and Vietnamese. Within these groups are further distinctions of ethnicity, religious affiliations associated with ethnicity or class, different colonial histories, and regional origins.[1] Each group has different health care issues and needs, different culturally appropriate ways of dealing with illness, and vastly different patterns of disease. Add to this the complexities of gender expectations and immigration histories, and it is obvious that generalizations cannot be easily made about Asian/Pacific Americans.

In this chapter, we examine the sociodemographics and immigration patterns of Asian/Pacific American women. Then we present case studies on health issues of Japanese American and Southeast Asian American women to illustrate the importance of addressing specific sociocultural contexts.

Sociodemographics

According to the Census Bureau, 7,273,663 Asian/Pacific Americans lived in the United States in 1990, forming 2.9 percent of the population. This number represents an increase of 107.8 percent since 1980, largely as a result of immigration, the largest growth of any group in the country (U.S. Bureau of Census 1990).[2] The ten-year increase for the nation as a whole was 10 percent: whites 6 percent, blacks 13 percent, Native Americans 38 percent, and Hispanics 53 percent.

Among Asian/Pacific Americans, the six most populous groups are Chinese (1,645,472), Filipino (1,406,770), Japanese (847,562), Asian Indian (815,447), Korean (798,849), and Vietnamese (614,547).[3] Fifty-six percent live in the West, and 40 percent live in California. Of those who live in California, 42 percent live in Los Angeles and Orange Counties (U.S. Bureau of Census 1990).

Nationally, Asian/Pacific Americans have the highest median household income ($36,784) compared with whites ($31,435), Latinos ($24,156), Native Americans ($24,156), and blacks ($19,758). This gross figure obscures complexities. Many Asian/Pacific Americans have large households with many more workers (in some cases several families) contributing to a single household income. Consequently, the amount of money available for each individual is reduced. The per capita income for Asian/Pacific Americans in Los Angeles County illustrates this: the Asian/Pacific American household income exceeded the white household income by about $450, but per capita Asian/Pacific Americans made only seventy-one cents for every dollar a white American made (Hubler 1992).

Slightly more women (51%) than men (49%) are of Asian/Pacific ancestry: 3,715,624 women to 3,558,038 men (U.S. Bureau of Census 1990). This is a vastly different sex ratio from the initial period of Asian American immigration beginning in the mid-nineteenth century when the immigrants were almost all male.

History

Given the large numbers of foreign-born Asian/Pacific Americans, it is easy to overlook the fact that Asians have been in the United States officially for over 140 years and unofficially for over 225 years. Some Asians have been in this country for more than seven generations. Pacific Americans, of course, represent the indigenous populations of Hawai'i, American Samoa, and Guam.

Early Immigration

The immigration of women and the establishment of families differed tremendously among early pioneer Asian American groups: Chinese, Japanese, Korean, and Filipino.

Chinese Immigration

The first major Asian immigration began with the Chinese in the mid-nineteenth century. Like all early Asian immigrant groups, it was almost exclusively male. In 1880 the Chinese male-female sex ratio was 27:1. These men were imported as labor for the agricultural fields of California and Hawai'i. The bulk of the early Chinese immigration occurred between 1849 and 1882, when the first of many anti-Asian exclusion acts was passed. The 1882 act prevented the immigration of Chinese laborers and prohibited the naturalization of Chinese. Early Chinese immigrants were often married in China and came over as sojourners, leaving their wives and sometimes unseen offspring in China assuming they would someday return. Chinese wives of laborers were barred from entering the United States in 1884. In 1924, all Chinese ancestry women were barred. Therefore, Chinese Americans could not establish families in any number until after 1943 (when the Exclusion Acts were repealed allowing for renewed immigration from China) and after World War II (when immigration restrictions were eased for the foreign-born wives and offspring of U.S. veterans of Chinese ancestry).

Japanese Immigration

Male Japanese immigrants were recruited to fill the void left by the 1882 exclusion of Chinese laborers. Japanese women began emigrating to the United States in 1900. Twenty-four years later, immigration quotas were installed "excluding aliens ineligible for citizenship," and Japan was given a quota of zero. Most Japanese women immigrants who arrived before 1924 were the so-called picture brides (Ichioka 1980). These women were not chosen out of a photo catalog of available, nubile women. These were marriages arranged by families and strictly regulated by the Japanese government. Photographs were exchanged between families of prospective grooms and brides. A more precise referent to this system would be "photo marriages," which is the actual translation of the Japanese term. This practice was voluntarily halted in 1919 by the Japanese government following pressure from the U.S. government. This left 43 percent of the Japanese men in the United States unmarried. Antimiscegenation laws prevented them (and other Asian ancestry men) from marrying white American women. The Japanese male/female sex ratio at the time was 6:4.

Barriers to Female Immigration

The Cable Act, enacted in California in 1922, prevented American citizens from marrying those ineligible for citizenship. This act was primarily aimed at male Japanese and Chinese aliens (who were legally barred from citizenship) and at American citizens who might marry them. If an American woman did marry an alien ineligible for naturalization, the woman's citizenship was revoked. An added racial dimension was that if an immigrant Japanese or Chinese husband of a white American woman died or was divorced, she would regain her citizenship, but if either of those situations occurred to an American woman of Asian ancestry, she would not regain her citizenship (Osumi 1982).[4] Such laws were passed to prevent the establishment of families and a second generation of U.S. citizens of Asian ancestry.

Korean Immigration

The first Korean immigrants arrived in 1903. An early group of Christians left Korea because of persecution, and a second group fled the Japanese occupation and annexation of Korea. Both groups were relatively small, and most immigrants initially settled in Hawai'i as agricultural laborers. By 1920, almost five thousand Koreans lived in Hawai'i and over twelve hundred had settled on the U.S. mainland. Nearly all were men.[5]

In the period 1905–10, only 613 out of 7,296 Koreans were women (a 10:1 male/female ratio). From 1910 to 1924, between 600 and 800 picture brides arrived, nearly doubling the population of Korean women in Hawai'i and reducing the sex ratio to 5:1 (Yang 1984). A culturally important institution for these pioneer women was the *gye* (or *kye*), a rotating credit system where a group of women pooled their money and established a lending and repayment plan. They would draw on these monies to help establish a business or to pay for school fees for their children.

Filipino Immigration

Filipino American immigration followed the earlier patterns, beginning in 1924 with young single men. Filipinos filled the agricultural labor vacuum created by the exclusion of the Japanese by the National Origins Act, which lasted until 1934. Because the Philippines was a U.S. territory, Filipinos carried U.S. passports and were not affected by the National Origins Act of 1924. After 1934, U.S. legislation limited Filipino immigration to fifty people a year. Following Philippine independence in 1946, only 100 immigrants were allowed into the United States each year until U.S. immigration laws changed in 1965. A substantial female immigration period never occurred. Cultural and religious restrictions on travel by unaccompanied women, particularly single women, was a major restraint. The United States also was considered too dangerous for Filipino women. There was no cultural system such as picture marriages or governmental support to provide an infrastructure. The distances and expenses prevented men from traveling back to the Philippines and returning to the States with brides. Most men planned to return to the Philippines, but few succeeded. The Filipino male/female ratio in 1940 was 7:1 (Osumi 1982), and most Filipino men from this early immigrant phase were fated to spend their entire lives as single migrant workers.

Gender Roles

Early restrictive immigration and antimiscegenation laws influenced the structure and the establishment of Asian American families. For example, first-generation Chinese, Japanese, and Korean women were able to develop much more egalitarian marital relationships and more independence than they would have had in their homelands. One of the critical factors was the absence of a mother-in-law to dominate the household, as would have been the case in Korea, Japan, or China. Also, many of the women were younger and healthier than their older, more weathered husbands and could take more control of the household and family business as their husbands aged. Glenn discusses how domestic work gave first-generation Japanese American women some measure of financial and physical independence from their husbands. In small family businesses they became partners, working as a team in laundries and restaurants or sometimes becoming the primary operators of rooming houses and stores (Glenn 1983, 1986).

Gender changes occurred early in Asian American history. In evaluating present-day family and marital relationships, one cannot assume a passive female and a dominant male as the Asian/Pacific model (Howard 1974; Yanagisako 1985). Another consideration is the developmental pattern of marital relationships. Howard discovered that the pattern of male-female dominance between Hawai'ian couples changed as a marriage developed and children were born. Initially the men dominated and confronted their wives, but this pattern reversed itself with the birth of children and establishment of a household and as the women became more secure in their position and hence more confrontational and dominant.

Therefore, there is considerable variability both within and across the different early Asian/Pacific American groups. Although current descendants of these early arrivals are highly acculturated and most likely monolingual English speakers, cultural differences and patterns are still clearly discernible.[6]

Recent Immigration

After the National Origins Act was repealed in 1965, a new wave of immigrants arrived. Quotas per country were replaced by policies that favored family reunification and certain skilled occupations. Initially, many new Asian/Pacific immigrants came under the preference for skilled occupations. Subsequently, using the preference for family reunification, many were able to bring other family members to the United States. Many post-1965 immigrants, for example, Koreans and Filipinos, were accustomed to American culture and medicine through their countries' long association with the American military and U.S. corporations. Broadcast of American TV shows and music also familiarized immigrants with American culture before their arrival.

Southeast Asian Immigration

After 1975, when North Vietnamese troops and insurgents overthrew the South Vietnamese government and further turmoil engulfed the region, Southeast Asians arrived in the United States as refugees. The first group of Vietnamese and a small group of Cambodians were generally well educated, familiar with American culture, and spoke some English. The period from 1978 to the present is marked by a second group of the so-called boat people and land people from Vietnam, Laos, and Cambodia, including ethnic Chinese from Vietnam and rural Hmong from Laos. The boat people were primarily Vietnamese headed for Thailand or the Philippines, Malaysia, or Hong Kong. Land people were Cambodians, Hmong, and other Laotians who traveled through jungles to reach refugee camps along the eastern border of Thailand. Although most second-wave immigrants were rural, poor, and often illiterate, many of the ethnic Chinese in this group were well educated and middle class (Tabayas and Pok 1983).[7] Many more of these boat and land people are entering through the immigration preference for family reunification (rather than the preference for skilled occupations).[8]

Disease and Illness

Medical sophistication among Asian/Pacific Americans is varied. It includes highly acculturated third- and fourth-generation Japanese Americans; medically and pharmacologically knowledgeable urban Taiwanese who combine Western medicine with the beliefs and practices of traditional Chinese medicine; Hmong folk and herbal practitioners; and some Filipinos who use both Western medicine and faith healers.

In medical anthropology, it is important to distinguish between disease and illness. Disease is the biophysiological disturbance of body organs and systems. Illness is the personal experience, evaluation, understanding, and interpretation made by those who suffer the disease. "To state it flatly, patients suffer 'illnesses'; physicians diagnose and treat 'diseases'" (Eisenberg 1977:11). Therefore, anthropologists are interested not only in rates of diseases but also in cultural interpretations of illness.

Disease

A major problem in studying disease rates for Asian/Pacific Americans is the lack of adequate data. Asian/Pacific Americans do not exist in large enough numbers in data banks at the National Center for Health Statistics, so they rarely appear in ethnic breakdowns of health parameters or disease prevalence. Nor has there been a continuous body of research on any one health topic or disease of particular relevance to Asian/Pacific Americans. This dearth of data on the incidence or prevalence rates makes it difficult to develop a coherent picture of Asian/Pacific American health and disease.

Available aggregate data on Asian/Pacific Americans obscure specific health and disease profiles of particular groups. For example, Hawai'ian women have the highest incidence of breast cancer and mortality rates of any ethnic/racial group in the country: an incidence rate of 111 per 100,000 and a mortality rate of 33.3 per 100,000.[9] In comparison, Filipino women have the lowest incidence rate (43.4/100,000) and mortality rate (8.0/100,000) for breast cancer of all ethnic/racial groups with the exception of Native American women (see chapter 2).

National data also suggest that positive health models might be identified by investigating the sociocultural lifestyles of Asian and Pacific Americans. For example, infant, neonatal, and postneonatal mortality rates for Asian and Pacific Americans are the lowest of all U.S. groups. Is there something in the postnatal (or prenatal) environment that encourages such positive outcomes?[10]

One area of health concern for Asian Americans, particularly Asian immigrant women, is a high prevalence of hepatitis B. Chronic hepatitis B surface antigen carriers are at risk for chronic liver disease and liver cancer; these women can infect other family members, particularly their newborn infants (Stevens et al. 1985).

The health problems of Southeast Asians run the gamut from posttraumatic stress disorders (PTSD) and depression to malnutrition and tuberculosis. A California study of 2,700 Southeast Asian refugees found over 40 percent had a moderate to severe need for mental health treatment and over 16 percent were diagnosed as having PTSD (Gong-Guy 1986).

The rate of tuberculosis for Southeast Asian refugees is 250 per 100,000 as opposed to 9 per 100,000 for the total U.S. population. Illustrative of poor nutrition during formative years, a small study of thirty-six refugee children ages one to twelve found 22 percent were below the weight-for-height index as opposed to 5 percent of Asian Americans and 3 percent of white American children. In addition, 47 percent were below the height-for-age index, as opposed to 24 percent of Asian Americans and 8.5 percent of white Americans (U.S. General Accounting Office 1990:33–35).

Illness

Although aggregate health statistics are difficult to interpret, qualitative research on the health of specific Asian/Pacific American groups reveals many complexities. In an ethnographic study conducted on Asian Americans and health care, culturally distinct patterns of illness interpretation were found between women of Chinese, Japanese, and Filipino origin living in Los Angeles (Ito 1982). All were highly acculturated and almost exclusively used allopathic medicine to treat their diseases, but cultural patterns suggested differential interpretations of etiology, personal control, and responsibility.[11]

Chinese Americans appeared to view health skeptically and as problematic. Good health was an uncertainty. Even if a person looked healthy and had good medical care and health habits, one never knew when sudden death, severe illness, or psychological problems would develop. Attempts to maintain good physical health focused on particular attention to food and cooking styles with emphasis on Chinese cooking as "better for you" and "healthier." But unexpected maladies remained of concern.

The Japanese Americans interviewed saw health as a matter of will. Dwelling on oneself or even preventive monitoring was self-indulgent and reprehensible: "If you think about getting sick, you will." Prevention took the form of ignoring symptoms and performing daily duties and work: "Pretty soon you'll forget about feeling sick." Here the mind-body relationship was important for health maintenance and illness prevention.

Filipino Americans seemed to consider health as a moral statement about the correct fulfillment of social (particularly kin) obligations. Prevention appeared less secular than in the other two groups. Religious devotion and faith in God was a leitmotif in the lives of these Filipino Americans. For example, a characteristic phrase was *"Bahala na,"* which means trusting in God or that some event is God's will. Unlike Japanese Americans, Filipino Americans believed that an important relationship for health maintenance and illness prevention existed between body and soul rather than between body and mind.

The definition of illness (rather than disease)—what causes illness, when one decides one is sick, and what one decides to do about it and when—is largely related to our concepts of self, our understanding of our place in the world, and our relationships to others. Being sick estranges or reaffirms social and metaphysical relationships; it threatens, sustains, or reorganizes one's self-concept and culpability. Health care providers must concern themselves not only with the disease that ails the patient but with these critical elements of illness that concern the person.

Cases

The next two sections will focus on two Asian American groups and health problems specific to each. The first group, Japanese Americans, has the highest percentage of native-born members whereas the second group, Southeast Asians, has the highest percentage of foreign-born members, giving a picture of health problems for both an established Asian American ethnic group and the most recent group to arrive. The first section will be on Japanese Americans and cancer. The importance for health care professionals to understand cultural interpretations of meaning and self-concept will be discussed. The subsequent section will focus on Southeast Asian Americans and their physical and mental health problems. Many of the problems this group faces are a complex mix of physical, mental, and social problems that pose unique difficulties and barriers to care.

Japanese American Women: Coping with Cancer

Disease

Until recently, data collected on women's health focused primarily on maternal and child health. This pattern is no different for Asian/Pacific American women. There are few studies on the prevalence of disease among Asian/Pacific American women. However, California data on cancer reveal that breast cancer is by far the most commonly occurring cancer among California Asian/Pacific American women; the second is lung cancer, and the third is cervical cancer (California Department of Health Services 1990). Reasons for different breast and cervical cancer rates between the various Asian/Pacific Americans have not been adequately studied. But, as with other groups, these differences are likely attributed to differences in relevant elements of lifestyles such as diet and smoking as well as variability in health education exposure about the need for early screening and prevention techniques. For example, in the groups of Asian/Pacific Americans where the prevalence of these three cancers was the highest, basic education was limited and early detection procedures were rarely available. One study found that two-thirds of Asian female immigrants had never had a Pap smear and 70 percent had never had a mammogram (Asian Pacific Island California Statewide Health Steering Committee 1991). There also is evidence of late diagnosis and high cancer recurrence rates in Japanese American and Filipino American women (Saunders 1989).

Illness

As previously stated, being sick or injured threatens one's ideas of mortality and wholeness. In spite of suffering the same disease, people display different illness reactions. In this section, some differences in illness reactions to the disease of cancer by Japanese Americans and European Americans will be presented. The details of how each group reacts to the disease and the differences in self-concept and emotional support needs illustrate how health care providers must take into account cultural differences even with members of characteristically acculturated ethnic groups.

Japanese Americans offer a unique comparative population with European Americans as they are the only Asian/Pacific American group with primarily one immigration period (1880 to 1924) with little subsequent immigration. Japanese Americans are considered one of the most acculturated of the Asian/Pacific American groups with the attainment of a stable middle class largely composed of white-collar workers and professionals, although there is a "persistence" of ethnicity despite structural assimilation (Fugita and O'Brien 1991).

Cancer Coping Strategies

In 1988, one of the authors compared Japanese American and European American cancer patients and their coping patterns (Kagawa-Singer 1988). The sample consisted of twenty-five Japanese Americans and twenty-five European Americans: eighteen women and seven men in each group. The median age was sixty-seven. The men and women in the sample had various types of cancers.

The first step in coping with the cancer diagnosis reported by both groups was the acceptance of the diagnosis as a reality. Over 80 percent of both Japanese and European Americans reported the importance of this first step. However, they differed in their responses to this "acceptance." European Americans reported that acceptance required them to accept that it was fate that they should have cancer. Japanese Americans perceived cancer as one's karma or destiny.[12] Although these two concepts appear similar, each group's acceptance led to different emotional and behavioral responses. The emotional response of the European Americans to one's fated diagnosis was acknowledgment or resignation but not capitulation. Their behavioral response was to resist the onslaught of the disease and fight a heroic and valiant battle against a tenacious but beatable adversary. In contrast, the Japanese Americans' emotional response was acceptance of their responsibility in causing the disease and their behavioral response was to accommodate and bear the necessary onslaught of pain and suffering with silent, internal strength and dignity (gaman). Both were active and strong responses but qualitatively different forms of "acceptance."

Emotional Responses

The psychosocial literature on emotional responses to cancer focuses on patients' anger and denial as a response to cancer. In this study, rather than anger, the common response of both groups was sadness coupled with disappointment and fear. The sadness was for the loss of what might have been. As for denial, patients did not completely deny their situation but used "denial-like processes" of avoidance and suppression (Lazarus 1983). There were cultural differences in the manner of denial. Japanese Americans used denial in the form of avoidance and deflection. They would resist learning too much detail about their disease or prognosis: "Don't ask, then you don't have to deal with the new information," or "I don't want to know, so I don't ask." The European American patients demonstrated denial through optimism and will: "I just have to keep a positive attitude," or "I won't allow myself to be down."

Maintaining Social Roles

Both groups expressed concern that the disease and its treatment would interfere with fulfilling roles that provided them with a sense of self-worth and satisfaction, roles in which they felt they were competent. Interestingly, European American males and Japanese American females appeared to experience the greatest difficulties in coping with cancer. For both, the disruption of daily life and their competency was the most difficult part of the cancer experience. Both European American males and Japanese American females experienced the most "somatic distress" or side effects from the treatments. Eighty-three percent of the European American men and 64 percent of the Japanese American women suffered greater distress than the European American women (31%) and Japanese American men (33%). In addition, for the European American men these side effects infringed on their job performance and feelings of competence and productivity. For the Japanese American women it was an infringement on their independence and self-sufficiency, as well as on their role competence as the manager and emotional center of the family. (See also Glenn 1986; Yanagisako 1977.) Nisei Japanese American women were raised to fulfill the dependency needs (*amae*) of their husbands and children largely through their own self-sacrifice.

Japanese American men reported experiencing the least disruption to their lives, perhaps secure in the knowledge that their wives would meet their physical and emotional needs. It is a telling example that one of the Japanese American men left his wife upon her cancer diagnosis, perhaps in reaction to the possible role reversal required of him to provide the emotional and physical support for her.

Communication about Cancer Condition

The pattern of communication about their disease condition was more direct and open for the European American patients than for the Japanese Americans. For example, one European American woman, Mrs. Hamil, told her family all she knew of her disease and how she felt about it.[13] She felt it was best to have everything out in the open. In contrast, the Japanese Americans emphasized their desire not to talk about the cancer. Mrs. Oishi felt that as long as she could keep the facade of "normality" for her children, they would feel that everything was fine. She felt that was her role. She denied anything was wrong in order not to disrupt her family and to keep their lives on course. No one could talk with her about her disease. A charade ensued where the family then went along for her benefit (Long and Long 1982).

Japanese American wives of cancer patients may act as buffers against their husbands' acknowledgment of their diagnosis. In one case, a seventy-six-year-old man did not "know" he had cancer. He and his wife spoke to the interviewer in not so subtle allusions about his situation. When asked by Kagawa-Singer what disease he had, Mr. Takei replied, "Don't know. Doctor didn't tell me anything. He didn't tell me cancer." His wife inserted that the doctor told the family, but "he [referring to her husband listening in the same room] doesn't know." After some discussion by both husband and wife about famous people who had cancer, Mrs. Takei said, "But, uh, us, you know, common people, it's more comfortable. Then you are getting well. Then you have cancer. Then his mind is getting—" Her husband interjects: "More shock!" "Yeah, more down," adds his wife. He continues, "I'm not like famous man, see? [laughs] So if I die, it's okay. I die." His wife, surprised, says, "Oh, yeah?" "Yeah," he responds, "die, no writing or something. Just wife and kids worry, ne [right]? And anyway, Mama [his wife] take care of me." This last comment poignantly emphasizes the wife's role as caretaker of a husband's emotional and physical needs.

The reluctance to express one's feelings to others does not mean that one is unaware of the feelings, but feelings are suppressed rather than repressed (Lebra 1984). Mrs. Kanagai used a cultural form of writing to express her innermost feelings.

> Used to write, I hate to talk to anybody about my troubles—so I put in my life and make a story. I do that for a long time now, for twenty-five years, began when I was a child and lived with my aunt and uncle in Japan. I had nobody to talk to about my feelings, so I began writing Tanka poetry [a Japanese literary form]. When I came back from [internment] camp, I brought back a lot of newspapers, and chronicles and things, and records I had kept, but anyway, I was working and I never wrote them up or finished. So all that was wasted. [laughing] I was going to write something. Lot of things. Can't write now. No energy.

Cultural Considerations for Interaction

The rule for interpersonal interactions, particularly for Japanese American women, is that the "other" is always the center of one's concern. The Japanese American women in this study knew that their families worried and grieved for them, but perhaps they felt their families could not share or acknowledge this grief because it might intensify the suffering of the family and place the self-effacing patient uncomfortably in the spotlight. Therefore, the ultimate sacrifice one could make would be to leave as gracefully as possible without complaining, continuing to maintain self-sufficiency and showing gratitude for the things they had. They would not unduly burden their loved ones with inconsolable sorrow. It would be easier to maintain the illusion of having completed one's responsibilities without causing undue hardships on anyone. Mrs. Nawata's remarks personify this attitude:

> Most of the people, you know, are really surprised that I take it all so calmly, but not really. Inside I'm like this [indicating tied up in knots]. But like I said, I hate to put burden on somebody else if it's my problem. I feel everybody has their own problems. Other people can't solve it for you, I figure. What's done is done, and I have to face it. I've done that all my life, so that's the way I do it, I guess.

Forcing these patients to talk about their feelings can be not only counterproductive but destructive. One of the Japanese American women, a fifty-year-old mother of three, had been in family counseling because of a son's drug problems. She felt extremely uncomfortable talking about family problems, conflicts, and her own unstated emotions. Her remarks illustrate a distinctly cultural response:

> I would feel worse to complain and confront. I haven't gotten to the point where I could complain and not feel bad about it. . . . I worry too much on what effect it would have on the guy who had to listen to it! I've said stuff that I thought shouldn't be heard or anything—and then I just feel so AWFUL afterwards. It didn't make me feel any better. So it's better if I don't say [anything]—but maybe, like family stuff—if someone doesn't do something they should have, maybe if I could learn to handle it—then everybody would know exactly where I stand. But, you know, we were taught not to speak badly of anyone. I just feel terrible afterwards. It's not worth it! We tried it a couple of times as a family. But I guess I REALLY didn't want to do it—to sit there and *confront*. So we never did. We did a couple of times, but IT'S JUST NOT NORMAL.

Culturally Relevant Cancer Care

The objective for health care workers is to relieve suffering and assist the individual to obtain, maintain, or regain physical and emotional integrity. However, to achieve these ends, the interventions must be tailored to individual and cultural differences in the meaning of the illness, the side effects created by the cancer, and its treatment and effect on the communication patterns in the family.

Most Asian cultures require a period of acquaintance before members will discuss private, personal matters. They rarely discuss such matters with a stranger. Further, divulging private information may be difficult to do with a health care provider who is viewed as an authority figure. Many Japanese Americans defer to authority figures and will not wish to "make trouble" by telling them personal problems. Therefore, the health care worker must have the patience to build rapport to nurture a sense of trust. Health care providers need to negotiate with the patient *and* family (recognizing the designated decision maker in the family may not be the patient) about the desired outcome and plan of care.

Negotiation is a relatively new American concept between patient and practitioner, and for more traditionally raised Asians, negotiating as an equal with a physician is an alien concept. Among Japanese Americans, particularly first-generation Issei and second-generation Nisei, deference to authority figures rather than negotiation would be the preferred interaction approach. It is unlikely that negative comments or confrontation will be made by patients or family members. Rather, nonadherence is often the means for expressions of disagreement with the health care plan, although adherence is often high for the more acculturated Asian patient. It will take time to educate the patient and family about expectations of discussion and negotiation, but this method ensures a higher likelihood that the patient and family will adhere to the decisions made.

Sontag's work on illness as metaphor (in spite of the author's protestations) conveys the power of the symbolic meaning of cancer (1977) and the potency of illness interpretation over the biophysical elements of disease. The comparative study of cultural and gender responses to cancer illustrates the need for cultural sensitivity toward the very different illness interpretations and coping patterns regarding a single disease, even for an Asian/Pacific American group that is among the most acculturated.

Southeast Asian American Women: Mental Health Needs

The mass exodus of Southeast Asian refugees from their homes in Cambodia, Laos, and Vietnam to escape war, genocide, political turmoil, and famine resulted in an estimated 900,000 Southeast Asian refugees resettling in the United States (Rumbaut 1990).[14] The age distribution is skewed toward the young (median age of 23.9 years) and roughly evenly divided between men (56%) and women (44%) (U.S. Committee for Refugees 1984). Although Southeast Asian refugees have settled in every state in the United States, this population is concentrated in California, Texas, and Washington.

Physical Health

Most of the literature on Southeast Asian refugees has focused on psychological adjustment; there is little research on physical health issues. However, the refugees have been found to experience not only psychiatric symptoms and disorders but also neurologic disorders and a host of physical disorders and infectious diseases (Catanzaro and Moser 1982; Hoang and Erickson 1985; Mollica and Jalbert 1989; Mollica, Wyshak, Coelho, and Lavelle 1985).[15]

A large percentage of women have undergone abortions as a result of the high incidence of rape and sexual abuse. Both women and men have been found to experience sexual dysfunction and mutilation of their genitalia (Mollica and Jalbert 1989).

Psychological Problems

Southeast Asian refugees, especially women, have been categorized as a high-risk group for developing serious psychiatric disorders because of their traumatic premigration experiences (Lin, Tazauma, and Masuda 1979; Mollica and Lavelle 1988; Mollica, Wyshak, and Lavelle 1987; Rumbaut 1990). Traumatic events are divided into three periods of premigration: the war and active genocide, the escape process, and the refugee camp experience (Mollica and Lavelle 1988). Many refugees experienced multiple traumas including physical and psychological torture. Cambodians have been found to have had more traumatic events during these three periods than other Southeast Asian groups. The final relocation (or "migration") trip to the eventual host country is not generally associated with serious personal and physical injury in itself, but it is considered "ecologically traumatic." This discussion will focus on women's experiences during the premigration and the resettlement periods.

Common psychiatric disorders found among Southeast Asian refugees are depression, anxiety, and post-traumatic stress disorders (PTSD) (Kinzie et al. 1984; Kinzie and Manson 1983; Mollica et al. 1987; Mollica and Lavelle 1988). Many also experience demoralization, powerlessness, hopelessness, despair, poor concentration, low energy, decreased appetite, and sleep disorders (Mollica and Jalbert 1989; Mollica and Lavelle 1988). These findings are not surprising considering the level and degree of traumatic events this group has suffered: torture, imprisonment, the witnessing of executions, and being forced to commit atrocities themselves.

Premigration Trauma

Refugee women in the United States have reported higher levels of psychological distress than their male counterparts (Chung and Kagawa-Singer 1993; Mollica, Lavelle, and Khoun 1985). Three of the most serious premigration traumas for refugee women were rape or sexual abuse, widowhood, and the loss of children. Many women experienced all three traumas.

Rape and Sexual Abuse. There have been numerous reports of sexual abuse of Southeast Asian women during the war, in the overcrowded refugee camps, and during their escape. For example, pirate attacks on the boat people have been well documented by the popular media. An estimated 77 percent of the refugee boats were attacked (U.S. Committee for Refugees 1984). Some of the boats were buried or destroyed by pirates after robbery, murder, abduction, and rape of the women. Women of all ages were victimized in these attacks, and few were spared. Many experienced multiple rapes, with some individuals reportedly suffering ten to thirty rapes. Most of the rapes were described as brutal, leading to deformation or mutilation of the genitalia. Many of the victims were then kidnapped and/or sold into prostitution (Burton 1983).

In Southeast Asian cultures, women typically blame themselves for the rape, and only a few seek help. They are engulfed by shame and guilt, by the loss of their self-respect and honor, and how they have dishonored their family. Most attempt to bury or repress their feelings. Many rape victims do not dare tell their husbands, because husbands often will leave them if they have been sexually violated. These women are perceived as having been "used," "violated," or "left over" by the rapist. For example, a Cambodian woman was raped by a soldier while she was gathering firewood in the jungle at a refugee camp. Following this incident, her husband regularly beat her, haunted by memories of her rape whenever he made love to her (Mollica and Son 1989). A Vietnamese proverb brutally summarizes these sentiments: "Someone ate out of my bowl and left it dirty."

The social consequences of rape include community rejection, family disownment, divorce, and even murder of the rape victim by family members. In a culture where virginity is viewed as a "prized possession" for single women with a strong emphasis on fidelity for married women, rape victims are blamed and punished for destroying their family's honor. Many victims are unable to turn to family members and friends for support due to their fear of the social and cultural consequences of revealing the rape. Therefore, sexual trauma is a deeply held secret kept from everyone; the woman suffering in isolated silence. Some have committed suicide by hanging or poisoning because of the shame, stigma, and lack of support (Mollica and Son 1989).

In addition to the psychological effects of rape (anxiety over unwanted pregnancies, the reduced chance for a good marriage, depression, insomnia, nightmares, impaired concentration, identity problems, sexual problems, phobias, and difficulties in interpersonal relationships), severe physical conditions also can occur. These include venereal disease, HIV infection, mutilation of the female genitalia, infertility, miscarriage, menstruation disorders, and severe and chronic abdominal and pelvic pain.

Widowhood. Another group of women who are at risk for developing serious psychological disorders are refugees widowed during the premigration period. Many of these women witnessed their husbands' murders. In general, women experienced a greater frequency of spousal loss than men, with Cambodians having the highest rate of spousal loss among refugee women (Gong-Guy 1986; Mollica, Lavelle, and Khoun 1985).[16] These women have exhibited depression, anxiety, and PTSD.

Child Loss. Women have reported witnessing their babies being beaten to death against trees because they were weak or sickly, children being torn limb from limb, or children starving to death (Ponchaud 1978; Szymusiak 1986). Many women who lost their children through such unnatural means also have consequent psychological problems. Again, Cambodian women lost more children than other Southeast Asian groups. For example, in the California Statewide Needs Assessment of Southeast Asian Refugees, 53 percent of the Cambodian women in the sample reported the loss of their children through such traumatic means as compared with 11 percent of Laotian and Vietnamese women (Gong-Guy 1986). As with the other two groups the most common psychological problems of these women who lost children during premigration are depression, anxiety, and PTSD.

Resettlement Issues

Rape and Sexual Abuse. Abuse can continue during the resettlement period. Shame and secrecy may create social disruption. For example, a Vietnamese adolescent was adopted by a Vietnamese family in the United States. A stepuncle raped her several times a night. This continued for over a year. When a concerned teacher spoke to the girl about her tendency to fall asleep in class every day, she discovered the pattern of sexual abuse. The teacher reported the matter to the police. After the police investigation made the rapes public knowledge, the victim's family was so humiliated and "tainted" in the Vietnamese community that they were forced to move to another state where the family could maintain the teenager's secret (Chung 1988).

Employment. During the resettlement phase, women must cope with a host of new problems: they are expected to care for their families and contribute to the new life in a productive way (Davison 1981). Unemployment or underemployment of refugee men commonly forces women to work to support their families. Most Southeast Asian refugee men have not been able to find work commensurate with their education and training in their homeland. Physicians, academics, and former military officers have been reduced to taking low-paying unskilled jobs. Women, whose primary role in their home country was as unpaid labor as a homemaker or in a family business or farm, find work in the United States in sewing factories, as assemblers of computer components, or other such unskilled work. Women's work sometimes provides the only household income.

Those who work in factories or assembly companies often work twelve-hour days, seven days a week. Recognizing the frequency of layoffs, they try not to miss any days, and they work hard to impress their employers to be kept on the payroll. Obviously, such individuals find it impossible to keep medical appointments or adhere to a course of treatment for serious diseases.

Gender Roles. Ironically, whereas many refugee men have experienced downward mobility, many women have experienced a kind of upward mobility through paid employment. The resulting changes in gender roles have placed severe pressures on marital relationships. Researchers have found that the increase in spousal abuse and divorce is a direct result of this tension (Luu 1989).

Previously unknown opportunities and freedom for women also can bring desires for more professional advancement and life enhancement such as an education. In a recent tragedy, a wife's desire to get an education and a job was vigorously opposed by her husband. She separated from him, stating her intentions to obtain a divorce and custody of the children. The distraught husband set fire to their home, killing himself and their four children. Before this, the family had seemed an exemplary case of adjustment to American life. They were devout Catholics, they had close, extended family members in the area, the husband was employed, and all four children were born in the United States (Dizon and Le 1992). Although this is an extreme and unusual case, it illustrates the strength and volatility of emotions even within seemingly stable families with solid social support systems.[17]

Child-Rearing Expectations. Language barriers coupled with cultural differences add to refugee women's problems. Refugee women have been accused of child neglect and abuse because of misunderstandings by Americans about cultural practices. For example, "coining," where the edge of a coin or spoon is rubbed firmly over places of the body to correct a systemic imbalance in the body's hot/cold equilibrium, often leaving welts or bruises, has been mislabeled as child abuse (Nguyen, Nguyen, and Nguyen 1987).[18]

Many refugee women lack family members to help with child care. Some who have left their children unaccompanied or with older siblings out of necessity have been accused of child neglect.

Psychosomatic Disorders. Some older Cambodian women in the United States have displayed nonorganic or psychosomatic blindness in response to the severity of their premigration traumas. The degree of subjective visual impairment has been found to be significantly related to the number of years the women were interned in the camps and also the degree and level of traumatic events they witnessed. A common explanation given by these women was this: "I started crying hard for a long time. . . . Later when I finally stopped crying I could not see" (Rozee and Van Boemel 1989).

Support and Strength

What is not publicized is the special strength many refugee women possess. In some cases they have been found to cope better than men during the resettlement period (Davison 1981; Gellerman 1980). Highly traumatized women appear to obtain the greatest benefit from professional treatment. What is striking is their dramatic ability to use clinics as a source of support. Many reportedly experienced a major reduction of symptoms as well as marked improvement in social functioning (Mollica, Lavelle, and Khoun 1985). Some display amazing courage, strength, and will power to overcome their traumas and to rebuild their lives. It is important to acknowledge the strengths of Southeast Asian refugee women as well as the disadvantages they face. Also, it is vital to provide treatment and support for those who desperately need help.

Culturally appropriate community-based programs can assist sexually abused women. For example, new Buddhist rituals and rites for "cleansing" sexually abused women are needed. Buddhist nuns can be trained to provide counseling for rape victims. Education programs should be developed to teach both male and female refugees about preventive medicine, primary health care, family planning, support groups, acceptance of both male and female sharing roles within the household, sanitation, and infant and child care. These programs should be held in or close to residential areas, community centers, and commercial centers. Active outreach programs must be established to reach isolated women in their homes and places of work. Recruitment of bilingual/bicultural personnel for all services is crucial. Finally, although Southeast Asian women have been discussed as a group, vast differences within this group of histories, cultures, languages, and education must be taken into account to plan appropriate programs and health care.

Summation

Although Asian/Pacific Americans make up only 3 percent of the nation's population, they are the fastest growing group in the country. Furthermore, there is a population concentration in the western states, particularly in California, where 40 percent live, forming 10 percent of that state's population. But there are Asian/Pacific Americans in every state, each one of them entering the health care system at some time in his or her life. The sheer complexity of this ethnic collection must not obscure human variability. Both the group complexity and individual differences must be recognized and incorporated into programs and people's consciousness to provide culturally sensitive and appropriate service for everyone, from the long established American-born groups such as Japanese Americans to the most recent arrivals such as Southeast Asians.

It has become a bit of a cliché to note that not only must the disease be cured but the patient, too, must be healed. But that makes it no less of a truism. In that regard, we must be sensitive to the cultural dynamics of comfort and care not only for Asian/Pacific Americans but for all people.

NOTES

Thank you to the Women, Health, and Healing Program at the University of California, San Francisco, for the generous support that made this chapter possible.

1. Examples of these complexities include Hindu Tamils and Buddhist Sinhalese in Sri Lanka; Cantonese speakers in Hong Kong and the primarily Mandarin Chinese speakers in adjacent China; Western and American Samoa; and Vietnamese Buddhists and Catholics.

2. Census materials were generously provided, often on short notice, by Jerry Wong, information services specialist of the U.S. Census Bureau.

3. These national census figures do not include write-in responses for such groups as Cambodian, Thai, Laotian, or Fijians. Although these groups are included in the sample tabulations, the 100 percent tabulations do not represent a full count for Asian/Pacific Americans. Further, it is felt that Asian Americans were drastically undercounted in the census. One particular group of note is the Vietnamese. In addition to problems of literacy, mobility, multiple-family households, language, and nonreturn of forms, many Vietnamese who are ethnically Chinese identified themselves as Chinese and not Vietnamese.

4. See Cheng and Cheng 1984:9–10 for what appears to be a Chinese American case of lost citizenship caused by the Cable Act.

5. This early Korean immigration was considered by the American and Japanese governments as part of Japanese immigration and jurisdiction, despite vigorous protestations by Koreans in the United States.

6. For example, see Johnson (1974) and Fugita and O'Brien (1991) for cultural continuity among Japanese Americans extending into the third generation.

7. One of the best compilations on the backgrounds, traumas, and family struc-

tures of these various Southeast Asian groups is a 1983 handbook published by the Asian American Community Mental Health Training Center in Los Angeles called *Bridging Cultures: Southeast Asian Refugees in America*. It had a limited distribution but is available through libraries.

8. Even more recently there is a special nonimmigrant, nonrefugee class of public interest parolees who were largely "reeducation" camp detainees in Vietnam. But the majority of Southeast Asians still arrive as refugees and are therefore eligible for certain government support programs.

9. See the special issue of *Social Process in Hawaii* on the health of native Hawai'ians (Wegner 1989) for more details. A recent report released by the National Cancer Institute on the average annual incidence and mortality rates of cancer from 1988 to 1992 is one of the first to report data for various ethnic groups by sex. In this most comprehensive report on cancer incidence and mortality for minority groups, data are provided on Chinese, Filipino, Hawai'ian, Japanese, Korean, and Vietnamese men and women. Data are also presented for Alaska Natives, American Indians (New Mexico), blacks, Hispanics (total), white Hispanics, and whites. Hawai'ian women ranked fourth in average annual incidence (321/100,000), behind Alaska Native women (348/100,000), white women (346/100,000), and African American women (326/100,000). However, Hawai'ian women tied with African American women for the second-highest mortality rates (168/100,000), behind Alaska Native women (179/100,000). White women ranked next with a mortality rate of 140/100,000 (Wright 1996). In addition, Hawai'ian women had the second-highest incidence rate of breast cancer (105.6/100,000), as compared to whites (115.7), blacks (95.4), and Japanese (82.3); while Vietnamese women had an astonishing 43.0/100,000 incidence rate for cervical cancer, as compared to the next-highest incidence rates among white Hispanic (17.1), Hispanic (16.2), Alaska Native (15.8), and Korean women (15.2) (Miller et al. 1996). This may indicate differential access to early testing and treatment or cultural barriers to testing and treatment for minority women.

10. A considerably different pattern of infant mortality rates exists in Hawai'i, where the 1980–86 rates per 1,000 were 9.3 of the entire state's population, 6.6 for whites, 7.3 for Japanese, 14.1 for Hawai'ians, 8.8 for Filipinos, 7.7 for Chinese, and 9.3 for others (Bell, Nordyke, and O'Hagan 1989).

11. The first author wishes to thank the National Institute of Mental Health grant No. Ro1MH33038 for funding of this research, "Health Care Alternatives of Asian American Women."

12. Karma in Buddhism and Hinduism is a belief that one's previous lives affect one's current state: "Suffering and hardship must be accepted with resignation [because of one's predestination]. . . . Things are considered irreversible once they have taken place. It is silly, therefore, to regret [things that have taken place] . . . because no amount of regret can reverse the course of events" (Lebra 1976:165–66).

13. Pseudonyms are used throughout.

14. Note that this amount is considerably above the official U.S. Census Bureau count but may be more accurate.

15. Common physical ailments in Southeast Asian refugees are skin diseases, gum and teeth diseases, respiratory infections, urinary tract infections, ear and eye

infections, pneumonia, nutritional disorders, cardiovascular disorders, hepatitis, tuberculosis, heart disease, diabetes, and infectious diseases. These medical problems have been found to be related to malnutrition and the shortage of water during premigration. Neurologic disorders, such as head injury, have been associated with severe beatings and torture (Mollica and Jalbert 1989).

16. The California Statewide Needs Assessment of Southeast Asian Refugees (Gong-Guy 1986) reported 22 percent of the Cambodian women in the sample were widows as compared with 2 percent of Cambodian men, 3 percent of Lao women, 5 percent of Lao men, 11 percent of Vietnamese women, and 9 percent of Vietnamese men.

17. Thank you to Nghia Trung Tran, executive director of the Vietnamese Community of Orange County, Inc., for providing not only this example but the Orange County news coverage of this event as well.

18. This practice is based on a layperson's interpretation of Chinese medical practices. The rubbing releases the excess of heat in one's system, as evidenced by the red marks, and is usually done to remedy minor illnesses such as sore throats or cold/flus. See Pokert 1976 for a brief summary of Chinese medicine and the importance of maintaining equilibrium for good health. See Veith 1966 [1949] for an introduction to and translation of the classic and oldest known document of Chinese medicine, the *Nei Ching*.

REFERENCES

Asian Pacific Island California Statewide Health Steering Committee
 1991 Position Paper on Cancer. Unpublished paper.
Bell, Bella Zi, Eleanor C. Nordyke, and Patricia O'Hagan
 1989 "Fertility and maternal and child health." Social Process in Hawaii 32:87-103.
Burton, Eve
 1983 "Surviving the flight of horror: the story of refugee women." Indochinese Issues 34:1-7.
California Department of Health Services
 1990 "California behavioral risk factor survey." Unpublished data.
Catanzaro, Antonio, and Robert J. Moser
 1982 "Health status of refugees from Vietnam, Laos and Cambodia." JAMA 244(2):2748-49.
Cheng, Lucie, and Suellen Cheng
 1984 "Chinese women of Los Angeles: a social historical survey." Pp. 1-26 in Linking Our Lives. Los Angeles: Chinese Historical Society of Southern California.
Chung, Rita Chi-Ying
 1988 Unpublished interviews.
Chung, Rita Chi-Ying, and Marjorie Kagawa-Singer
 1993 "Predictors of psychological distress among Southeast Asian refugees." Social Science and Medicine 36(5):631-39.

Davison, Lani
  1981   "Women refugees: special needs and programs." Journal of Refugee Re-
          settlement 1(3):16–26.
Dizon, Lily, and Thuan Le
  1992   "Father and four children die in fire." Los Angeles Times, 4 August.
Eisenberg, Leon
  1977   "Disease and illness." Culture, Medicine and Psychiatry 1(9):9–23.
Fugita, Stephen, and David J. O'Brien
  1991   Japanese American Ethnicity: The Persistence of Community. Seattle:
          University of Washington Press.
Gellerman, Randy
  1980   "Towards understanding Third World womanhood: Vietnamese women,
          their men, their children, and their lives." Paper presented at the Asso-
          ciation of Asian Studies Annual Conference. Washington.
Glenn, Evelyn Nakano
  1983   "Split household, small producer, and dual wage earner: an analysis of
          Chinese-American family strategies." Journal of Marriage and the Family
          45(1):35–46.
  1986   Issei, Nisei, War Bride. Philadelphia: Temple University Press.
Gong-Guy, Elizabeth
  1986   The California Southeast Asian Mental Health Needs Assessment. Oak-
          land: Asian Community Mental Health Services.
Hoang, Giao N., and Roy V. Erickson
  1985   "Cultural barriers to effective medical care among Indochinese patients."
          American Review of Medicine 36:229–39.
Howard, Alan
  1974   Ain't No Big Thing: Coping Strategies in a Hawaiian American Com-
          munity. Honolulu: University of Hawaii Press.
Hubler, Shawn
  1992   "'80s failed to end economic disparity, census shows." Los Angeles Times,
          17 August.
Ichioka, Yuji
  1980   "Amerika Nadeshiko: Japanese immigrant women in the United States,
          1900–1924." Pacific Historical Review 48:339–57.
Ito, Karen L.
  1982   NIMH Final Report: Health Care Alternative of Asian-American
          Women. Grant No. Ro1MH33038.
Johnson, Colleen Leahy
  1974   "Gift giving and reciprocity among the Japanese Americans in Hono-
          lulu." American Ethnologist 1(2):295–308.
Kagawa-Singer, Marjorie
  1988   "Bamboo and oak: differences in adaptation to cancer between Japanese
          American and Anglo-American patients." Ph.D. diss., University of Cal-
          ifornia, Los Angeles.

Kinzie, David, and Spero Manson
> 1983 "Five years' experience with Indochinese refugee psychiatric patients." Journal of Operational Psychiatry 14(3):105-11.

Kinzie, David, R. H. Frederickson, Rath Ben, Jenelle Fleck, and William Karls
> 1984 "Post-traumatic stress disorder among survivors of Cambodian concentration camps." American Journal of Psychiatry 141:645.

Lazarus, Richard S.
> 1983 "The costs and benefits of denial." Pp. 1-30 in Shlomo Breznitz (ed.), The Denial of Stress. New York: International Universities Press.

Lebra, Takie Sugiyama
> 1976 Japanese Patterns of Behavior. Honolulu: University of Hawaii Press.
> 1984 "Nonconfrontational strategies for management of interpersonal conflict." Pp. 41-84 in Ellis S. Krauss, Thomas P. Rohlen, and Patricia G. Steinhoff (eds.), Conflict in Japan. Honolulu: University of Hawaii Press.

Lin, Keh-Ming, Laurie Tazauma, and Minoru Masuda
> 1979 "Adaptational problems of Vietnamese refugees." Archives of General Psychiatry 36:955.

Long, Susan, and Bruce D. Long
> 1982 "Curable cancer and fatal ulcers: attitudes toward cancer in Japan." Social Science and Medicine 16:2101-8.

Luu, Van
> 1989 "The hardships of escape for Vietnamese women." Pp. 60-72 in Asian Women United California (eds.), Making Waves: An Anthology of Writing by and about Asian-American Women. Boston: Beacon Press.

Miller, B. A., L. N. Kolonel, L. Bernstein, J. L. Young Jr., G. M. Swanson, D. West, C. R. Key, J. M. Liff, C. S. Glover, and G. A. Alexander
> 1996 Racial/Ethnic Patterns of Cancer in the United States, 1988-1992. NIH Publication No. 96-4104. Bethesda, MD: National Cancer Institute.

Mollica, Richard F., and Russell R. Jalbert
> 1989 Community of Confinement: The Mental Health Crisis on Site Two: Displaced Persons' Camps on the Thai-Kampuchean Border. Boston: Committee on World Federation for Mental Health.

Mollica, Richard F., and James Lavelle
> 1988 "Southeast Asian refugees." Pp. 262-303 in L. Comas-Diaz and E. E. H. Griffith (eds.), Clinical Guidelines in Cross-Cultural Mental Health. New York: Wiley.

Mollica, Richard F., and Linda Son
> 1989 "Cultural dimensions in the evaluation and treatment of sexual trauma." Psychiatric Clinics of North America 12(2):363-79.

Mollica, Richard F., James Lavelle, and Fran Khoun
> 1985 "Khmer widows at highest risk." A paper presented at the Cambodian Mental Health Conference: A Day to Explore Issues and Alternative Approaches to Care. New York.

Mollica, Richard F., Grace Wyshak, Rosemarie Coelho, and James Lavelle
   1985   The Southeast Asian Psychiatry Patient: A Treatment Outcome Study.
          Boston: Indochinese Psychiatric Clinic.
Mollica, Richard F., Grace Wyshak, and James Lavelle
   1987   "The psychosocial impact of war trauma and torture on Southeast Asian
          refugees." American Journal of Psychiatry 144:1567.
National Cancer Institute
   1996   Racial/ethnic patterns of cancer in the United States, 1988–1992. Sur-
          veillance, Epidemiology and End Results (SEER) Program Monograph.
          Bethesda, MD: NCI.
Nguyen, Nga, Phouc H. Nguyen, and Loc H. Nguyen
   1987   "Coin treatment in Vietnamese families: traditional medical practice vs.
          child abuse." Unpublished manuscript.
Osumi, Megumi Dick
   1982   "Asians and California's anti-miscegenation laws." Pp. 1–37 in N.
          Tsuchida (ed.), Asian and Pacific American Experiences. Minneapolis:
          University of Minnesota Asian/Pacific American Learning Resource
          Center.
Ponchaud, Francois
   1978   Cambodia: Year Zero. New York: Holt, Rinehart and Winston.
Porkert, Manfred
   1976   "The intellectual and social impulses behind the evolution of traditional
          Chinese medicine." Pp. 63–76 in C. Leslie (ed.), Asian Medical Systems.
          Berkeley: University of California Press.
Rozee, Patricia D., and Gretchen Van Boemel
   1989   "The psychological effects of war trauma and abuse on older Cambodian
          refugee women." Women and Therapy 8(4):23–50.
Rumbaut, Reuben G.
   1990   "The agony of exile: a study of the migration and adaptation of Indochin-
          ese refugee adults and children." Pp. 53–91 in F. L. Ahearn and J. Garri-
          son (eds.), Refugee Children: Theory, Research, and Practice. Baltimore:
          Johns Hopkins University Press.
Saunders, L. Duncan
   1989   "Differences in the timeliness of diagnosis, breast and cervical cancer, San
          Francisco 1974–1985." American Journal of Public Health 79:69–70.
Sontag, Susan
   1977   Illness as Metaphor. New York: Random House.
Stevens, Cladd E., Pearl T. Toy, Myron J. Tong, Patricia E. Taylor, Girish N. Vyas,
Prem V. Nair, Madhu Gudavalli, and Saul Krugman
   1985   "Perinatal hepatitis B virus transmission in the United States." JAMA
          253:1740–45.
Szymusiak, Molyda
   1986   The Stones Cry Out: A Cambodian Childhood, 1975–1980. New York:
          Hill and Wang.

Tabayas, Theresa, and Than Pok
  1981   "The Southeast Asian refugee's arrival in America: an overview." Pp. 3–14 in Social Work with Southeast Asian Refugees (eds.), Bridging Cultures: Southeast Asian Refugees in America. Los Angeles: Asian-American Community Mental Health Training Center.
U.S. Bureau of Census
  1990   Summary Tape File 1A and unpublished census files.
U.S. Committee for Refugees
  1984   Vietnamese Boat People: Pirates' Vulnerable Prey. Washington: American Council for Nationalistic Services.
U.S. General Accounting Office (GAO)
  1990   Asian-Americans: A Status Report. Gaithersburg, MD: General Accounting Office.
Veith, Ilza
  [1949] Huang Ti Nei Ching Su Wen: The Yellow Emperor's Classic of Internal
  1996   Medicine. New ed. Berkeley: University of California Press.
Wegner, Eldon, ed.
  1989   "The Health of Native Hawaiians: A Selective Report on Health Care Status and Health Care in the 1980s." Social Process in Hawaii 32 (special issue).
Wright, Walter
  1996   "Hawaiians rank no. 1 in cancer death rate." Honolulu Advertiser, 1 May.
Yanagisako, Sylvia J.
  1977   "Women-centered kin networks in urban bilateral kinship." American Ethnologist 5(1):15–29.
  1985   Transforming the Past: Tradition and Kinship among Japanese Americans. Stanford: Stanford University Press.
Yang, Eun Sik
  1984   "Korean women of America: from subordination to partnership, 1903–1930." Amerasia Journal 11(2):1–28.

[13]

Issues in Latino Women's Health:
Myths and Challenges

SUSAN C. M. SCRIMSHAW, RUTH E. ZAMBRANA,
AND CHRISTINE DUNKEL-SCHETTER

These scholars' qualitative research on pregnancy behaviors of Puerto Rican women in New York City and Mexican American and Mexican immigrant women in Los Angeles illustrates how cultural misconceptions held by hospital personnel can negatively influence the quality of medical care provided. Their recommendations for how to offer more culturally appropriate care provide a model of how qualitative research can be used to reshape the behavior of health workers, not just that of patients.

Historically, the medical and public health communities have largely ignored ethnic and class differences among populations they served. The underlying assumptions guiding these professional communities have been that the technology of biomedicine is applicable to all consumers of health services, irrespective of individual social, cultural, and class variations. Although the last twenty years have witnessed an increased awareness of ethnic and class differences, particularly in the areas of reproductive health, there is still limited recognition and knowledge among health care providers of the influence of sociocultural behaviors on doctor-patient relationships, the use of health services, and health status. Researchers and health care providers can make incorrect assumptions about these different subgroups. They may fail to understand why people do not seek medical care, why medical advice is not followed, and why treatments don't work. Among Latino women, particularly with respect to reproductive health issues, misconceptions regarding culturally shaped behaviors are common and often negatively influence the quality of the delivery of health care services. Thus it is essential to challenge existing assumptions and to clarify the meaning of health behaviors to improve the existing delivery of services in our pluralistic society.

The purpose of this chapter is threefold: to present and discuss some common behaviors related to pregnancy among Latino women, to address a set of misconceptions held by health care providers regarding these cultural behaviors, and to offer some recommendations regarding the provision of appropriate health services to Latino women. The data presented here are based on systematic observations and on empirical studies conducted in obstetrical facilities in New York City with Puerto Rican women and in Los Angeles with Mexican American and Mexican immigrant women.

Background

There is a lack of empirical work on the particular health needs of Latino women and their families. It has only been during the decade of the 1980s that specific systems for identifying members of the Latino subgroups have been put into operation in national data collection systems. In fact, there is an ongoing controversy over whether *Hispanic* or *Latino* should be the national umbrella term (Hayes-Bautista 1980; Trevino 1987). *Hispanic* is more acceptable among national government organizations and in the eastern and southern United States, whereas *Latino* is preferred in the West and Southwest. Unless we are citing published work that uses the word *Hispanics*, we will use the term *Latino* in this chapter.

At present, there are about 20 million Latinos living in the United States, of which 60 percent are Mexican American, 14 percent Puerto Rican, 6 percent Cuban, and 20 percent other Hispanics, mainly Central Americans. It is projected that Latinos will constitute the largest minority population in this country by the year 2000 (Bean and Tienda 1987). In California, it has been projected that Latinos will constitute 50 percent of the population by the year 2010 (Hayes-Bautista, Shink, and Chapa 1988). There are distinct differences between Latino subgroups with respect to country of origin, geographic concentration, English language proficiency, years in the United States, socioeconomic status, and health risk factors. Despite these variations, Latino families tend to be younger, poorer, and less educated than the norms for the U.S. population, which reflect a much higher proportion of individuals born and raised in this country. Youth, poverty, and lower levels of education correlate with less access to health care for Latinos (U.S. Dept. of Commerce 1993). This lack of access is exacerbated by low levels of health insurance. McCarthy and Valdez (1986) estimate that one-third of the Latino population lack health insurance. These characteristics influence the health of women, children, and their families.

Current data are not adequate to identify the most significant health problems for Latinos, although a few government reports, such as the Black and Minority Health Volumes (U.S. Department of Health and Human Services 1986) and Children's Defense Budget (1986), have begun to identify specific health needs of Hispanic subpopulation groups. Two major questions need to be addressed: How do Latino subgroups (as defined above) relate to overall health indicators? And how do their health profiles and needs compare with the services available in the existing structure of the health system? These questions are most critical in the areas of maternal, child, and adolescent health, because the Latino population tends to be young with a high number of women of childbearing age and a high fertility rate (Bean and Tienda 1987; Molina and Aguirre-Molina 1994; Wingard, chapter 2, this volume).

These questions about health profiles and their relationship to services take on a new complexity in the context of both class and culture. Culture includes norms, behaviors, and their meanings, and these may vary with the Latino subgroups but still make up a pattern distinct from other cultures in this country. Class refers primarily to socioeconomic status. Often, it is difficult to tell whether a behavior such as low utilization of health services is due to socioeconomic obstacles or cultural beliefs about the degree of need for health care. It is important to understand how the role of culture for United States Latinos is interrelated with socioeconomic status and other attributes. Specifically, among Mexican origin and Puerto Rican groups, these attributes consist of lower educational levels, less knowledge of health care services and health promotion activities, less experience with large bureaucratic health care systems, more reliance on extended family support, and more traditional beliefs regarding gender roles (Perales and Young 1987; Zambrana 1987; Zambrana and Ellis 1995).

Our research at UCLA on Latino pregnancy and childbirth addresses some of these questions. The data emphasize the importance of challenging the assumptions that guide health care programs and practices in the United States.

Origins of the Research Projects on Latino Women's Reproductive Health

The authors have had a long-standing history of work on the reproductive health needs of Latino women. Two of the authors began working in New

York City in the 1970s with Puerto Rican and other minority groups. Some issues discussed here were raised first when the first author was observing obstetrical residents in a New York hospital in order to understand the socialization of physicians. The obstetrical patients in that hospital were low-income women, predominantly from three ethnic groups: Puerto Rican, Haitian, and American blacks. It was very clear from observations that women in the three groups coped with labor differently and evoked different reactions from hospital staff. For example, the Haitian women made rhythmic sounds, even in early labor. This was regarded as a bid for attention by the staff, who were scornful: "She's only in early labor." In fact, labor chants are a part of labor management in Haiti and might be seen as the Haitian equivalent of Lamaze. Certain sounds are made (such as ooo . . . ooo), whereas others are considered cowardly (such as ow). The sounds may vary with the stage of labor. When this was pointed out to the medical staff, resentment toward "hypochondriacal" Haitians dissipated and was replaced by fascination. Staff tried to guess a woman's stage of labor by her chanting patterns. The most frustration expressed by obstetrical staff, however, was not with the Haitian women but with the Puerto Rican women, who were viewed as excessively noisy and bothersome during labor. Seeing the change in attitude toward the Haitian women when the cultural meaning of the sounds they made was understood raised questions about the need for similar information on Latinos.

Hurst and Zambrana (1980) found that these low-income Puerto Rican women had negative obstetrical experiences with providers and that they were viewed as noncompliant patients. Their study suggests that, for these women, the lack of familiarity with the health care system and their poor treatment by providers was a result of providers' lack of understanding of the women's needs and sociocultural behaviors. The next opportunity to examine issues surrounding birth for Latina women emerged in Los Angeles.

Pilot Research on Myths and Stereotypes about Pregnancy and Birth in Latinos

In 1977, the first author began to explore the opportunities to increase medical professionals' understanding of birth in Latino women in the Los Angeles area. The first myth about Latino women was identified when several departments of obstetrics and gynecology were approached about the possibility of research on Latino women and childbirth. Staff at UCLA agreed to allow a pilot study with the expectation that they would receive help in solving a problem. Latino women, they said, came to the hospital in early labor or not in labor at all (but merely having experienced some of the uterine contractions that often occur in late pregnancy). When told that labor had not yet begun, or that true labor was hours or days away, and that they needed to go home, these women were described by staff as reacting tearfully and argumentatively. The staff asked for help in facilitating an understanding by patients and their families regarding the need to return home. In response to this request, we gathered ethnographic data by observing and interviewing fifty women during labor and delivery and the postpartum hospital stay. This work quickly revealed that women's views of the birth process and their definitions of labor differed greatly from those of the physicians and nurses. Because there is no word for labor in Spanish, only the word for pain, the concept of a long process with distinct stages was absent (Scrimshaw and Souza 1982).

To improve communication between staff and patients regarding the onset of labor, a booklet entitled *Understanding Labor* was developed on the basis of the ethnographic data, supplemented by interviews and discussion groups with additional prenatal patients. This booklet was tested through postpartum interviews with women who had not received the booklet and a comparable number of women who had received it during the last month of pregnancy. All women were asked how many trips they made to the hospital before they were able to stay and deliver. The myth that Latino women were the most likely to come to the hospital repeatedly before true labor was disproved. In fact, it was the Caucasian women having their first babies who were the most frequent early visitors to the hospital because they thought they were in labor. The staff had thought the Latinos came more often because their interactions with them were more salient and memorable. However, the Caucasians were more likely to understand and accept the concepts of false and early labor (due to higher rates of prenatal education and a common language with staff) whereas the Latinos were more likely to protest the decision that it was not yet time to be admitted to the hospital (Scrimshaw and Souza 1982).

Other views of labor based on the pilot study revealed a second set of issues. Latino women experiencing their first birth discovered that their expectations regarding the onset of labor and the subsequent sequence of events differed from the actual process. Figure 13.1 shows a typical example

Figure 13.1 Actual Places, Events and Their Interrelationships in Intended Hospital Births

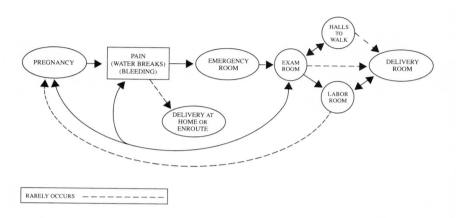

RARELY OCCURS — — — — — — — —

of locations and events in most intended hospital births. A pregnant woman gets some sign, usually pain, that the birth is imminent. She goes to the emergency room of a local hospital, where she is examined for signs of labor. From there, she may be sent home because it is too early, sent to a labor room, or sent to walk the halls because labor has begun and walking will help it along. Once she is ten centimeters dilated and the baby has been pushed through the birth canal until its head is visible (crowning), she goes from the labor room to the delivery room. Very rarely, labor moves quickly and the woman delivers at home or on her way to the hospital (as indicated by the dotted lines). It is possible for a woman to suspect labor and make the trip to the hospital several times before she is actually admitted.

Figure 13.2 shows the perceptions of this process held by many of the Latino women studied in the pilot research. Rather than the feedback loops in figure 13.1, where the process of going to the hospital may occur repeatedly, the process is seen as linear. A woman is pregnant, has pains, goes to the emergency room and then to the room where the baby is born. Delivery at home or on the way to the hospital is seen as a likely and frightening prospect. The idea of going to the hospital and being told it is too early is not present. Given these varied perceptions of the process, it is not surprising that the staff and patients had difficulties.

Figure 13.3 shows how some of these concepts translate into a woman's perceptions of her "job" during labor. Many of the Latino women

Figure 13.2 Common Perceptions Held by Primiparous Latino Women of the Sequence of Places and Events in Intended Hospital Births

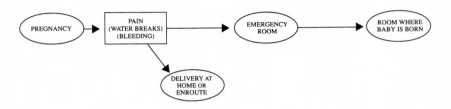

studied felt that their task was to get to the hospital and to have the baby. Getting to the hospital was complicated for most by not having a car. Because most felt the baby would come soon after pains started, the concept of a long labor with various stages was absent. Meanwhile staff members (dotted line) were already at the hospital and not necessarily aware of the effort it took to get there. They saw the woman's "job" as "being a good lady" during the early stages of labor and then later to push. Because the doctor "performed" the delivery, the woman's main effort was

Figure 13.3 Comparison of Primiparous Latino Women's and Provider's Perception of Woman's Effort in the Birth Process

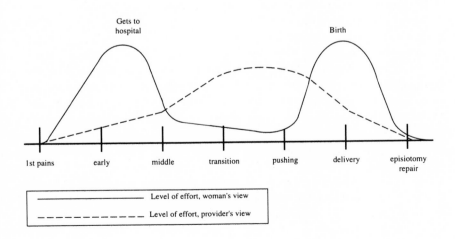

Figure 13.4 Provider versus Patient Perceptions of Danger during Childbirth

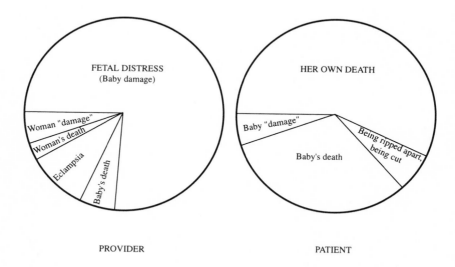

PROVIDER   PATIENT

seen as the pushing. Again, staff and patient views of the process diverged with the potential for misunderstanding.

Finally, health care providers and patients differed in their perceptions of danger (figure 13.4). Hospital staff, who were aware of the relatively low risks of childbirth in a tertiary care center in the United States, are most concerned with a delivery process and a baby free of any complications, however minor. Latino women, who often come from rural villages where they knew someone who died in childbirth, are most afraid that they will die and leave their babies motherless. Their second concern is that their baby will die, which is not so far-fetched, because many babies who are saved with dramatic modern medical techniques would not survive in rural Latin America. The women's fear of childbirth and particularly of the possibility of her own death was not fully appreciated or understood by staff in general.

Following the pilot project that identified key issues, these figures, along with classification systems contrasting provider and patient breakdowns of the word *birth* (Scrimshaw and Souza 1982), were developed and presented to staff. They reacted with fascination and increased appreciation of their patients' experiences and needs.

The UCLA Birth Project

From July 1980 through September 1982 we studied cultural and medical aspects of birth in primiparous women of Mexican origin and descent who were delivering in two Los Angeles hospitals.[1] We interviewed 291 low-risk primiparous women once in the last six weeks of pregnancy and again during their postpartum stay in the hospital.[2] This group is referred to as the *longitudinal sample*. Another 227 women who met the study criteria were interviewed only postpartum, although a few relevant questions from the prepartum questionnaire were also asked. These latter women were not located in the prenatal clinics serving the two hospitals, although, as will be seen, most had received prenatal care of some kind. This group is referred to as the *postpartum sample*. We collected data on the medical course of their labor and delivery for both samples from the women's medical charts for the total sample of 518 women. In addition, a subsample of forty-five women were observed throughout labor and delivery for a total of 273 hours of observation.

Fifty physicians and forty-four nurses affiliated with the labor and delivery services of the two study hospitals answered questions about their attitudes toward patients (Zambrana, Mogel, and Scrimshaw 1987). In particular, we asked them to describe and compare the women in the different ethnic groups they served.

The primary research questions addressed by the study were these: What beliefs, behaviors, and expectations do women bring to the birth process? Do these vary by levels of acculturation? How do these interact with the biological realities of childbirth? This project produced data that challenged other myths and stereotypes regarding Latino women. Before discussing these, the women studied are briefly described below.

Ninety-five percent (N = 518) of the total sample were born in Mexico. Eighty-nine percent of the women had been in the United States seven years or less, and 25 percent had been in the United States one year or less. Eighty-five percent of the women declared a preference for receiving explanations in Spanish. Forty-three percent of the sample were under twenty years of age (range thirteen to thirty-eight years, mean age twenty-one). Most of the women in the study were married (64 percent). Most (82 percent) of the unmarried women stated that the baby's father was planning to help support the baby. The mean years of schooling was eight (range birth to eighteen years). Forty-seven percent of the women described themselves as housewives with no personal income. The others had worked in factories, offices, and stores or had cleaned homes and cared for children. Only 3 percent had professional skills. Both occupation and level of education indicate that most were of low socioeconomic status, in keeping with our selection criterion of clinic patients only.

Confronting Additional Myths and Stereotypes

Prenatal Care. Staff at the hospitals involved as well as other health professionals in the Los Angeles area frequently stated that many women of Mexican origin in Los Angeles did not obtain prenatal care at all or sought it late in pregnancy and made relatively few prenatal visits (Norris and Williams 1984; Williams and Chen 1981). We found, however, that 76 percent of the entire sample reported being in their first trimester at the time of their first prenatal visit. By the fourth month of pregnancy, 86 percent had initiated some prenatal care. Only 4 percent initiated care in the third trimester, and only four women, less than 1 percent of the sample, did not seek prenatal care. These data are biased in that all the women studied had delivered in a hospital, so that women in the community who did not have a delivery in one of the two hospitals studied would not be picked up in our sample. Still, the proportion of women receiving prenatal care is high even for a sample of women delivering in hospitals. Also, the staff who felt many Latino women received no prenatal care were talking about these same women, the ones delivering in their hospitals. The mean number of visits (8.7 for the longitudinal sample and 7.4 for the postpartum-only sample) was also adequate by medical standards.

It seems likely that the staff perceptions of late or no prenatal care for Latinos were incorrect in part because of their methods for obtaining information about prenatal care. Staff tend to look for medical records of prenatal care. If a woman received care in Mexico or in another part of California or in another state, as some did, this would not show up in the records. Also, if women's records from Los Angeles County or the study hospital clinics were not immediately available, they might be labeled incorrectly as women who had not obtained prenatal care. Often, the women are not asked about prenatal care in other settings or their replies are not trusted. The possibility that prenatal care use is often underreported for this population should be considered.

We also must point out that this sample consisted of women having their *first* births, who are more likely to seek prenatal care than women who have already had a successful pregnancy. Nevertheless, many Latinos do appear to make a strong effort to obtain prenatal care. In a culture that highly values pregnancy and children and that places a strong emphasis on self-care in pregnancy, this is not surprising. The figures reported by Wingard (chapter 2) and other researchers (e.g., Norris and Williams 1984) indicate that there may be an important gap between trying to obtain prenatal care and actually obtaining it in an effective, consistent manner. Given some of these divergent findings on prenatal care for Latino women, it is hard even to identify the magnitude of the problem. A better tracking system is needed so that women's records are available to labor and delivery staffs during labor when they are needed to provide appropriate care during the birth process. In addition, researchers would do well to triangulate their results by collecting information from the women as well as from the medical and birth records to obtain more accurate data.

Because most of the 518 women in the sample were recent immigrants, it was important to explore whether concerns about citizenship status were an obstacle to prenatal care for these women in particular. To keep anxiety to a minimum, we asked an indirect question: "Based on your citizenship, are you concerned about your ability to receive health care?" Forty-five percent expressed some degree of concern. Those who did were asked *how* they felt their citizenship affected their ability to receive health care. Women responded with concerns about their immigration status ("They treat you as a noncitizen"), their ability to communicate in English, and their ability to pay. Twelve percent (60) said they had no money for health care and could not get public assistance because they were not citizens.

Social Support. Another stereotype about pregnancy is that social support for pregnancy and delivery comes primarily from the baby's father. This belief by staff is based on middle-class Caucasian ideas about family structure, social support, and childbirth education. Birth project results showed that social support from the baby's father and from the woman's family were both important and had different correlates. Support from the baby's father was significantly related to the time of initiation of prenatal care and the number of prenatal visits (Engle et al. 1990) and duration of breast-feeding (Scrimshaw et al. 1987). During prenatal visits the baby's father sometimes accompanied the woman, making it easier for her to make the trip. In the case of breast-feeding, father support was correlated with when a woman returned to work, which in turn was related to the duration of breast-feeding. Financial support from a man meant she could delay the return to work longer.

On the other hand, family social support was correlated with lower levels of anxiety, a higher degree of acculturation, less desire for pain medication during labor, expectations for a more active role during labor, and greater knowledge of childbirth. In addition, the women observed during labor often preferred to have their mother or sister in the labor and delivery room with them rather than the baby's father. Staff assumptions that the baby's father is the most important led, for example, to the rule in one of the study hospitals that only the father could accompany the woman in labor. The other hospital let the woman choose her source of support and even permitted family members to take turns in the labor room.

Breast-feeding. The hospital staff also believed that Latino women are not very interested in breast-feeding. In our population 74 percent initiated breast-feeding while still in the hospital; 26 percent planned to breast-feed at least three months, and 44 percent planned to nurse at least four to six months whereas 30 percent planned to nurse more than six months. There was a difference between the two hospitals in the percentage who initiated breast-feeding postpartum, although prepartum women's intentions were the same irrespective of where they planned to deliver. The hospital with a higher proportion of women nursing in the recovery room and with a chance for mother and baby to share a room had the highest rate of initiation of breast-feeding. If given the opportunity, many women will breast-feed. This is probably due in part to the high value placed on breast-feeding in Mexico and the fact that so many of our sample were recent immigrants (Scrimshaw et al. 1987).

Medication and Control during Labor and Delivery. An additional stereotype encountered was that Latino women do not want natural childbirth but instead want to be medicated. This belief was enhanced by the fact that most (over 90 percent) of these women did not receive childbirth education, where the management of labor pain is taught. This appeared to result from language differences between patient and childbirth educator, difficulty in going out in the evenings when most classes are held, and fear of the birth process. In the latter instance, women appeared to prefer not to think about the birth process before it happened and to rely on hospital staff to look after them once labor had begun.

These women might fear delivery, but 63 percent said they did not want pain medication. Childbirth, including some pain, was seen as a woman's right and an honorable duty. Medication was viewed as bad for the baby. Our observations of labor showed that, although women sometimes requested pain medication, more often the staff suggested it. In fact, during both the pilot phase and the main study, women commented that they would have refused medication offered near the end of the cervical dilation stage of labor if they had known this is usually the most painful period and that pushing, which follows, is more comfortable. A typical comment was: "I knew I could handle the pain I had, but I didn't think I could handle more. Since I thought the worst pain was when the baby's head came out, I took the medicine."

Another stereotype, frequently mentioned by staff, is that Latino women are likely to scream during labor. Observation notations included a seven-point scale of noise level completed by the observer for a sample contraction in every five-minute period. When those data were compiled, it was clear that most Latino women made low or moderate sounds and only a few were very loud. It is likely that a few were influencing the way the group as a whole was perceived. It would be interesting to repeat these observations with other ethnic groups to compare actual and perceived noise made during labor.

Interviews with the fifty obstetricians serving the study hospitals in Los Angeles obtained data on these physicians' views of the ideal patient and the difficult patient. Physicians revealed that their ideal patient was one who was informed, knowledgeable, and compliant during the labor and delivery process. Their perception of Latino patients clearly showed that they were stereotypically viewed as nice but "out of control" (noisy and loud) and uninformed. The data revealed that only 13 percent of the providers viewed Mexican Americans as compliant (Zambrana, Mogel, and Scrimshaw 1987).

Cesarean Birth. A search did not uncover any literature on ethnic differences in attitude toward cesarean birth before the publication of results from this project, but it is well known that women in general fear and dislike this method of birth. Contrary to this, the Latino women in this study tended to regard cesareans as "normal," and 6 of the 57 women who underwent cesarean sections (of the 518 women we interviewed) thought they provided advantages over vaginal births. Most of the women in the sample who gave birth by cesarean did not regard it as an unsatisfying, psychologically negative experience. In fact, some reported feeling lucky to have avoided labor (Cummins, Engle, and Scrimshaw 1988). Latino women apparently suffer greater anxiety about childbirth than other American women.

Patient-Provider Communication. Another impression held by staff was that they had to speak Spanish to effectively communicate with their Latino patients. Many staff members berated themselves for their poor Spanish. In fact, when the patients were polled about staff qualities, Spanish ability was tied for fifth in the list of desired attributes. Ninety percent of the patients said that providing explanations was very important, 89 percent said it was important to know a lot about medicine, 73 percent valued friendliness, 76 percent wanted staff to be understanding and sympathetic, 63 percent wanted them to be polite, and an equal proportion wanted them to speak Spanish. Essentially, Mexican and Mexican American women wanted what most patients want from medical staff: information, professional competence, and courtesy. During the labor and delivery observations, there were many instances of staff who communicated with smiles, a few words of fractured Spanish, gestures, and touch, and these were greatly appreciated by patients. Given the choice, women appeared to prefer an empathic non-Spanish speaker to a less supportive Spanish speaker.

Preferences for Sex of Children. Another commonly held myth was that Latino women prefer male children, especially for their firstborn. A detailed look at sex preferences for this sample revealed that sons and daughters were equally desired by the mother except when she was in a poor relationship with the baby's father. In that case, she had a slight preference for a boy. We attributed this to her feeling that the baby's father would prefer a son and that having one would help improve the relationship (Engle, Scrimshaw, and Smidt 1984).

Summary

The research described here revealed some misleading conceptions about Latino women. Our conclusions regarding common behaviors relating to pregnancy among Latino women are as follows:

1. Latino women do not come to the hospital before the onset of true labor more often than other women.
2. Latino women hold concepts of the labor and delivery process unlike those of labor and delivery staff.

3. Latino women do not understand the low risks of labor in a modern U.S. hospital and are very worried about birth.

4. The primary source of social support for a pregnant woman is not necessarily the baby's father. The woman's family is also very important during pregnancy and birth.

5. Latino women, unlike most women in the United States, do not all feel negatively about a cesarean section. Some women regard it as an advantageous method of delivery.

6. Latino women are interested in breast-feeding, and most will breast-feed, especially if given opportunity and encouragement during the postpartum period.

7. Many Latino women want to avoid medication in labor and want to be in control during labor and delivery.

8. Latino women are not all noisy in labor.

9. It is highly desirable, but not essential, to speak Spanish to work well with Latino women. Other aspects of communication such as nonverbal empathy and support are important substitutes for Spanish skills and should be employed as much as possible.

10. Latino women want a healthy child of either sex for their firstborn, and they value both daughters and sons.

11. Assertions about late or no prenatal care or relatively few visits for Latino women must be interpreted with caution. The primiparous Latino women in this sample obtained appropriate prenatal care in terms of the trimester they began the care and the total number of visits. These rates are higher than others reported for Latino women and may reflect extra attention to prenatal care in the first pregnancy. All the women we studied had hospital deliveries, and several sources (women's statements and clinic records) were used to establish prenatal care use. Other studies may underreport prenatal care use because records on care sought from multiple sources may not have been obtained.

The fact that the women we studied tended to differ from these stereotypes indicates that research on women and health must look at ethnicity and sociocultural behaviors that influence women's health in addition to biomedical and other behavioral variables. Generalizations that ignore ethnicity and socioeconomic status cannot and should not be made (Molina and Zambrana 1994).

Challenges and Directions for Future Research

The myths in the public health community regarding Latino women and complex realities displayed by the UCLA Birth Project and the studies that led to it point to the need for further description and analysis of cultural and socioeconomic variations relevant to women's health. Following the UCLA Birth Project, the Stress in Pregnancy Study[3] looked at high- and low-risk women having either first or subsequent births and representing a variety of ethnic groups. It examines issues of perceived stress, coping, and social support in relation to pregnancy risk status and pregnancy outcome. Ethnicity, class, and cultural factors are considered along with the biomedical and psychological variables. The Birth Mediators Study (1987–90)[4] examined determinants of pregnancy outcome in newly arrived Mexicans, women of Mexican descent, blacks, and a small sample of Caucasians. This project attempts to explain variations in pregnancy outcome as measured in weeks of gestation, birthweight, and complications of childbirth. These outcomes are better for some ethnic groups (particularly Latinos) than others, even when all women studied are of a similarly low socioeconomic status and could be expected to have similar rates of adverse outcomes. Cultural factors may be influencing behaviors such as prenatal care use, alcohol, tobacco and drug use, and perceived stress and social support. Understanding sociocultural factors may provide the keys to differences in birth outcomes and the bases for pregnancy interventions to improve outcomes for women in all ethnic groups (Zambrana, Scrimshaw, and Dunkel-Schetter, forthcoming).

It is essential that women be seen as individuals and as members of their cultures and not just as a uniform group of patients or, worse, as behaving in strange ways that often cause them to be incorrectly labeled as "difficult." We tread a fine line when we say that reproductive health research must record, analyze, and discuss diversity, yet must avoid labeling and stereotyping. The effort must be made to provide information for health professionals that will allow them to provide more appropriate programs and to understand the women they serve as they really are. More cross-cultural, interdisciplinary research is needed that combines cultural, socioeconomic, biomedical, behavioral, and psychological information. In addition, health care providers must begin with an appreciation for cultural diversity and the willingness to learn from the people they seek to serve. By considering the whole woman, rather than a part of her anatomy or a biological process such as pregnancy, caring, humanistic, and more effective health care can be achieved.

NOTES

This chapter, which summarizes many of the results of the UCLA Birth Project, carries with it our gratitude to Dr. Charles Brinkman and Ms. Lauren Kartozian. As head of obstetrics at UCLA and head of the obstetrical nurses, Charlie and Lauren stepped outside of conventional medical boundaries and let an anthropologist, a psychologist, and public health students into the labor and delivery rooms. Then they listened to and implemented many of our findings. We also wish to acknowledge the multiple contributions made by Patricia Lee Engle, co-principal investigator of the UCLA Birth Project and coauthor of many of the articles discussed in this chapter.

1. The UCLA Birth Project was supported by a grant from the National Institute of Child Health and Human Development #RO1-HD13796-01A1.

2. Between twenty-four and forty-eight hours postpartum for vaginal deliveries and between forty-eight and seventy-two hours postpartum for cesarean section deliveries.

3. Psychosocial Mediators of Stress in Pregnancy in Relation to Pregnancy Outcome. Christine Dunkel-Schetter, P.I., Susan Scrimshaw, Co-P.I. March 1984–February 1986. March of Dimes Foundation.

4. Mediators of Birth Outcome among Three Low-Income Ethnic Groups. Ruth E. Zambrana, P.I., Susan Scrimshaw, Co-P.I., Christine Dunkel-Schetter, Co-Investigator. 1987–1990. National Institute for Health Services Research.

REFERENCES

Bean, F. D., and M. Tienda
    1987   The Hispanic Population of the United States for the National Committee for Research on the 1980 Census. New York: Russell Sage Foundation.
Children's Defense Budget
    1986   An Analysis of the Fiscal Year 1987 Federal Budget and Children. Washington: Children's Defense Fund.
Cummins, Laura H., Patricia L. Engle, and Susan C. M. Scrimshaw
    1988   "Views of cesarean birth experience among primiparous women of Mexican origin." Birth 15(3):164–70.
Engle, Patricia L., Susan C. M. Scrimshaw, and Robert Smidt
    1984   "Sex differences in attitudes towards newborn infants among women of Mexican origin." Medical Anthropology 8(2):27–45.
Engle, Patricia L., Susan C. M. Scrimshaw, Ruth E. Zambrana, and Christine Dunkel-Schetter
    1990   "Prenatal and postnatal anxiety in women of Mexican origin and descent giving birth in Los Angeles." Health Psychology 9(3):285–99.
Hayes-Bautista, David E.
    1980   "Identifying 'Hispanic' populations: the influence of research methodology upon public policy." American Journal of Public Health 70(4):353–56.

Hayes-Bautista, David E., and Jorge Chapa
    1987   "Latino terminology: conceptual bases for standardized terminology."
           American Journal of Public Health 77(4):61-68.
Hayes-Bautista, David E., Werner Shink, and Jorge Chapa
    1988   The Burden of Support. Palo Alto: Stanford University Press.
Hurst, Marsha, and Ruth E. Zambrana
    1980   "The health careers of urban women: a study of East Harlem." Signs 5(3),
           Pt. 2, 112-26. Reprinted, pp. 109-23 in Catherine R. Stimpson, Elsa
           Dixler, Martha J. Nelson, and Kathryn B. Jatrakis (eds.), Women and the
           American City. Chicago: University of Chicago Press.
McCarthy, Kevin F., and Robert B. Valdez
    1986   Current and Future Effects of Mexican Immigration into California.
           RAND Corporation R-3365-CR. May.
Molina, Carlos, and Marilyn Aguirre-Molina, eds.
    1994   Latino Health in the U.S.: A Growing Public Health Challenge. Wash-
           ington, D.C.: American Public Health Association.
Molina, Carlos, and Ruth E. Zambrana
    1994   "The influence of culture, class and environment on health care." Pp.
           23-24 in Carlos Molina and Marilyn Aguirre-Molina (eds.), Latino
           Health in the U.S.: A Growing Challenge. Washington, D.C.: American
           Public Health Association.
Norris, Frank D., and Ronald L. Williams
    1984   "Perinatal outcomes among Medicaid recipients in California." American
           Journal of Public Health 74(10):1112-17.
Perales, C. A., and L. S. Young, eds.
    1987   Women, Health, and Poverty. New York: Haworth Press.
Scrimshaw, Susan C. M., and Ruth Souza
    1982   "Recognizing active labor: a test of a decision-making guide for pregnant
           women." Social Science and Medicine 16:1473-82.
Scrimshaw, Susan C. M., Patricia L. Engle, Lola Arnold, and Karen Haynes
    1987   "Factors affecting breast-feeding among Mexican women in Los Ange-
           les." American Journal of Public Health 77(4):467-70.
Trevino, Fernando M.
    1987   "Standardizing terminology for Hispanic populations." American Journal
           of Public Health 77(1):69-72.
U.S. Department of Commerce, Bureau of the Census
    1993   Persons of Hispanic Origin in the United States. 1990 Census of the
           Population. Current population survey CP-3-3. Washington, D.C.: U.S.
           Government Printing Office.
U.S. Department of Health and Human Services
    1986   Report of the Secretary's Task Force on Black and Minority Health:
           Infant Mortality and Low Birthweight. Vol. 4. Washington, D.C.: U.S.
           Department of Health and Human Services.
Williams, R. L., and P. M. Chen
    1981   "Identifying the sources of the recent decline in perinatal mortality rates

in California." Paper presented at the annual meeting of the Western Society for Pediatric Research.

Zambrana, Ruth E.
1987   "A research agenda on issues affecting poor and minority women: a model for understanding their health needs." Women and Health (Winter) 1987:137-60.

Zambrana, Ruth E., and Britt Ellis
1995   "Contemporary research issues in Hispanic/Latino Women's Health." Pp. 42-70 in Diane L. Adams (ed.), Health Issues for Women of Color: A Cultural Diversity Health Perspective. Thousand Oaks, CA: Sage.

Zambrana, Ruth E., Wendy Mogel, and Susan C. M. Scrimshaw
1987   "Gender and level of training differences in obstetricians' attitudes towards patients in childbirth." Women and Health 12(1):5-24.

Zambrana, Ruth E., Susan C. M. Scrimshaw, and Christine Dunkel-Schetter
forth- "Prenatal care and medical risk in low-income primiparous Latino and coming African-American women." Families, Systems and Health 14.

[PART V]

Intersections of Race, Class, and Culture

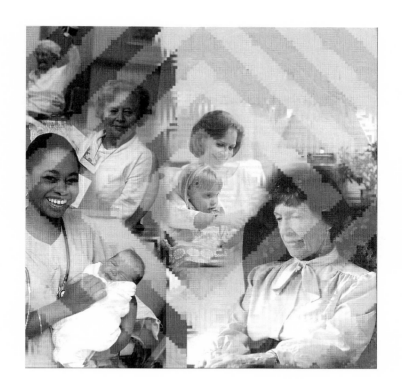

Social, cultural, and biological factors interact to produce different patterns of health and illness in groups that share certain characteristics. In part 5, contributors address some of the specific patterned ways in which race/ethnicity, class (often termed socioeconomic status), and culture interact and combine over the life cycle to produce patterned differences in health status, caregiving, and social control over goods and services that sustain or undermine women's health.

Why do some women become sick while others remain healthy, even under adverse conditions? What are the relationships between mental/emotional and physical health? Such concepts as "host resistance" to disease have not been adequately studied for women or for men. Nor do we yet know enough about the ways in which race/ethnicity, social class, and culture intersect with gender to produce distinct patterns of physical and emotional/mental health. Overall, socioeconomic status and education, which tend to be related, are directly associated with health status. Women in the lowest socioeconomic groups have the poorest health status whereas women in the highest socioeconomic groups have the best health status. This social class gradient in health status is well known in public health, but it is often ignored in social action. In health statistics, these gradients are often presented simply as "differences." Other observers describe patterned differences between social groups as disparities—inequities in health status that warrant remediation.

In chapter 14 Nikki Franke emphasizes how disparities in health status between black and white women reflect the cumulative consequences of differential exposure to life stressors as well as diseases. This theme is echoed in chapter 15 by Weber, Hancock, and Higginbotham, who focus on women's mental health. Women have traditionally suffered from mental illnesses at higher rates than men. Weber and her colleagues emphasize the negative impact of inequalities of power and privilege on

351

women's mental health and the ways in which multiple factors can affect women simultaneously and even contradictorily. The complexity of intersections of race, class, and gender statuses are well illustrated by these scholars' research on depression and other mental disorders in managerial women.

Women's social statuses and relationships also shape caregiving. Women who care for others—either informally in the home or in hospitals, clinics, and agencies—are important health resources. Not only is their labor valuable in terms of the care they provide but this personal caring in terms of advice, concern, and attention often produces and facilitates health in others. Women's own health is also a resource, yet extraordinary resourcefulness is required of women to navigate difficult social and economic situations that affect health throughout the life cycle.

As Virginia Olesen points out in chapter 16, women's resourcefulness in caring for children and sick family members is understood but seldom rewarded. The costs and consequences of caretaking take new directions for many elderly women who have insufficient funds of their own or from a spouse to maintain their health late in life. The growing ranks of elderly women whose health is fragile also affect women as caregivers. Women continue to provide most of the care, both paid and unpaid, for the elderly.

For all women, income acquired throughout life and particularly in retirement is consequential for older women's health, including life expectancy, risk of illness, access to care, and opportunities to participate in society. Family members' health is also of concern to older women. Vida Jones and Carroll Estes elaborate on these themes in chapter 17, presenting a chilling picture of the challenges that we all face in a rapidly aging society. How will we balance the needs of women in different life circumstances for resources that are important for health and well-being over the entire life cycle? How will we, as a society, manage the intersections of race, class, and gender in planning for a future in which economic resources may be increasingly scarce? What kinds of family relationships, communities, and social institutions will support or undermine women's health and well-being? Will differences and disparities in health status widen or narrow?

[14]

African American Women's Health:
The Effects of Disease and Chronic Life Stressors

NIKKI V. FRANKE

Taking a public health perspective, Nikki Franke focuses
on disparities in health status between black and white
women and the particular hardships faced by low-income
urban women. Although she calls for improvements in
medical care, Franke argues that classism, racism, and sexism in all American institutions, not just medical care,
must be redressed to improve African American women's
health.

In this chapter I examine many of the key health problems that disproportionately affect African American women. These include several
chronic illnesses, violence, AIDS, drug addiction, and daily life stressors
that result in differential life expectancy and mortality rates. I shall discuss
how these problems have negatively affected the health of African American women and that of their families. I have taken a holistic view of black
women's health because their health cannot be regarded as separate from
that of their families or from the health of their communities.

African American women throughout the United States face myriad
health problems that in many ways reflect their unique position in our
society. Taking a broad definition of health, many factors disproportionately affect black women. Primarily because they are black, female, and
often of limited economic independence, some of these factors are unique.
Cultural practices, personal health habits, family background, socioeconomic status, education, and lack of access to quality health care all
influence black women's health status. In addition, racism, sexism, classism, and the reduction of funding for a variety of programs that were
intended to reduce inequities in the health care system cannot be ignored
as issues that negatively influence the health and well-being of black
women today (Davis 1990).

The poor treatment of many African American women by the health
care system only mirrors the negative treatment they have consistently

received in American society. As long as sexism, institutional racism, and discrimination limit their opportunities, they will continue to exhibit poorer health than other groups of American women. Limited opportunities for better education, jobs, adequate housing, and improved health services will prevent many African American women from improving their overall health status and quality of life.

The Diversity of African American Women

African American women share many beliefs, attitudes, traditions, and habits. However, many differences also exist, reflecting varied life conditions and past experiences. These differences affect black women's health status and their need for specific types of disease prevention and health promotion programs. Because African American women have widely varying health problems, concerns, and priorities, generalizing about their needs is problematic.

No single image accurately characterizes black women; they are truly diverse. They come from all socioeconomic groups. Their cultural values and habits have been influenced by parents and grandparents possibly raised in very different settings, ranging from northern industrial cities to the rural South to the Caribbean. Today they are wives as well as single heads of households. They live in rural as well as urban areas, are homosexuals as well as heterosexuals, and are homemakers as well as working women. Health care professionals and researchers must remember not to view them as just a single group of women, but as members of several different subcultures within the black community.

African American women's varied backgrounds and living conditions shape their individual health concerns and priorities. For example, although violence related to increasing drug use and access to lethal weapons may be a primary health concern for many urban women, mere access to a health facility is a primary concern for some rural women. For working mothers, the difficulty of finding quality and affordable child care may be a major health stressor compounding the everyday difficulties of parenting. For many, who must contend with fulfilling basic daily needs such as adequate food and shelter for their families, concern about their own longevity and the use of preventive health services is far from a high priority. For these women, health becomes a concern only when it interferes with their ability to fulfill more essential needs. This does not mean, however, that efforts to provide quality preventive health services and screening programs should be abandoned for these women. It just means that health care providers must be sensitive to these other pressing concerns when planning health interventions.

Along with the many African American women who feel they cannot afford to make their own health a high priority, there are also many who are concerned about their health and the quality of their lives. Health care professionals must be careful not to ignore this group and mistakenly form a stereotype, assuming that all black women are unconcerned about their health. This type of overgeneralization is detrimental and can easily be used as a justification to provide only limited funding for preventive health services and screenings in black communities. Due to the disproportionate number of health problems and life stressors that negatively affect black women, health professionals must work diligently to find creative ways to offer quality health services, including preventive care, that are accessible and sensitive to the varied needs of all black women.

Disparities in Health Status

African American women and their families suffer disproportionately from health problems compounded daily by racism, sexism, and classism. Persons outside the black community often fail to recognize how these factors contribute to black women's poor health status. For African American women, the discrimination that results in lack of quality health care, inaccessible mental health services, and inhumane and disrespectful treatment by some health care providers is just one of the significant barriers to their good health (Davis 1990).

Lack of adequate medical coverage in some states for those living below the poverty level, inability of the working poor to pay for health insurance, lack of health insurance following job loss, poor quality health care when it is available, and underutilization or delay in the use of existing health services when they are needed—all contribute to the poorer health status of many black women (Walker 1992). The degree to which health problems are self-inflicted through negative habits that result from the inherent problems of dysfunctional families or are externally induced by a society that is both racist and sexist is somewhat irrelevant to black women. The fact is that both institutional and behavioral barriers have detrimental effects on African American women's mental, physical, and emotional well-being. Health administrators must consider all these factors when formulating effective health policies.

Health literature rarely identifies the various subcultures found in black communities. General statistical comparisons are still consistently made between blacks and whites, but these statistics are not entirely accurate. These analyses may, however, help to give a clearer picture of the significant racial differences that exist. These statistics may also be useful because they help to portray the human price paid by African Americans as a result of the disparities that exist in the health care system and other social institutions. One must still remember, however, the diversity that exists in black communities. Health data for the various subcultures need to be carefully studied because these groups may differ significantly from each other as well as from the national norms.

For many African Americans, the significant differences in health status that exist between blacks and whites are the consequence of a long history of institutional racism in a health care delivery system that often does not adequately serve black communities. The health care system, like other institutions in the larger society, does not value the lives of blacks the same as it does those of whites. This is evident in the lack of research involving women of color, disparity in treatments, and inadequate funding for preventive health education programs and early screening services for African Americans.

Although the health of all Americans has generally improved over the last several decades, a significant gap still exists between the health status of black women and white women (René 1987). Health professionals must become more sensitive to the diversity in African American communities and the distinct needs and concerns of its various subgroups. They must begin to work with community leaders to effect change and help empower residents to adopt more positive health behaviors.

Differential Health Objectives

The quality of life for African Americans has been ignored for so long that what to do about it is itself controversial. For instance, conflict over public policy approaches has mounted recently concerning the lack of visibility of many African American concerns in the national health objectives put forth by the U.S. Public Health Service. The first national health objectives issued, to be met by 1990, were designed to direct national health policy to satisfy specific goals, such as reducing the number of smokers or increasing the number of women who received baseline mammograms (U.S. Department of Health, Education, and Welfare

[HEW] 1979). The 1990 objectives did not specifically identify goals for some of the health care problems of particular concern in black communities, and they were not well received by many professionals working in these communities.

In an attempt to address the significant differences found between black and white health status, different goals were established for "special high-risk populations" for the Healthy People 2000 Objectives. The establishment of these different targets was an attempt to "narrow the gap between the total population and those special population groups that experience above average incidence of death, disease, and disability" (U.S. Department of Health and Human Services [DHHS] 1991a:29).

How ethical is it to identify different health status goals based solely on ethnicity? Is it ethical to accept an infant mortality rate of 11 per 1,000 births for blacks while seeking a rate of 7 per 1,000 births for whites? Given that black infant mortality rates are more than twice that of whites, how realistic is it to expect that within one decade these significant differences can be eliminated entirely? Is it meaningful to set a common target rate for all groups? Do different official goals for different groups legitimize health status differences and lead us to accept some health problems as unavoidable or inevitable? Do these differential targets allow for or excuse inadequate and/or inequitable services for black communities? What level of disparity does the Public Health Service or society find acceptable? Who should make that decision? These are crucial questions for African Americans as well as for health care policymakers to address. We must be careful not to use these different "special population" targets to avoid aggressively attacking serious health problems. Significant inroads can and must be made to change the clear disparities that exist. To avoid this responsibility will cost thousands of lives each year.

Lifestyle Issues

Some health status differences are related to unhealthy lifestyles found in many African American communities: smoking, poor nutrition, violence, alcoholism and drug abuse (especially among women of childbearing age), as well as the underutilization of preventive health services when they are available. In addition, the high levels of daily stress that are uniquely part of the black experience in America can clearly have a negative effect on black women's health. Given the limited financial or other resources many black women possess for managing life stresses, it

TABLE 14.1
Life Expectancy at Birth by Race and Sex, 1900-1992

Year	Black Female	White Female	Blacks: Both Sexes	Whites: Both Sexes
1900	33.5	48.7	33.0	47.6
1970	68.3	75.6	64.1	71.7
1980	72.5	78.1	68.1	74.4
1984	73.6	78.7	69.5	75.3
1989	73.3	79.2	68.8	75.9
1992	73.9	79.8	69.6	76.5

Source: National Center for Health Statistics, 1994.

should not be surprising to find a higher incidence of severe mental and emotional health problems (Bennett 1988). Despite this, however, little research has specifically addressed the relationships between lifestyle, daily stressors, and the health status of African American women. The lack of research addressing this problem, as well as the lack of quality interventions and services designed to help people change negative health behaviors and manage daily stresses, underscores the devaluation of black women's health by the larger society.

Life Expectancy

One way of analyzing the health status of a particular population is to examine life expectancy rates, which have continuously improved since 1900 for both blacks and whites. The gap between them, however, actually widened between 1984 and 1992 (see table 14.1). In 1984, life expectancy at birth for all African Americans reached 69.5 years, by 1989 it had dropped to 68.8 years, and in 1992 it was 69.6 years. During this same period, the life expectancy for whites rose from 75.3 to 76.5 years (Collins et al. 1994; National Center for Health Statistics 1995; U.S. Dept. of Health and Human Services 1991; Women of Color Partnership 1991). For black women, the life expectancy in 1992 was 73.9 years compared with 79.8 years for white women. Tragically, this means that, on average, a black baby born in 1992 began life with almost seven fewer years to live than the average white baby born the same day, possibly even in the same hospital.

TABLE 14.2
Age-Adjusted Death Rates by Gender and Race, 1992

Causes of Death	White Females	Black Females	Relative Risk
Heart disease	98.1	162.4	1.7
Cancer	110.3	136.6	1.2
Stroke	22.5	39.9	1.8
Accidents	16.1	19.3	1.2
Diabetes	9.6	25.8	2.7
Homicide	2.8	13.0	4.6
Cirrhosis	4.6	6.9	1.5
AIDS	1.6	14.3	8.9

Source: National Center for Health Statistics, 1994.

Note: Death rates based on number of deaths per 100,000 in population.

Identifying the factors that explain this seven-year difference is crucial for developing policies and programs to reduce such a significant disparity. Until the causes of these differences in life expectancy are well researched and clearly understood, efforts to improve life expectancy will not successfully address the real health problems of black communities. The lack of attention paid to these disparities again raises questions about the commitment on the part of the public and private health care sectors to promote improvements in the health status of African Americans.

Health Problems of African American Women

Leading Causes of Death

Specific health problems that contribute to disparities in life expectancy are shown in table 14.2. Overall, heart disease is the leading cause of death for African American women in the United States. Cardiovascular disease killed about 65 percent more black than white women in 1992, and this gap has not narrowed since 1960 (Jones and Rice 1987). In fact, during the 1980s, the gap actually widened (Hale 1992).

Cancer is the second leading cause of death for black women. Over the past thirty years, mortality rates for breast, respiratory, and pancreatic cancer have increased for black women (Baquet et al. 1991; Jones and

Rice 1987). Only the mortality rate for uterine cancer has declined. Overall, black women in 1992 had a 20 percent greater chance than white women of succumbing to cancer (HEW 1983; National Center for Health Statistics 1995). Although incidence rates for some cancers (i.e., breast, uterine) are lower for blacks than for whites, blacks are more likely to die from these cancers (Collins et al. 1994; White 1990). For all cancer sites combined, blacks have a 30 percent lower five-year survival rate than whites (Baquet et al. 1991; Leigh 1994). These differences in mortality may result from later diagnosis, lack of financial resources for adequate long-term care, poor quality primary health care, lack of knowledge about the early warning signs, improper diet, smoking, and hazardous occupational exposures.

Stroke is the third leading cause of death among black women (Hale 1992). Although deaths caused by cerebrovascular disease have been steadily decreasing over the past several decades, in 1992, the mortality rate for black women was still 80 percent higher than that for white women. In addition, according to Jones and Rice (1987:48), "strokes occur at a younger age in blacks than whites, are more debilitating, and result in death more often." They add that the significant drop in the number of strokes among African American women in the 1970s (from 108 to 62 per 100,000) was directly related to a decline in the use of oral contraceptives. During this same period, routine hypertension screenings in black communities also helped to reduce the number of African Americans with uncontrolled high blood pressure, a major cause of stroke.

The other leading causes of death for black women are diabetes, accidents, pneumonia, influenza, homicides, and AIDS (National Center for Health Statistics 1993). In 1992, homicide was the leading cause of death for black women between the ages of fifteen and twenty-four, and it ranked second for black women ages twenty-five to thirty-four. The incidence of HIV and AIDS is also growing rapidly among African Americans. Women, especially black women, have become the fastest growing group at risk for HIV infection. From 1990 to 1992, new AIDS cases increased by 50 percent among black women. In 1992, HIV was the leading cause of death for African American women between the ages of twenty-five and thirty-four. In 1993, black women, who constitute 12 percent of the total female population, accounted for 57 percent of the HIV/AIDS cases in women over age thirteen and were nine times more likely to die from HIV infection than white women (Leigh 1994; National Center for Health Statistics 1995; Schneider and Stoller 1994).

Maternal Death Rates

Black women constitute approximately 40 percent of all maternal deaths in the United States. In 1992, the maternal death rate for black women was 20.1 per 100,000 live births compared with only 4.7 per 100,000 live births for white women. Although maternal death rates have declined dramatically over the last fifty years, they are now rising for black women (National Center for Health Statistics 1995). Why do black women die four times as often as white women from complications surrounding childbirth? Contributing factors include the lack of early prenatal care, education, quality health services, health insurance, and decent housing. Poor nutrition and other negative health behaviors, as well as increasing rates of teenage pregnancy, also contribute to maternal mortality. Comprehensive programs for pregnant women are essential to reduce maternal as well as infant mortality rates and improve the quality of African American women's lives and those of their children.

Infant Mortality

Along with maternal death rates, black women have significantly higher infant mortality rates than white women. According to Jones and Rice (1987), infant mortality rates have declined almost two-thirds since 1940. However, the black/white infant mortality ratio has continued to widen because mortality has declined more rapidly for whites than for blacks. In 1992, the infant mortality rate for blacks was more than twice that for whites (16.8 vs. 6.9 deaths per 1,000 live births). The gap is now larger than it was thirty years ago (see figure 14.1).

Today, African American women have the highest infant mortality rate of any ethnic group in the United States. Low birthweight (under 5.5 pounds) is the leading cause of infant mortality, and in 1992, 13.3 percent of black infants born were underweight as compared with only 5.8 percent of white infants. Low birthweight infants are forty times more likely to die in their first month of life than babies born weighing more than 5.5 pounds (National Center for Health Statistics 1995).

Although the overall health status of white Americans has improved in recent decades, black health status is declining. The rates of infant mortality and low birthweight show how the health care system and other social service agencies have not adequately addressed the special needs of many pregnant black women. Although early prenatal care is essential for

Figure 14.1 U.S. Infant Mortality Rates by Race of Mother, 1960-92

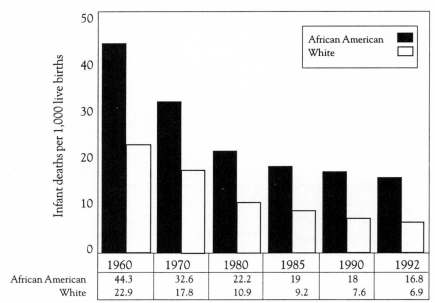

	1960	1970	1980	1985	1990	1992
African American	44.3	32.6	22.2	19	18	16.8
White	22.9	17.8	10.9	9.2	7.6	6.9

Source: National Center for Health Statistics (1994).

increasing birthweights and reducing infant mortality, only 64 percent of African American women received prenatal care in their first trimester of pregnancy in 1992 (National Center for Health Statistics 1995). This is only slightly higher than the 62.4 percent in 1980. Well-planned and implemented programs for early prenatal care, nutrition education, childbirth and parenting education, as well as support systems to meet the special needs of teenage parents must be established. Programs such as the "Healthy Start" initiative (which provides communities with the highest infant mortality rates comprehensive services for pregnant women) may well be a step in the right direction to improving infant and maternal mortality rates.

Drug Use and Maternal/Infant Mortality

The number of infants born to mothers who have abused alcohol and/or other drugs during pregnancy is increasing. A 1988 study of thirty-six hospitals conducted by the National Association for Perinatal Addiction Research and Education found that one out of every eleven infants were born to women who used illegal drugs during pregnancy. Although it has been reported that white women are more likely to use drugs during pregnancy than black women, the increasing number of pregnant women in the black community using drugs is still significant (Floyd 1992). This is an alarming trend and poses serious problems for health, educational, and social service agencies. Some of these infants must undergo treatment for drug withdrawal at birth and will develop chronic illnesses. Many must remain in the hospital for extended periods to receive necessary treatment whereas others will remain in the hospital because they have been abandoned by addicted mothers who cannot care for them. Still other infants may have no one at home capable of caring for them given their possible health and developmental problems. Unfortunately, some of the "lucky" newborns who are taken home are at increased risk for child abuse and/or neglect. This is especially true if the infant is sent home with a drug-addicted mother. As Regan, Ehrlich, and Finnegan (1987) have shown, the high incidence of abuse and violence experienced by pregnant, drug-dependent women also increases the likelihood that they will abuse their own children. It is clear that increased numbers of drug treatment programs must be developed to meet their specific needs.

Women's increasing use of crack cocaine is especially troubling because of its easy availability and affordability. In Philadelphia, for example, from 1991 to 1992, 70 percent of the 5,300 women admitted to addiction treatment programs used cocaine as their drug of choice (Uniform Data Collection System for Philadelphia 1992). Cocaine-related emergency room episodes have been steadily increasing for women since 1990. The highly addictive characteristic of crack makes it difficult for women to stop using it, even when they understand its detrimental effects. Many women addicted to crack become so focused on their addiction that little else matters. They become extremely apathetic about many aspects of their lives, including their children (Battle 1990). Many of these women are products of dysfunctional families themselves, and even those who were part of a supportive family network, after several years of addiction, in all likelihood have alienated themselves from their families. After many attempts to help addicted daughters, granddaughters, and sisters, many family members feel frustrated, angry, and helpless. The addicted woman has often used everyone who has ever cared about her until they have had to abandon her for their own sanity and survival. This tragic family situation becomes even worse when addicted women become pregnant. Because many have severed all family ties before their pregnancy, extended family members who normally would try to help these newborns are often not even aware of their existence or location.

Occasionally, family members are contacted or come forward to assume responsibility for the children of an addicted family member. However, their burden is tremendous. Social welfare agencies are increasingly aware of the need to support these extended family members, but bureaucratic processes make obtaining medical and financial support difficult. Therefore, most relatives must care for these infants without financial support from either the child's parents or governmental agencies. An older grandparent living on a fixed income will struggle, as will a younger grandparent still in the workforce who must now find and pay for quality child care services. Medical expenses pose still another problem. Recent research shows that crack babies may exhibit long-term physical and psychological problems that require extensive and costly treatment (Women of Color Partnership 1991). As drug abuse continues to plague many sectors of the black community, such problems will overburden families, social workers, educators, and health care providers.

The data on infant and maternal mortality show that not only is health status not equitable for black women but that it may actually be getting worse. More must be done to help improve the plight of black women, particularly low-income women, who are at highest risk. Unhealthy women shorten their own lives and unavoidably compromise the births and quality of life of their children. For far too many African American families, the expected beauty and joy of childbirth too often ends in tragedy, creating additional stresses on the entire family and the community.

Coping Strategies for Survival

What price survival? There are many things African Americans feel they must do just to survive in the United States. Some are positive responses to daily stressors, and others are negative. Many types of coping behaviors are exhibited throughout black communities. For example, although the suicide rate among African Americans is the lowest of all ethnic groups in the United States, other forms of self-destructive behavior such as drug addiction and violence are increasing. For a segment of the population, these negative behaviors are seen as a way to cope with the inhumane conditions and stresses they encounter daily. But for others, more positive means of coping are sought. The focus, however, for both groups is still very much one of survival. Often, the health outcome of their behavior is not the primary reason for the way they choose to confront their daily life stressors.

When family, spiritual, and other support systems don't succeed, some women seek professional help. Outpatient mental health services, when they are available, are utilized more by women than by men (Taylor 1992). Because African American women are more likely to be poor and to be subjected to racism and sexism, their need for mental health services may be greater than that of other groups (Bennett 1988). Seeking help can be difficult yet essential. Inadequate as they often may be, mental health services are a critical lifeline for many black women who often face extraordinary stresses and problems daily.

Religion also plays a key role in their lives. The church has always been a strong institution in the African American community, especially for women. It is a place that makes the unbearable bearable, where women hope to find the energy and determination needed to make it through another day. The church promises that if one lives the "good life" on earth there will be rewards in the afterlife. Christians learn from the Bible of God's promise that, in heaven, those on earth who were first will become last and those who were last will become first. This deep faith in the life hereafter enables many to cope with the hatred, injustice, and discrimination that they face daily. In short, for many black women, the church provides the hope that they desperately need and gives meaning to their existence when there are so few tangible rewards available to many of them.

Religious leaders have always been among the most visible leaders in the black community and can be an important resource. They are a pipeline to the community, important allies whom health professionals have not utilized well in the past. Through black churches, a great many people, especially women, can be reached and helped.

The Changing Family

Historically, one of the strengths of the African American community has been the existence of the "extended family," a structure that has been critical to the survival of African Americans in this country. The extended family was essential during slavery when the nuclear family unit could be thrown into turmoil at the whim of a slave owner. The physical and emotional support system that the extended family, as well as the black church, provided was second to none. Today, with the increasing number of young single mothers, the need for extended family support is escalating. But fewer and fewer mothers and grandmothers of these young women are homemakers or are retired and available to help care for these youngsters. Many grandparents are still in the workforce themselves or live in distant cities. Young single mothers, many of whom are at greater risk for many sociomedical problems, are placing inordinate demands on a shrinking extended family support system. This is truly a significant loss in black communities.

Historical Role of Women in the Family

Any attempt to understand the African American family and women's roles must take a historical perspective. Throughout history, institutional racism has been pervasive in the development of policies that were intended to destroy the black family. These policies were especially aimed at weakening the role of black men by eroding their position in the family and in society. This lessened their perceived threat to white America by rendering them powerless in many ways. Economically, black men have been denied equal access to quality education, jobs, housing, and training. The media and politicians have consistently portrayed black men in a negative light. The welfare system for many years limited a family's eligibility for Aid to Dependent Children if there was a father present in the home, thus discouraging black men from remaining with their families. This led many to abandon their families because there were limited opportunities to find work to support them. Although racial discrimination prevented equality in education, training, and employment for black men, society still expected them to provide adequately for their families. Under such financial and emotional strains, many marriages inevitably suffered and disintegrated. Often, either choice that was made by these men, to stay or to leave, further eroded their image and self-respect, increased their frustration and anger with society and with their own families, and increased the emotional and physical stresses on black women and their children.

Female-Headed Households

The number of female-headed households in the United States is rising. One reason is the increased number of divorces. In 1993, 12 percent of black women were divorced as opposed to just 5 percent in 1970 (U.S. Bureau of the Census 1994). Forty-four percent of all black households in 1990 were supported by women who were single parents (Leigh 1994). Although decreasing numbers of marriages are often cited as an explanation for the increasing number of female-headed households, increasing divorce rates also contribute.

Another reason for the high number of black female heads of households is the sex and age ratios. In 1992, women outnumbered men. In 1980, the average black woman was just under twenty-seven years of age, whereas the average black man was only twenty-four (Johnson 1987; U.S. Bureau of the Census 1989). Therefore, black women not only outnumbered black men but were also, on average, older. This sex ratio difference is further exacerbated by the number of young black men who are incarcerated, addicted to drugs, and under- or unemployed, all of which decrease the number of African American men who are available and/or considered "desirable" as marriage partners.

A growing proportion of African American women who are heads of households have never been married. In 1993, 35 percent of all black women (and 41 percent of black men) had never been married (U.S. Bureau of the Census 1994). This indicates that for some, the single lifestyle is not necessarily one of choice but has been dictated to some degree by the number of African American men available as "suitable" partners. Many black women who do wish to marry find that by the time they are ready, their "Prince Charming" just doesn't exist. And the longer they delay marriage, the more difficult it becomes to find a mate and the more likely it is that they will never marry. This is true not just for poor women but for well-educated women as well.

As heads of households, African American women have constantly struggled with the negative portrayal of them as strong "black matriarchs"—domineering, overbearing, emasculating. This is an image portrayed not only by the media but also by many historians and researchers. Attempts to systematically destroy the black family have often forced women into the role of primary provider and protector of their children. However, the social and economic realities of American life for blacks has made it difficult to successfully fulfill this role. The fact that unemployment and underemployment are higher for African American women than for any other group in this country increases the economic and emotional strain on families (Carrington 1980). In 1993, 58 percent of female-headed households with children in the black community had incomes below the poverty level (U.S. Bureau of the Census 1992; National Center for Health Statistics 1995). Being strong has not been easy or as much of a "choice" for black women as it has been a necessity for survival. By taking on this role, however, African American women have been criticized and singled out as "the problem" with the black family, a classic example of "blaming the victim."

The stresses of motherhood are often magnified by the additional stresses of being poor and alone. Many black women who are heads of households are solely responsible for providing physically, emotionally, and economically for their families. This is especially difficult for mothers who are relegated to low-paying jobs or unemployment as a result of poor education, racism, and sexism (Bennett 1988). The constant struggle to provide for one's children is a chronic life stressor that is seldom recognized by health professionals or medical researchers. As a significant factor that contributes to black women's poor physical and emotional health, it needs to be studied (Zambrana 1987).

As researchers and practitioners attempt to examine the black family and understand the dynamics of the many segments of the black community, they must realize that much can be learned by identifying family strengths as well as weaknesses. What factors have contributed to its survival over the years, despite tremendous obstacles? What support mechanisms were created that worked and what is needed to further strengthen the family? These are some of the questions that need to be addressed.

Changing Image of Female Heads of Households

The negative image of black female heads of households has begun to diminish recently as a direct result of the increased number of white female heads of households. The negative image of the "black matriarch" is diminishing with the adoption of a much more positive label for these women—that of the "single mother." This term has been used by many white women as a badge of honor, indicating that they have somehow managed to gather the strength and resources necessary to raise a family on their own. For this, they argue, they should be congratulated, not condemned, for "choosing" the lifestyle that many black women have been forced to accept and have long been criticized for accepting. The "single mother" of today is not regarded nearly as negatively by society as the "black matriarch" of the past. White female heads of households, unlike their black counterparts, are not viewed by most researchers as the primary "cause" of problems within the white family.

Changing attitudes toward single parents as well as increased social support services may very well help African American female heads of households view themselves and be viewed by others more positively. With increased understanding from society regarding the difficulties of raising children alone, as well as improved support services and increased economic opportunities for all women, the health of black women and their children, as well as the quality of black family life, may be greatly enhanced.

The Economics of Health

"Socioeconomic status is one of the major factors influencing minority health status" (DHHS 1992:8). Poverty brings with it poor housing, lack of quality health care, stress, lack of health insurance, and poor nutrition among other problems. In 1990, the median household income for blacks was 55 percent that of whites. In 1993, 33 percent of blacks had incomes below the poverty level compared with only 12 percent of whites (Hale 1992; Lee and Estes 1990; National Center for Health Statistics 1995; Women of Color Partnership 1991). The percentage of black families living below the poverty level in 1992 was the highest it had been since 1983 (U.S. Bureau of the Census 1994).

The increasing number of single-parent households has contributed to the increasing number of black families living in poverty. For many African American women, a two-salaried family is their primary means of escaping poverty and obtaining middle-class status. In 1990, 36 percent of black women lived in poverty. This is larger than any other group of U.S. women. In addition, 48 percent of black families with a female head lived in poverty (Leigh 1994; DHHS 1992). For black women, the nonexistence or loss of a partner can throw a family into poverty and inflict tremendous stress. Because a two-salaried household is often crucial to make ends meet, the loss of a spouse can be not only a devastating emotional blow but a severe economic one as well. Because black women outnumber and on average outlive black men, even those who do marry are likely to be widowed before retirement, renewing the threat of poverty in their lives and prolonging their need to work. This increases their stress and undoubtedly affects their emotional and physical well-being.

Life Stressors

Problems that affect people on a consistent basis for prolonged periods of time may be considered life stressors. These stressors occur not necessarily because of something negative people have done but simply as they attempt to carry out their daily activities. Life stressors may not always be the most prominent concern on someone's mind, but their presence is always felt both physically and psychologically.

Many of the unique problems African American women encounter add to the list of daily problems and stresses that all women face. Stress levels are high not only for single, African American women who are poor and heads of household but for every segment of the black community (Carrington 1980). Maintaining middle- and upper-class status is also stressful for black women. Because they seldom come from wealthy or even middle-class families, they often do not have a sizable bank account to fall back on and may indeed be living from paycheck to paycheck. If for some reason those paychecks were to stop, their relatives would seldom have the financial resources to help "tide them over." All too often, they are the "successful" ones in the family who are counted on to help everyone else in emergencies.

For example, N.S. has loaned each of her siblings money in the past, knowing it will never be repaid. Yet, she also knows that if she were in trouble and needed financial help, although they'd want to help her, none are in the financial position to do so. Even when her grandmother died recently, her family, including her mother, depended on N.S. to help with the burial costs. The stress of knowing they could lose everything they have worked for with just one major illness or one pink slip is frightening for many successful black women. They can never feel totally secure in what N.S. calls the "illusion" of being middle class.

This feeling was echoed by L.W., a city employee whose husband is the only African American in his company, which is downsizing. The loss of his job would not only mean they would have to struggle to pay their mortgage. They would also have a medical crisis on their hands because one of their children has sickle cell anemia and must receive transfusions several times each month. If her husband were to lose his job, they would be forced to use a less comprehensive health plan that their physician doesn't accept. This would not only cause them major financial problems but could also jeopardize their child's health. This fear has produced a constant stressor in their lives.

Other unique life stressors that exist for middle- and upper-income black women include fewer available black men as mates, especially at similar social and economic levels, constant challenges to their authority from both black and white males in the workplace, cultural alienation, loss of income and, consequently, health benefits, racism, and isolation. In addition, for those who have "made it" and are also married, divorce rates increase with level of education and economic independence (Cope and Hall 1987). Such conflicts contribute to the health problems that "successful" women report, including hypertension, weight gain, depression, and alcoholism. (Weber and her colleagues discuss these issues in greater depth in chapter 15.)

Stresses of Teen Pregnancy

The long-term effects of pregnancy on a teenager and her family are tremendous. For both black and white women, birth and fertility rates have decreased by almost one-third since 1950. However, in 1992 blacks ages ten to fourteen had a birthrate six times that of whites (4.7 vs. 0.8 births per 1,000). Blacks between the ages of fifteen and seventeen gave birth almost three times as often as whites (81.3 vs. 30.1 per 1,000), and blacks between eighteen and nineteen gave birth almost twice as often as whites in this same age group (157.9 vs. 83.8 per 1,000) (National Center for Health Statistics 1995).

Half of nonwhite girls ages fifteen to nineteen keep their babies (Furstenberg 1987; DHHS 1991b). Most do not marry, and tremendous additional responsibilities as well as emotional and economic stresses fall on them and their families. Because less than 5 percent of African American teenage mothers are actual heads of households, many of their babies are partially, if not almost completely, raised by their grandmothers (Women of Color Partnership 1991). Therefore, when working with teen mothers, health professionals must not only be concerned with the problems of the teenage mother and her child but must also be sensitive to the additional stresses placed on the infant's grandparents. Additional strain on the grandmother-mother relationship can also contribute to poor physical and mental health. Even under the best of circumstances, mother-daughter relationships during the teen years are often turbulent. These difficulties are compounded by pregnancy and child-rearing issues.

Teenage mothers add to the growing proportion of black women who are poor with few if any job skills and who consequently have little hope of escaping poverty and its ramifications (Wattleton 1990). Although Furstenberg (1987) found that the majority of African American teenage mothers he studied completed high school, Avery (1992) found that 80 percent of the pregnant teens she studied did not graduate. Continuation of a teen's education must be a primary concern of health professionals. For those who do not finish high school, the chance of leading healthy, economically productive lives is greatly reduced. Among black adults who did not have a high school diploma, 44 percent lived below the poverty level as opposed to 20 percent of whites in 1992. For those who did finish school, it was still difficult to succeed in the job market. In 1992, 28 percent of black adults with a high school diploma, compared with only 8 percent of whites, lived in poverty (U.S. Bureau of the Census 1994). As mentioned earlier, health status is directly related to socioeconomic status.

Stresses of Violence

Violence is another life stressor and significant health risk for many African American women. In 1992, homicide was the leading cause of death among all blacks between the ages of fifteen and twenty-four (DHHS 1992). From 1990 to 1992, the homicide rate for black women between fifteen and forty-four was five times that for white women: 41 deaths vs. 8.1 per 100,000. However, it is not just black women's own risk of harm that is threatening and stressful in their lives. There is also the potential risk to their sons, husbands, lovers, brothers, and fathers. From 1990 to 1992, the homicide rate for black men was almost eight times greater than that for white men: 69.7 vs. 9.2 deaths per 100,000 (National Center for Health Statistics 1995). These statistics are alarming, and something must be done to reduce them. Our society, both black and white, cannot afford economically or morally to allow this number of premature deaths to occur. Health and social service agencies need to do more to help people reduce violence in our society. Reversing this rising health threat will take more than just building new prisons. We must attack its true causes, which include poverty, unemployment, drugs, easy access to guns, and an overwhelming feeling of hopelessness among black youth (Mercer 1994; Rodriguez 1992). Prevention, not just increased punishment, is the long-term answer.

Black women must also contend with abuse at the hands of spouses, partners, and/or family members (Roberts 1994; Ross 1994; White 1990).

Neither law enforcement nor public health agencies have successfully addressed this problem until recently. Minimizing its existence in black communities has been a significant barrier to its being recognized as a serious health problem. Until agencies successfully address domestic violence, far too many women and their children will have to live with the daily stress of being "at risk." (For further discussion of domestic violence see chapter 19.)

Stresses of Child Rearing: Socialization of Sons

Increasing violence (homicides, assaults, gang-related violence, police violence, and drug-related deaths) among young black males also adds stress to the lives of black women. They must be concerned not only with their own safety but also with that of their families. A black mother's concern for her son begins not when he first reaches fifteen and falls into the age group at greatest risk for homicide. It begins the first time he ventures out into society. Black mothers are constantly faced with the special dilemma of how to protect their sons from the negative influences of the community as well as from the devastating effects of the racism and discrimination they will undoubtedly encounter. Mothers also must equip their sons with the skills they will need to survive as men both in the black community and in white America. Mothers must strive to maintain a delicate balance in socializing their sons. If their sons become too assertive (a behavior often rewarded in white males), they are often deemed threatening and "aggressive" by whites, and consequently they find it difficult to advance in school or in the workplace. On the other hand, if they are not assertive enough or if they lose sight of their own culture, they will find it difficult to interact and survive with other black men. Learning how to live in one world yet survive in another becomes even more difficult in a female-headed household. If there are no positive male role models within the extended-family network for young adult men to interact with on a regular basis, they are particularly susceptible to peer influences as they search for their place in society.

Stresses of the HIV/AIDS Epidemic

Although AIDS was originally viewed primarily as a white gay male disease, its increasing prevalence in the African American community has forced health providers and policymakers to reexamine educational efforts and treatment programs. In 1991, 28 percent of Americans diagnosed with AIDS were black, yet blacks constituted only 12 percent of the U.S. population (Jenkins 1992). In addition, although the majority of people with AIDS are white, blacks with AIDS generally do not live as long as whites: 8 months for blacks versus 18–24 months for whites (Schneider and Stoller 1994; Women of Color Partnership 1991). This difference may be caused by delayed diagnosis and treatment, inadequate medical treatment, lack of knowledge about AIDS, inadequate health insurance, poorer health status before contracting AIDS, and institutional racism and discrimination in the health care system toward both blacks and AIDS patients.

Nearly 20 percent of African Americans with AIDS are women. Of special concern to the African American community is that although only 11 percent of AIDS sufferers are women, 53 percent of all women with AIDS are black. It is estimated that nearly half of black women with AIDS were infected through IV drug use, whereas nearly one-third contracted the disease through heterosexual contacts (Avery 1992; Fullilove et al. 1990; Schneider and Stoller 1994).

The number of AIDS cases in the black community continues to rise despite the increased efforts of AIDS educators. Black women are affected by this growing health problem not only as its victims but also as the mothers, wives, lovers, and sisters of the many people with AIDS. Few families in the black community today have not been touched by this fatal disease in some way.

AIDS also permeates deeply into the African American community by affecting its children. In New York, the state with the most AIDS cases, the majority of African Americans with AIDS are heterosexual, and 57 percent of the children born with AIDS are black (Wharton 1986). Nationally, in 1993, 61 percent of children with HIV infection were black. In 1992, AIDS was the leading cause of death for black women between the ages of twenty-five and thirty-four (National Center for Health Statistics 1995). As mothers die or become too ill to care for their children, the burden passes on to others. The black community has not systematically addressed the problem of AIDS and consequently has not developed a strong support system for AIDS patients and their families, as has the white gay community. Nor has the African American community become a strong political force lobbying for AIDS services. As a result, social services for babies and children with AIDS are extraordinarily scarce. (For more about women with AIDS see chapter 18.)

Conclusion

African American woman face myriad health problems that are unique to them because of their peculiar position in American society. These problems, and a lack of adequate resources to cope with them, all contribute to a higher incidence of many physical, mental, and social ills. If health professionals are serious about improving the health status of black women in this country, it is important to take a holistic view of African American women and the wide range of social factors and stressors that affect their lives, their health, and the health of their families. We cannot address inaccessibility to quality health care, poor nutrition, alcohol and drug addiction, smoking, the need for affordable health insurance, and lack of prenatal care without also examining the many chronic life stressors that affect black women daily. We cannot afford to think that improvements in their health can be accomplished without addressing the underlying issues of classism, racism, and sexism in all American institutions, not just in the health care industry. American institutions have historically provided inferior services to African Americans and the poor and have placed little value on their lives. All of these factors contribute to the significant disparities between white and black mortality and morbidity.

One of the major problems faced by health professionals is how to improve the health of African American women and provide health education and quality health care services at a time when cost containment and budget cutbacks are the order of the day. The current trend is to cut back on the poor's utilization of health services. There also seems to be little concern by some politicians for the marginally poor who are ineligible for Medicaid yet cannot afford even inferior health services. This must change.

Health professionals must become more sensitive to the diversity within black communities and work with community leaders to effect change and empower residents to improve their health status. Change begins with each of us being concerned about those who suffer the most and attempting to do something about it. Women, and black women especially, are at the bottom of the economic ladder. Until opportunities for women increase, many health problems and life stressors that are compounded daily by poverty and larger societal problems will not change. The various segments of black communities must band together to take charge of their lives and their health. They must define their own health concerns and priorities and not depend solely on health professionals outside of their communities. However, concerned community members cannot improve conditions alone. They must work along with dedicated health professionals and government agencies to address what are narrowly viewed by some as strictly "black health problems." We cannot lose sight of the many health problems that disproportionately affect black communities. We need increased resources for research, additional programs for early diagnosis and treatment, more trained black health professionals, and viable programs and services that are culturally sensitive and holistic in nature. Many gaps that exist between the health status of blacks and whites can only be closed through genuine commitment, proper planning, adequate funding, and community involvement. All too often, those most affected by policy decisions are not included in the decision making process. African Americans must expect and demand more from the health care system.

A challenge for health professionals is to improve the health care system in black communities and encourage all African Americans to make good health a priority. One particular challenge is finding ways to persuade black Americans to utilize available health care services, even though these services are provided by a system that historically has mistreated and at times abused them. Because they are the largest ethnic group in the United States, we must improve the health status of African Americans if we are to improve the health status of the nation. We must continue to seriously address those issues that affect the well-being of African American women, their families, and the black community as a whole. We must work toward educating the community and improving the quality of direct patient care and make significant changes in the racist and sexist attitudes and practices of the larger society. In the final analysis, these are the issues that affect longevity as well as the quality of not only African American women's lives but the lives of all Americans.

REFERENCES

Avery, Byllye Y.
    1992   "The health status of black women." Pp. 35–51 in Ronald L. Braithwaite and Sandra E. Taylor (eds.), Health Issues in the Black Community. San Francisco: Jossey-Bass.

Baquet, C. R., J. W. Horm, T. Gibbs, and P. Greenwald
    1991   "Socioeconomic factors and cancer incidence among blacks and whites." Journal of the National Cancer Institute 83:551–57.

Battle, Sheila
    1990   "Moving targets: alcohol, crack and black women." Pp. 251–56 in Evelyn C. White (ed.), The Black Women's Health Book. Seattle: Seal Press.

Bennett, Maisha B. H.
   1988   Afro-American Women, Poverty and Mental Health: A Social Essay. New York: Haworth Press.
Carrington, Christine H.
   1980   "Depression in black women: a theoretical appraisal." Pp. 265–71 in La Frances Rogers-Rose (ed.), The Black Woman. Beverly Hills, CA: Sage.
Collins, Karen, Diane Rowland, Alina Salganicoff, and Elizabeth Chait
   1994   Assessing and Improving Women's Health. Washington: Women's Research and Education Institute.
Cope, Nancy R., and Howard R. Hall
   1987   "Risk factors associated with the health status of black women in the United States." Pp. 43–56 in Woodrow Jones and Mitchell F. Rice (eds.), Health Care Issues in Black America. Westport, CT: Greenwood Press.
Davis, Angela Y.
   1990   "Sick and tired of being sick and tired: the politics of black women's health." Pp. 18–26 in Evelyn C. White (ed.), The Black Women's Health Book. Seattle: Seal Press.
Floyd, Virginia Davis
   1992   "Too soon, too small, too sick: black infant mortality." Pp. 165–77 in Ronald L. Braithwaite and Sandra E. Taylor (eds.), Health Issues in the Black Community. San Francisco: Jossey-Bass.
Fullilove, Mindy Thompson, Robert E. Fullilove, Katherine Haynes, and Shirley Gross
   1990   "Black women and AIDS prevention: a view towards understanding the gender rules." Journal of Sex Research 27:47–64.
Furstenberg, Frank F.
   1987   "Race differences in teenage sexuality, pregnancy, and adolescent childbearing." Milbank Quarterly 65:381–403.
Hale, Christiane B.
   1992   "A demographic profile of African Americans." Pp. 6–19 in Ronald L. Braithwaite and Sandra E. Taylor (eds.), Health Issues in the Black Community. San Francisco: Jossey-Bass.
Jenkins, Bill
   1992   "AIDS/HIV epidemics in the black community." Pp. 55–63 in Ronald L. Braithwaite and Sandra E. Taylor (eds.), Health Issues in the Black Community. San Francisco: Jossey-Bass.
Jones, Woodrow, and Mitchell F. Rice
   1987   "Black health care: an overview." Pp. 3–20 in Woodrow Jones and Mitchell F. Rice (eds.), Health Care Issues in Black America. Westport, CT: Greenwood Press.
Lee, Philip R., and Carroll L. Estes
   1990   The Nation's Health. Boston: Jones and Bartlett.
Leigh, Wilhelmina A.
   1994   The Health Status of Women of Color. Washington: Women's Research and Education Institute.

Mercer, Joye
  1994   "Dr. Deborah Prothrow-Smith: these kids are made, not born." Health
          Quest 5:43–45.
National Center for Health Statistics
  1993   "Advance report of final mortality statistics, 1991." Monthly Vital Sta-
          tistics Report 42 (2) suppl. Hyattsville, MD: Public Health Service.
  1995   Health, United States, 1994. Hyattsville, MD: Public Health Service.
Regan, Dianne O., Saundra M. Ehrlich, and Loretta P. Finnegan
  1987   "Infants of drug addicts: at risk for child abuse, neglect, and placement
          in foster care." Neurotoxicology and Teratology 9:315–19.
René, Antonio A.
  1987   "Racial differences in mortality: blacks and whites." Pp. 21–41 in Wood-
          row Jones and Mitchell F. Rice (eds.), Health Care Issues in Black Amer-
          ica. Westport, CT: Greenwood Press.
Roberts, Tara
  1994   "When violence hits home." Health Quest 5:50–53.
Rodriguez, Roberto
  1992   "Understanding the pathology of inner-city violence." Black Issues in
          Higher Education, 23 April:18–20.
Ross, Sonya
  1994   "Jesse Jackson: a call to disarm." Health Quest 5:32–35.
Schneider, Beth E., and Nancy E. Stoller, eds.
  1994   Women Resisting AIDS: Feminist Strategies of Empowerment. Philadel-
          phia: Temple University Press.
Taylor, Sandra
  1992   "The mental health status of black Americans: an overview." Pp. 20–34
          in Ronald L. Braithwaite and Sandra E. Taylor (eds.), Health Issues in
          the Black Community. San Francisco: Jossey-Bass.
Uniform Data Collection System for Philadelphia
  1992   Coordinating Office for Drug and Alcohol Abuse Programs. Philadelphia.
U.S. Bureau of the Census
  1989   "Projections of the population of the United States, by age, sex, and race:
          1988–2080." Current Population Reports, ser. P-25, no. 1018. Washing-
          ton: Government Printing Office.
  1992   The Black Populations in the United States: March 1991. Current Pop-
          ulation Reports, ser. P-20, no. 464. Washington: Government Printing
          Office.
  1994   Statistical Abstract of the United States, 1994. 114th ed. Washington:
          Government Printing Office.
U.S. Department of Health, Education, and Welfare (HEW)
  1979   The Surgeon General's Report on Health Promotion and Disease Preven-
          tion. Washington: Government Printing Office.
  1983   Health, United States, 1983. Washington: Government Printing Office.
U.S. Department of Health and Human Services (DHHS)
  1991a   Healthy People 2000: National Health Promotion and Disease Preven-

tion Objectives. DHHS Pub No. (PHS) 91-50212. Washington: Government Printing Office.

1991b   Health Status of Minorities and Low-Income Groups, 3d ed. Washington: Public Health Service.

1992   Health Statistics. Report of the Public Health Service Task Force on Minority Health Data. Washington: Government Printing Office.

Walker, Bailus

1992   "Health policies and the black community." Pp. 315-20 in Ronald L. Braithwaite and Sandra E. Taylor (eds.), Health Issues in the Black Community. San Francisco: Jossey-Bass.

Wattleton, Faye

1990   "Teenage pregnancy: a case for national action." Pp. 107-11 in Evelyn C. White (ed.), The Black Women's Health Book. Seattle: Seal Press.

Wharton, Carla L.

1986   AIDS in the Black Community: Urban League Black Papers. New York: Urban League.

White, Evelyn C.

1990   The Black Women's Health Book: Speaking for Ourselves. Seattle: Seal Press.

Women of Color Partnership

1991   Reproductive Health among Black Women in the United States: A Fact Handbook. Washington: Women of Color Partnership Program, Religious Coalition for Abortion Rights.

Zambrana, Ruth E.

1987   "A research agenda on issues affecting poor and minority women: a model for understanding their health needs." Women and Health 12(3-4):137-60.

[15]

Women, Power, and Mental Health

LYNN WEBER, TINA HANCOCK,
AND ELIZABETH HIGGINBOTHAM

These sociologists argue that power and privilege
significantly influence women's mental health as do
events that occur in women's social networks. Their research, comparing mental health problems in black and
white managerial women from different social class backgrounds, suggests new avenues for understanding how
race, class, and social mobility intersect and produce mental health problems.

Mental health, like physical health, is strongly shaped by inequalities of
power and privilege in society. Power and privilege promote mental health
both directly, by reducing stressors that challenge health, and indirectly,
by increasing access to the resources that may reduce stress.

Economic Position and Stress

Think about what happens, for example, when a teacher calls a mother
to tell her that her daughter has become ill and needs medical attention.
First, the mother must identify where the child needs to go and see that
she gets there. If the mother is a *highly paid professional,* she most likely
has many options to get the child to treatment: call another family member, leave work herself, send her secretary, or pay a child-care worker to
see that she gets medical attention. If the mother is a *middle-class homemaker,* she can most likely take the child herself. But if the mother is
working class and is employed in the kitchen at McDonald's, the problem
is more complicated. Unless she has family or friends who can step in, she
may not be able to leave her job without serious consequences. If the
mother is a *welfare recipient,* she may not be working, but she is also less
likely to have transportation available for the trip.

Second, these mothers must pay for the medical visit. The highly paid professional and the middle-class homemaker are more likely than the others to have medical insurance to cover the visit. The McDonald's employee is likely to have neither medical insurance nor Medicaid. The welfare recipient may have Medicaid, which ensures care but restricts her choice in where to get that care. Finally, for the working-class or welfare mother, this stressful life event—her daughter's illness—may become a larger crisis if the mother's having to leave work precipitates the loss of income or if the child's illness is exacerbated by a delay in obtaining care. Even though all four women experienced stress, who experienced more stress at the end of the day: the professional, the homemaker, the McDonald's employee, or the welfare mother?

Gender and Stress

Gender inequality in roles and institutional structures produces systematic obstacles to obtaining and maintaining mental health. Think about these four women again. One thing they share—whether married or not, whether employed or not, whether wealthy or not—is primary responsibility for child care. And they are each rearing children in a society that places little value on child rearing. To confirm this gender bias, we need only think about the meager wages paid to most day-care workers, the low wages paid to school teachers relative to other professionals, and the lack of workplace programs or policies that facilitate caring for a sick child.

Research on women's mental health shows that women are more affected than men by "network events"—life events that happen to someone in a person's social network (family and/or friends) (McLeod and Kessler 1990). And women with small children, especially single parents, are more likely to experience depression than any other group (Weber Cannon, Higginbotham, and Guy 1989; Weissman and Klerman 1987).

These four mothers illustrate how everyday parenting issues can provoke great stress, especially for women. Their lives also show how class differences among women produce tremendous diversity in the stressors they face, the resources they have for coping with stressors, and the ultimate mental and/or physical effects of that stress.

Race, ethnicity, social class origin, current social class, socioeconomic status (income, education, prestige), sexual identity, age, citizenship or immigration status, and other socially structured hierarchies of power and privilege—all influence women's mental health.

Oppression and Mental Health

To understand the processes through which social structural inequalities affect mental health, we must understand what is meant by both oppression and mental health. Privileged groups in society have power and control over socially valued resources in three realms: the economic—material resources, the political—rights and privileges, and the ideological—belief systems (Collins 1990; Poulantzas 1975; Vanneman and Weber Cannon 1987). Control over the economic, political, and ideological bases of a society enables powerful groups to maintain their privileges by denying full participation and self-determination to members of oppressed groups. Although these forms of denial are sometimes very subtle, they can be very effective.

Economic Oppression

In the economic realm, the labor power of women, people of color, the poor, and the working classes is exploited by restricting job access for the vast majority to sectors of the labor force that are characterized by low skill levels, low wages, high turnover, few benefits, and high risk—such as domestic work or work in the fast growing service sector in hotels and restaurants.

As a result of their economic position, everyday life is stressful for the poor because they lack the resources to meet basic human needs. For example, based on his observations of the daily life of a welfare mother, Alex Kotlowitz argues in *There Are No Children Here* (1991) that many young people today are denied a childhood. These are the children who grow up with hunger, violence in the streets and in their housing projects, racist treatment from the police, and fear for their personal safety in schools.

Political Oppression

Through political oppression people are denied access to society's basic rights and privileges. U.S. civil rights laws, for example, give every citizen the right to vote. But patterns of discrimination such as cumbersome registration regulations, gerrymandering of districts, and low literacy rates among some groups limit full access to political participation. Without access to political power, oppressed people are not able to shape their own destinies. Consider the national debate that has focused for some time on welfare issues such as government's obligation to poor women and children, reductions in funding, and changing eligibility requirements (e.g., to require schooling and work). The one group conspicuously absent from the debate and unable to shape its direction is the welfare recipients themselves. Women on welfare today receive approximately 27 percent less in real dollar benefits than they did in 1972 (DeParle 1992). As a consequence, these women have few economic resources with which to face the challenges of raising children in a declining economy.

Ideological Oppression

It is perhaps in the struggle to control how groups are defined—the ideological realm—that the relationship between oppression and mental health is most clearly seen. Negative stereotyped images of women, members of different racial and ethnic groups, gays and lesbians, and other subordinate groups pervade the media and institutions such as education and the law. The objective of a stereotype is not to reflect or represent a reality but to function as a disguise or mystification of actual social relations. Stereotypes are invoked to make racism, sexism, and other forms of oppression appear to be natural, normal, and inevitable parts of everyday life (Collins 1990). Because of the pervasiveness of group stereotypes, members of oppressed groups routinely face difficulties when people in positions of power act to limit their life options based on stereotypes of them as less competent, less capable, less worthy—in short, as less than fully human.

Defining Mental Health

The term *mental health* was originally intended to reflect psychological well-being and resilience—in essence, a satisfactory if not optimal state of being (Vega and Rumbaut 1991:355). Arising in the 1950s, this definition was reinforced by the community mental health movement of the 1960s, which focused attention on entire communities and away from images of bleak institutions housing the severely mentally ill. But as a nation we continue to focus more on mental illness than on mental health. In fact, the very definition of mental health or of mental illness is contested in the public arena by groups that occupy different locations in the social hierarchy.

Contested Definitions of Mental Health

In 1973, for example, the American Psychiatric Association removed homosexuality from its list of mental illnesses. Before 1973, the American Psychological Association—the primary professional group given the social power to define mental illness—defined people who expressed a homosexual orientation as mentally ill. Such definitions affected how gay men and lesbians were treated not only in psychotherapeutic settings but also in all major social institutions—from their own families, to the courtroom, to schools, to the job market.

In a now classic study, Broverman et al. (1970) asked mental health professionals to identify the characteristics that defined mentally healthy adults, mentally healthy men, and mentally healthy women. These mental health professionals' definition of a mentally healthy adult was the same as their definition of a mentally healthy man. As a result, women are—by definition—unhealthy. And women faced a double bind: They could not be seen as feminine (and therefore desirable to men) by acting assertively and decisively to shape their own lives.

Resisting Oppression

Although this research, now over twenty years old, focused on challenging negative views of women that were held by privileged groups and were disseminated through the media and educational systems, it also emphasized the ways in which women are victimized by the images and actions of men. But the relationship between oppression and mental health is dynamic—oppression does not simply, uniformly, and directly create women victims. Nor do male psychologists' views of women as unhealthy make all women see themselves as mentally ill.

Some recent scholarship acknowledges women's involvement in creating their environments and focuses on their resistance to oppression in the ideological as well as in the economic and political realms. These women who resist are not passive victims of structural discrimination doomed to poor mental health. Rather, they actively resist unfair treatment and negative images, and that resistance is a part of the process of being mentally healthy.

Other recent scholarship focuses on the relationship of social structural location and mental health, linking high status to a sense of competency, mastery, and self-esteem that results from a belief in one's ability to control good and bad outcomes (Mirowsky and Ross 1990; Rosenfield 1989; Wheaton 1990). But although high status provides access to resources and options that increase one's sense of control, members of disadvantaged groups can also access opportunities for personal and social change and act effectively to solve problems. This topic, though not yet central to mainstream mental health literature, is a recurrent theme in the writings of oppressed groups, most notably women of color (Collins 1990; Gilkes 1980; Scott 1991).

In *Black Feminist Thought*, Collins (1990) describes the dialectic relationship between oppression and activism that is necessary to ensure personal as well as group survival, for mental health among oppressed groups is created and maintained in the psychological struggle for self-definition and positive valuation in the face of powerful negative and limiting stereotypes. Specifically, the struggle of these groups for mental health is a struggle against internalized oppression: the internalization of structural limitations and of self-blame and negative self-images.

At the psychological level, empowerment is a process of becoming aware of the ways that one has internalized negative images and of actively rejecting those powerless and devalued definitions of self (Rose 1990). Collins discusses the ways in which black women's empowerment involves rejecting the dominant view of reality, including the pervasive cultural stereotypes of black women as subjugated and devalued persons in American society. Collins describes the creation of a separate reality for black women as they confront and dismantle controlling, negative images of themselves as matriarchs, mammies, welfare mothers, physically unattractive women: "When Black women define themselves, we clearly reject the assumptions that those in positions granting them the authority to interpret our reality are entitled to do so. Regardless of the actual content of Black women's self-definitions, the act of insisting on Black females' self-definition validates Black women's power as human subjects" (Collins 1990:106–7).

Dominant versus Subordinate Group Definitions of Mental Health

Collins's articulation of black feminism helps us to understand that self-definition and racial validation in opposition to dominant culture messages that devalue women of color should be viewed as mental health strengths. This view is very unlike popular culture's and the traditional mental health professions' conceptions of psychological well-being as "adjustment to reality." An empowerment perspective raises the question: Whose reality—the dominant group's or the subordinate group's?

This concept of personal empowerment implies that what constitutes good mental health in oppressed populations must be viewed differently from commonly held views of what constitutes good mental health in dominant, mainstream populations (Gutierrez 1990). Strong ego boundaries, for example, that separate self from other and that therefore set the stage for competitive effort and individualist orientations to achievement and success are characteristics typically associated with the dominant white middle class. And from the dominant perspective, these characteristics are associated with high levels of ego functioning in our society.

These same traits in women of color may not only be unrealistic but may serve to impede collective efforts to survive in a racist and sexist society. The traits that we see in women of color may in fact reflect a strong "other" orientation, including fluid self and family boundaries that permit assumption of responsibility for non-kin children in the black community (Collins 1990) and that encourage sharing and swapping of personal resources within a low-income black community network (Stack 1974).

Physical Health and Mental Health

The struggle for mental health is not purely a psychological struggle. Physical health problems pose great threats to mental health. Thomas LaVeist (1992) argues that the political empowerment of minority communities is an important determinant of their health. When, for example, people of color are elected to city councils, their presence can affect the community's health in at least two ways. First, council members can direct to minority communities resources that improve their health (e.g., health clinics). Second, the council members can divert projects that might threaten community health (e.g., toxic waste dumps). Thus political empowerment to dismantle structural systems of oppression is essential to everyone's long-term physical and mental health.

Toward a Wider Perspective

Although the women's movement has helped to highlight mental health issues, much of the focus in research has been on exploring the stresses and strains experienced by white middle-class women to the exclusion of women of color and other oppressed groups (Comas-Diaz and Greene 1994; Greenspan 1983). In addition, most feminist treatment models have tended to focus on one-to-one therapy, often overlooking the need for approaches that utilize the collective experiences and issues of racial and ethnic women. At this time little mental health research seeks to address the ways that race, class, and gender intersect to shape mental health outcomes for women.

The Memphis Study: "Race, Social Mobility, and Women's Mental Health"

To begin to identify some of the dynamics of these relationships, we undertook a study of social mobility, race, and mental health among professional and managerial women in the Memphis, Tennessee, area. Before our research most scholarship on women's mobility focused on marriage as women's only viable mobility channel. That approach was based on white women's experiences in the 1940s and 1950s and has become inappropriate for women born after World War II, many of whom have secured higher educational credentials and have assumed primary responsibility for their social class positions (Higginbotham and Weber Cannon 1988). Our research sought to unravel the interlocking dynamics of the relationship between social structural inequality as represented in race, class, and gender systems; the intervening influences of resources/supports and stressors; and mental health outcomes, including depressive symptoms and general well-being.

We studied Memphis women who were

— "baby boomers" (born between 1945 and 1960)
— college graduates who went directly from high school to college or went within two years of high school graduation
— full-time employed professionals, managers, or administrators.[1]

To examine the simultaneous influence of race, class, and gender on their lives, we conducted life history interviews with two hundred women:

— 100 black and 100 white
— 100 from working-class backgrounds and 100 from middle-class backgrounds
— 100 in female-dominated and 100 in male-dominated professional and managerial jobs.

Mobility as a Collective Process

To shed light on the meaning of family to women's well-being, our study examined race and class differences in women's relationships with their families of origin and in their connections to the community (Higginbotham and Weber Cannon 1992). Focusing on the topic of upward social mobility, we investigated how race and class shaped the mobility process for black and white women and the roles their families played in this process.

Education. Education was stressed as important in virtually all of the families of these middle-class women. But the upwardly mobile women, both black and white, received less emotional and financial support for college attendance than did women in middle-class families.

Career and Marriage. Black and white women received different messages from family about what their lives should be like as adults. Black women were told that they needed an occupation to succeed in life and that marriage should be a secondary concern. Julie Barnes, a black junior high school teacher, said: "My father would always say, 'You see how good I'm doing? Each generation should do more than the generation before.' He expects me to accomplish more than he has."

The messages that white upwardly mobile women received were not as clear. Only half said that their parents stressed the need for an occupation to succeed, and 20 percent said that their parents stressed marriage as the primary life goal. The most common message these women got was that because marriage could not be counted on to provide economic survival, an occupation was necessary. But having a career could be detrimental to adult happiness. This was the case with Elizabeth Marlow, a public interest attorney from a working-class background: "My parents assumed that I would go to college and meet some nice man and finish, but not necessarily work after. I would be a good mother for my children. I don't think that they ever thought I would go to law school. Their attitude about my interest in law school was, 'You can do it if you want to, but we don't think it is a particularly practical thing for a woman to do.'"

Commitment to Community. Many black women, whose educational and occupational attainment involved crossing racial barriers as well as class barriers, expressed a sense that their mobility was connected to an entire racial uplift process, not merely to an individual journey. Lillian King, a high-ranking city official who was raised working class, discussed her current commitment to the black community: "Because I have more opportunities, I've got an obligation to give more back and to set a positive example for black people and especially for black women. I think we've got to do a tremendous job in building self-esteem and giving people the desire to achieve."

Role of Family and Friends. The roles that family and friends played for these women varied. Black women were especially likely to express the feeling that they owed a great debt to their families for the help they received. Black upwardly mobile women were also much more likely to feel that they currently give more than they receive from kin. Once they achieve professional managerial employment, their sense of debt combines with their greater access to resources to put them in the position of being asked to give more to both family and friends. White upwardly mobile women, on the other hand, felt that they had accomplished mobility alone and were less likely to feel indebted to kin.

The sense of connectedness accompanied low rates of depressive symptoms among black upwardly mobile women, and the isolation of white working-class women accompanied high rates of depressive symptoms.

Depressive Symptomatology

One of the ways power is wielded to perpetuate race, class, and gender bias is through continued reliance on individual versus social structural explanations of mental health problems. Conventional thinking in the mental health arena, for example, dictates that depression be defined and treated as an individual, psychological disorder of an emotional and cognitive nature. But even though the disorder occurs twice as frequently in women as it does in men, the social dynamics of gender relations are not addressed in traditional explanations of the causes of and treatments for depression (Weissman and Klerman 1987). Indeed, the eighties and nineties have witnessed an even stronger entrenchment of organic (physiological) and genetic theories of depression (Vega and Rumbaut 1991). Viewed, however, from a social structural perspective, depression can be seen as a logical outcome of societal arrangements in which women are restricted from access to social, economic, and political power.

Economic, Political, and Ideological Power and Depression

When people lack *economic power*, they face financial obstacles to meeting basic human needs, and those obstacles produce stress. Women still have little control over the labor market and the larger economy. They routinely face wage and job discrimination, often struggling in educational institutions to secure the credentials for well-paid jobs.

When women lack *political power*, both the community's access to resources and women's sense of efficacy—the sense that what they do matters—are restricted. The sense of efficacy enhances self-esteem. Women are not well represented in elected offices and appointed positions at the city, county, state, or federal level.

This lack of representation was dramatically demonstrated during the Anita Hill/Clarence Thomas hearings, where fourteen white male senators listened to Hill's testimony of sexual harassment and none exhibited any concrete understanding of the female experience on the job. This situation is duplicated regularly in other political arenas and in the criminal justice system, where people with little awareness of gender inequality shape the laws and regulations that govern women's lives.

Finally, in the *ideological realm*, establishing a positive self-definition is difficult in the face of media images that devalue women and over which women still wield little control. Pervasive images of women as childlike or as sex objects, for example, serve to keep the economic and political systems of oppression intact. These images also have a detrimental impact on a woman's fight to achieve positive mental health in a society that devalues women.

Relationship of Race and Class to Depression

The Memphis study examined the role of race and class background in producing depressive outcomes among middle-class managerial and professional women. Because power relationships are central to oppression, we were interested in discovering how women's mental health is affected by holding or not holding power (supervisory versus nonsupervisory responsibilities) in the workplace. What does it mean if women have the power to define work, to hire and fire employees, and to set the pace of work? Might the supervisory relationship have a different meaning for women of different racial and class backgrounds? We expected, for example, that women from middle-class backgrounds would be more comfortable with the power inherent in managing or supervising others and that this relationship would produce some strain for women from the working class who wield power over others in the ranks these women came from themselves.

We found that race, class background, and supervisory status do interact to influence depressive symptomatology for the women (Weber Cannon, Higginbotham, and Guy 1989). As expected, upwardly mobile women in supervisory positions and women raised middle class in nonsupervisory positions had higher levels of depression than either upwardly mobile women who were not supervisors or women raised middle class who were. For women raised working class, exercising control over others was stressful and, for some, produced depression. In contrast, women raised in middle-class families with the expectation that they would be in positions of control were more likely to be depressed when they lacked supervisory power.

Nonsupervisors Raised Middle Class. In the life of Jean Cameron, a white clinical social worker, we can see how unmet achievement expectations can be a source of distress, particularly for women from middle-class families. When asked about her chances for promotion, Jean was frustrated by the sexism she experienced: "The executive director has an extreme bias in favor of males and against women. He put a man who is much less experienced and doesn't know beans in a position way ahead of what he was ready for. They'll let me advance in terms of the kind of clinical work that I do, but in terms of upper management, no."

The failure to move up and be in a position of supervisory power and control was especially frustrating in light of Jean's goals based on her middle-class upbringing: "I certainly am similar to my father in career being the dominant thing in my life and the central driving force. And I'm sure I got a great deal of that from him as well as the desire to have my own business and not work for somebody else—and to resent the money that someone else makes off of me."

It hardly seems surprising that Jean also said, "I don't get along with my supervisor." Yet even though she identified sexism outside of herself for her inability to move up, she also blamed herself for the fact that she doesn't earn the income she would like: "My parents, even now, buy me things I can't afford that they think are expected for a person to have. And I feel badly that in some ways they're still paying for me. I want to get myself in a better situation financially, but that doesn't come as easy to me as it does to my father. *Maybe because I'm not willing to make the sacrifices.*" This sense of self-blame for failed mobility can contribute to depressive symptoms. When asked about how she feels before she goes to work, Jean said, "Currently, my attitude is sort of perfunctory, just grind it out, get through the day."

Supervisors Raised Working Class. In contrast to this middle-class woman's sense of failure relative to her family expectations, women from working-class backgrounds have achieved well beyond their parents' means and often beyond their expectations. The working-class women who were depressed were instead more likely to be supervisors and to find the relationships with their subordinates stressful.

For some of these women, one of the ways they had achieved their own upward mobility was by being strongly self-disciplined and motivated, being "perfectionist" and pushing themselves hard to achieve. These very qualities sometimes created stress when they expected them of their subordinates. For example, when asked about what is difficult about supervising, Jan Brady, a black Equal Employment Compliance Specialist from a working-class family, said: "Making the time for that individual. I'm not a very—I can't say structured—but the person who works under me has to be self-disciplined and self-motivated. I just don't have the time to crack the whip or stay on them. You know, I think when you're at that level that should not be necessary." When asked about her greatest weakness as a supervisor, Jan replied, "Impatience. I'm a perfectionist, and I think a lot of times, instead of delegating work, I'll do it myself because I know how I want it to be done. Instead of having to explain."

It is not surprising that with such high expectations and with the failure to work out the relationship with subordinates in a satisfactory way, Jan feels overloaded: "I'm overloaded right now. I've had, even though I supervise one person, I've had three people in that position over the last year. So when that position is vacant, I have to pick up the slack. So I might have some feelings of being overworked at times. And I'm unable to resolve problems or complaints as quickly as I would like." Jan indicated that she has been seeing a counselor in part to deal with "bouts with lack of confidence."

Single Women and Parent Nonsupervisors. Two other groups of women also displayed significantly higher levels of depressive symptoms than their counterparts: parents and single women in nonsupervisory positions. The lack of intimate support that comes from having a spouse or partner and the demanding gender role of parent were likely to produce depression among this group of middle-class women only when they also lacked supervisory power at work.

Shirley Day, a black educational specialist raised middle class who is married with one child, illustrates how combining parenthood and work in nonsupervisory positions contributed to stress and depression. When asked if she felt she held the position she deserved at work, Shirley said, "No, because I would like to be better—sometimes. Then sometimes I want to be at home and not work at all. . . . I'm about to burn out. I'm tired and I want to do something else, and I think I have greater potential in other areas than the one I'm working in now." When asked about her current career goals, Shirley said, "I want to be a mother. And that's not a career. I just want to stay at home with my daughter and still draw a salary." Shirley was conflicted and depressed as she faced a job where she was "burned out," mobility barriers to changing jobs, and the desire to care for her young child. These cases demonstrate that social structurally derived sources of power such as occupying a supervisory position on the job play an important role in women's psychological health.

Race and Class Background and Depression. Race and class produced different mental health outcomes. Black women from middle-class backgrounds and white women from working-class backgrounds expressed higher levels of depressive symptoms than either black women from working-class or white women from middle-class backgrounds (Weber Cannon, Higginbotham, and Guy 1989). As noted above, black upwardly mobile women were especially likely to feel close to kin, whereas white women from the working class were more isolated from family support.

It is also true that both groups exhibiting higher symptom rates may be thought of as "hidden populations": most black women currently in the middle class have been upwardly mobile from the working class, and most white middle-class women were raised in middle-class families. Groups that differ from their racial norm—black women raised middle class and upwardly mobile white women—face more stress, possibly because co-workers and others are likely to make inaccurate assumptions about their lives. Further, their smaller numbers may provide them with less access to support groups.

Interestingly, our data also reveal that the group most visible in the media and public discourse on women—that is, white women managers from middle-class backgrounds—is actually at least risk for depressive symptoms of all middle-class women. When this group is used as a standard, important mental health issues for the majority may be completely overlooked or distorted.

Further Issues in Mental Health and Diversity

As in other research on women's health issues, attention to diversity is key to understanding women's mental health. *Power and privilege* have dramatic implications for people's day-to-day lives. *Race and ethnic group membership* form unique contexts in which people confront common obstacles to their development. *Current social class and class background* are also dimensions of experience that produce another complex web of stressors and resources. Given that power relations are so critical to mental health, age is another important dimension. As children we are powerless, but as we grow up, we expect to become powerful. Instead, many of us remain powerless. But as we face stressors that threaten our mental health, we also gain options that can expand our resources for handling the stresses of life. Finally, in a society that remains committed to privileging heterosexual identity, *sexual orientation* is also a critical factor: Lesbians experience unique material, social, and psychological stressors.

This complex and intersecting web of social relationships based in race, ethnic group, social class, age, sexual orientation, and other dimensions of experience challenge and/or support women's mental health. Teenage parenthood, for example, is typically seen as producing problems for females because it pushes them into adult roles before they have completed their own social and emotional development. Yet not all pregnant teenagers bring the same resources to their situation. The most common pattern in the black community is for the pregnant daughter to remain at home, where she has access to an extended family network. In contrast, pregnant Puerto Rican teens are more likely to marry and start their own households.

Only when we acknowledge the importance of this diversity and of power and privilege in shaping all aspects of life will we fully understand the threats to women's mental health and the resources necessary to confront them.

NOTE

1. We recognize that our study is focused on only a small section of the ethnically and racially diverse population of women that reside in the United States today. We

cite the data here, however, to illustrate some ways that intersecting social structures of race, class, and gender shape mental health outcomes for women. For rationale on the study selection criteria see Weber Cannon et al. (1988, 1989). As is the case with many studies of special categories of women, we had no way to randomly sample the population to fit the above study parameters. Instead, we employed a quota sample stratified by three dimensions of inequality: race and class background of the respondents and the gender composition of her occupation. Each dimension was operationalized into two categories: black and white, raised working class/upwardly mobile and raised middle class/middle class stable, and female dominated and male dominated. Data were gathered from two hundred women in the Memphis area. Twenty-five cases were selected of the eight cells of this 2 x 2 x 2 design so that the cells would be large enough to allow statistical estimates of the relationship of the major independent variables with our dependent variables. (For more details on the sampling procedures see Weber Cannon, Higginbotham, and Leung 1988.)

REFERENCES

Broverman, I. K., D. Broverman, F. E. Clarkson, P. S. Rosenkrantz, and S. R. Vogel
    1970   "Sex-role stereotyping and clinical judgments of mental health." Journal of Consulting and Clinical Psychology 34:1–7.

Collins, Patricia Hill
    1990   Black Feminist Thought. New York: Routledge.

Comas-Diaz, Lillian, and Beverly Greene, eds.
    1994   Women of Color: Integrating Ethnic and Gender Identities in Psychotherapy. New York: Guilford.

DeParle, Jason
    1992   "Why marginal changes don't rescue the welfare system." New York Times, 1 March, E3.

Gilkes, Cheryl Townsend
    1980   "Holding back the ocean with a broom: black women and community work." Pp. 217–30 in La Frances Rodgers-Rose (ed.), The Black Woman. Beverly Hills, CA: Sage.

Greenspan, Miriam
    1983   A New Approach to Women and Therapy. New York: McGraw-Hill.

Gutierrez, Lorraine
    1990   "Working with women of color: an empowerment perspective." Social Work 35:149–53.

Higginbotham, Elizabeth, and Lynn Weber Cannon
    1988   "Rethinking mobility: towards a race and gender inclusive theory." Research Paper No. 8, Center for Research on Women, Memphis State University, Memphis, TN.
    1992   "Moving up with kin and community: upward social mobility for black and white women." Gender and Society 6 (September):416–40.

Kotlowitz, Alex
    1991   There Are No Children Here. New York: Doubleday.
LaVeist, Thomas A.
    1992   "The political empowerment and health status of African Americans: mapping a new territory." American Journal of Sociology 97:1080-95.
McLeod, Jane D., and Ronald Kessler
    1990   "Socioeconomic status differences in vulnerability to undesirable life events." Journal of Health and Social Behavior 31:162-72.
Mirowsky, John, and Catherine Ross
    1990   "Control or defense? depression and the sense of control over good and bad outcomes." Journal of Health and Social Behavior 31:71-86.
Poulantzas, Nicos
    1975   Classes in Contemporary Capitalism. Translated from French by David Fernbach. London: New Left Books.
Rose, Stephen
    1990   "Advocacy/empowerment: an approach to clinical practice in social work." Journal of Sociology and Social Welfare 17(2):41-51.
Rosenfield, Sarah
    1989   "The effects of women's employment: personal control and sex differences in mental health." Journal of Health and Social Behavior 30:77-91.
Scott, Kesho Yvonne
    1991   The Habit of Survival. New Brunswick, NJ: Rutgers University Press.
Stack, Carol B.
    1974   All Our Kin: Strategies for Survival in a Black Community. New York: Harper and Row.
Vanneman, Reeve, and Lynn Weber Cannon
    1987   The American Perception of Class. Philadelphia: Temple University Press.
Vega, William A., and Reuben G. Rumbaut
    1991   "Ethnic minorities and mental health." Pp. 351-83 in W. Richard Scott and Judith Blake (eds.), Annual Review of Sociology. Palo Alto, CA: Annual Reviews.
Weber Cannon, Lynn, Elizabeth Higginbotham, and Rebecca Guy
    1989   "Depression among women: exploring the effects of race, class and gender." Working Paper #9. Center for Research on Women, Memphis State University, Memphis, TN.
Weber Cannon, Lynn, Elizabeth Higginbotham, and Marianne Leung
    1988   "Race and class bias in qualitative research on women." Gender and Society 2:449-62.
Weissman, Michaele M., and Gerald L. Klerman
    1987   "Gender and depression." Pp. 3-15 in Ruth Formanek and Anita Gurian (eds.), Women and Depression: A Lifespan Perspective. New York: Springer.
Wheaton, Blair
    1990   "Life transitions, role histories, and mental health." American Sociological Review 55:209-23.

[16]

Who Cares? Women as Informal
and Formal Caregivers

VIRGINIA L. OLESEN

Caring for the elderly, disabled, or ill children or adults
involves several types of women caregivers. Informal caregivers work without pay to help sick family members,
often in highly stressful situations. Specific social and economic factors may increase or reduce their burdens.
Women formal caregivers working for pay in health care
institutions are largely clustered in the lower levels of the
health care pyramid. Their responsibilities and opportunities reflect changing trends in medical economics and
practice.

This chapter examines two major types of caregiving, informal and formal.
Informal caregivers are unlicensed and unpaid individuals, sometimes
called "unaffiliated providers" (Abel and Nelson 1990:8). They work outside institutional settings, usually in the home and often with relatives.
Formally licensed, trained, and remunerated caregivers include certified
nurse's aides, licensed vocational nurses, registered nurses, and physicians.
They usually work in hospitals, clinics, nursing homes, or agencies.

The chapter also briefly mentions two other types of caregivers: (1)
formally trained and paid "alternative" caregivers such as chiropractors,
not usually included in western biomedical domains but within formal
caregiving systems, and (2) culturally designated care providers, i.e., spiritual healers, granny midwives, rootworkers, and *curanderas*, who provide
care, sometimes for pay, sometimes not, but almost always outside the
formal health care system.

Informal Caregiving

A curious contradiction arises around women as care providers: on the
one hand, women are expected to give informal care. On the other hand,

there has been considerable reluctance to prepare women and admit them to elite care provider roles in medicine. There has also been only grudging recognition of provider professions, such as nursing, in which women predominate.

Feminists disagree on whether women are "natural" care providers: some criticize this view as "essentialist," meaning that a characteristic has been attributed to women as inherent in being female, rather than socially acquired or attributed or constructed in specific contexts (Scheper-Hughes 1992). Some have pointed out that thinking about caring as "natural" or "essential" to women obscures the complexities within caregiving (Fisher and Tronto 1990:39), which blends many seemingly opposed attributes such as autonomy and nurturance, reason and emotion, public and private (Abel and Nelson 1990:5). Others, although agreeing that essentialism is an erroneous way to view women's actions, nevertheless argue effectively for "maternal thinking," an attribute they claim can be found in either men or women (Ruddick 1983).

Most feminist writing on informal care has not assumed that women have a natural tendency to do caregiving. Instead, the view here is that cultural demands in women's lives in the everyday world place them, much more frequently than men, in the job of informal caregiver or direct provider to the disabled, ill or elderly. In general, other than physicians, very few males undertake direct caregiving roles, especially not in the home.

Feminist Concern with Informal Caregiving

Feminists interested in women's health have gradually recognized informal care as an important activity done by women, but they have been slow to recognize the many differences among women doing informal care. Otherwise stimulating examinations of household tasks (Berk 1985) or emotions in a domestic setting (Hochschild 1987) did not include caregiving. British feminists began examining the gendered nature of informal care and its place in society (Finch and Groves 1982; Graham 1985; Ungerson 1983). They clarified the idea that, although caregiving was a labor of love, it was also *work* that could be analyzed in ways that would recognize women's labor. American feminist scholars quickly developed a parallel body of work that deepened the issues (Abel 1990a; Abel and Nelson 1990; Fisher and Tronto 1990; Glazer 1990) and extended the discussion to matters of ethics and moral boundaries (Larrabee 1993; Tronto 1993).

However, these early feminist analyses of caregiving generally were based on married, able-bodied, middle-class white women with extended kin, a view that hid important features of caregiving in many women's lives. Early formulations of caregiving left no room for analysis of the caregiving experiences of women of color, disabled women, or lesbians (Graham 1993). Indeed, some researchers have questioned whether inferences about primary care providers based on the experiences of able-bodied white American women are applicable to women in nonwhite racial or ethnic groups (Hatch 1991).

Informal Care of the Elderly Infirm

Much of what is known in the social sciences about informal health care providers comes from studies on care of the elderly done by researchers in gerontology, public health, social welfare, nursing, medical sociology, and medical anthropology. This work reflects scholars' and policymakers' concerns about the aging American population (see chapter 17).

That literature shows that not only are most elderly Americans female, but most of those who care for the male and female elderly are also female. More than 70 percent of caregivers to the elderly are wives and adult daughters, though sisters and daughters-in-law are also frequently involved (Coward and Dwyer 1990). Paid providers in nursing homes deliver some of this care to ill, elderly females, but informal or hidden providers at home provide a substantial amount. One study found that the incidence of informal caregiving was highest among minority women (Montgomery and Datwyler 1990), which reflects the fact that frail, elderly women of color are underrepresented in nursing home populations (Abel 1990b:74).

The emotional, financial, and physical burdens of informal caregiving are heavy for all women. Some single women give up social relationships in order to provide care (Burnley 1987). Other caregivers find that having to take charge of a frail parent or parents poses stressful issues of role reversal. One caregiver who has responsibilities for both her mother and mother-in-law commented: "With children you have more control. With a parent, you're only halfway in control, and I don't want to be in control of my mother. When we find ourselves in a position where she's forced to relinquish control, it makes everybody uncomfortable." Her sister added: "There's an emotional/psychological thing about role reversal that's very hard" (Beth Witrogen McLeod, *San Francisco Examiner*, 2 April 1995,

A16). Not the least of the burdens, aside from physical care, are the endless search for assistance, adequate, safe, and economically feasible day-care or residential care facilities, management of the elder person's sometimes diminishing economic resources, and continuing struggles with the complexities of Medicare or Medicaid and other insurance companies.

Some informal caregivers often are also raising dependent children (Brody 1990). The strains of feeling rushed, frustrated, anxious, and/or isolated are enlarged for these women in the "sandwich generation" (Walker, Martin, and Jones 1992). A single mother raising two teenagers and also caring for her disabled parents and an aunt remarked: "One of the hardest things about this is that there are so many different needs from so many different people, it's like spinning all the plates in the air, and no matter which one you turn to, somebody else's need is starting to spin down and drop on the floor. . . . It's sort of an endless episode of guilt: while you're doing something for one guy, you're letting the other one go. . . . There are not many thank-yous" (Beth Witrogen McLeod, *San Francisco Examiner,* 16 April 1995, C4). The burden is especially heavy for disabled women who struggle with their own physical limits as they care for others (Hillyer 1993).

Sources of support and of strain differ among women, but relatively little is as yet known about such differences. One inquiry found that some black caregivers have more support than white caregivers (Smerglia, Deimling, and Barresi 1988). Others have noted that contrary to assumptions about elaborate extended families, some Asian women lack such support (Goodman 1990). Concerning support systems, church attendance is more likely to predict informal support patterns for black caregivers than it is for white caregivers (Hatch 1991).

Sources of strain may also differ. A study of black and white daughter caregivers found that both groups experienced conflicts between caregiving and their personal and social lives which related to strain, though black women reported less role strain overall (Mui 1992). For black women, poor perceived health and the lack of respite support also pointed to strain, whereas for white women the poor quality of relationship with their parents and conflicts with their paid work were sources of strain. Another comparison of employed women caring for frail parents found that interferences with their work (late arrival, early departure, unscheduled days off) predicted more poor mental health for white caregivers and more fragile physical health for black caregivers (Lechner 1993).

The few comparative studies of male and female caregivers show some striking differences which reveal some of the distinctive pressures on female caregivers. Having a job lessened the time spent caregiving for males, but did not do so for employed female caregivers (Stoller 1983). Further, men perform caregiving differently. Among men and women who gave care after their spouse had cardiac surgery, men were able to find more resources and to get others to help more easily than were women (Rankin 1988; Miller 1990). One interpretation is that men approach informal caregiving instrumentally (in terms of tasks) rather than expressively (in terms of emotion or personal relationships). Moreover, friends and relatives, noting the unusual situation of a male being in the caregiving role, may be more likely to offer help (Horowitz 1985).

This and other studies also show that male caregivers report less emotional strain and stress than do female caregivers (ASPE-HCFA 1982:42; Chang and White-Means 1991; Montgomery and Datwyler 1990).[1] Cultural expectations around gender not only influence who becomes the caregiver, but such expectations also shape how the caregiver performs informal care and his or her emotional response to the work.

Could more men become informal caregivers (Kaye and Applegate 1990)? Increasing male participation in informal caregiving would depend in part on expanded work leave policies which would provide such for employed males beyond what is now possible under the Family Leave Act. Equally significant, cultural expectations for both males and females would have to change considerably.

Sick Children and Family Members

Even in households where there is no care of an elderly person, women provide a great deal of informal care to household members, especially children. This is particularly problematic for large numbers of women who work outside the home. In 1993 almost 60 percent of all mothers with preschool children (under the age of six) were in the labor force, compared with only 32 percent in 1970 (Current Population Survey 1993). This dramatic increase holds for single, married, divorced, and widowed mothers (U.S. Bureau of the Census 1994:402).[2] There are about 9.6 million working women with preschool-aged children. About 11.5 million preschoolers and 27.1 million children ages six to seventeen have mothers in the labor force (Current Population Survey 1993).

Women workers may use their sick leave or vacation time to do caregiving, inflating women's sick leave use rates and giving the impression that

women themselves are "sicker" than men. Women workers take off between 5.6 and 28.8 days annually to take care of sick children (Landis and
Earp 1987). This means that women utilize paid sick leave for their children, risking inadequate sick leave for their own illnesses. Estimates of the
value of the time that employed women spend just taking children for medical visits range from $572 million to $1.1 billion (Carpenter 1980). Fathers
are much less likely, or in some instances less able, to take time off to care
for sick children. Working mothers' informal care of sick or handicapped
children is part of the larger problem of child care in contemporary American society, which lags far behind other industrialized nations in the availability of adequate, safe child care.

The Family Leave Act of 1993 provided up to twelve weeks of
unpaid leave each year for both female and male employees of public
agencies or businesses with fifty or more employees to care for newborn
or adopted children, themselves, or immediate family members with a
serious medical condition. Unlike such laws in other countries it does
not provide coverage of salary (England and Naulleau 1991). Moreover,
many workers still do not have access to such leave because they work
in smaller firms not included under the law. In the early eighties, 88
percent of U.S. businesses had fewer than twenty employees (U.S. Bureau of the Census 1984).

The care of nonelderly adults who are ill or injured also often falls to
the women in the household or to female kin. Caregiving for persons
suffering from AIDS-induced illnesses is, for example, a largely invisible
service given by women kin and friends of the afflicted person (Schiller
1993) as well as by gay males (Turner and Pearlin 1989).

Productive Aspects of Informal Health Care

Informal caregiving has two productive aspects, which are frequently
overlooked or underestimated: the value to society of the care given and
the importance of creating good health.

If "free" or unpaid services in the care of the noninstitutionalized
elderly were to be replaced with waged work, the cost would be $9.6
billion (Paringer 1983). Much of these dramatic costs come from the
informal care of the elderly who are ill. In fact, this figure probably underestimates the value of informal care, for it does not reflect the value of
lost wages to women who relinquish paid work to care for an elderly
person. Not surprisingly, more women than men give up paid work to care

for the elderly or take time off from work to do so and, if employed outside the home, to seek part-time jobs (Boaz and Muller 1992), which will mean diminished income in old age as a result of decreased Social Security benefits and/or pensions (Estes, Gerard, and Clarke 1984).

Most scholarly and policy discussions treat informal health caregiving as the provision of service and assistance during an actual illness. However, there is another side to the productive aspect of informal care. The informal caregiver often produces healthy (or unhealthy) conditions for the family by preparing meals, cleaning, and offering health advice to both children and adults in the home (DeVault 1991; Graham 1985). Thus the informal provider is a key figure in how children and other adults are taught to be healthy or not. But very few (Campbell 1975; Carpenter 1980; Cunningham-Burley and Irvine 1987; Mechanic 1964; Prout 1988) have looked at this important communication. Most other studies take a developmental approach that neglects parents' part in childhood socialization to health and illness. This merits much more attention if the complexities and implications found in this part of informal caregiving are to be fully understood.

The informal care provider is also a significant participant in both the informal and formal health care systems as illness or recovery occurs. She may informally discuss the process with family, friends, colleagues, or acquaintances and in that sense influence how others participate in the illness or recovery trajectory (Furstenberg and Davis 1984). She is an important negotiator and interpreter of health care activities (Graham 1985). Because these productive activities of informal caregivers are not included in the estimated value of informal caregiving noted above, women's informal caregiving is a much more valuable resource than is commonly acknowledged.

Underexplored Issues

Black, disabled, and lesbian feminist writing has urged the decentering of white experiences in women's health and pointed to important differences among caregivers, deriving from race, disability, and sexual orientation (Asch and Fine 1992; Bair and Cayleff 1993:15; Stevens 1992). Yet there is still limited understanding of "how cultural variations in household structure and meanings of family responsibilities alter the caregiving experience" and, indeed, the very meaning of caregiving (Abel 1990b:74).

The few studies done provide glimpses of important issues worthy of further research:

— How strain and support systems differ among caregivers is still unknown yet crucial to fully understanding different care contexts. Differentiating caregiving obligations and tasks, as has been done in a study of black and white caregivers, would advance understanding (Horwitz and Reinhard 1995).

— The few studies about support and strain suggest that conditions under which support is received and from whom merit attention, including the contested issue of domestic service.[3]

— Such questions as why and under what circumstances do men provide informal care and how is it different from that done by females have only barely been explored, yet they may contain important leads for the recruitment of men to caregiving.

— How cultural themes about illness and health play a part in informal care also needs to be explored: e.g., the importance of the concepts of nervios (nerves) and fallo mental (mental failure) for Hispanics caring for a mentally ill family member (Guarnaccia et al. 1992).

Trends That Have an Impact on Informal Care

Examination of these underexplored issues will become more urgent because a number of trends will increase the importance of informal caregiving at the same time material resources for support of caregivers will remain relatively unchanged (Alford-Cooper 1993) or perhaps even diminish.

Social Trends. More men and women will live longer. Between the years 2030 and 2050 the population age 85 and older will be five times larger than it was in 1995; about half will need help with routine activities (Selker 1993). No one knows whether there will be enough younger women to care for this population (Foulke, Alford-Cooper, and Butler 1993). Among other factors, large numbers of black, white, and Latino women, even those with young children, will continue to enter the labor force as they find more work opportunities and/or as the cost of living dictates the necessity for two family incomes and/or as the number of single mothers increases. In 1993, 58 percent of the civilian labor force were women, but by 2005 this percentage is expected to rise to 63.6 (U.S. Bureau of the Census 1994:395). This means that along with the emotional, physical, and occupational costs noted in this chapter, pressures on women caregivers who themselves are aging will also continue.[4]

Economic trends. Federally mandated reimbursement practices of dismissing very ill patients after shorter hospital stays shift the burden of care once given in clinics or hospitals to the household (Glazer 1990). Not only is the patient sent home early, but often complex care technologies (respirators, dialysis, and certain drugs) move from hospitals or skilled nursing facilities to private homes along with the patients. There untrained and technically unskilled caregivers are forced to assume the responsibility of giving safe care after only brief training in using the technology. These technologies, challenging even for professional caregivers (Kaye and Reisman 1991), are daunting for unskilled, informal caregivers. For dialysis patients and their informal caregivers, this relationship is fraught with anxiety and considerable strain as they attempt to normalize an unusual situation, a process which is by no means smooth and orderly for all such couples (Gerhardt and Brieskorn-Zinke 1986).[5] People who live alone are particularly vulnerable in such situations.

Disease Trends. Reported AIDS cases among American women increased 5.7 times between 1981 to 1985 (1,098) and 1992 (6,312). AIDS in men increased 2.7 times, from 14,466 cases reported between 1981 and 1985 to 39,160 cases in 1992 (U.S. Bureau of the Census 1994:139). Although AIDS affects all social and racial groups, women of color have been particularly affected: in 1994, 77 percent of female AIDS patients were black or Latino. It is the fourth leading cause of death in women ages 25-44 and the leading cause of death among black women in that age group (Centers for Disease Control 1995). As the disease progresses, many of these women will be unable to care for children or elderly parents and will require care themselves. (For a detailed discussion of women and AIDS, see Stoller's analysis in chapter 18.)

A further and poignant problem arises: there was a fourteenfold increase in AIDS cases reported among children under the age of thirteen between 1981 and 1991 (U.S. Bureau of the Census 1994:125). The burden of pediatric AIDS care disproportionately affects black and Latino women. Between 1981 and 1993, of the 4,710 cases of AIDS in children under thirteen, 2,574 were black, 1,146 Latino, 942 white, 21

Asian-Pacific Islander, 15 American Indian/Alaskan Native, and 12 un-known (Centers for Disease Control 1993).

To the worries of child-rearing are added additional burdens for informal care during the stressful illness (Bonuck 1993; Strauss et al. 1991). Mothers are not the only relatives involved in caring for AIDs-infected children: grandmothers who may have provided long-term care to a son or daughter dying of AIDS are increasingly being called upon to care for their orphaned grandchildren (Lee 1994; Ward 1993). They are part of a national trend. In 1992, 865,000 children were raised by grandparents; in 1993 that number grew to over one million (*New York Times*, 21 November 1994). (For an extended discussion of grand-parents' care of children in the black communities, see Jones and Estes, chapter 17.)

What will these trends—an increasing older population, more women in the labor force, reduction of patient time spent in institutional care facilities, growing reliance on use of care technology at home, increases in cases of maternal and pediatric AIDS—mean for women as informal caregivers? Obdurate cultural pressures on women to provide "free" infor-mal care will continue. Deeper exploration of differential sources of strain and support for the many diverse contexts in which women do informal care is requisite. Until such differences are clarified, the processes of in-formal caregiving will not be fully understood, nor will policies on such caregiving be aptly framed to recognize or facilitate women's extensive and undervalued work of informal caregiving. An example of policy mind-ful of differences that could be articulated at all levels where caregiving policy is formulated would be to fine-tune leave taking in small and large work contexts to accommodate issues of sexual orientation, gender, ethnicity, color, and disability.

Formal Care

"Formal caregivers" here refers to those who are licensed by the state to deliver care to patients or recovering patients in offices, clinics, hospitals, and at home. Their work is psychosocial, supportive, curative, and tech-nical. Because many formal caregivers work in all three modes simulta-neously (Butter et al. 1987:135–36), this chapter discusses caregivers without drawing the distinction made in much of the literature between caring and curing. For example, a physician can give supportive care, assess the patient technically via tests, and prescribe all in five minutes.

In return, these caregivers receive fees or salaries, whereas informal care-givers' labor, though valuable and time-consuming, is rarely remunerated.

Although this chapter focuses on female caregivers within the health care system, it is important to remember that there are many other care-givers, some formally trained and licensed, some not, from whom women from diverse economic, cultural, and social contexts seek help, sometimes at the same time they receive care from formal health care providers.[6] Licensed, trained practitioners include chiropodists, chiropractors, ho-meopaths, osteopaths, acupuncturists. As is true of medicine and dentistry, relatively few women, including women of color, are found in the ranks of these "alternative" or "concurrent" caregivers. Unlicensed healers and caregivers occupy recognized, culturally designated roles, such as *parteras* (Mexican American midwives) (Spector 1991), lay and granny midwives (Davis and Ingram 1993; Holmes 1990), rootworkers (Snow 1974), and spiritual healers (Fontenot 1993; Fox 1989; McGuire 1988; Singer and Garcia 1989). Aside from these cultural roles there are herbalists, vitamin therapists, masseuses, and biofeedback therapists who are licensed in some states. All are socially and culturally situated in many ethnic/racial groups and social classes. These caregivers may have come to their work through spiritual inclination or accumulated experience. They may learn their trade as apprentices or through a formal course of instruction. Primarily female, they have long provided significant care. Sometimes this care can be more sensitive to different women's situations than that offered by scientific medicine in the health care system precisely because it emerges from and recognizes specific cultural and social aspects of those diverse situations. A good deal of research remains to be done on women's use of alternative practitioners and on the practitioners themselves.

Feminist Views of Physicians and Nurses

Although feminist scholars early analyzed the situation of women in medicine (Lorber 1975), they were slower to examine or even recognize nursing as a possible topic for feminist analysis. Some feminists in the 1960s deemed nursing inappropriate for "liberated" women: they saw "maleness" as the standard for useful work, a perspective which ruled out nursing because of the diverse nurturing, caring aspects and the fact that most nurses are female (Lewin 1977).[7]

Later feminist historical analyses (Melosh 1982; Reverby 1987), as well as work by nurse scholars (Cleland 1971), and social scientists (Lewin and

Olesen 1980), shifted away from such androcentric thinking to examine nursing's many complexities as a caregiving profession and the experiences of nurses in a "female" profession. As was the case with feminist analyses of informal care, recognition of the history and particular situation of non-white nurses was also slow. Hine's (1985, 1989) history of black nurses documented the long struggle for recognition and equitable treatment within the profession and more generally in the health care field.

The Formal Caregiving Pyramid

The distribution of formal caregivers takes the shape of a pyramid with very few women at the top, where the largest salaries are found, and a great many women at the bottom, where salaries are modest.

1. Physicians occupy the top level. Eighty percent are white males, with a smaller number of women, also mostly white (U.S. Bureau of the Census 1994:407). As is true in all levels, even in this highly paid sector of the health care system, women earn only 59 percent of what men receive (Butter et al. 1987:144).

2. A much larger middle level comprises primarily registered nurses, mostly white females with a few women of color. In 1988, 7.1 percent of employed registered nurses were black and 2.4 percent were Latino (U.S. Bureau of the Census 1994:392). Also here are licensed allied health personnel, such as nurse midwives, physical therapists, and dietitians who are primarily white females (Muller 1994:189). Salaries here are much lower. But again, men receive higher remuneration than women. For instance, 71.5 percent of physical therapists are women, but they earn only 67.4 percent of what male therapists receive (Butter et al. 1987:144).

3. The bottom and largest level consists mostly of licensed vocational nurses, licensed practical nurses, and health aides. Almost a third of these women are black or Latino (Hart-Brothers 1994:206). Their work is critical, particularly for hospitalized women or those residing in a skilled nursing care facility. Again, men earn more than women in these positions.

Changes and Their Implications

The general shape of the pyramid of health caregivers has remained the same since the American health care system began to diversify and include such roles as aides and LVNs early in this century. However, some changes have occurred within various levels where numbers of women or women of color have increased.

Looking first at the top level of physicians, in recent decades more women have entered medical school and are now practicing. Women applicants increased from 28.3 percent in 1979 to 41.8 percent in 1992–93. In 1969–70, 9.2 percent of enrolled medical students were women. By 1992–93 this number had risen to 39.4 percent. The increase in practicing women physicians has also been dramatic: in 1970 7.6 percent of physicians were women; in 1992 this rose to 18.1 percent and is expected to reach 29.4 percent by 2010 (Bickel and Kopriva 1993:141–42).

Numbers of women of color have also increased in medicine. In 1988, for instance, 65 percent of black medical students were women. Predictions are that 39.3 percent of black and 22.8 percent of Latino physicians practicing in 2000 will be women (Hart-Brothers 1994:210–13).

Looking at changes in other levels in the pyramid, over the decade of the 1980s there were small increases in numbers of women of color enrolling in and graduating from nursing programs that lead to becoming a registered nurse (university or four-year college baccalaureate programs, community college associate of arts programs, and hospital programs) (Hart-Brothers 1994:211).[8] Black women enrolled in such programs in larger numbers than any other minority group (National League for Nursing 1991:113). Although their numbers were small, they were also the largest minority group studying for graduate degrees or doing postdoctoral work (American Association of Colleges of Nursing 1995:18).[9]

These changes in the general shape and composition of the pyramid are positive but minor. Most women of color will continue to be found at the bottom in the rapidly growing health aide category. Diminishing funding for baccalaureate nursing programs further depresses possibilities for poor women to enter at this level, thus perpetuating the racial and class differences in the profession (Glazer 1991; Manley 1995).[10]

Women Caregivers' Diverse Experiences

Irrespective of the profession, many women preparing for and practicing in formal caregiver roles experience situations in which racial and/or sexual issues demean or discriminate against women. Two general types of situations occur. The first is interactional. Here discrimination ranges from verbal behavior such as slurs or sexually tinged comments to invidious statements about competence or their very presence in the health care system on through physical behaviors such as unwanted physical contact or the request for sexual favors in return for grades or promotion. (See Britton in chapter 19 on sexual harassment.) The second is structural and institutional. Here discrimination includes being overlooked or neglected for promotion or receiving a salary less than males or whites in the particular level. (The shape and nature of the pyramid of care attests to this second type.)

Looking first at interactions, speaking of her experiences as a medical student, Vanessa Northington Gamble, a black physician, remembered the doubly painful experience of racial and sexual slurs (1990:59): "Wearing a lab coat and carrying a stethoscope, I walked into a patient's room . . . and introduced myself as a student doctor. . . . Later the white male intern came out of the patient's room. 'You know what that guy asked me,' he laughingly announced. 'Why didn't that girl clean up while she was in here?' My being mistaken for a maid became a joke on the ward team, all of whom, other than myself, were white and male."

Cheryl M. Killion, a black nurse doctorally prepared in anthropology now at the University of Michigan School of Nursing, recalled from her student days that many patients could not believe that a black woman was studying to become a registered nurse (1990:244). One problem for students who experience these regrettable incidents is that there are still very few female role models or mentors from underrepresented groups on faculties of health professional schools, though minority faculty should not be the only faculty responsible for counseling and supporting students after such events.[11]

Between 1990 and 1992, 60 percent of women medical school graduates reported sexual harassment (Lenhart 1993:155). One woman stated: "The incident which made me angriest (and I do not anger easily) was when, at the conclusion of the afternoon rounds, the chief resident stated that I could now come and 'service' him and the third-year resident in the call room. This was not said in a flirtatious manner: it was very derisive in tone. It was obviously meant to anger me and it did" (Silver and Glicken 1990:530). This statement, a type of verbal rape, erases the woman as medical student and reduces her to sexual object. Female medical school faculty have also experienced sexual harassment, such as Dr. Frances Conley's widely publicized resignation from the Stanford University Medical School Department of Neurosurgery in 1991. Some reforms have occurred with new procedures for reporting and handling such complaints.[12]

Problems of institutional discrimination against women in medicine reflect biases among key decision makers, group dynamics, and sexual stereotypes (Lenhart 1993:156). Women are overlooked for promotion, refused maternal or family leave, excluded from important professional contacts and referral, and given salaries smaller than males at their level. These often result in high stress and low morale. As Sharyn Lenhart wrote, "It is remarkable that so many women physicians persist, excel and succeed" (159). Nurses, too, experience discrimination both in practice and academic settings, often complicated by their subordinate status.

Issues to Be Explored

The extent to which education for medicine and nursing are gender and diversity sensitive is a major research question which bears on both would-be caregivers undergoing professional socialization and the very act of caregiving once in practice. The extent to which concerns about women's issues have entered professional school curricula varies. Since the early 1980s, baccalaureate and graduate nursing education has included materials in some required and some elective courses on women's health that go beyond a maternal and child focus.[13]

Not surprisingly because of turf struggles among and between medical specialties and medicine's orientation to women patients, medical curricula have not advanced to the same extent. A small movement in this direction has recently emerged in a struggle among feminist medical educators over the utility of a new women's health specialty. Though the American Medical Women's Association drafted a core curriculum for such a specialty in 1992, it remains a contested possibility and not widely found in medical schools (Johnson 1992; Wallis 1992, 1994). Proponents argue that training in such a specialty would avoid the biologized view of women common in medicine and encourage taking the woman patient as a whole person, resulting in better care. In an era of economic reform where services are fragmented, it would offer a better chance for integrated care for all women in various subgroups (Hoffman and Johnson 1995; Johnson 1992; Johnson and Hoffman 1994). Others sympathetic to the problems of adequate health care for women fear that such a new specialty would become marginalized and argue instead for "mainstreaming" women's health issues in all the medical curriculum or for an interdisciplinary (nonmedical) master's degree in women's health (Harrison 1992, 1994). Internists, now at the helm of primary care, are quickly expanding their practices to include routine gynecological services such as Pap smears and birth control prescriptions.

Regarding racial, ethnic and cultural diversity in professional curricula, the extent to which these materials enter nursing and medical curricula also varies. Where medical anthropologists or sociologists have been influential for medical school curricula, materials reflecting diversity appear, but these are not widespread instances. Nursing, which includes a number of nurses doctorally prepared in anthropology and sociology and has generally been more receptive to social scientists, has moved farther in this respect. But even here critics urge greater cultural sensitivity in education and in research training (Barbee 1993; Jackson 1993).

With respect to sensitivity to both gender and diversity, thoughtful research on medical and nursing curricula, with concurrent attention to increasing the now small numbers of female faculty from minority groups, seems imperative if future formal caregivers are to be well prepared to deliver sensitive care.

Trends and Their Implications

Many of the trends noted in the section on informal caregiving will also influence formal caregivers. Of particular interest is the emphasis on cost cutting in health care delivery because it intersects with the growing numbers of women in medicine.

More physicians in general now end up in health maintenance practices (see discussion on HMOs in chapter 8) or other group practice, rather than solo practice. This trend will continue and even grow. One commentator even boldly predicted that women physicians could well be the salvation of the health care system because they accept less pay and more subordinate roles (Butter et al. 1987:148). Cost containment emphases could also lead to utilization of other less highly paid caregivers, such as nurse practitioners, particularly those specialized in areas where many women seek care: family, primary medicine and ob-gyn. This is now the case in many HMOs. How exactly the growth in number of female physicians relates to the growing popularity of nurse practitioners is a question which turns on the tensions between economic reform and quality (see chapter 23). Whatever the case, it is clear that women formal caregivers, as women so often have been, are regarded as an economic element in the nation's struggles for health care reform.

The related question, and one of deep concern in this book, is whether and how increased numbers of women, including women of color, as physicians and nurses, will make a difference in terms of providing care sensitive to the needs of diverse women patients. This question carries within it hints of the essentialist view of women's nature discussed at the outset of this chapter, that women by nature are more caring and humane. It also overlooks diversities in practice settings as well as cultural, structural and economic realities in care delivery. Yet it also acknowledges the deeply gendered nature of social life.

The evidence thus far is equivocal on whether increased numbers of women physicians will make a difference, a question which seems to assume that humanizing practice lies solely with the doctor and is not a shared responsibility or an organizational issue. By the end of medical school there were no gender differences around humanistic or psychosocial issues, even though women students had indicated greater interest at the outset (Dufort and Maheux 1995). One study, however, found that in practice settings there was no difference between men and women regarding technical care, but women seemed to communicate sensitivity and caring more effectively (Arnold, Martin, and Parker 1988). Other evidence indicates that women patients are more likely to get mammograms and Pap smears if the physician is a woman (Lurie et al. 1993).

Longtime observers of medicine have argued that not until there is a critical mass of women physicians (a larger numerical aggregate) with authority and power and interested in aligning with others such as nurse practitioners to reform the system rather than perpetuate professional dominance will the full impact of a caring or humanistic view be felt (Lorber 1984, 1985; Stacey 1988). Whether women physicians will chose locations where they work with underserved populations is a related question of interest. Many of the settings where women physicians have chosen to work to date are those which provide care to these populations (Bowman and Gross 1986). It is likely that women physicians, including women of color, will be providing much of this care. Women graduates of one medical school tended to work in impoverished areas more than their male colleagues (Hart-Brothers 1994:207).

Conclusions

Informal and formal caregiving stand as equally important sectors in health and illness where women of all social classes, racial and ethnic groups, ablebodied and disabled, and of different sexual orientations make crucial contributions as yet not recognized. Differentiating and acknowledging those contributions, so critical to humane care of the suffering and decent care of the well, are critical tasks for feminists in an era of increasing differences.

NOTES

1. That men and women differ in their responses to and management of informal caregiving in no way suggests that such care is without strain for male caregivers. One man reported: "As time went by they [his parents] needed more and more help. . . . So I gave up my job in Mountain View and moved to my parents' place. I was naive enough to think I could take care of my parents myself—a big, big mistake. I would have become seriously ill had it continued" (Beth Witrogen McLeod, *San Francisco Examiner*, 9 April 1995, A17).

2. In 1993 the percentages of working mothers with children between the ages of six and seventeen had increased for single mothers to 70.2 percent, for married mothers to 74.9 percent from 39 percent in 1960 and for divorced or widowed mothers to 78.3 percent from 65.9 percent in 1960. (The 1960 figures for single mothers is not available.) Increases for working mothers whose children were under six were: single mothers—47.4 percent in 1993 (1960 not available); married mothers—59.6 percent in 1993 from 18.6 percent in 1960; divorced or widowed mothers—60.0 percent in 1993 from 40.5 percent in 1960 (U.S. Bureau of the Census 1994:402).

3. Some feminists have argued that employment of domestic servants constitutes exploitation of women by other women, whereas others rejoin that this work provides paid employment. Paid domestic services can be a means of support for informal caregivers who can afford them. In other cases, paid domestic service constitutes the informal care. The percentage of women of color who work as domestic servants is disproportionate relative to their numbers in the population (53.3 percent are black or Latino) (U.S. Bureau of the Census 1994:407). Women of color and white women who do domestic work themselves often are without back-up for informal care needs in their own families (Collins 1990; Graham 1991; Nakano Glenn 1980; Palmer 1990; Rollins 1985).

4. Anticipated increases in numbers of home health aides (estimated to be between 128.7 percent and 140.6 percent between 1992 and 2005 (U.S. Bureau of the Census 1994:639) probably will not provide relief. Many women caregivers could not afford such paid services because of their low earnings, which remain considerably less than men's. In 1993 median weekly earnings for males and females were: white males, $531, white females, $403; black males, $392, black females, $349; Latino males, $352, and Latino females, $314 (U.S. Bureau of the Census 1994:429).

5. Quite aside from the transfer of the technology of care, medical technology creates other problems in informal caregiving. Utilization of medical technology to save or extend lives of endangered newborns can increase informal caregivers' burdens. Such infants are often multiply handicapped and require extensive care, which puts substantial stress on vulnerable families (Morse 1979). Use of such technology creates a different caregiving problem for disabled women. Among disabled women's groups,

divisions occur between those who object to technological preselection of "defective fetuses" and mothers of disabled children who argue that their lives are consumed by the care of these children. One feminist critic, herself the mother of a disabled child, has observed that the sometimes overwhelming difficulties of rearing such a child can impede the caregiver's own struggles for independence (Hillyer 1993).

6. A poll done in the San Francisco Bay area in April 1995 showed that 46 percent of all women surveyed had tried an alternative practitioner in the past year. (*San Francisco Chronicle*, 17 May 1995, A12).

7. This uninformed feminist view failed to recognize complexities in nursing and the fact that many women find highly satisfying careers in this work. It was particularly curious given the commitment of nurses to feminist causes: nursing leaders in the 1920s strongly supported the suffrage movement, and the American Nurses' Association early endorsed the Equal Rights Amendment.

8. In 1980-81, 6.6 percent of RN students were black and 2.6 percent were Latino. By 1989-90, 10.3 percent were black, 3.0 Latino, 2.6 Asian/Pacific Islander, and 0.5 American Indian (Hart-Brothers 1994:212). (Figures were not given for Asian/Pacific Islanders and American Indians in 1980.)

9.In 1994, 8.9 percent of baccalaureate students, 6.1 percent of master's students, and 5.3 percent of doctoral students were black—compared with Asian women who were 3.1 percent of master's students, 3.1 percent of doctoral students, and 3.6 percent of postdoctoral scholars or Latino women who were 2.5 percent of master's students, 1.6 percent of doctoral students, and 3.6 percent of postdoctoral scholars. Less than 1 percent of students in the master's and doctoral programs were Native Americans (American Association of Colleges of Nursing 1995:18).

10. However, the demand for skilled baccalaureate nurses, which has created a surge of registered nurses with diplomas or associate of arts degrees entering programs where they can become prepared at the baccalaureate level, may increase numbers of minority nurses at the baccalaureate level. Seventy-seven colleges have programs designed to bring LPNs to the associate or bachelor's degree level, and 542 have programs to take RNs through the baccalaureate degree. Enrollment in RN-baccalaureate programs has steadily increased: 20.7 percent in full-time students and 4.7 percent in part-time students in 1994 (American Association of Colleges of Nursing 1995:1, 6).

11. Though the numbers of full-time women medical school faculty doubled between 1980 (7,171, or 15.9 percent) and 1992 (15,475, or 22.2 percent), the percentage of women from underrepresented minority groups was still less than 10 percent of all women faculty (Bickel and Kopriva 1993:142).

In 1990 less than 6 percent of all full-time nursing faculty were black, less than 2 percent were Asian, and less than 1 percent were American Indian or Latino (National League for Nursing 1991:212).

12. Dr. Conley was later rehired. In spring 1995 Stanford University took disciplinary action against two medical school professors for sexual harassment (*San Francisco Chronicle*, 23 April 1995).

13. There are 190 nurse practitioner programs that offer master's level preparation in family, ob-gyn, or women's health practitice, and 110 programs that give post-master's

work in these areas (American Association of Colleges of Nursing 1995:40–41). In the mid-1980s when the editors of this book directed three national summer institutes on faculty development in women, health, and healing, the majority of enrollees were faculty from community colleges and collegiate nursing programs.

REFERENCES

Abel, Emily K.
    1990a   "Informal care of the disabled elderly: a critique of recent literature." Research on Aging 12:139–57.
    1990b   "Family care of the frail elderly." Pp. 65–91 in Emily K. Abel and Margaret K. Nelson (eds.), Circles of Care: Work and Identity in Women's Lives. Albany: State University of New York Press.
Abel, Emily K., and Margaret K. Nelson
    1990   "Circles of care: an introductory essay." Pp. 4–34 in Emily K. Abel and Margaret K. Nelson (eds.), Circles of Care: Work and Identity in Women's Lives. Albany: State University of New York Press.
Alford-Cooper, F.
    1993   "Women as family caregivers: an American social problem." Journal of Women and Aging 5:43–57.
American Association of Colleges of Nursing
    1995   1994–95 Enrollments and Graduations in Baccalaureate and Graduate Programs in Nursing. Washington: American Association of Colleges of Nursing.
Arnold, Robert M., Steven C. Martin, and Ruth M. Parker
    1988   "Taking care of patients: does it matter whether the physician is a woman?" Western Journal of Medicine 149:729–33.
Asch, Adrienne, and Michelle Fine
    1992   "Beyond pedestals: revisiting the lives of women with disabilities." Pp. 129–71 in Michelle Fine (ed.), Disruptive Voices: The Possibilities of Feminist Research. Ann Arbor: University of Michigan Press.
Assistant Secretary for Planning and Evaluation (ASPE) and Health Care Financing Administration (HCFA), Department of Health and Human Services
    1982   National Survey of Long-Term Care/National Survey of Caregivers. Washington: Government Printing Office.
Bair, Barbara, and Susan Cayleff, eds.
    1993   Wings of Gauze: Women of Color and the Experience of Health and Illness. Detroit: Wayne State University Press.
Barbee, Evelyn L.
    1993   "Racism in U.S. nursing." Medical Anthropology Quarterly (n.s.) 7:346–62.
Berk, Sara Fenstermaker
    1985   The Gender Factory: The Apportionment of Work in American Households. New York: Plenum.

Bickel, Janet, and Phyllis R. Kopriva
  1993   "A statistical perspective on gender in medicine." Journal of the American Medical Women's Association 48:141-44.
Boaz, R. F., and C. F. Muller
  1992   "Paid work and unpaid help by caregivers of the disabled and frail elders." Medical Care 39:149-58.
Bonuck, Karen A.
  1993   "AIDS and families: cultural, psychosocial, and functional impacts." Social Work in Health Care 18:75-89.
Bowman, Margery, and March Lynn Gross
  1986   "Overview of research on women in medicine: issues for public policymakers." Public Health Report 101:513-21.
Brody, E. M.
  1990   Women in the Middle: Their Parent-Care Years. New York: Springer.
Burnley, Cynthia S.
  1987   "Caregiving: the impact of emotional support for single women." Journal of Aging Studies 1:253-64.
Butter, Irene H., Eugenia S. Carpenter, Bonnie J. Kay, and Ruth Simmons
  1987   "Gender hierarchies in the health labor force." International Journal of Health Services 17:133-49.
Campbell, J. D.
  1975   "The child in the sick role: contributions of the age, sex, parental status, and parental values." Journal of Health and Social Behavior 8:83-95.
Carpenter, Eugenia
  1980   "Children's health care and the changing role of women." Medical Care 18:1208-18.
Centers for Disease Control and Prevention
  1993   HIV/AIDS Surveillance Report (July). National Center for Infectious Diseases. Atlanta: Public Health Service.
  1995   HIV/AIDS Surveillance Report (July). National Center for Infectious Diseases. Atlanta: Public Health Service.
Chang, Cyril F., and S. I. White-Means
  1991   "The men who care: an analysis of male primary caregivers who care for frail elderly at home." Journal of Applied Gerontology 10:343-58.
Cleland, Virginia
  1971   "Sex discrimination: nursing's most pervasive problem." American Journal of Nursing 71:1542-47.
Collins, Patricia Hill
  1990   Black Feminist Thought. Boston: Unwin Hyman.
Coward, Raymond T., and Jeffrey W. Dwyer
  1990   "The association of gender, sibling network composition, and patterns of parent care by adult children." Research on Aging 2:158-81.
Cunningham-Burley, Sarah, and Sandy Irvine
  1987   "'And have you done anything so far?' An examination of lay treatment of children's symptoms." British Medical Journal 19:700-702.

Current Population Survey
  1993   Marital and Family Characteristics of the Labor Force. Bureau of Labor
         Statistics, Department of Labor.
Davis, Sheila P., and Cora A. Ingram
  1993   "Empowered caretakers: a historical perspective on the roles of granny
         midwives in rural Alabama." Pp. 191-201 in Barbara Bair and Susan E.
         Cayleff (eds.), Wings of Gauze. Detroit: Wayne State University Press.
DeVault, Marjorie
  1991   Feeding the Family. Chicago: University of Chicago Press.
Dufort, Francine, and Brigitte Maheux
  1995   "When female medical students are the majority: do numbers really make
         a difference?" Journal of the American Medical Women's Association
         50:4-6.
England, Suzanne E., and Beatrice T. Naulleau
  1991   "Women, work, and elder care: the family and medical leave debate."
         Women and Politics 11:91-107.
Estes, Carroll L., Lenore Gerard, and Adele E. Clarke
  1984   "Women and the economics of aging." International Journal of Health
         Services 14:55-67.
Finch, Janet, and Dulcie Groves
  1982   "By women for women: caring for the frail elderly." Women's Studies
         International Forum 5:10-15.
Fisher, Berenice, and Joan Tronto
  1990   "Towards a feminist theory of caring." Pp. 35-62 in Emily K. Abel and
         Margaret K. Nelson (eds.), Circles of Care: Work and Identity in
         Women's Lives. Albany: State University of New York Press.
Fontenot, Wonda Lee
  1993   "Madame Neau: the practice of ethnopsychiatry in rural Louisiana." Pp.
         41-53 in Barbara Bair and Susan E. Cayleff (eds.), Wings of Gauze.
         Detroit: Wayne State University Press.
Foulke, S. R., F. Alford-Cooper, and S. Butler
  1993   "Intergenerational issues in long-term planning." Marriage and Family
         Review 3/4:73-95.
Fox, Margery
  1989   "The socioreligious role of the Christian Science practitioner." Pp. 98-
         114 in Carol Shepherd McClain (ed.), Women as Healers. New Bruns-
         wick, NJ: Rutgers University Press.
Furstenberg, Anne, and Linda J. Davis
  1984   "Lay consultation of older people." Social Science and Medicine
         18:827-37.
Gamble, Vanessa Northington
  1990   "On becoming a physician: a dream not deferred." Pp. 52-64 in Evelyn
         C. White (ed.), The Black Women's Health Book: Speaking for Our-
         selves. Seattle: Seal Press.

Gerhardt, Uta, and Marianne Brieskorn-Zinke
  1986   "The normalization of hemodialysis at home." Vol. 4, pp. 271-317 in
          Julius A. Roth and Sheryl Burt Ruzek (eds.), Research in the Sociology
          of Health Care. Greenwich, CT: JAI Press.
Glazer, Nona Y.
  1990   "The home as workshop: women as amateur nurses and medical care
          providers." Gender and Society 4:479-99.
  1991   "'Between a rock and a hard place': women's professional organizations
          in nursing and class, race and ethnic inequalities." Gender and Society
          5:351-72.
Goodman, Catherine C.
  1990   "The caregiving roles of Asian American women." Journal of Women
          and Aging 2:109-20.
Graham, Hilary
  1985   "Providers, negotiators, and mediators: women as the hidden carers." Pp.
          20-30 in Ellen Lewin and Virginia Olesen (eds.), Women, Health, and
          Healing: Toward a New Perspective. London: Tavistock Methuen.
  1991   "The concept of caring in feminist research: the case of domestic service."
          Sociology 25:61-78.
  1993   "Social divisions in caring." Women's Studies International Forum
          16:461-70.
Guarnaccia, P. J., P. Parra, A. Deschamps, G. Milstein, and N. Argiles
  1992   "Si dios quiere? Hispanic families' experiences of caring for a seriously men-
          tally ill family member." Culture, Medicine, and Psychiatry 16:187-215.
Harrison, Michelle
  1992   "Women's health as a specialty: a deceptive solution." Journal of
          Women's Health 1:101-6.
  1994   "Women's health: new models of care and a new academic discipline."
          Pp. 79-90 in Alice J. Dan (ed.), Reframing Women's Health: Multidis-
          ciplinary Research and Practice. Newbury Park, CA: Sage.
Hart-Brothers, Elaine
  1994   "Contributions of women of color to the health care of America." Pp.
          205-22 in Emily Friedman (ed.), An Unfinished Revolution: Women
          and Health Care in America. New York: United Hospital Fund.
Hatch, Laurie Russel
  1991   "Informal support patterns of older African American and white women:
          examining effects of family, paid work, and religious participation." Re-
          search on Aging 13:144-70.
Hillyer, Barbara
  1993   Feminism and Disability. Norman: University of Oklahoma Press.
Hine, Darlene Clark
  1985   Black Women in the Nursing Profession. New York: Garland.
  1989   Black Women in White: Racial Conflict and Cooperation in the Nursing
          Profession, 1850-1950. Bloomington: Indiana University Press.

Hochschild, Arlie R.
  1987   The Second Shift: Working Parents and the Revolution at Home. New York: Avon Books.
Hoffman, Eileen, and Karen Johnson
  1995   "Women's health and managed care: implications for training of primary care physicians." Journal of the American Medical Women's Association 50:17–19.
Holmes, Linda Janet
  1990   "Thank you Jesus to myself: the life of a traditional black midwife." Pp. 98–106 in Evelyn C. White (ed.), The Black Women's Health Book. Seattle: Seal Press.
Horowitz, Amy
  1985   "Sons and daughters as caregivers to older parents: differences in role performance and consequences." Gerontologist 25:612–17.
Horwitz, Allen V., and Susan C. Reinhard
  1995   "Ethnic differences in caregiving duties and burdens among parents and siblings of persons with severe mental illness." Journal of Health and Social Behavior 36:138–50.
Jackson, Eileen M.
  1993   "Whiting out the difference: why U.S. nursing research fails black families." Medical Anthropology Quarterly (n.s.) 7:363–85.
Johnson, Karen
  1992   "Women's health: developing a new interdisciplinary specialty." Journal of Women's Health 1:95–99.
Johnson, Karen, and Eileen Hoffman
  1994   "Women's health and curriculum transformation: the role of medical specialties." Pp. 27–39 in Alice J. Dan (ed.), Reframing Women's Health: Multidisciplinary Research and Practice. Newbury Park, CA: Sage.
Kaye, L. W., and Jeffrey S. Applegate
  1990   "Men as elder caregivers: building a research agenda for the 1990s." Journal of Aging Studies 4:289–90.
Kaye, L. W., and S. I. Reisman
  1991   "Life prolongation technologies in home care for the frail elderly: issues for training, policy, and research." Journal of Gerontological Social Work 16:79–91.
Killion, Cheryl M.
  1990   "Service without subservience: reflections of a registered nurse." Pp. 240–50 in Evelyn C. White (ed.), The Black Women's Health Book. Seattle: Seal Press.
Landis, Suzanne E., and Jo Anne Earp
  1987   "Sick child care options: what do working mothers prefer?" Women and Health 12:61–77.

Larrabee, Mary Jeanne
    1993   An Ethic of Care: Feminist and Interdisciplinary Perspectives. London: Routledge.

Lechner, Viola M.
    1993   "Racial group responses to work and parent care." Families in Society 74:93–103.

Lee, F.
    1994   "AIDS toll on elderly: dying grandchildren." New York Times, 21 November, A1, A11.

Lenhart, Sharyn
    1993   "Gender discrimination: a health and career development problem for women physicians." Journal of the American Medical Women's Association 48:155–59.

Lewin, Ellen
    1977   "Feminist ideology and the meaning of work: the case of nursing." Catalyst 10/11:78–103.

Lewin, Ellen, and Virginia Olesen
    1980   "Lateralness in women's work: new views on success." Sex Roles 6:619–29.

Lorber, Judith
    1975   "Women and medical sociology: invisible professionals and ubiquitous patients." Pp. 35–50 in Marsha Millman and Rosabeth Moss Kantor (eds.), Another Voice. New York: Anchor.
    1984   Women Physicians. London: Tavistock.
    1985   "More women physicians: will it mean more humane health care?" Social Policy 14:50–54.

Lurie, Nicole, J. Slater, M. McGovern, J. Ekstrum, L. Quan, and K. Margolis
    1993   "Preventive care for women: Does sex of the physician matter?" New England Journal of Medicine 329:478–82.

Manley, Joan E.
    1995   "Sex-segregated work in the system of professions: the development and stratification of nursing." Sociological Quarterly 36:297–314.

McGuire, Meredith
    1988   Ritual Healing in Suburbia. New Brunswick, NJ: Rutgers University Press.

Mechanic, David
    1964   "The influence of mothers on their children's health attitudes." Pediatrics 33:444–53.

Melosh, Barbara
    1982   The Physician's Hand. Philadelphia: Temple University Press.

Miller, Baila
    1990   "Gender differences in spouse management of the caregiver role." Pp. 92–104 in Emily K. Abel and Margaret K. Nelson (eds.), Circles of Care: Work and Identity in Women's Lives. Albany: State University of New York Press.

Montgomery, Rhonda J. V., and Mary McGlinn Datwyler
 1990 "Women and men in the caregiving role." Generations 14:34–38.
Morse, Joan
 1979 "A program for family management of the multiply handicapped child: TEMPO as a clinical model." Rehabilitation Literature 40:134–35.
Mui, A. C.
 1992 "Caregiver strain among black and white daughter caregivers." Gerontologist 32:203–12.
Muller, Charlotte
 1994 "Women in allied health professions." Pp. 177–203 in Emily Friedman (ed.), An Unfinished Revolution: Women and Health Care in America. New York: United Hospital Fund of New York.
Nakano Glenn, Evelyn
 1980 "The dialectics of wage work: Japanese American women and domestic service, 1905–1940." Pp. 345–72 in Ellen Carol Dubois and Vickie L. Ruiz (eds.), Unequal Sisters: A Multicultural Reader in U.S. Women's History. New York: Routledge.
National League for Nursing
 1991 Nursing Data Review 1991. New York: National League for Nursing Division of Research.
Palmer, Phyllis
 1990 Domesticity and Dirt: Housewives and Domestic Servants in the United States, 1920–1945. Philadelphia: Temple University Press.
Paringer, Lynn
 1983 "The forgotten costs of informal long-term care." Washington: Urban Institute.
Prout, Alan
 1988 "'Off school sick': mothers' accounts of school sickness absence." Sociological Review 36:765–89.
Rankin, Sally
 1988 "Gender, age, and caregiving: mediators of cardiovascular illness and recovery." Ph.D. diss. dissertation, Department of Family Health Care Nursing, University of California School of Nursing, San Francisco.
Reverby, Susan
 1987 Ordered to Care: The Dilemma of American Nursing, 1885–1945. Cambridge: Cambridge University Press.
Rollins, Judith
 1985 Between Women: Domestics and Their Employers. Philadelphia: Temple University Press.
Ruddick, Sara
 1983 "Maternal thinking." Pp. 213–20 in Joyce Trebilcot (ed.), Mothering: Essays in Feminist Theory. Totoway, NJ: Rowan and Allanheld.
Scheper-Hughes, Nancy
 1992 Death without Weeping: The Violence of Everyday Life in Brazil. Berkeley: University of California Press.

Schiller, Nina Glick
    1993   "The invisible women: caregiving and the construction of AIDS health services." Culture, Medicine, and Psychiatry 17:487–512.

Selker, Leopold G.
    1993   "Psychosocial support needs of older women care-givers and older women living alone: implications for allied health professionals." Loss, Grief, and Care 7:21–30.

Silver, Henry K., and Anita Duhl Glicken
    1990   "Medical student abuse, incidence, severity, and significance." Journal of the American Medical Association 263:527–32.

Singer, Merrill, and Roberto Garcia
    1989   "Becoming a Puerto Rican esperitista: Life history of a female healer." Pp. 157–85 in Carol Shepherd McClain (ed.), Women as Healers. New Brunswick, NJ: Rutgers University Press.

Smerglia, Virginia L., Gary T. Deimling, and Charles M. Barresi
    1988   "Black-white family comparisons in helping and decision-making networks of impaired elderly." Family Relations 37:305–9.

Snow, Loudell
    1974   "Folk medical beliefs and their implications for care of patients." Annals of Internal Medicine 81:82–96.

Spector, Rachel E.
    1991   "The use of parteras in the Rio Grande Valley, Texas." Pp. 277–302 in Rachel Spector (ed.), Cultural Diversity in Health and Illness. East Norwalk, CT: Appleton and Lange.

Stacey, Margaret
    1988   "Regulating the Professions in the UK: Nurses, Doctors, and Others." 1988 Lucile P. Leone Distinguished Lecture, Department of Social and Behavioral Sciences, School of Nursing, University of California, San Francisco.

Stevens, Patricia E.
    1992   "Lesbian health care research: a review of the literature from 1970 to 1990." Health Care for Women International 13:91–120.

Stoller, Eleanor
    1983   "Parental caregiving by adult children." Journal of Marriage and the Family 45:851–58.

Strauss, Anselm L., Shizuko Fagerhaugh, Barbara Suczek, and Carolyn Wiener
    1991   "AIDS and health care deficiencies." Society 28:63–73.

Tronto, Joan C.
    1993   Moral Boundaries: A Political Argument for an Ethic of Care. London: Routledge.

Turner, Heather A., and Leonard I. Pearlin
    1989   "Issues of age, stress, and caregiving." Generations 13:56–59.

Ungerson, Clare
    1983   "Women and caring: skills, tasks, and taboos." Pp. 62–77 in Eva Garmarnikov et al. (eds.), The Public and the Private. London: Heinemann.

U.S. Bureau of the Census

1984   County Business Patterns. Washington: Department of Commerce.

1994   Statistical Abstract of the United States. Washington: Department of Commerce.

Walker, A. J., S. S. Martin, and L. L. Jones

1992   "The benefits and costs of caregiving and care receiving for daughters and mothers." Journal of Gerontology 43:S130–39.

Wallis, Lila

1992   "Women's health: a specialty? Pros and cons." Journal of Women's Health 1:107–8.

1994   "Why a curriculum on women's health?" Pp. 13–26 in Alice J. Dan (ed.), Reframing Women's Health: Multidisciplinary Research and Practice. Newbury Park, CA: Sage.

Ward, Martha C.

1993   "A different disease: HIV/AIDS and health care for women in poverty." Culture, Medicine, and Psychiatry 17:413–30.

[17]

Older Women:
Income, Retirement, and Health

VIDA YVONNE JONES AND CARROLL L. ESTES

Vida Jones and Carroll Estes use their sociological approach to studying aging and health policy to identify
critical issues and trends in aging women's health situations. Social policies affecting older women's health need
careful scrutiny and redesign to reduce gender discrimination, especially for women of color who remain disproportionately disadvantaged in terms of economic
resources in old age.

It is always simpler to categorize and make general assumptions—identifying
groups of people with certain views, images, and characteristics—than it
is to address existing and complex heterogeneity. Women, racial and ethnic groups, and the elderly are often categorized. The real world is not
that simple, however, and people do not fit neatly into homogeneous
groups.

The United States is aging. In 1940, 9 million Americans (6.8%)
were over 65. By 1980 the number had risen to 25.7 million (11.3%), and
Rice (1989) projects that by the year 2030, 64.6 million Americans (20%)
will be 65. Older African Americans' chances of surviving past 65 are
much lower than those of Caucasians. Native Americans and Alaskan
Natives in reservation states are also less likely than white Americans to
survive to age 65 (U.S. DHHS 1991). Women generally outlive men. In
1992, life expectancy was 73.2 years for white men, 79.8 for white women,
65.0 for black men, and 73.9 for black women (National Center for
Health Statistics [NCHS] 1996). As a result, we have more elderly women
than elderly men.

The elderly population exhibits a stunning diversity: people who are
over 65 (the young old), those over 85 (the old-old), those who are
healthy and active, those who live with chronic illness and disability,
those who are frail and institutionalized, those who live independently in
their own homes or within residential and other care settings, those who

still work, those who are retired, those who are dissatisfied and resist retirement, those who welcome retirement, those who are economically secure, and those who live in poverty.

This chapter focuses on older women, particularly on their retirement income and how it affects their health. Caregiving in traditional and extended family structures will be addressed, and we will analyze the ideological framework upon which are based current public policies that affect older women.

Income or Retirement Benefits and Health

The strength of social class as a predictor of health and longevity has been underscored in the United States and in virtually all other western industrialized nations. As Butler and Lewis (1982:11) have observed, "Demographic data show conclusively that an increasing life expectancy follows in the wake of increasing income and status." The Black Report (Black et al. 1982) is the classic text on the persistence of class differences in health as well as the difficulties in eradicating these deep inequalities in health, even with the provision of universal health coverage such as the British National Health Service.

Certainly, income is one of the most important dimensions of social class in predicting health status. Poor older people are twice as likely as older people with moderate or high incomes to report health problems (44% versus 22%; NCHS 1987b). Similarly, data from the 1995 health interview survey show an inverse relationship between family income (age adjusted) and limitations in activity due to chronic conditions (NCHS 1995).

Income is a factor in work disability. Approximately half (45.2%) of women with work limitations are poor, and of people who have work disability, 42.5 percent receive Social Security retirement disability benefits (LaPlante, Miller, and Miller 1992). Rose Gibson (1989) calls midlife African Americans who receive disability payments in government programs the "unretired-retired," workers who leave the workforce for reasons of physical disability rather than for traditional retirement. Given the shorter life expectancy of African Americans, particularly men, Gibson raises the question of whether age-based policies in general are inappropriate for them. She contends that retirement should be added to the list of critical life events that occur earlier for many blacks. These events include the birth of the first child, onset of disability, loss of a

TABLE 17.1

Median Income of People Ages 65+ by Age, Race, Hispanic Origin, and Sex, 1989

Race and Hispanic Origin	Both Sexes			Men			Women		
	65+	65–69	70+	65+	65–69	70+	65+	65–69	70+
All races	9,420	10,722	8,936	13,024	15,273	12,022	7,508	7,584	7,476
White	9,838	11,323	9,305	13,391	15,680	12,410	7,816	7,977	7,756
Black	5,772	6,552	5,517	8,192	10,464	7,224	5,059	5,235	5,032
Hispanic[a]	5,978	6,664	5,715	8,469	10,240	6,816	4,992	4,640	5,112

Source: "Aging America: Trends and Projections, 1991," U.S. Senate Special Committee on Aging. As taken from U.S. Bureau of Census, unpublished data from the March 1990 *Current Population Survey.*

[a]Hispanic people may be of any race.

spouse, and death. This differential timing of major life events suggests an earlier social aging, and it is critical to the extent that benefits are provided too late in life spans that are truncated by death rates in midlife and affected by the earlier onset of disability.

Not only is low income a risk factor in health but reductions in income are associated with increased risk of mortality (Kaplan and Haan 1989). The effect of income is also observed on lifestyle behaviors related to health. Amir (1987) reports data showing a positive relationship between income and preventive health behaviors among older persons in Scotland, a finding consistent with studies on the North American continent (Norman 1985).

Although the proportion of the older population living below the poverty line has declined (to 12.4% in 1986), nearly one-third (28.0%) of the elderly are poor or "near-poor"—that is, living within 150 percent of the poverty line. The oldest old (those 85 or older) experience the highest poverty rates (17.6%) of all older groups, almost twice the 10.3 percent rate of those 65 to 74 (U.S. Bureau of Census n.d.; U.S. Senate 1988:44-45). Poverty among elderly African Americans and Hispanics and among a substantial proportion of older women is pervasive and unrelenting (table 17.1). Members of minority groups experience two to three times the poverty rate of whites, with 71 percent of all aged blacks being poor or "economically vulnerable"—that is, within 200 percent of

Figure 17.1 Percentage of Elderly Living below the Poverty Level by Selected Characteristics, 1989

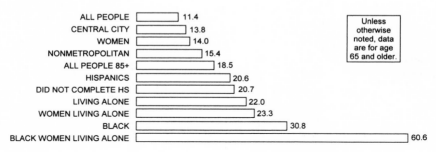

Source: U.S. Senate Committee on Aging, "Aging America: Trends and Projections, 1991." As taken from U.S. Bureau of the Census, "Money Income and Poverty Status in the United States: 1989," Current Population Reports Series P-60, No. 168 (September 1990) and unpublished data from the March 1990 *Current Population Survey.*

the official poverty line (Villers Foundation 1987:25). Almost half of old white single women and 80 percent of old black single women live at or near the poverty level (Villers Foundation 1987). Figure 17.1 illustrates the dramatic numbers of elderly women, particularly black women, who are living below the poverty level. With these statistics, the connection between health and longevity is not surprising.

Racial differences are found in various chronic conditions and activity limitations (NCHS 1996). Older blacks have poorer health status than whites, according to both indicators. Furthermore, women, persons with lower incomes, and members of minority groups have the highest rates of activity limitations due to chronic illness (NCHS 1987a). In a study of the relationship of social support networks and support network function to the health status of older widowed black females, Charlotte Perry (1991:96) found that "older widows' health status is largely a function of personal characteristics, network structure, network function, and network adequacy. Of these variables, income was most important to instrumental activities of daily living. This finding suggested that older black widows who had higher incomes had maintained adequate health care over the years, and perhaps this resulted in good health."

Additionally, women who provide care and who often outlive their potential caregiving family members have a higher prevalence of disability and higher rates of institutionalization at most ages than men (Soldo and Manton 1985). Overall, women, older people, black people, and people of low income have relatively high rates of functional limitations. Low-income households are more likely to have persons with functional limitations and severe limitations. According to Mitchell LaPlante and colleagues (1992:2), "Four out of ten people in the lowest income groups were functionally limited, against only one out of ten in the highest income group." It is important to understand why many older women have lower incomes and are thereby at risk for poorer health.

Women's Paid Work and Low-Benefit Work across the Life Span

As Beeson (1975) noted, women and women's experiences have been ignored or underemphasized in the study of aging. The same can be said for people of color. A historical examination of the work experiences of the current cohort of older women in general and of older women of color is necessary to illustrate the connection between lifetime work patterns and current retirement income and health.

Two world events influenced the workforce experiences of women: the Great Depression and World War II. Public policy in the 1930s and 1940s also reflected this shift in values in response to economic conditions. The development of Social Security, retirement, and work programs in the 1930s signaled a change in attitude away from the primacy of reliance on individualism and the family and set a precedent for the state's role in helping individuals. Public policy, nevertheless, incorporated traditional gender-based assumptions that (1) women are economically dependent on their husbands and (2) women's participation in the workforce should be regarded as supplemental and intermittent (Zones, Estes, and Binney 1987). During the Depression, women were often forced into the paid labor market for the first time to help deprived households make ends meet (Elder 1974:82). Nearly half of the women in hard-pressed families were working outside the home at some point in the 1930s, with many continuing to hold jobs during the war when male labor was reduced and production demands were high (Elder 1982).

After the war, women returned (sometimes involuntarily) to their traditional roles, the primacy of the nuclear family. This strongly affected their Social Security benefits in that women who entered the workforce during the Depression or war and then left it for more than the allowed "five years out" have additional "nonworking" years averaged into their earning base upon which Social Security benefits are calculated. As a result of their episodic work histories and lower pay, these women now receive Social Security benefits that are considerably lower than men's. In many cases it is more advantageous for married women—working or not—to receive half of their spouse's benefits than to receive their own (Zones, Estes, and Binney 1987).

Overall, the income of working women relative to men is virtually unchanged over the past 50 years (Hewlett 1986; Grune 1981), at less than 70 cents for every dollar a man earns (U.S. Bureau of Census 1991). For some women, the steep rise in divorce rates and the no-fault divorce (Fuchs 1986; Weitzman 1985) have had devastating effects on women's income, assets, opportunities for social mobility, and even maintenance of social class position. Some have predicted that future generations of women will perhaps arrive at old age even poorer than in the past because of the dramatic growth in female-headed households, impoverishment earlier in the life course, and the growing number under 65 who have no health insurance (Estes and Arendell 1986).

As noted earlier, events of the 1930s and 1940s pulled women into the paid, skilled workforce. Significantly, however, this was not true for black women who had experienced a lifetime of low-paying jobs without Social Security and other retirement benefits. Reviewing black women's work experiences between World Wars I and II, Algea Harrison (1989) found that black women did not match the occupational gains of white women. The new technological and skilled jobs were occupied by white women. Most black women continued to work as domestic servants, and their labor market role remained basically the same. When men entered the armed services, white women filled the void and black women could not enter the defense industries because of racial discrimination and their ensured cheap labor as domestic servants.

Paula Giddings (1984) described how the chief opposition to the employment of black women came from local housewives who feared losing their low-benefit laborers (maids, cooks, etc.) and from women employed in factories who did not want to work with blacks. When black women did enter the defense industries, they generally were assigned, like black men, to custodial positions. Their type of work simply moved from private residences to the business sector.

Although many older women of color find divorce a disruptive life event, other economic issues that prevail in their earlier years, such as low-benefit wages that do not provide Social Security benefits and that lack adequate retirement benefits and plans, are extremely significant to their income in old age, as it is to men of color. Black women and men, for example, who are generally lifetime workers, have similar discontinuous work patterns (Gibson 1988).

Many older Mexican Americans have also had a lifetime of employment discrimination and low-benefit labor, with intermittent periods of unemployment, which has influenced retirement income (Markides and Mindel 1987). For older Mexican American women, cultural issues related to familism have also helped shape their participation in the workforce. Elisa Facio (1987) shows how gender has historically placed Chicana older women in low-benefit labor, affecting their retirement benefits. The cultural patriarchal concepts, combined with the effects of class and race, continually limit Chicana women. However, the low-benefit employment and disadvantaged economic status of Mexican American or Chicano men greatly influence their lives as well.

The same is true of Native Americans, who as a group were displaced from their land as their economies were destroyed. Historically, Native American women were strong influences within their diverse communities. This was, however, affected by colonization and the imposition of traditional American sex role differentiation that was developed and encouraged on the reservation (Wittstock 1980). Older women have suffered disadvantaged health and economic status as a result of being removed from their land and their traditional work and forced to settle on reservations or relocated to urban areas where they are also marginalized (Markides and Mindel 1987).

Women's Unpaid Work: Income and Health Consequences of Caregiving

A caregiver is someone who provides unpaid assistance to another person on a regular basis, including the care of the elderly, adult children who are disabled or ill, grandchildren, great-grandchildren, and other extended family members. Caregiving is generally considered woman's work, as reflected in the fact that 75 percent of the caregivers of persons 50 and older are women (AARP 1988). These caregiving activities of women directly and negatively affect their retirement income and health.

Caregiving, Income, and Retirement

The economic costs of caregiving are both direct and indirect. This and other structural conditions contribute to women's lower socioeconomic status. For the women who care for their disabled spouses, there is a drain on savings and assets acquired during the marriage, particularly for those who must "spend down" in order to receive necessary medical care and, eventually, public assistance. For the caregiver of an elderly parent, spouse, or physically or emotionally compromised child or grandchild, there are often additional financial costs of supplementing that person's already inadequate resources (Arendell and Estes 1987).

Because family care is not valued by the government in terms of dollars, the services provided simply go unvalued. In other words, family labor—more precisely, women's unpaid labor—is viewed as free labor if recognized as labor at all. Yet, according to Feldblum (1985:220), "over 40 percent of adult offspring participating in one survey reported that the time spent on caregiving tasks was equivalent to the time required by a full-time job." There are also the economic costs of caregiving for the women who forego employment in order to provide care, who end their paid work, or who reduce their employment in order to better accommodate their caregiving demands. There is not only the loss of immediate wages but also long-term loss of wage-related benefits. For example, women who reduce their paid labor activities are likely to jeopardize or lose disability and health insurance while also losing Social Security credits. Women caregivers are often called upon to quit work altogether before reaching age 65 or 67, incurring significant penalties in their Social Security benefits (a decline of 20% to 30%). Women who spend time out of the workforce raising children, those who are unmarried, those who work at low-benefit jobs, those who retire early to caregive, and those who are not eligible for a dependent's benefit are particularly disadvantaged. Women, on average, spend 11.5 years out of the workforce compared with 1.3 years for men (Older Women's League 1992). As caregivers, women find themselves in a no-win situation: they are expected to provide care to their husbands and other relatives, yet public policy penalizes them economically for doing do. Because the majority of older women's economic situations are precarious at best, the added costs of caregiving are significant (Arendell and Estes 1987).

Health Consequences of Caregiving

Caregiving carries high physical health risks (Bader 1985; Brody 1985). Physical labor, sometimes excessive, is part of caregiving, and disabled persons need various kinds of assistance. Because more than 60 percent of caregivers themselves are old or approaching old age (Stone, Cafferata, and Sangl 1987), they too are vulnerable to the chronic ailments experienced by care recipients. If the care recipients are children, there are additional stresses and demands that are damaging to the caregiver's physical and psychological health. Older women have greater chronic health problems to manage than do older men (Rice and Estes 1984; Verbrugge 1983, 1984), yet it is women who do most of the caregiving work. Additionally, there are somatic outcomes of high levels of stress: high blood pressure, fatigue, and greater susceptibility to physical illness (Verbrugge 1985). Lack of respite and relief from responsibilities, lack of assistance in performing physical tasks, and emotional fatigue and overload thwart a caregiver's recovery from illness (Corbin and Strauss 1985). Caregivers' physical health may also be endangered by a lack of preventive health care, resulting from inadequate financial resources, time, or attention to the onset of disabilities (Brody 1985; Bader 1985). Caregivers may postpone attending to their own medical needs because of the demands placed on them by a care recipient, and many do not have adequate funds to obtain timely health care (Arendell and Estes 1987).

Older Women Providing Primary Care for Grandchildren

Drug addiction affects a broad spectrum of the population, cutting across class, race, and gender boundaries. Communities with the fewest resources and highest rates of poverty are those most devastatingly affected. The black community has been hit hard. In the tradition of responding to social and economic crises in creative and often self-sacrificing ways, older black women and men are developing strategies to ensure that children are protected in the homes of relatives. They do this by becoming primary caregivers for grandchildren and even great-grandchildren who are inadequately cared for because of the illness or death of a parent addicted to drugs, most commonly crack cocaine.

It is important to emphasize that this is not the grandparenting role for a majority of black grandparents. Such generalizations are too often made regarding women, people of color, and older people. This is one important and diverse segment of the black as well as Hispanic and white grandparent community. However, this discussion focuses on black older women because of the very limited information that does exist for this particular population (Poe 1992; Burton 1991; California State Assembly 1989). This form of caregiving is different from grandparents rearing grandchildren during economic crises when adult children are off seeking employment opportunities or when they assist single parents with child care following divorce or other changes in family structure. These children have particular physical and psychological health needs that add an unusual burden to a traditional form of extended family support.

The experience of black grandparents rearing grandchildren is not new. This is simply a contemporary variation of extended family traditions in place since slavery. Historically, the extended family functioned as a means of pooling limited resources during periods of devastating economic hardship (Staples 1986). Black grandparents were an important part of this structure. E. Franklin Frazier's (1939) study of the black family described grandmothers as "the guardians of the generations" whose role was considered vital to the survival of the black family. Older women cared for the children when the parents were forced to leave for economic or other reasons associated with slavery and racism, not out of a matriarchal desire to control the family but out of necessity (Burton 1991). Other studies have shown that black grandparents still serve as an anchor for their grandchildren, taking on the functions and responsibilities of personal welfare agencies for children when parents do not provide this care (Jackson 1986).

Economic and Health Consequences

This caregiving by grandparents of children exposed to crack cocaine is not likely to be done without devastating risks to their economic viability and health. The economic costs of caring for grandchildren with special health problems are astounding for older and midlife grandmothers. In a study of black grandparents, Lenora Poe (1992) found that the financial demands of caregiving were the primary burden, with many in her sample already on medical disability or retired when they assumed their unpaid work of rearing grandchildren. They often had to return to work to supplement their income, or they had to quit their jobs when grandchildren required sensitive, closely supervised attention.

Nonexistent or inadequate state and federal policies related to foster care exacerbate the financial burden incurred by these caregivers. Selected foster parents who are not relatives and elect to care for children affected by the drug crisis are eligible for monthly stipends commensurate with the psychological and physical health needs of the child. No such benefits exist for grandparents because they are relatives and because they "choose" to intervene when they observe abuse or neglect of the children. Current federal policy will consider basic foster care stipends for relatives if the abuse and neglect of the children require them to become adjudicated dependents of the court or if they are taken from the parent by court order. Grandparents fear that by the time the bureaucracy notices a neglected child, it may be too late, and they do not wait to bring the children into their home. State policy provides foster care dollars for children who are placed with nonrelatives. The frustration experienced by grandparents is illustrated in this statement by an older woman taking care of her grandchildren:

> When I first took over these children in March 1988, I was a very angry, still angry, very resentful, and very frightened grandparent, mainly because I had thought that I had reached the stage of my life where I would not have to reassume this type of responsibility. I had recently retired, and I thought that these were going to be my golden years, and all the good things that come along with retirement were going to come along for me. However, I found that not to be the case. The thought of parenting two children over again was just overwhelming. I really didn't know how I could or how I would be able to handle it at this point of my life. I knew that I was the only person that would be able to pick up these two children and help them grow and develop in a better environment than what they had been in for the past six or seven months. (California State Assembly 1989:10)

The age and health of grandparents can range from age 40, with the grandparent in good health and employed, to a frail older person 70 and over, managing multiple and serious chronic conditions such as diabetes and hypertension on limited incomes. Without the support given to non-relatives, older women are forced to take their own meager retirement resources to meet the needs of their grandchildren or, if at all physically possible, return to work. Black women have often worked regardless of their health status and forced themselves to work when it has been demanded by the situation, which may explain some of the dismal morbidity and mortality data (Edmonds 1990).

It is clear that if they are to continue rendering this difficult yet extremely important unpaid labor they need support from policymakers and social service agencies (Burton 1991). This demands an intergenerational approach that considers the issues important to children, adults living with addictions, and the older women engaged in caregiving.

Public Policy and Older Women

An Antifemale Ideological Framework

The issues of old age in America are directly related to the situation of older women in contemporary health policy. Both are understandable in the context of ideological shifts occurring during the 1980s. As we have argued elsewhere (Estes 1991), the focus of U.S. discourse on social policy in the 1980s successfully shifted from activism and improvement to crisis and budget cutting (Edsall 1988). This was accomplished with the support of an ideological revolution that reinstated the primacy of the economy as the driving rationale for state action and sought to impose a romanticized notion of individualism and the family as the justification for shifting responsibility from the state to the private sector. As the primary providers of care to the family throughout their life span, women are primarily affected by this romanticized notion of forcing the family to endure the burden of responsibility.

Medicare and Medicaid

For most older women, Medicare and Medicaid are the predominant sources of public health insurance and health care services, although many also purchase supplemental private insurance to cover costs that Medicare does not. Private health insurance is costly for older women. Women in midlife (41–50) pay 28 percent more for private health insurance than men of the same age (Older Women's League 1992). Women ages 65 and over spend approximately 28 percent of their $8,044 median annual income on health care alone, and almost 24 percent of older women and 20 percent of older men spend a fifth or more of their after-tax income on acute health care (Older Women's League 1992).

Medicare is the program of public insurance for acute care that pays primarily for doctor and hospital bills. Medicaid is the federal state program for the poor (aged and nonaged), blind, and disabled. The 1980s also brought a tightening of Medicaid eligibility and cuts. Approximately twice as many midlife and older women have health insurance under Medicaid, with minority women even more heavily dependent on this form of insurance.

The percentage of the poor covered by Medicaid declined from 63 percent to 46 percent between 1975 and 1985 (Darling 1986). Although Medicaid was designed to provide health protection for the poor and to reduce out-of-pocket medical costs, only one-third of the disadvantaged elderly and only one-tenth of the near-poor (those with incomes ranging from $6,000 to $12,000 per year) have Medicaid coverage (U.S. Senate 1991). Since 1981, federal budget tightening aimed at Medicaid has pressed states to curtail eligibility and utilization while also producing greater variability among the states in Medicaid access and services. The burden on the poor has increased (Holahan and Cohan 1986).

As the only health program that finances long-term care, Medicaid is particularly important to the aged in its coverage of nursing-home care, but only for those who "spend down" to (or below) the poverty level, using up all their personal monies. Only 36 percent of the old poor are on Medicaid (Villers Foundation 1987). Most are older women in nursing homes. Medicaid is described as a policy that promotes both impoverishment and dependency for the aged. Medicare's acute-care emphasis is clearly mismatched with the needs of the older population in a society characterized by increasing life expectancy and growing "population frailty" (Verbrugge 1989).

Of serious consequence to the millions of female caregivers of elders, the hospital cost containment strategy produced immediate reductions in the average length of hospital stay for Medicare patients, shifting more than 21 million days of care from the formal hospital care system to the informal care of home and family, care traditionally provided by women in the first year of the Prospective Payment System (PPS) (Stark 1987). Simultaneously, Medicare restricted its already limited home health benefits. These changes occurred in the context of other austerity policies that had reduced the already meager social service funding, produced higher out-of-pocket costs, and increased women's caregiving responsibilities.

Dominant Effects of Policies on Health Care for Older Women

Most important for older women are the effects of public policies in health and social care during the 1980s and 1990s, particularly (1) the growth of for-profit medical care and medicalization of care for the aging in ways that stimulate the expansion and cost of the medical-industrial complex (Estes and Binney 1988); (2) the continuing refusal of the state to provide meaningful long-term care benefits to the elderly and disabled, forcing women to continue to provide a substantial amount of unpaid informal care; (3) the declining ability of a beleaguered network of traditionally nonprofit home and community-based health and social service providers to provide social supportive services to those who cannot pay for them privately (Estes, Wood et al. 1986); and (4) the use of policy to increase family responsibility and dependence on the work of women through the increased informalization of care as very sick and very old patients are discharged earlier than ever before to save hospital costs.

These and other efforts to restore and regulate family life are congruent with the deep concerns of the state and corporate sector to minimize their respective costs for the elderly and the intentions of the New Right to restore patriarchal family arrangements to ensure a continuing supply of free female labor essential to the reproduction and maintenance of the workforce (Abramovitz 1988:349–79).

Social Struggles

Older women are caught in the middle between (1) the dual interests of the state and corporate sectors, each of which is attempting to constrain and reduce its own costs and neither of which is particularly concerned about inequities in gender, race, health status, or access to care and (2) contradictions between the shared goals of the state and part of the elements of the corporate sector that want to reduce medical care costs versus the corporate sector that is the medical-industrial complex, which wants the state to continue to subsidize a strong and profitable market in medical care. The results have been a costly and deeply stratified health care system for all Americans, with particularly deleterious effects on women, minorities, and the poor.

Other recent policies have fueled gender struggles. Neoconservative ideology has laid the effective base for increased pressures on women in terms of family responsibility. Three other social trends have further heightened the latent gender tensions in relation to eldercare: (1) the increase in family responsibilities for posthospital care of the elderly as a result of Medicare's hospital prospective payment system, (2) the demographics of a rapidly growing aging population accompanied by what demographers label a "baby dearth" and a growing proportion of females in the workforce, and (3) the continuing lack of public financing for social policy alternatives of formal long-term care in support of the elderly. Each of these trends presses American women to return home to meet the rising burden (and expectations) of providing extensive free care.

Racial and ethnic struggles continue in the 1990s with the racial divisiveness that was present at the beginning of the century also prevalent today. In 1903, W. E. B. DuBois wrote that the major problem of the twentieth century is the color line (Miller 1987). Discussions of the color line and the conditions that keep the races apart and prevent everyone from participating in the mainstream of the American economy are still relevant. Black workers, for example, are said to form 10.1 percent of the workforce yet receive only 8.0 percent of the earnings (Hacker 1992). Class struggles persist as well. The "new class war" first described by Piven and Cloward (1982) is exemplified in the widening income gap between rich and poor and in the dramatic rise in the number of Americans who are uninsured for health care in the United States.

Social policy for the aging as well as for other segments of the population is shaped largely by requirements of the economy, the power of business, and the politics surrounding both. Women's position as workers, caregivers, and beneficiaries of public policies continues to be systematically unequal to that of nonminority men. By failing to address these structural inequities, social policy perpetuates, both directly and indirectly, the disadvantaged economic and health status of older women, particularly minority women, throughout old age.

Necessary Changes

The economic and health situation of older women requires deep structural and policy changes to redress inequities and provide access to basic resources, including Social Security, housing, nutrition, health, and long-term care and broad-based social reforms to end the life course social and economic inequities experienced by women. The attendant economic and health issues confronted by aging and minority women challenge the very structure of our social institutions. Women's income issues are an essential part of the health policy debate. Policies are needed to abridge and compensate for the gendered division of labor and lifelong discrimination that women and people of color experience.

Efforts geared toward necessary policy changes to improve the lives of older women who are economically disadvantaged must also take into consideration the life course experience and sociocultural patterns of other disadvantaged groups, regardless of age, race, or gender. As the discussion of older women who work as unpaid caregivers to grandchildren illustrates, older people live age-interconnected lives, and what affects their children, grandchildren, and other family members often affects them. These changes will require an ideological shift that encourages U.S. policies, particularly retirement policies, to effectively take into consideration the lifetime work experiences of the many diverse groups within society and the structural impediments to gender justice within these groups.

REFERENCES

Abramovitz, Mimi
    1988   Regulating the Lives of Women. Boston: South End Press.
American Association of Retired Persons (AARP) and Travelers Insurance Companies Foundation
    1988   National Survey of Caregivers: Summary of Findings. Hartford, CT: AARP and Travelers.
Amir, D.
    1987   "Preventive behavior and health status among the elderly." Psychology and Health 1(4):353-71.
Arendell, Terry, and Carroll L. Estes
    1987   "Unsettled future: older women, economics and health." Feminist Issues 7(1):3-24.
Bader, Jeanne E.
    1985   "Respite care: temporary relief for caregivers." Women and Health 10(2-3):39-52.
Beeson, Diane
    1975   "Women in aging studies: a critique and suggestion." Social Problems 21(1):52-59.
Black, Douglas, J. N. Morris, C. Smith, and Peter Townsend
    1982   "The Black report." In Peter Townsend and Nick Davidson (eds.), Inequalities in Health. Harmondsworth, Middlesex: Penguin.
Brody, Elaine
    1985   "Parent care as a normative family stress." Gerontologist 25(1):19-29.

Burton, Linda M.
  1991   "Everyday life in two high-risk neighborhoods: caring for children."
          American Enterprise (May-June):34–37.
Butler, R. N., and M. L. Lewis
  1982   Aging and Mental Health: Positive Psychosocial and Biomedical Ap-
          proaches, 3d ed. Columbus, Ohio: Merrill.
California State Assembly, Human Services Committee
  1989   Hearing on Drug Exposed Infants: The Role of Grandmothers as Care-
          takers. San Francisco: State of California Human Services Committee.
Corbin, Juliet, and Anselm Strauss
  1985   "Issues concerning regimen management in the home." Ageing and So-
          ciety 5(3):249–65.
Darling, Helen
  1986   "Role of the federal government in assuring access to health care." In-
          quiry 23:286–95.
Edmonds, Mary McKinney
  1990   "The health of the black aged female." Pp. 205–20 in Zev Harel, Edward
          A. McKinney, and Michael Williams (eds.), Black Aged: Understanding
          Diversity and Service Needs. Newbury Park, CA: Sage.
Edsall, Thomas Byrne
  1988   "The Reagan legacy." Pp. 3–50 in Sidney Blumenthal and Thomas Byrne
          Edsall (eds.), The Reagan Legacy. New York: Pantheon Books.
Elder, Glen H., Jr.
  1974   Children of the Great Depression. Chicago: University of Chicago Press.
  1982   "Historical experiences in the later years." Pp. 75–107 in T. Hareven
          and K. Adams (eds.), Aging and Life Course Transitions. New York:
          Guilford Press.
Estes, Carroll L.
  1991   "The Reagan legacy: privatization, the welfare state, and aging in the
          1990s." Pp. 59–83 in John Myles and Jill Quadagno (eds.), States, Labor
          Markets, and the Future of Old-Age Policy. Philadelphia: Temple Uni-
          versity Press.
Estes, Carroll L., and Terry Arendell
  1986   "The unsettled future: women and the economics of health and aging."
          Presented at UCLA conference "Who Cares for the Elderly?"
Estes, Carroll L., and Elizabeth A. Binney
  1988   "Toward a transformation of health and aging policy." International Jour-
          nal of Health Services 18:69–82.
Estes, Carroll L., Juanita B. Wood, et al.
  1988   Organizational and Community Responses to Medicare Policy: Conse-
          quences for Health and Social Services for the Elderly. Final Report. 3 vols.
          San Francisco: Institute for Health and Aging, University of California.
Facio, Elisa
  1986-87 "The interaction of age and gender in Chicana older lives: a case study

of Chicana elderly in a senior citizen center." Renato Rosaldo Lecture Series 4.

Families USA Foundation
1992   The Health Cost Squeeze on Older Americans. Washington: Public Welfare Foundation.

Feldblum, C.
1985   "Home health care for the elderly: programs, problems, and potentials." Harvard Journal on Legislation 22(1).

Frazier, E. Franklin
1939   The Negro Family in the United States. Chicago: University of Chicago Press.

Fuchs, Victor R.
1986   "Sex differences in economic well-being." Science 232:459-64.

Gibson, Rose C.
1988   "The work, retirement, and disability of older black Americans." Pp. 304-24 in James S. Jackson (ed.), The Black American Elderly. New York: Springer.
1989   "Blacks in an aging society." Pp. 389-406 in Reginald L. Jones (ed.), Black Adult Development and Aging. Berkeley, CA: Cobb and Henry.

Giddings, Paula
1984   When and Where I Enter: The Impact of Black Women on Race and Sex in America. New York: Morrow.

Grune, J., ed.
1981   Manual on Pay Equity: Raising Wages for Women's Work. Washington: Conference on Alternative State and Local Policies.

Hacker, Andrew
1992   Two Nations: Black and White, Separate, Hostile, Unequal. New York: Scribner.

Harrison, Algea O.
1989   "Black working women: introduction to a life span perspective." Pp. 389-406 in Reginald L. Jones (ed.), Black Adult Development and Aging. Berkeley, CA: Cobb and Henry.

Hewlett, S. A.
1986   A Lesser Life. New York: William Morrow.

Holahan, John F., and Joel W. Cohan
1986   Medicaid: The Trade-off between Cost Containment and Access to Care. Pp. 5-31, 33-52. Washington: Urban Institute.

Jackson, Jacqueline
1986   "Black grandparents: who needs them?" Pp. 186-94 in Robert Staples (ed.), The Black Family: Essays and Studies. Belmont, CA: Wadsworth.

Kaplan, George A., and Mary N. Haan
1989   "Is there a role for prevention among the elderly?" Pp. 27-51 in Marcia G. Ory and K. Bond (eds.), Aging and Health Care: Social Science and Policy Perspectives. New York: Routledge.

LaPlante, Mitchell P., Shawn Miller, and Karen Miller
  1992   Disability Statistics Abstract, No. 4. Washington: Department of Educa-
          tion, National Institute on Disability and Rehabilitation Research
          (NIDRR).
Markides, Kyriakos, and Charles H. Mindel
  1987   Aging and Ethnicity. Newbury Park, CA: Sage.
Miller, S. M.
  1987   "Race in the health of America." Milbank Quarterly 65(2):500–531.
National Center for Health Statistics (NCHS)
  1987a   Health Statistics of Older Persons, United States, 1986. Vital Health
          Statistics. Series 3, no. 25. DHHS Pub. No. (PHS) 87-1409. Washington:
          Government Printing Office.
  1987b   The Supplement on Aging to the 1984 National Health Interview Sur-
          vey. Series 1, no. 21. DHHS Pub. No. (PHS) 87-1323. Washington:
          Government Printing Office.
  1995   NCHS Current Estimates from the National Interview Survey, 1994.
          Series 10, no. 193. December.
  1996   NCHS Vital Statistics of the United States. 1992 Life Tables. Vol. 2, sec.
          6. April. Washington: Government Printing Office.
Norman, R.
  1985   The Nature and Correlates of Health Behavior. (Health Promotion Stud-
          ies, No. 2). Ottawa: Health Promotion Directorate.
Older Women's League
  1992   1992 Mother's Day Report—Critical Condition: Midlife and Older
          Women in America's Health Care System. Washington: Older Women's
          League.
Perry, Charlotte Marie
  1991   The Relationship of Social Support Network Function to the Health
          Status of Older Widowed Black Females. Ph.D. diss., University of North
          Carolina at Greensboro.
Piven, F., and R. Cloward
  1982   The New Class War. New York: Pantheon Books.
Poe, Lenora Madison
  1992   Black Grandparents as Parents. Berkeley, CA: Author.
Rice, Dorothy
  1989   "Health and long-term care of the aged." American Economic Review
          79:343–47.
Rice, Dorothy, and Carroll L. Estes
  1984   "Health of the elderly: policy issues and challenges." Health Affairs
          3(4):25–49.
Soldo, Beth, and Kenneth Manton
  1985   "Changes in the health status and service needs of the oldest old: current
          patterns and future trends." Milbank Quarterly 63(2):286–323.

Staples, Robert
    1986   The Black Family: Essays and Studies. Belmont, CA: Wadsworth.
Stark, F. H.
    1987   Introductory Remarks to Hearing on Medicare Hospital DRG Margins. Washington: House of Representatives, Subcommittee on Health of the Ways and Means Committee.
Stone, Robyn, Gail Lee Cafferata, and Judith Sangl
    1987   "Caregivers of the frail elderly: a national profile." Gerontologist 27(5):616-26.
U.S. Bureau of the Census
    n.d.   Current Population Reports. Series P-60, consumer income, no. 161. Unpublished, data from March 1988 Current Population Survey. Washington.
    1991   Statistical Abstract of the United States. Washington: Department of Commerce.
U.S. Department of Health and Human Services (DHHS)
    1991   Health Status of Minorities and Low-Income Groups, 3d ed., 283-90. Washington: Public Health Service, Human Resources and Services Administration (HRSA).
    1992   Health, United States, 1991, and Prevention Profile. Washington: Public Health Service, Center for Disease Control, National Center for Health Statistics.
U.S. Senate Special Committee on Aging
    1968   Developments in Aging. Pp. 335-411. Washington: Congress.
    1985   Developments in Aging: 1984. Washington: Government Printing Office.
U.S. Senate Special Committee on Aging, the American Association of Retired Persons, the Federal Council on Aging, and the U.S. Administration on Aging
    1988   Aging America: Trends and Projections, 1987-88 ed. Washington: Department of Health and Human Services.
    1991   Aging America: Trends and Projections, 1991 ed. Washington: Department of Health and Human Services.
Verbrugge, Lois M.
    1983   "Women and men: mortality and health of older people." Pp. 139-74 in Matilda White Riley, Beth B. Hess, and Kathleen Bond (eds.), Aging in Society: Selected Reviews of Recent Research. Hillsdale, NJ: L. Erlbaum.
    1984   "A health profile of older women, with comparisons to older men." Res. Aging 6:291-322.
    1985   "An epidemiological profile of older women." Pp. 41-64 in M. R. Haug, A. B. Ford, and M. Sheafor (eds.), The Physical and Mental Health of Aged Women. New York: Springer.
    1989   "Recent, present, and future health of American adults." Pp. 10:333-62 in J. E. Breslow, J. E. Fielding, and L. B. Lave (eds.), Annual Review of Public Health. Palo Alto, CA: Annual Reviews.

Villers Foundation
    1987   On the Other Side of Easy Street. Washington: Villers Foundation.
Weitzman, L.
    1985   The Divorce Revolution. New York: Free Press.
Wittstock, L. W.
    1980   "Twilight of a long maidenhood." In Beverly Lindsay (ed.), Comparative
            Perspectives of Third World Women: The Impact of Race, Sex, and
            Class. New York: Praeger.
Zones, Jane Sprague, Carroll L. Estes, and Elizabeth A. Binney
    1987   "Gender, public policy, and the oldest old." Ageing and Society 7:275–
            302.

[PART VI]

Power and Social Control

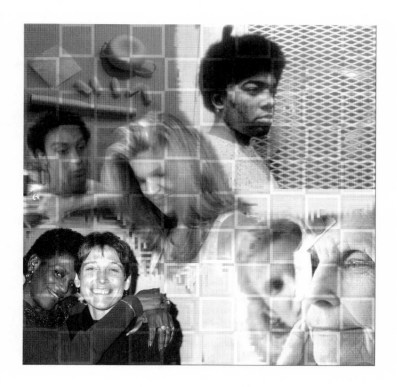

Social control is an element of social life that takes many forms: it is found in interpersonal expectations for behavior in others; it is located in formal rules and regulations that guide many aspects of everyday life from driving a car to submitting an income tax form; it is also evident in differences in power between groups or individuals who are members of particular groups. Power in this context refers to situations in which individuals, groups, or social institutions can require and enforce certain behaviors, thoughts, or actions or limit the choices and options of other individuals and groups.

How are power and social control intertwined, and how do they affect women's health? In chapter 18, Nancy Stoller shows how the powerful relegate the powerless to inadequate health care, particularly when stigma and marginality make the inadequacies of care invisible. The dynamics of power and social control can also be seen in violence against women in both domestic and public situations, violence which too often has tragic consequences. In chapter 19, Britton, Lempert, Von Schulthess, and Pickels highlight the many ways in which social and cultural arrangements shape both the extent and subjective experiences of violence. From the most intimate to the most public places, violence touches women's lives. As the essays in this section highlight, violence against women takes many forms. Yet as Lempert and Clarke point out in their introductory essay, these various forms have many distinct features that cannot be subsumed by a global view of violence. In addition, women themselves disagree about what causes violence and what might be done to stem it in American society.

Social control can take many other forms, including the curtailment of reproductive rights. In recent years, questions have emerged over the slow development of new contraceptive technologies. Controversies over social control and the safety of new contraceptives are really new versions of old issues. In chapter 20, Cheri Pies puts some of the recent conflicts and controversies in the development of long-lasting contraceptives into its broad historical and reproductive rights perspective.

Looking toward the future, what strains and tensions in society may lead to conflict or reconciliation around social control issues? How are ongoing debates over health and welfare, both at the national level and in local communities, struggles over social control? How will these struggles be addressed in an increasingly diverse and complex society marked by growing social inequities?

[18]

Responses to Stigma and Marginality:
The Health of Lesbians, Imprisoned Women, and Women with HIV

NANCY E. STOLLER

Nancy Stoller uses the sociological concepts of stigma and marginality to show how devalued social identities, as well as economic disadvantage, can result in inadequacies in health care. To do this she looks at problems faced by three very different groups of women—lesbians, prisoners, and women with HIV. Although each group has its own health needs, the social response of both patients and providers is shaped by perceptions of the social valuation of these women.

A major dynamic affecting health is stigma. In his groundbreaking work on this topic, Erving Goffman discussed the role of "spoiled identity" in social interaction. Stigmatized persons are avoided, rejected, and seen as a source of contamination. In the institutional worldview, their self-identities are excluded, rephrased, distorted, and/or relatively devalued. In a medical setting, the devaluation is often associated with experimentation, being a training opportunity (e.g., for residents and medical students), and the exoticization of one's characteristics.

Although not all marginalized people become stigmatized, nor is institutional marginality always a result of stigma, the two phenomena often occur together. Marginality can generate signs of inadequacy, spoilage, and danger, and stigmatized individuals are often purposely kept at the margins of institutions in order to protect those viewed as morally acceptable and to make the institutional boundaries more explicit. Fear of the contamination of the "innocent" through social contact with the stigmatized is an important key to understanding the treatment of lesbians and women with HIV. It also helps explain the aversions that women in prison sometimes display toward each other.

In most if not all societies, certain groups and individuals are situated at the edges of the dominant and institutionalized activities—they are marginalized. An individual can choose to be central to one group and marginal to another—for example, a research scientist who is centrally located in her profession but chooses marginality in her university's bureaucracy. But some people, because of their social identity, find themselves marginalized regardless of their choice. They are then excluded from normal interaction; they can be given the dregs and leftovers. In economic language, they may be called the lumpen proletariat, the final recipients of "trickle-down" capitalism. Formally and informally they mark the boundaries of inclusion in normal social life.

Within a health care system, people with marginal status are likely to face some or all of the following problems: (1) difficulty in gaining access to services, (2) services that are delivered through the lowest tier in any multitiered system, and (3) access to services that are located at the geographical, social, and temporal margins of larger institutions.

For example, they find care in publicly financed clinics (instead of major medical centers or profitable private systems), after regular hours, or only after very long waits. They may also find care in unofficial or extramedical settings, such as in pharmacies or from unlicensed providers. In general, their care is delivered at the periphery of the health system.

Many groups of women and men perceived as marginal, such as the homeless, prostitutes, and drug users, receive lower quality health care. Their marginality goes beyond gender, race, or class discrimination—although these categories are often relevant and do interact, creating multiple marginality, for example, an African American, homeless, alcoholic woman. In an analogy to the Marxist concept of "the superexploited," we can say that these populations are "supermarginalized." They cluster at and beyond the identified margins of the American health care system.

Lesbians, women in prison, and women with HIV infection are marginal not only in the broader society but also in the worlds of feminist health consciousness. Their needs are often forgotten. As a result, they have been approached by women's health movements in a complex manner: they have been seen as exotic, repulsive, appealing, dangerous, expendable, dependent, and occasionally useful to promote the ends of the movement. In this chapter, we will see them as they are—socially stigmatized and marginalized women struggling for survival.

Linkages among These Groups

The health care experiences of these women are linked in several ways. Members of all three groups are routinely stigmatized and marginalized because of their social identities. Lesbian identity is associated with sexual choice. Women with HIV are linked by a disease. And women in prison are marked by their common legal and "residential" status. But in all three cases, their public identity results in stigma and marginalization, which in turn result in inferior services and care.

These groups of women are further linked by common demographics. For example, women with HIV disease and women in prison usually share many background characteristics, the most prominent of which are their racial-ethnic backgrounds and poverty. In many ways, these two groups overlap. Of all women in prison, African Americans are most over-represented, followed by Latinas (primarily Puerto Ricans and Chicanas). Whites and Asians are found in jail in disproportionately fewer numbers than would be expected by direct population projections. The ethnic/gender distribution of AIDS diagnoses and HIV infection rates among women follows the same ethnic/gender pattern (Schneider and Stoller 1994). Indeed, studies of HIV and AIDS in correctional settings indicate that many women with HIV move in and out and back to jail or prison.

The demographic background similarities between women with HIV and women in prison are associated with similar health needs. These needs are primarily the result of poverty and—not surprisingly in the American context—racism. Poverty may generate physical and emotional problems ranging from malnutrition to maternal deprivation. Racism exacerbates these difficulties and hinders access to treatment. Racism also concentrates social and health problems—such as the scourge of drug addiction and drug sales—in neighborhoods and ghettos inhabited by people of color. Illegal drug systems, prostitution, and other underground and illegal economies are the prime reasons that women are in prison and jail. Such economies flourish where access to legal economies is impaired, as is the case in the areas where African Americans, Puerto Ricans, Chicanos, and Native Americans live. Because the drug economy is illegal, possession of its paraphernalia is also illegal in most states. Illegal—and therefore usually unsanitary—hypodermic needles are the most common means of heroin and cocaine consumption. Consequently, racism, the drug economy, social marginality, HIV infection, and incarceration are inextricably linked in the United States.

These connections mean that a woman who is in prison and has HIV disease is in many ways less alone, or less different from other prisoners, than she—and her health care providers—may think. In fact, it might be her similarity to the vast majority of other prisoners that has in many institutions generated considerable fear among inmates and a tendency by staff to quarantine and isolate HIV-identified women. In the close and inescapable confines of prison, the fear of catching a disease known to be both infectious and deadly can lead to psychological panic and a desire to mark and isolate the carrier of the virus.

But how do lesbians fit into this HIV and prison story? First, lesbians are inextricably linked both politically and socially to HIV disease. This is true no matter where they are found (in or out of prison—and the majority are outside) or how they feel about their connection to gay men or to the epidemic. This unavoidable political connection is partly the result of a common (but incorrect) idea that because both lesbians and gay men are called "homosexual" and many male homosexuals have HIV, then many female homosexuals must also have high infection rates. The political connection has been intensified by recent increases in homo-phobic violence (see Britton, Lempert, and von Schulthess in chapter 19) and legislation, which harm women as well as men. The 1980s rise in homophobia is generally interpreted as linked to the AIDS epidemic, both by its perpetrators and by those who oppose it. Additional social-psychological connections arise between lesbians and HIV from lesbian friendships with gay men, participation in mixed male-female gay-identified organizations, and identification as a member of a gay commu-nity or subculture. To the extent that some lesbians are actively involved with women's issues, including health issues, they may also find them-selves involved in the work of the epidemic because of their identifica-tion as women.

The second linkage of lesbians, women with HIV, and women in prison is found in the fact that most incarcerated women are in single-sex institutions. Even when co-ed facilities exist, the majority of an inmate's time is spent with other women. Many women in prison are "situational" lesbians emotionally, affectionally, and in many cases sexually. Although many return to heterosexuality on release, a significant number continue to seek primary emotional and sexual relationships with women after they leave. Still others arrive as lesbians and in most institutions find an open lesbian subculture.

Lesbian health in prison (or to put it another way, the health of women in prison who are living lesbian lifestyles) is a topic that has scarcely been studied. Nevertheless, the demographic issues already noted in discussing HIV rates and incarcerated women also apply to the incar-cerated lesbian: she is likely to be poor, black or Latina, to have partici-pated in the drug culture and/or economy, and to have a good chance of exposure to HIV.

In addition to their common marginality and their occasionally over-lapping demographic similarity and institutional location, the women in these three groups sometimes find themselves together in other ways. The same individual can carry all three identities. And each stigma—incarceration, disease, sexual deviance—operates both independently and cumulatively. In jail, the incarcerated woman (who is most likely poor, black, and in bad physical and emotional health on her arrival in jail) must struggle to get basic care in a limited service system. If she has HIV, she must also live with her marginalization from mainstream AIDS services as well as the in-prison stigma associated with HIV. And if she is a lesbian, she will confront additional homophobia and misunderstanding.

These three groups of women also have unique health issues. As the following discussion indicates, some issues arise from the group's demographic composition or its social position. The level of health care and the quality of medical research provided for each group are functions of the degree of organization and political influence of the group and the extent to which services for the group are seen as also benefiting others outside the group. For example, much of the research about and education for women with HIV infection can be seen as a result of a concern for men and infants who might be infected by the women rather than explicit concern for the women per se. Similarly, because lesbians are perceived as connected to no one but themselves, their health needs are generally ignored by the medical establishment. And the primary occasions for interest in the health of women or men in prison are when they are seen as possibly passing on a health problem to someone outside, such as a spouse or a child.

Contemporary Lesbian Health Issues

Before the gay liberation movements of the late 1960s and early 1970s, most twentieth-century writing on lesbian health was focused on lesbian sexual identity and behavior as the sole health or medical problem of the female homosexual. The authors, many of them physicians and therapists, sought the roots of the "problem" of lesbianism in biological and/or psychological disturbance. Treatments were also focused on these realms and on such behavior modification strategies as marriage (Hitchcock 1988). With the birth of the gay and lesbian political movement of the late 1960s came a redefinition of normality and the beginning of a drive by lesbians and gay men to examine and describe their own realities, including their own views of what their "health" issues are.

A new wave of research on lesbian health issues occurred as a direct result of this political movement and the consequent emergence of more public lesbian communities and lesbian research agendas. Especially in larger cities, conferences, workshops, clinics, and nonprofit agencies that were primarily focused on women or on the male and female gay community have developed lesbian-specific services as well (Haas 1994). Lesbian consciousness has changed to include a new sense of entitlement to a full reproductive and family life and an increasing awareness of the emotionally damaging results of stigma (Bradford and Ryan 1988). This combination has provided the basis for both research and social change. Although much of the serious research and writing about lesbian health in the 1970s was the work of nonprofessional lesbian health activists and health care providers (O'Donnell et al. 1979), increasingly in the 1980s it has been conducted by lesbian and (occasionally) heterosexual academics and physicians (Haas 1994; Stevens 1992). This reflects both the greater legitimacy of the topic and the increased numbers of openly lesbian scholars.

An array of lesbian health issues has been defined as salient by feminists, the lesbian community, or the medical/academic establishment. Primary areas of lesbian concern in which work has recently been done are chronic disease and disability (including HIV and cancers), substance abuse, domestic violence, mental health, and gynecological and reproductive health. In many cases the activists have a broader focus than lesbians—for example, women or disability—but they have also focused a part of their attention specifically on lesbians within the broader category.

Chronic Disease

Within the area of chronic disease, major areas of concern have been cancer, HIV disease, chronic fatigue syndrome, and the consequences of disability. These concerns result from the invisibility that lesbians face in health care and legal systems. Most women's health care is delivered through heterosexual institutions. For example, primary access to inexpensive Pap smears and breast exams by professionals is through ob/gyn services, Planned Parenthood, and local health department family planning clinics, where the focus is on heterosexual sex. There are no parallel state-funded services directed at lesbians. In such settings, which are sometimes the only source of Pap smears for those without money, lesbians are explicitly or implicitly forced to receive birth control counseling in order to obtain routine gynecological testing. Such restrictions may be one reason lesbians have a lower-than-average rate of Pap smears. Approximately 50 percent in the National Lesbian Health Care Survey had been examined in the previous year, compared with a national average of 72 percent for all women (Bradford and Ryan 1988; Robertson and Schachter 1981). Regular Pap smears are the best way to prevent or detect cervical cancer early on so that it can be treated. The extent to which lesbian needs are invisible during cancer recovery has been poignantly documented by Audre Lorde in *The Cancer Journals* (1980).

Lesbians are almost invisible in AIDS statistics. Although the sexuality of men is prominently categorized and the relevance of ethnicity, region, drug use behavior, age, education, and other cultural factors is frequently explored in AIDS epidemiology, lesbians are rarely identified in official epidemiological statistics collected and presented by federal agencies. Except where they have insisted on incorporation, lesbians are also absent as targets of AIDS outreach and education programs. I once spent five months negotiating printing permission for a brochure for lesbians from my own AIDS education agency, when other proposed brochures received a turnaround of about a week. The argument given for not printing this brochure was that lesbians were "not at risk for AIDS." The legal and social denial of lesbian relationships further interferes with the ability to protect and/or care for one's lover when she is disabled (Hunter, Michaelson, and Stoddard 1992; Simkin 1991; Thompson and Andrzejewski 1988). In these ways, the exclusion of lesbian existence from the consciousness of health care providers leads to a greater risk of chronic disease and additional difficulties in treatment and recovery.

Substance Abuse

Use of and addiction to alcohol and other drugs have been increasingly identified as problems in lesbian and gay communities (Bradford and Ryan 1988). Historically, bars and other settings with alcohol were primary locations for gay people to gather. Following the development of alternative social institutions in the 1970s, and increasingly since health consciousness grew in the 1980s, various programs have been developed to encourage sobriety and provide drug- and alcohol-free environments. Within the gay community, these environments are contrasted to, and sometimes seen as supplements to or replacements for, a previously limited range of gathering places.

Discrimination, homophobia, and other forms of gay oppression have also been identified as sources of the desire for escape through alcohol or drugs. Beyond programs developed within the gay and lesbian community itself, there is little evidence of sensitivity in publicly funded or private services for people with addiction and/or substance abuse problems.

Domestic Violence

Domestic violence is a hidden feature of some lesbian relationships. In a national survey of 1,925 lesbians, Bradford and Ryan (1988) found that 8.3 percent had been physically abused by a lover, 4.3 percent by a husband, and 15.8 percent by an adult when they were still children. Both lack of awareness and sensitivity about publicizing such "unacceptable" behavior have resulted in limited development of services concerning violence within the lesbian community (White and Levinson 1993). In addition, there is considerable argument about appropriate models for understanding violence between women. Is violence "male" behavior? How useful is a heterosexual family model in counseling lesbian partners? Where does sadomasochism (a form of consensual sexuality that includes pain and is practiced by some lesbians) fit in all this?

Meanwhile, many battered women's shelters actively exclude lesbians and censure "lesbian behavior" among clients and/or staff (see Britton, Lempert, and von Schulthess in chapter 19). This combination of denial and rejection in both lesbian and heterosexual services has left both lesbian batterers and battered lesbian partners even more isolated and invisible.

Mental Health

In the area of mental health, lesbian needs are associated with common concerns of all women: money problems, job or school worries, problems with lovers, too much work responsibility, family matters, depression, and so on. Bradford and Ryan (1988) found, as one might expect, that the intensity of these concerns varied with demographic factors of race, income, employment status, and age. But the women in their survey also gave evidence of the unusual intensity with which these problems might be felt. Over 17 percent had attempted suicide, and 73 percent had received some sort of mental health counseling. The most common reason for seeking counseling was depression—50% percent—followed by problems with a lover, problems with family, anxiety, personal growth, homosexuality, and loneliness. Further strains on lesbian mental health include the stresses of confronting heterosexism and homophobia, the special needs of lesbians living with children, and the broad range of difficulties associated with the legal and social invisibility of lesbian relationships.

To meet these needs, lesbian mental health services have developed at a faster rate than many other health services for this population. Many metropolitan areas have feminist and/or gay mental health services with explicit programs for lesbians and an extensive literature in the area has begun to develop (Boston Lesbian Psychology Collective 1987).

Gynecological and Reproductive Health

The most serious difficulties encountered by lesbians in terms of reproductive health are their invisibility and their fears of stigmatizing treatment by health care providers if they do identify themselves. Many women who identify as lesbians are, or have been, sexually active with men. In 1978, Bell and Weinberg found that 75 percent reported sex with men, and Bradford and Ryan (1988) concluded that about half their 1985 sample had done likewise. Therefore, when thinking of lesbian gynecological health, one must be aware of both past and present and of the possibility that a given patient may be, or may have been, sexually active with both men and women. The most important gynecological and obstetrical issues for lesbians are sexually transmitted disease (generally much less common for lesbians than for heterosexual women) (Robertson and Schachter 1981), diseases of the reproductive organs, and pregnancy (increasingly common via artificial insemination) and childbirth.

The lesbian response to exclusionary practices has been to develop alternative lesbian health clinics, research projects, self-help groups, insemination services, and parenting organizations. An extensive counterculture of lesbian-oriented health activities and institutions in these areas has modified the impact of heterosexist reproductive and sexual health services and has given lesbians who have access to them a nonstigmatized route to these types of health care. However, the movements have had little impact on mainstream services, except where feminist and lesbian providers have become part of dominant institutions. Even then, the changed reception for the patient is usually limited to the provider herself and not to the service institution of which she is a part.

Women in Prison

Health needs and medical problems of women in jail and prison have also received little study. During the 1970s, waves of prison litigation and feminist activism with roots in the civil rights movement coincided. Some progress was made in acknowledging and redressing the grievances of women prisoners, especially inadequate living conditions and health care. Since the 1980s, however, jail and prison conditions have badly deteriorated throughout the United States, and the suffering of both men and women has increased. A review of women's needs on entering correctional systems, the subsequent impacts of incarceration, and the roles of both prisoners and professionals in addressing these needs will illuminate this situation.

Health on Arrival: The Impacts of Gender, Race, and Class

Although this essay deals primarily with women, correctional systems are organized for male inmates because 80–90 percent of all incarcerated persons are men. In prison health, female differences from men are crucial: the female reproductive system, including its different response to sexually transmitted diseases; women's ability to be pregnant, give birth, and nurse; women's greater tendency to become obese; gender differentials in rates of certain illnesses, such as lung cancer, breast cancer, and hemophilia; the greater likelihood that women have been victims of physical and sexual abuse and incest; and the different experiences men and women have with the health care system.

Poverty, powerlessness, and racism are basic facts of life for women who end up in prison. National studies indicate that from 50 to 75 percent have been on welfare shortly before incarceration, and they are overwhelmingly black and Latino (Glick and Neto 1976; Henriques 1972; McCall, Shaw, and Casteel 1985). The offenses that bring them to prison are the crimes of poverty: drug offenses, drunkenness, prostitution, and vagrancy (Wyrick and Owens 1977). When women arrive at jail, they show the health effects of such lives. Common ailments are drug addiction, psychiatric illness, hypertension, respiratory ailments, sexually transmitted diseases, and untreated reproductive tract abnormalities (Chapman 1980; Glick and Neto 1976). One study found that 17 percent of women admitted to the New York City jail system showed evidence of recent physical trauma (Anno 1977; McCall et al. 1985; Novick et al. 1977). In 1989 20 percent of New York State women inmates were estimated to be HIV positive (New York City AIDS Surveillance Unit 1989).

The Pains of Imprisonment

The combination of poor prison conditions, minimal rights, and grossly inadequate health care intensifies the suffering of women inmates. This leads to further psychological and physical mortification of the body, a loss of reproductive freedom, physical deterioration, and overuse of psychotropic medication.

Basic prison conditions include far-reaching invasion into personal life, ranging from internal pelvic searches and individually dispensed sanitary napkins to severe overcrowding with four women in a space designed for one, locked down for days and sharing an open toilet in a small cell. Women's fears of contagion are exacerbated by the sense of close contact with stigmatized others, for inmates too can share others' repulsions about criminals. And there are real epidemics of diseases in prisons, caused by overcrowding, poor sanitation, and inadequate medical attention (Anno 1977; Anno and Lang 1978). Consequently, many inmates feel that their bodies are defiled, damaged, and endangered.

Reproductive choices are almost completely removed from the inmate's control. Even in co-correctional settings and in short-term jails, most prisoners are denied birth control on the grounds that sex is forbidden. If a woman is pregnant, abortion may be legally available but routinely delayed beyond practical usefulness to the point of forced childbearing. Diet, work conditions, exercise, continuity of care, and access to normal pregnancy monitoring are usually far below community standards. Except for a few small programs scattered among the states, there is no routine way for a woman to be with her child after a prison birth, beyond a few days in the hospital. Not only is nursing impossible, therefore, but the bonding that provides a base for a strong parent-child relationship is also prohibited.

Physical deterioration in the form of weight gain is common, resulting in obesity for many women (Shaw 1985). Studies of both men and women in prison have indicated that, following incarceration, health deteriorates over time (Jones 1976; McCall et al. 1985). Further complicating the picture is the use of inappropriate medication, including psychotropics. The medical practice of higher prescription rates of psychotropic medication for women than men is replicated in prison settings (Resnik and Shaw 1980; Shaw, Browne, and Meyer 1981). Although the major scandals concerning overuse of psychotropic medication in women's prisons took place in the 1970s, monitoring continues to be thin and institutions have become more crowded. Both conditions are highly conducive to the prescribing of tranquilizers and other psychotropics.[1]

Responses

If one were to rank groups of health care consumers by their evident power to effect change, women in jail and prison would appear near the bottom, perhaps just above female mental patients. Disenfranchised by gender, class, race, and legal status, they bring few obvious resources to their situation beyond an ability to stay alive.

Yet in many prisons, women inmates have responded collectively to their marginalization. In most cases, the response is mutual assistance, which can be as limited as the sharing of home remedies or food. Sometimes they band together informally to pressure staff to respond to a woman with an untreated health problem. In other institutions, they have arranged for health education programs. They have also joined in suits challenging the denial of adequate care (Resnik and Shaw 1980).

Some of the most significant long-term changes in prison health care have arisen from such litigation. During the 1970s, the basic right of all prisoners to a standard of care that matched that of the broader community was secured, only to be eroded in the 1980s, as the federal courts became increasingly conservative. A second professional approach has been the development of accreditation programs. Jail and prison health care accreditation programs emerged in the early eighties, partly in response to successful litigation. Accreditation for those institutions that met detailed minimum standards was promoted by both the American Public Health Association and the American Medical Association. The AMA's program was eventually transferred to the American Correctional Health Association (which the AMA had helped start) and became the primary accreditation system. Although many correctional systems have pursued accreditation primarily as a strategy for avoiding litigation, it has nevertheless improved the basic care in most institutions in which it has been used. This includes health care for women prisoners (Resnik and Shaw 1980). Still, the level of care prescribed by accreditation and pro-tected through litigation does not include the sorts of health monitoring, "well health" emphases, or protections of reproductive rights that most people would consider basic to women's needs.

Consciousness and activism concerning both lesbian and prisoners' health have been developing since the early seventies. The health of these two marginalized and stigmatized groups came into focus within the political and social activity of broader liberation movements. In the case of lesbians, members of the stigmatized group themselves led the way to alternative per-spectives, services, and institutions. For incarcerated women, these tasks were primarily accomplished by outside advocates in cooperation with the marginalized women.

Women with AIDS/HIV

The third marginalized group to be discussed in this article—women with HIV infection—has a somewhat different story. "Women with AIDS" is a new social category because AIDS itself was unknown before 1981. Could such a group and an identity appear, be marginalized, and be the object of a political destigmatizing response, all within a few years? The answer is clearly yes, and the reasons are found in both the multiple identities of women with HIV and in the already established and new political movements and institutions that have sought to include these women in their own bases of legitimacy and representation.

During the first few years of the AIDS epidemic, there was no con-sensus on the cause of the disease. It was labeled a syndrome of "acquired immune deficiencies" and was defined by differential diagnosis—that is, by excluding other causes of the illnesses that made up the AIDS syn-drome. The term *AIDS-related complex* (ARC) was then applied to a set of illnesses that were clearly related to the syndrome but less severe or not yet definitively diagnosed. After the discovery of the human im-munodeficiency virus (HIV) and its linkage to AIDS in 1983 came the development of inexpensive tests for an antibody to the virus. A new language with terms such as *HIV disease* and *positivity* became prominent. Following this change, AIDS itself was relegated to the role of the "end stage" of HIV disease, and interest shifted increasingly to the spectrum of health and illness associated with earlier stages of infection. As knowledge about the virus and its effects has grown, new treatments have changed the potential life expectancy of those infected. It is against this background of changing knowledge and new potentials for individual and collective survival of the epidemic that the following discussion of women and HIV must be understood.

Demographics

AIDS is a reportable illness in the United States. AIDS statistics, collected by the Centers for Disease Control, have been used to provide a somewhat accurate, if time-lagged, picture of the population affected by HIV. Studies based on HIV antibody testing generally support the argument that the infection pattern is similar to the pattern of AIDS diagnoses. According to CDC reports, women constitute slightly less than 10 percent of people with AIDS. The women are overwhelmingly African American (51%) and Latina (Puerto Rican and Chicana primarily) (20%). (African American women and Latinas have been estimated to have a risk of infection that is twelve to thirteen times that of white women.) Most women with AIDS are of reproductive age (79% are between 13 and 39) with a significant number in their twenties. This indicates that many were infected when they were teenagers. The most common source of infection is intravenous drug use, followed by heterosexual transmission (Guinan and Hardy 1987).

HIV infection studies in the late 1980s found continuing transmission in the already identified populations with the most rapid spread among the poor, the illiterate, IV drug users (especially African Americans), non-English-speaking persons, and teenagers. HIV testing in prisons and among Army recruits has also shown an increasing number of women to be infected with the virus.

Health Consequences of Infection

Untreated HIV infection gradually causes a loss of immune system effectiveness. Among women, the first signs of HIV disease may be gynecological infections that will not respond to treatment, even repeated treatment, such as chronic vaginitis and pelvic inflammatory disease. Other opportunistic infections commonly found in women with HIV disease include herpes, toxoplasmosis, cytomegalovirus infections of the urinary tract and/or genitals, tuberculosis, septicemia (a generalized severe infection), syphilis, chronic obstructive pulmonary disease, and Pneumocystis carinii pneumonia. Kaposi's sarcoma, a rare skin cancer whose sudden appearance in 1981 helped raise awareness of AIDS, is rarely seen in women. In some cases women discover their HIV positivity through pregnancy and childbirth, either because a child is born infected and becomes ill or because the hospital or physician orders HIV testing.

Correct diagnosis and appropriate treatment are two major issues confronting women with HIV infection. A 1989 study by the New York City AIDS Surveillance Unit compared life expectancies of men and women with AIDS diagnoses in California, Miami, and New York, the three areas with the most cases of men and women with AIDS. The Unit concluded that women had significantly shorter life expectancies than men.

Three reasons may account for this. First and foremost is poverty. Poverty's impact is felt in everything from hospital waiting-room delays and lower quality care to delays in and denials of treatments, medications, food supplements, housing, and other services. All are hard to find for people dependent on Medicaid, welfare, and other forms of public assistance. Typically, women with HIV are also unconnected to any private sources of assistance beyond extended family networks of other poor women. Poverty is also associated with delayed diagnosis of AIDS. Women who are diagnosed late in their illness are sometimes too ill for effective treatment, even when such treatments are available. Another source of delayed diagnosis is misdiagnosis, when health workers do not realize that a woman's symptoms are related to HIV.

Second, women with HIV disease often develop life-threatening opportunistic infections (OIs), such as tuberculosis and chronic obstructive pulmonary disease, some of which do not meet the existing CDC definition of AIDS, which has been based on male symptomology (see Narrigan et al. in chapter 21). Although the women are seriously ill, they often lack an AIDS diagnosis and are consequently ineligible for some services and treatments linked to the diagnosis. When they finally meet the diagnostic criteria, they are already exhausted from multiple bouts of "non-AIDS" illness. In contrast, the male survival statistics are enhanced by the presence of men who have Kaposi's sarcoma, a disease whose existence fulfills diagnostic criteria for immune system breakdown and AIDS but whose progress is relatively slow and less damaging initially than many other OIs.

The social consequences of gender make it a third factor shortening the life expectancy of HIV-infected women, especially the health impacts of women's social roles as mothers and nurturers. Quite often a woman with HIV has a child or children as well as a male partner. One or more of them may also be infected or ill. But the woman is usually the primary caregiver, and her own health takes a backseat. Without special assistance, such women are more likely to miss their own medical appointments and be unable to follow prescribed treatment regimens (Macks 1988).

Another unique aspect of the gender and AIDS life expectancy relationship has been the explicit rejection of women "of childbearing potential" as research subjects. According to FDA guidelines in effect in 1989, women of childbearing age were to be excluded from all Phase I (toxicity) trials and from early Phase II (dose range and efficacy) trials unless "adequate information on efficacy and relative safety have been amassed" (U.S. Department of Health, Education, and Welfare 1977). At the time this regulation was in effect, however, almost all drugs with potential for treating HIV infection were in Phase I or II trials. In some cases, where the exclusion was not explicit, de facto exclusion occurred regardless because of trial locations, charges to participants, and locations of trials in the private medical sector. For the poor—almost all women with HIV are poor—participating in public access research protocols has been the only route to potentially effective treatment. People with more financial resources and/or gay community contacts have been able to obtain the drugs through underground suppliers, foreign distributors, and/or private physicians involved in parallel track studies or research. Some used all these approaches to test and combine treatments. But such avenues have essentially been closed to women by cost, location, and/or lack of effective publicity. Not surprisingly, women have had shorter life spans as a result.

Social-Psychological Issues

Psychological issues of HIV infection for women include a sense of physical contamination and dirtiness. These feelings can be especially intense in the presence of chronic gynecological infections. There are also feelings of parental failure and, if a child is also infected and/or ill with HIV, there may be a continuing sense of guilt—even if the woman was unaware of her health status when she was pregnant. Other issues include frequent loss of contact with children; stress associated with substance abuse or other addictions; isolation caused by the small numbers and great diversity of women with HIV illnesses and by a lack of women-focused services; loss of pre-infection sexuality; and difficulties in adjusting to the dangers of, or loss of, reproductive function and role (Maier 1987). On a social level, a woman may lose employment and housing and may even face physical violence when her HIV status becomes known. Many women lie about their HIV status and their current health to protect themselves and their children.

Becoming "a person with HIV" means taking on a stigmatized identity, both internally and externally. The societal response to this identity is most typically exclusion and marginalization, both of which further reinforce stigma and isolation. Although discovery of infection may initiate a sense of crisis followed by a stabilizing period of adjustment, the onset of symptoms (AIDS or ARC) produces a new crisis. Additional symptoms and illnesses produce further health crises and further adjustments, which can themselves produce emotional exhaustion and a sense of hopelessness (Dilley 1984). A growing fear of death, pain, and abandonment may set in. For women, their social roles of primary parent and nurturer to the family produce additional emotional, social, and legal issues. Although sick herself, the woman with AIDS must arrange care for children during her own daily and weekly illnesses. She may also have to care for an ill child or partner, and she must address the inevitable issues of adoption and/or foster care after she dies.

Programs and Development

Early in the 1980s, few physicians were knowledgeable about the manifestations of AIDS in women and children. As medical, social, psychological, and legal services developed for people with AIDS in the United States, they were structured according to a male model. The AIDS patient was treated by the medical profession as if he or she were a single, white, gay male with no dependents. Volunteer and community programs, which supplemented public and private services, were primarily based in the gay community. They also assumed the gay male as their primary client. But many people with AIDS were not gay, white, or male. Responding to this exclusion, AIDS advocacy movements for women, African Americans, Latinos, Asians, and Native Americans exploded in the mid-1980s. Gradually programs emerged to meet the needs of patients with drug dependencies and/or children. Services and education began to be provided in more neighborhoods, in a greater variety of languages, and with new cultural emphases. Some hospitals opened women-centered HIV clinics, and social services for

HIV-positive women and their families were designed. In terms of preven-tion, AIDS programs began to include such strategies as women's work-shops to teach effective skills for negotiating safer sexual encounters. But both treatment and prevention programs are few, and they function more as models for appropriate care than at the full level of services needed. Most women with HIV are from ethnic minority communities that are histori-cally and currently underserved in terms of all kinds of medical care. They cannot draw on the financial resources of the (predominantly white) gay community, which has helped many gay men survive longer with HIV and has humanized and destigmatized their experiences of the epidemic. Nor have they been able to force an adequate level of services from the govern-mental sector. Consequently, much of the activism for women's services has had a kind of "equal rights" perspective, focused on the argument that women need care that is just as good and as culturally relevant as that pro-vided to men.

Initially the pressure was on existing organizations (both public and private) to provide the services through specialized departments. In some cases an argument was made for separate funding—either to an organiza-tion serving women as a class (e.g., to a women's health clinic) or to an organization serving a particular group (African Americans, prostitutes, IV drug users, pregnant women). Increasingly, advocates for women's services have been addressing the overall issue of national health care and the struc-ture of the health care system, seeing the "problem" of women and AIDS as unsolvable without diagnosis and treatment of the problem of U.S. neglect and destruction of millions of its own citizens and permanent residents.

In some cases women with HIV have been active themselves in the advocacy movements. Their activism has been supported by organizations of people with AIDS and by feminist health activists. For many of the HIV-infected women arriving in the AIDS world with the low self-image of the poor, minority, female IV drug user, the discovery of other women like themselves through support groups and patient advocacy organiza-tions has been a first step toward personal and collective empowerment.

Conclusion

The history of activism and collective struggle in regard to women's health is as old as feminist consciousness. Sometimes this activism has been focused on the health needs or rights of all women (such as the absolute right to abortion and/or contraception). At other times, it has addressed the more specific needs of a particular economic class (public financing of abortion), ethnic group (preventing unwanted sterilization of Latinas), or set of health care consumers (the home birth and family-centered birth movement).

As we have seen, even women who are severely stigmatized and marginalized have mobilized to fight for their own health needs. The first step has often been the establishment of informal or formal support networks. For incarcerated women these networks have been overwhelmingly informal and/or modeled on the extended family. For lesbians such networks began informally but emerged as a wide variety of support and self-help groups. And for women with HIV they began as formal support groups established by advocates and service providers.

Out of the support groups and in connection with advocates and activists have come alternative organizations and political demands. The demands have been made on institutions ranging from hospitals, clinics, and local government funding agencies to the federal legal system. Yet all three groups of women remain marginalized despite their own efforts and those of their advocates. National health care may provide some medical hope for women with HIV. Greater access to community care and increased monitoring of prison health care delivery will help incarcerated women. And lesbians will probably benefit most from broad changes in public views on homosexuality. Until these types of changes occur, women in these groups will continue to receive second class care—or worse.

NOTES

The research for this paper was supported by the Faculty Research Funds of the University of California, Santa Cruz, and by a visiting scholar appointment at New York University. Editorial assistance from Adele Clarke, Lynn Jeffery, and Zoe Sodja is gratefully acknowledged.

1. California's primary state prison for women, built for 700, had a population of about 650 in 1974 and over 2,300 in 1989. The increase there and elsewhere is primarily the result of new and harsher sentencing laws.

REFERENCES

Anno, B. Jaye
    1977   Analysis of Inmate/Patient Profile Data: American Medical Association's Program to Improve Medical Care and Health Services in Jails. Washington: Blackstone.

Anno, B. Jaye, and Allen Lang
    1978   Analysis of Pilot Jail Post-Profile Data. Silver Spring, MD: B. Jaye Anno Associates.
Bell, Alan P., and Martin S. Weinberg
    1978   Homosexualities: A Study of Diversity among Men and Women. New York: Simon and Schuster.
Boston Lesbian Psychology Collective
    1987   Lesbian Psychologies. Urbana: University of Illinois Press.
Bradford, Judith, and Caitlin Ryan
    1988   The National Lesbian Health Care Survey (NLHCS). Washington: National Lesbian and Gay Health Foundation.
Chapman, Jane Roberts
    1980   "Criminal justice programs for women offenders." In Jane Roberts Chapman (ed.), Economic Realities and the Female Offender. Lexington, MA: Lexington Books.
Dilley, J. W.
    1984   "Treatment interventions and approaches to care of patients with acquired immune deficiency syndrome." Pp. 62–70 in Stuart Nichols and David Astrow (eds.), Psychiatric Implications of Acquired Immune Deficiency Syndrome. Washington: American Psychiatric Press.
Glick, Ruth, and Virginia Neto
    1976   National Study of Women's Correctional Programs. Washington: National Institute of Law Enforcement and Criminal Justice, Law Enforcement Assistance Administration, Department of Justice.
Guinan, Mary, and Ann Hardy
    1987   "Epidemiology of AIDS in women in the United States: 1981 through 1986." Journal of the American Medical Association 257(15):2039–42.
Haas, Ann Pollinger
    1994   "Lesbian health issues: an overview." Pp. 339–56 in Alice J. Dan (ed.), Reframing Women's Health: Multidisciplinary Research and Practice. Thousand Oaks, CA: Sage.
Henriques, Zelma
    1972   Imprisoned Mothers and Their Children. Lanham, MD: University Press of America.
Hitchcock, Jan
    1988   "Lesbian health." Women's Studies 17:61–73.
Hunter, N., S. E. Michaelson, and T. B. Stoddard
    1992   The Rights of Lesbians and Gay Men. Carbondale: Southern Illinois University Press.
Jones, David A.
    1976   Health Risks of Imprisonment. Lexington, MA: Heath.
Lorde, Audre
    1980   The Cancer Journals. San Francisco: Spinsters/Aunt Lute.

Macks, Judith
1988   "Psychosocial responses of people with AIDS/ARC." Pp. 49-61 in Angie
        Lewis (ed.), Nursing Care of the Person with AIDS/ARC. Rockville,
        MD: Aspen.
Maier, Catherine
1987   "Women with AIDS and ARC in San Francisco." Pp. 230-34 in Nancy
        Stoller Shaw (ed.), Women and AIDS Clinical Resource Guide. San
        Francisco: AIDS Foundation.
McCall, Carolyn, Nancy Stoller Shaw, and Jan Casteel
1985   Pregnancy in Prison: A Needs Assessment of Perinatal Outcome in Three
        California Penal Institutions. Sacramento: California Department of
        Health Services.
New York City AIDS Surveillance Unit
1989   Report. New York: City Department of Health.
Novick, Lloyd F., Richard Della-Penna, Melvin S. Schwartz, Elaine Remmlinger, and
Regina Loewenstein
1977   "Health status of the New York City prison population." Medical Care
        15(3):205-16.
O'Donnell, M., V. Loeffler, K. Pollock, and Z. Saunders
1979   Lesbian Health Matters! Santa Cruz, CA: Santa Cruz Women's Health
        Center.
Resnik, Judith, and Nancy Shaw
1980   "Prisoners of their sex: health problems of incarcerated women." Vol. 2,
        pp. 337-39 in Ira P. Robbins and Clark Boardman (eds.), Prisoners'
        Rights Sourcebook. New York: Clark Boardman.
Robertson, Patricia, and J. Schachter
1981   "Failure to identify venereal disease in a lesbian population." Sexually
        Transmitted Diseases 8:75-76.
Schneider, Beth E., and Nancy Stoller
1994   Women Resisting AIDS: Feminist Strategies of Empowerment. Philadel-
        phia: Temple University Press.
Shaw, Nancy
1985   "Eating more and enjoying it less: U.S. prison diets for women." Women
        and Health 10(1):39-57.
Shaw, Nancy Stoller, Irene Browne, and Peter Meyer
1981   "Sexism and medical care in a jail setting." Women and Health 6(1-
        2):5-24.
Stevens, P. E.
1992   "Lesbian health care research: a review of literature from 1970 to 1990."
        Health Care of Women International 13:91-120.
Thompson, Karen, and Julie Andrzejewski
1988   Why Can't Sharon Kowalski Come Home? San Francisco: Spin-
        sters/Aunt Lute.

U.S. Department of Health, Education, and Welfare

1977   General Considerations for the Evaluation of Drugs. HEW 77-3040. Washington: Department of Health and Human Services.

White, J., and W. Levinson

1993   "Primary care of lesbian patients." Journal of General and Internal Medicine 8:41-47.

Wyrick, J., and Charles Owens

1977   "Black women: income and incarceration." Pp. 85-92 in Charles Owens and Jimmy Bell (eds.), Blacks and Criminal Justice. Lexington, MA: Lexington Books.

[19]

"You Can Be Safer, But . . . ":
Different Women, Many Violences

Introduction

ADELE E. CLARKE AND LORA BEX LEMPERT

One of the major areas of feminist activism during the second wave has been violence against women. Year after year, starting in the late 1960s, different kinds of violence against women have been documented and placed on the agenda for discussion, analysis, and organized social action. To put some of the complexities of these issues in perspective, the following six minichapters speak to women's lived experiences of abuse and rape, issues in the battered women's movement, and the politics of rape, sexual harassment, and violence against lesbians.

Together the authors here offer their perspectives on violence against women, emphasizing the differences and complexities of women's health problems. Violence against women is not a singular phenomenon, but many different phenomena which, moreover, take place in many radically different contexts and situations. We no longer collapse women of color into a single category called "nonwhite" as was the case just twenty years ago. Nor do we even today collapse reproductive technologies (from contraception to artificial insemination to in vitro fertilization) together. Instead, we address them separately as they are technologies with different dynamics in terms of variously situated women. Similarly, we can no longer collapse the many kinds of violence against women together. The papers here address how differences of race, class, age, abledness, and sexuality are manifest in each form of violence against women and how women's experiences are similar.

Included here are two topics barely touched on elsewhere as yet. Britton powerfully assesses the battered women's movement in terms of race and class differences among both providers and clients that are agonizingly real to those involved. And von Schulthess addresses violence against lesbians, noting how it can link up with more generalized violence against women, especially in public places. Further, we have women's own voices presented by both Lempert and Pickels. All women's voices will never sound the same—even screaming. Nor should they, nor should our responses to them be the same.

Violence against women, and fears and threats of violence, are significant health and social problems that affect all social groups, all ages, and all races, including rural and urban women, heterosexuals, lesbians, bisexuals, rich and poor, abled and disabled. Dr. Helen Rodriguez-Trias, former president of the American Public Health Association, noted the magnitude of this problem in an editorial in the *American Journal of Public Health* (1992:663): "Assaults by husbands, ex-husbands and lovers cause more injuries to women than motor vehicle accidents, rape and muggings combined."

The different types of violence have various health consequences in terms of increased visits to physicians, physical and emotional trauma, and use of alcohol and drugs that can further disrupt women's physical and psychological health. For example, in this country a woman is battered every fifteen seconds, and one in five women probably experiences serious battering incidents each year (Worcester 1993). Violence is the second leading cause of injury to women of all ages and the leading cause of injury to women between the ages of fifteen and forty-four (Grisso et al. 1991). More than four thousand women are killed each year in the United States in "intimate assaults" (Royner 1991). Studies of hospital emergency department visits show that 22–35 percent of women were seeking services for acute consequences of partner abuse (Randall 1990). Ironically, it is trusted family members and partners who pose the greatest threats to women's health and safety (Council on Scientific Affairs 1992:3184; Flitcraft 1992). The most dangerous place for women is home.

Battery of pregnant women is particularly common. The 1985 National Family Violence Survey, for example, found 15 percent of pregnant women were assaulted by their partners in the first four months of pregnancy and 17 percent during the last five months (Helton et al. 1987). McFarlane (1991) reported 26 percent of pregnant teens were involved with a man who physically harmed them and 40–60 percent said that the assaults had begun or escalated with the pregnancy. Pregnant victims of partner violence face particularly serious medical risks including preterm labor, miscarriage, placental separation, antepartum hemorrhage, fetal fractures, and rupture of the uterus, liver, or spleen (Saltzman 1990).

Rape also has fundamental health consequences. Koss and colleagues (1990) found that rape victim visits to physicians increased 18 percent in the year of assault, 56 percent in the following year, and 31 percent in the year after. Today most cities and counties have some kind of antirape and victim assistance programs, often started by feminists. Most hospital emergency departments have developed rape protocols.

Recognizing that violence against women is routine and extensive, the medical profession has come to define it as a serious health problem. The June 1992 issue of the *Journal of the American Medical Association* was devoted to this problem. The AMA has also initiated a Physicians' Campaign against Family Violence to develop protocols for detection and management (Council on Ethical and Judicial Affairs 1992; Council on Scientific Affairs 1992; Flitcraft 1992; Novello 1992). Although improved medical attention to violence is important, some programs have also come under heavy criticism, such as forced reporting to police by medical personnel, which can seriously endanger women further when their partners find out or which may discourage women from seeking medical help in the first place (e.g., Stark and Flitcraft 1996).

The reduction of violent and abusive behavior has also become a major focus of the Healthy People 2000 objectives (U.S. Department of Health and Human Services 1991), and initiatives against all kinds of violence are proliferating. Because such violence continues at frightening levels in all spheres of American life, it will likely remain a national health issue for some time, costly in numerous ways, especially in women's suffering. But as we shall see, women also successfully resist violence of all kinds, and we are learning not only how to alleviate it but also how to heal from it.

REFERENCES

Council on Ethical and Judicial Affairs
> 1992 "Physicians and domestic violence: ethical considerations." Journal of the American Medical Association 267:3190-93.

Council on Scientific Affairs
> 1992 "Violence against women: relevance for medical practitioners." Journal of the American Medical Association 267:3184-89.

Flitcraft, Anne H.
> 1992 "Violence, values, and gender." Journal of the American Medical Association 267:3194-95.

Grisso, J. A., A. Wisher, D. F. Schwarz, B. A. Weene, J. H. Holmes, and R. L. Sutton
> 1991 "A population-based study of injuries in inner-city women." American Journal of Epidemiology 134:59-68.

Helton, A., J. McFarlane, and E. Anderson
> 1987 "Battered and pregnant: a prevalence study." American Journal of Public Health 77:1337-39.

Koss, Mary P., P. Koss, and W. J. Woodruff
    1990   "Relations of criminal victimization to health perceptions among women medical patients." Journal of Consulting Clinical Psychology 58:147-52.
McFarlane, Judith
    1991   "Violence during teen pregnancy: health consequences for mother and child." Pp. 136-41 in Barrie Levy (ed.), Dating Violence. Seattle: Seal Press.
Novello, Antonia C.
    1992   "From the Surgeon General." Journal of the American Medical Association 267:3132.
Randall, T.
    1990   "Domestic violence intervention calls for more than treating injuries." Journal of the American Medical Association 264:939-40.
Rodriguez-Trias, Helen
    1992   "Women's health, women's lives, women's rights." American Journal of Public Health 82:663-64.
Royner, S.
    1991   "Battered wives: centuries of silence." Washington Post, 20 August, 7.
Saltzman, L. E.
    1990   "Battering during pregnancy: a role for physicians." Atlanta Medicine 64:45-48.
Stark, E., and A. Flitcraft
    1996   Women at Risk: Domestic Violence and Women's Health. Thousand Oaks, CA: Sage.
Department of Health and Human Services
    1991   Healthy People 2000: National Health Promotion and Disease Prevention Objectives. DHHS Pub. No. (PHS) 91-50212. Washington: Government Printing Office.
Worcester, Nancy
    1993   "A more hidden crime: adolescent battered women." Pp. 15-20 in Nancy Worcester and Mariamne H. Whatley (eds.), Women's Health: Readings on Social, Economic, and Political Issues. Dubuque, IA: Kendall/Hunt.

Women's Lived Experiences of Abuse

LORA BEX LEMPERT

Abuse of women is simultaneously a political issue, a health question, a social problem, and a personal problem, as it typifies the social control of women, usually by men but also sometimes by female partners. Men in general have more social authority and power—physical, economic, and political—than women, which enables them to impose and enforce their interpretations of reality on others. Further, in abusive male-female situations, many elements—inability to escape, lack of economic independence, ineffective law enforcement policies, diminution in self-confidence—render women even more susceptible to male control (Gordon 1988).

Presented here are accounts from women who speak as experts of their own experiences of being physically, psychologically, and/or emotionally battered by their male partners. Their poignant stories, which narrate the evolution of abuse in intimate relationships problematically characterized by the *simultaneity* of love and violence, come from my research on wife abuse within heterosexual unions (Lempert 1992, 1994, 1995).[1] In the phenomenological sense, their voices serve as exemplars from whom we can learn and come to understand (Chamberlain 1990).

Language and Control

Lucinda, a white thirty-seven-year-old unemployed mother of two, echoes the experiences of others as she speaks retrospectively about authority in her former relationship:

> There was a whole lot of control going on that I really wasn't even aware of, or, how can I put it? I'd be aware of it sometimes, but he has such control and he was so good at it that I'd feel guilty for feeling like he was controlling me. Instead, I'd say, "No, wait a minute, you know he's not controlling me and I'm not doing enough," you know. It just sort of built up gradually until I couldn't quite, you know, figure out what was what. Um, the crazy, it's real crazy making. (Lempert 1992)

Abusers typically characterize their partners as cunts, whores, bitches, career woman hags, and so on. These epithets reflect broad social characterizations of women, but they are also particular attacks on individual women in their social locations vis-à-vis these men.

Husband-and-wife interactions, unlike most social roles with limited activity, cover wide varieties of continuous contact. Eating, sleeping, playing, and sexual activity are filled with unremitting intimacy. Even if women are employed outside the home, the potential for them to gain perspectives to counter those put forth by their abusers is limited if women's significant identities remain embedded in their relationships.

Because their partners are *the* significant others in their lives, the women in this study accord considerable legitimacy to the men's characterizations of them. These terms of derogation then become more than just features of women's lives with abusive men; they begin to constitute the contextual frames of their worlds. Publicly, most of the women acquiesce to the characterizations; privately, "deep down," they resist. The verbal control that abusive men assume, even as the women attempt to resist the denigrating characterizations, presages the overt physical violence that later permeates the couples' lives together.

In response to the characterizations and to the initial incidents of physical violence, women may consciously modify their usual actions to alter the men's characterizations thereby engaging in what Tifft (1993:33) has called "self-deconstructive behaviors." They act hesitatingly and they stop "activity in a lot of volunteer work and other community things," "friendships," "going to the gym," "taking the bus," "going to the store," and so on. Most do not report telling anyone about the abuse, and most do not report asking for help. Instead, they reconstruct violent episodes to make their realities and the abusers' actions correspond to their own expectations of love, marriage, and family.

Male partners are also reported to have defined both the verbal and physical assaults as nonviolent and as victim provoked. For reasons of personal safety, the women do not overtly contest the men's definitions; instead, they tacitly accept causal responsibility for the violence. Self-blame saturates their experiences, but it becomes increasingly untenable as the abuse continues. Rachel, a white forty-one-year-old landscape planner, articulates experiences reported by others:

> During that last year too I really tried to make it work. It was important to him that I cook dinner. So I made sure that I cooked dinner for him every evening. He'd come, he'd eat, he'd go back to the office which was, ah, two blocks away. So I really tried. I thought, well, it's me, I'm not pleasing him. So I tried to really be a good wife. I won't take as many classes. I'll really concentrate on making the marriage work. I'll keep the house really clean and I'll do his laundry and I'll cook him his meals and I'll do everything to make him happy so that he won't be unhappy anymore. And his problem will go away. And ha ha, you know, I mean it doesn't matter what you've done. They're still, they're still going to find something to explode about. (Lempert 1992)

Because violence ensures acquiescence, if not agreement, abusive males further attempt to impose their control over their intimate partners by preventing them from thinking critically about themselves as persons with separate identities (Tifft 1993; Lempert 1995). Lynette, a white forty-one-year-old fashion designer married to a foreign national, recounts the authority present in these control processes:

> And he came home and he walked in the door and he said, "What are you doing?" I said, "I'm drinking this can of Coke. I just finished cleaning the apartment." And whenever he said, "What are you doing?" there was a tone in his voice I knew I was in trouble, you know, it was like I knew it. And I couldn't figure out what I'd done. Immediately I go through this mental checklist—what did I do, am I wearing the wrong clothes, is something on the floor, is the cat in the wrong place, am I in the wrong place, you know, and I couldn't figure out what it was that I had done. I've done something. I don't know what it is. Well, it was the Coke. And he flew into a rage. "What a selfish, fucking asshole you are drinking the last Coke. How could you do that?" (Lempert 1992)

By focusing such intense criticism on the nonproblematic, taken-for-granted aspects of women's lives, abusive men effectively deny their partners safety, "sanity," and personhood.

Violence as Cause or Consequence

In trying to make sense of the violence that appears to be otherwise uncalled for (Johnson and Ferraro 1984), abused women ascribe motives for their partners' actions that include personal incompetencies imputed by their abusive partners, as well as the men's own situational difficulties, personal inadequacies, and unresolved personal issues. Yet such motivational explanations can also paradoxically be minimizing strategies (Mills 1985). That is, they can allow women to create potentially dangerous illusions of control and identities for themselves. Two such classic stories are "I am strong, he is weak" or "I can handle it" and that the violence will end if the situation causing it changes. In these constructions, the focus shifts away from violence as cause to violence as consequence of something else, that is, something that the women can remediate. ("I'll be a better wife." "I'll stop taking classes." "I'll stay home.")

As Lynette, Rachel, and Lucinda demonstrate, these minimizing strategies can also lessen women's control over their lives and lead to feelings of inadequacy, vulnerability, and incompetency (Baruch et al. 1983). Precisely because the problem of the men's violence is not addressed directly, either individually or socially, it is interpreted as both personal and idiosyncratic. ("I thought it was my fault." "I worked a full-time job, and he wasn't working." "He's a workaholic.") Abused women are caught between simultaneous, yet contradictory, beliefs. They see their partners as their sole sources of intimate love and affection, yet their partners remain the most dangerous persons in their lives. Alissa, a white thirty-four-year-old Air Force lieutenant in the process of divorce, movingly captures this contradiction: "He was, like, my best friend, you know—it's kind of like, beat the dog, and then pat it, you know—I don't know how you explain it, you know, it's like, he is your best friend, the person that you rely on for all the affection that you're gonna get" (Lempert 1992). Even after repeated violent episodes, abused women may continue to cling to their prior expectations of love and family. If they don't, the violence challenges the foremost assumptions of their lives, requires too much change too soon, and in the end they lose their identities. They are no longer loving wives but "victims." The men are no longer loving husbands but "assailants" (Denzin 1984). Darlene, a thirty-one-year-old African American administrative assistant, retrospectively illustrates the complex nature of this process:

> You still assume [after a violent event] that, that for the most part you are, your person is your own and that you are safe. And I, and I realize now that that's, that's a very essential survival instinct for most of us because if you don't think you're safe, you can't function. And that's what I couldn't do, I couldn't function, I couldn't. . . . I mean you can't, you can't function on a day-to-day basis and think that somebody's . . . maybe somebody's gonna come around the corner and still going to be as violently angry with you and do something to you. I felt, you know, like Bambi's mother. [laugh] I don't know. Don't walk out in the fields. (Lempert 1992)

Because American culture values the family as a kind, loving, and supportive haven (Mintz and Kellogg 1988), abused women initially represent their relationships as nonviolent and harmonious, what Tifft (1993) has called a "fiction of intimacy." Rachel explains the social shame motivating this masking process:

> Afterwards you feel ashamed that it happened. When you allow yourself to become a part of an abusive situation like that, you lose your identity. You become—your job is to be an extension of that person. And to help them deal with their problems and that's it. So I was ashamed of what had happened. I was ashamed that it was even going on. I wanted to pretend that it hadn't happened. I wanted to forget that it had ever happened. It was a mistake. It was just one of those things that happen in a marriage that was never going to happen again. (Lempert 1992)

Maintaining the invisibility of the violence is a face-saving strategy (Lester 1984), a way for abused women to maintain their social selves. Yet in preventing the men's abusive behavior from becoming public, the women simultaneously veil their own experiences of violence. Ironically, when women do begin telling others, they often find themselves trapped by their previous presentations. Their new descriptions are often challenged or denied by those who earlier accepted the "fiction of intimacy" (Tifft 1993).

Informal Help-Seeking and Help-Provision

A severe physical assault may unintentionally end this "fiction" as Rachel continues to explain:

> The first time I said anything to anybody was when he kicked me and hit me in the hip, when he kicked me in the hip, which really was the beginning of the end. I didn't go see [a doctor] right away. I thought it would just get better, and it did get better, but it didn't completely get well. And so I went to see him about a month and a half after it happened. And he was being funny when he entered the room and said to me, "Don't tell me your husband stepped on your foot again." And that was like the wrong thing to say because I just started crying. I just started crying. And he looked at me and he said, "You're having trouble with this guy, aren't you?" And I said yes. So then he knew. He knew. (Lempert 1992)

As the violence escalates from verbal to physical abuse, it becomes the most salient feature of these relationships. It may also become the catalyst for seeking help. For most women, seeking and receiving help from family and friends is taken for granted (Gerstel and Gross 1989; Belenky et al. 1986; Baruch et al. 1983; Hochschild 1983; Gilligan 1982). These interactions are only partly conscious and develop without deliberate attention unless they are unusual, repeated, and/or inconvenient. Seeking and providing assistance for a violent relationship involves precisely the unexpected, the recurrent, and the inconvenient.

When abused women do summon the courage to reveal their experiences to friends and family, they report that the experiences of violence become less "painful." Rhonda, a white thirty-two-year-old securities executive, articulates the effects of both abuser control and help from friends:

> One thing is that I don't think I really knew what was going on, and it really, there was so much anger inside of me that talking was a way to keep things on an even keel. Besides, he isolated me and always isolated me and always told me everything I did was wrong. And it helped to get feedback from other people to see that this man is the one who's doing it and not me. Because he really had me convinced that it was all me for a while there. (Lempert 1992)

Telling other people helps to end the invisibility and reduces the experiences of isolation and loneliness. The violent experiences are shared and reinterpreted, often in conformity with the women's own assessments. In seeking help, abused women want fundamental validation of their own perceptions of reality to counter their partners' continuous attempts to invalidate them. Affirmation by outsiders helps women to reinterpret the violence and the relationships.

Women often expect others to listen, to help them to interpret their experiences, but not to impose their own interpretations (Tannen 1990). Abused women, in particular, do not want to be defined by their experiences of violence. They do not want to be "battered wives," literally or figuratively (Denzin 1984; Loseke 1987). Abusive relationships are not *always* abusive. Violent partners are also described as warm, loving, nurturing, and romantic. It is this complexity and the contradictions inherent in simultaneous love and violence that are essential to understanding abuse in intimate relationships.

Helpers may unknowingly simplify these complicated relationships by reducing them to the incidents of violence and, consequently, reducing the women to "victims." Although they are victims of particular acts of violence, abused women are also actively evaluating, interpreting, negotiating, and perhaps loving their partners. Attributing victim status to the women leads helpers to view them as incapable of understanding or managing their own situations (Loseke 1992).

Friends, family, and coworkers are then justified in offering advice or stepping in to help them manage. As a consequence, abused women again lose control over the interpretations of their experiences and over their relationships with their partners (Loseke 1992; Loseke and Cahill 1984). This time the loss is to helpers instead of abusers. Celestine, a thirty-nine-year-old African American transit dispatcher, details the complicated effects of well-intentioned assistance as well as her own strategy for maintaining a measure of control:

> It wasn't helpful for her [cousin] to have me feel guilty, to lay some of the guilt trips on me that she did, and I think she was attempting, I think I understand why she did it, but it certainly didn't feel good. . . . She was trying to force my hand, and to her that was a good way of doing it, but it didn't serve me well at all to have her do that, and it didn't help to have people try to be therapists when they're not therapists. . . . I heard some of that and "you oughta," so I got all of these, you know, these bedside therapists, these shade tree therapists, who were telling me how to handle the situation that I was in, and I couldn't tell them, I didn't tell them everything that was going on, so they didn't know the whole story. (Lempert 1992)

When women can tell their stories to others who provide nonjudgmental support, they can begin to regain control of their lives and can make their own decisions regarding their future safety (Worcester 1992). Celestine continues:

> If I could bounce it off of somebody else who could listen and not be judgmental and not process me to the point of, God, I feel worse after talking to them because I'm feeling guilty. . . . I don't know how to get out of this relationship and just cut it off because I have some love—I love him and it's not good for me, it's not healthy . . . and I don't want to be controlled, and

yeah, yeah, and I don't want to commit to a man like that.
(Lempert 1992)

As Celestine and the others indicated, violent interpersonal relationships, like all others, are complex. Violence may be the context within which daily interactions occur, but it is not the only context. Abused women may hate the abuse but still love their abusers.

Conclusion

Abuse in intimate relationships creates simultaneous, yet contradictory, frames of love and violence. Abused women live in situations of competing interpretations where men assert their power to define and where violence ensures women's acquiescence, if not agreement. Women in these relationships struggle to understand the ambiguities of love and violence, that is, if he loves me, why does he hit me? As they accept responsibility, provide explanations, and/or deny the violence, they unwittingly participate in fictions that secure the violence in the relationships (Denzin 1984; Tifft 1993). Telling others shatters the fictions and facilitates reconstructions of the actions and of the relationships. Helping women to define themselves in more positive ways empowers them by validating their experiences and the meanings they attach to them.

NOTE

1. Insofar as abuse exists within homosexual unions and between generations, the processes outlined here of concurrent love and violence may sensitize concerned individuals to analogous practices in other intimate relationships. Clearly, more research is needed on these other contexts to understand and effectively assist all abused women.

REFERENCES

Baruch, Grace, Rosalind Barnett, and Carol Rivers
    1983   Lifeprints: New Patterns of Love and Work for Today's Women. New York: New American Library.
Belenky, Mary Field, Blythe McVicker Clinchy, Nancy Rule Goldberger, and Jill Mattuck Tarule
    1986   Women's Ways of Knowing. New York: Basic Books.

Chamberlain, D. F.
    1990   Narrative Perspective in Fiction: A Phenomenological Mediation of
            Reader, Text, and World. Toronto: University of Toronto Press.
Denzin, Norman K.
    1984   "Toward a phenomenology of domestic, family violence." American Jour-
            nal of Sociology 90:483–513.
Gerstel, Naomi, and Harriet Engel Gross
    1989   "Women and the American family: continuity and change." Pp. 89–120
            in Jo Freeman (ed.), Women: A Feminist Perspective. Mountain View,
            CA: Mayfield.
Gilligan, Carol
    1982   In a Different Voice. Cambridge: Harvard University Press.
Gordon, Linda
    1988   Heroes of Their Own Lives: The Politics and History of Family Violence
            in Boston, 1880–1960. New York: Penguin Books.
Hochschild, Arlie
    1983   The Managed Heart. Berkeley: University of California Press.
Johnson, John M., and Kathleen J. Ferraro
    1984   "The victimized self: the case of battered women." Pp. 119–30 in Joseph
            Kotarba and Andrea Fontana (eds.), The Existential Self in Society.
            Chicago: University of Chicago Press.
Lempert, Lora Bex
    1992   The Crucible: Violence, Help-Seeking, and Abused Women's Transfor-
            mations of Self. Unpublished dissertation. Department of Social and
            Behavioral Sciences, School of Nursing, University of California, San
            Francisco.
    1994   "A narrative analysis of abuse: connecting the personal, the rhetorical,
            and the structural." Journal of Contemporary Ethnography 22:411–41.
    1995   "The line in the sand: definitional dialogues in abusive relationships."
            Studies in Symbolic Interaction 18:15–20.
Lester, M.
    1984   "Self: Sociological Portraits." Pp. 18–68 in Joseph Kotarba and Andrea
            Fontana (eds.), The Existential Self in Society. Chicago: University of
            Chicago Press.
Loseke, Donileen
    1987   "Lived realities and the construction of social problems: the case of wife
            abuse." Symbolic Interaction 10:229–43.
    1992   The Battered Woman and Shelters. Albany: State University of New
            York Press.
Loseke, Donileen, and Spencer Cahill
    1984   "The social construction of deviance: experts on battered women." Social
            Problems 31:296–310.
Mills, Trudy
    1985   "The assault on the self: stages in coping with battering husbands." Qual-
            itative Sociology 8:103–23.

Mintz, Steven, and Susan Kellogg
    1988   Domestic Revolutions. New York: Free Press.
Tannen, Deborah
    1990   You Just Don't Understand. New York: Ballantine Books.
Tifft, Larry L.
    1993   Battering of Women. New York: Harper and Row.
Worcester, Nancy
    1992   "The unique role health workers can play in recognizing and responding
            to battered women." National Women's Health Network News
            (Mar./Apr.):1–5.

The Battered Women's Movement

BRANDY M. BRITTON

Hotlines for rape victims and shelters for battered women are common today in the United States, but such organizations are relatively new. Before the 1970s, the issues of woman battering and domestic violence received little public attention and there were few agencies to serve victims. Today's nationwide network of shelters, hotlines, and other services for battered women and rape victims resulted from women's coalition building and political organizing (Britton 1993; Schechter 1982; Tierney 1982). This is a brief history of the battered women's movement, the activists' struggles, and the problematics and challenges that activists face.

Although domestic violence, like rape, has existed for centuries, it has not always been considered a social problem. Historically, "wife" or partner abuse was tolerated and even encouraged as an effective and necessary means of "keeping women in line" (Yllo and Bogard 1988).[1] In the United States before the emergence of the battered women's movement, woman battering was generally tolerated or ignored, viewed as a "private" matter between a husband and wife and not as a public issue (Schechter 1982; Stark, Flitcraft, and Frazier 1979; Tierney 1982).

Rise of the Battered Women's Movement

During the 1970s through the efforts of the emergent battered women's movement, the issue of wife abuse began to receive widespread public attention in mass media.[2] For the first time in the United States, activists

joined with formerly battered women to establish services explicitly designed for victims of domestic violence and their children. Operating with
little money and staffed primarily by volunteers, crisis hotlines and shelters for battered women began to appear. The first known shelter in the
United States opened in Arizona in 1973. Five years later, 170 shelters
aided battered women, and by 1991, over 1,000 shelters were in operation
across the country.

Woman battering also captured researchers' attention. Activists' state
and national lobbying efforts pushed domestic violence into the policy
arena as well. Protective laws that made spouse abuse a crime and other
laws mandating the availability of temporary restraining orders to protect
victims were enacted through activists' efforts.

The battered women's movement had its roots in three social movements already under way that embraced women's autonomy and personal
freedom: the women's liberation, women's health, and antirape movements (Britton 1993; Tierney 1982). The battered women's movement
was able to draw on the other movements' established communication
networks and political organizations.

Problematics and Challenges

Although the battered women's movement has been successful in a number
of arenas, activists have also encountered resistance and disappointments.
Because the issue of domestic violence was framed as a "women's" issue and
because activists called for fundamental changes in gender relations, some
groups did not receive the movement well. Conservative groups and state's
rights actors such as the New Right and certain Republican Party representatives resisted and even actively campaigned against movement goals such
as shelters and the empowerment of women (Britton 1993; Davis and
Hagen 1988; Ryan 1992). These groups, which have gained political
strength since the 1980s, have sought to reinforce traditional gender relations rather than to empower women; their programs include assaults on
abortion rights, affirmative action legislation, and shelter funding.

Although many laws have been passed that make woman battering
illegal, police often refuse to arrest perpetrators, and in many cases they
arrest the victim instead to discourage them from seeking help through
law enforcement (Britton 1993, 1995). One activist in the battered
women's movement explained: "The police department here is trying to
teach us a lesson. Some of the officers don't agree with the mandatory

arrest policy, and they let us know by refusing to arrest or arresting the victim instead. One [police officer] told me, 'Hey . . . you want me to take someone in, I'll take someone in, but it's gonna be her.' We need the police on our side. . . . They still have a lot of decision making power in these situations" (Britton 1993:100).

Health care institutions and practitioners such as the medical profession and social workers have also proved problematic for battered women and for the movement. Although health care personnel finally began to take the issue of domestic violence seriously, the medical profession has also sought to control the "treatment" of battered women (Bowker and Maurer 1987; Kurz and Stark 1988; Stark, Flitcraft, and Frazier 1979). Some medical treatment for battered women includes medicating them with addictive sedatives and psychiatric intervention aimed at discovering common psychological pathologies among victims of domestic violence. Battered women's advocates criticize both "treatments": sedatives simply mask symptoms of abuse, and psychiatric treatment aimed at discovering personal characteristics of the victim that "caused" her to tolerate abuse indirectly blames her for her own victimization. Both deflect attention from the underlying social relations that create and perpetuate domestic violence. Thus both unwittingly legitimate violence against women as a means of social control of women.

Other challenges have come from within the battered women's movement itself, including conflicts over scarce resources (Britton 1993; Schechter 1982). Issues of diversities among women have also persistently plagued the movement. Which women will be allowed into one shelter? Are battered women who drink or use drugs to be automatically excluded, as many funding sources specify? Where *can* they go?

Further, women of color have critically noted the lack of attention to wife abuse in their communities. They point to the movement's failure to address women of color's issues of economic survival. Problems of economic survival are often magnified for immigrant and refugee women who are in abusive relationships. Language barriers and the undocumented status of these women make them particularly vulnerable during the help-seeking process. These women may fear deportation if they seek refuge in a battered women's shelter. Some shelters will not house these women because of restrictions imposed by shelter funding agencies (Family Violence Prevention Fund 1992).

Lesbian activists in the battered women's movement have faced homophobia and marginalization by other activists and by some of the battered women they serve (Britton 1993). Although lesbian women played a major role in establishing the movement, little attention has been given to the issue of battering in lesbian communities. Although violence between lesbians or "lesbian battering" is nowhere near as common as wife or partner abuse, services for victims in these situations are crucial, as there are few public institutions available to them for help of any kind (Kahuna 1990; Lobel 1986; Margolies and Leeder 1995). A lesbian activist with years of experience in the battered women's movement summarized the marginalization of lesbian battering and seeming lack of appreciation for lesbian activists' work:

> I know it [lesbian battering] is a tough issue for the movement, but ignoring it hasn't helped us any. Certainly it hasn't helped the victims, but it also hurts the movement. Lesbians become isolated and marginal to a movement that has been a big part of our community. We have a lot to offer, and have been around in the movement for a long time and have lots of experience with activism. And yet, some of us are feeling pushed out now, like we're not wanted anymore. "Thanks for the help," and when we ask for something in return, as women, as lesbians, of women—from our "sisters," we are turned away. (Britton 1993:233)

Class issues among activists have also led to strife within the movement. Increasing pressure from state and federal agencies that fund shelters to hire only women with college degrees to serve in these organizations led some activists with years of experience working in the movement to feel marginalized. One activist articulated this problem:

> It seems like things are going downhill in the [battered women's] movement in some ways. Things are getting more competitive and less cooperative with women. I know a woman who works in the movement at a different agency than mine. They told them they all had to get college degrees from now on to work there. . . . Her whole agency, they were required to get certain credentials to hold their positions. And she, after being there for several years, had to leave because she didn't have that credential. And this was a woman with tremendous experience in the movement . . . and she was a formerly battered woman . . . and she had to go. She was forced out. It makes me want to leave the movement myself. (Britton 1993:211)

As a result of these conflicts, the battered women's movement has increasingly adopted addressing issues of diversity among activists and among victims as a movement goal. The National Coalition Against Domestic Violence (NCADV), the main political organizing body for the movement in the United States, has made diversity a top priority and provides resources to facilitate implementing this (MacKenzie 1994). The sixteenth annual NCADV conference, "Many Voices, One Vision," was devoted to fostering diversity within the movement.

Women's shelters now reach out to underserved and historically marginalized groups of women, including African Americans, Asians, Latinas, and immigrants and refugees. Some shelters have also incorporated services for battered lesbians and for deaf and physically disabled women.

The battered women's movement has made tremendous strides toward redressing violence against women by advocating social change and by establishing services for victims of domestic violence. Attending to issues of diversity among activists and among victims will help to build stronger foundations from which to provide help to battered women and their children and to understand the underlying issues around male violence toward women in American society.

NOTES

1. In nineteenth-century England, for example, districts were named after the chosen method of disciplining one's wife. Severe beating, kicking, and burning were common and accepted practices (Stark, Flitcraft, and Frazier 1979). In fact, the common phrase "rule of thumb" originated in England as a "humanitarian" law to limit the severity of beatings inflicted upon wives by their husbands. A husband was not allowed to beat his wife with a switch any thicker than his thumb.

2. This growing attention included not only news but television movies and classic books such as Del Martin's widely acclaimed work *Battered Wives* (1977), *Violence against Wives* by Dobash and Dobash (1979), and *The Battered Woman* (1979) by Lenore Walker.

REFERENCES

Bowker, Lee H., and Lorie Maurer
    1987   "The medical treatment of battered wives." Women and Health 12:25–45.
Britton, Brandy M.
    1993   The Battered Women's Movement in the United States, c1973–1993: A

Micro-Macro Analysis. Ph.D. diss., Department of Social and Behavioral Sciences, School of Nursing, University of California San Francisco.

1995   "'So I ended up losing his baby': experiences of partner violence among pregnant drug addicts." Research presentation, University of Maryland, Baltimore County.

Davis, Liane V., and Jan L. Hagen

1988   "Services for battered women: the public policy response." Social Service Review (Dec.):649–67.

Dobash, Rebecca, and Russell Dobash

1979   Violence against Wives: The Case against Patriarchy. New York: Free Press.

Family Violence Prevention Fund

1992   "Domestic violence in the immigrant community." National Women's Health Network (July/August).

Kahuna, Valli

1990   "Compounding the triple jeopardy: battering in lesbian of color relationships." Women and Therapy 9:169–84.

Kurz, Demie, and Evan Stark

1988   "Not-so-benign neglect: the medical response to battering." Pp. 249–66 in Kersti Yllo and Michelle Bograd (eds.), Feminist Perspectives on Wife Abuse. Newbury Park, CA: Sage.

Lobel, Kerry, ed.

1986   Naming the Violence: Speaking Out about Lesbian Battering. Seattle: Seal Press.

MacKenzie, Eileen

1994   "Many voices: one vision." NCADV Voice (spring). Washington.

Margolies, Liz, and Elaine Leeder

1995   "Violence at the door: treatment of lesbian batterers." Violence against Women 1:139–57.

Martin, Del

1977   Battered Wives. San Francisco: Glide.

Ryan, Barbara

1992   Feminism and the Women's Movement: Dynamics of Change in Social Movement, Ideology, and Activism. New York: Routledge.

Schechter, Susan

1982   Women and Male Violence. Boston: South End Press.

Stark, Evan, Anne Flitcraft, and William Frazier

1979   "Medicine and patriarchal violence: the social construction of a 'private' event." Pp. 177–209 in Elizabeth Fee (ed.), The Politics of Sex in Medicine. Farmingdale, NY: Baywood Press.

Tierney, Kathleen J.

1982   "The battered women movement and the creation of the wife beating problem." Social Problems 29:207–20.

Walker, Lenore

1979   The Battered Woman. New York: Harper and Row.

Yllo, Kersti, and Michelle Bograd
    1988   Feminist Perspectives on Wife Abuse. Newbury Park, CA: Sage.

Rape

BRANDY M. BRITTON

Rape, like other forms of violence against women, has not always been considered a legitimate social problem. Although sexual assault of women was widespread in the United States before 1960, women's activism and antirape movements of the 1960s and 1970s brought rape into the public and political arena (Matthews 1995; Schechter 1982). Here are explored the incidence and prevalence of rape, the contexts within which women are most often assaulted, and the criminal justice response to rape and to victims. Also considered are the impacts that sexual assault has upon victims and theories about the social and cultural origins of rape.

Because definitions of rape vary within the legal community and lay public (Bourque 1989), there is no standard definition. Considerable variation exists in rape laws and in the interpretations and enforcement of statutes. The amount of force or coercion used, the relationship of the victim to the assailant, and the characteristics of the victim and of the assailant have each and all been factors in decisions concerning rape. Generally, rape includes any nonconsensual sexual activity. A more specific definition is "nonconsensual oral, anal, or vaginal penetration obtained by force, by threat of bodily harm, or when the victim is incapable of giving consent" (Koss 1993b:1062).

Although men can also be the victims of sexual assault, especially in prison, rape is a crime perpetrated primarily by men against women. Studies of both reported and nonreported rapes have found that more than 90 percent of rape victims in the United States are female (U.S. Department of Justice 1991a). Regardless of the sex of the victim, 97 percent of the assailants are male (U.S. Department of Justice 1991b). Cultural stereotypes dating back to slavery, which construct rape as a crime perpetrated by black men against white women (Collins 1993; Davis 1983), are not supported by research, which has found that 93 percent of sexual assaults are intraracial (U.S. Department of Justice 1988).

It is difficult to estimate the incidence and prevalence of rape in the

United States because many victims do not define the assault as rape per se and only 20–54 percent of all victims report the crime to the police (Koss 1993b; *New York Times* 1992; Warshaw 1988). Official statistics on the incidence of rape such as the FBI Uniform Crime Report include only those assaults reported to authorities.[1]

A recent study that relied on victims' accounts rather than on re-ported cases indicated that more than a million women are raped each year in the United States (National Victims Center 1992).[2] More than half of all rapes take place before the victim is eighteen years old, and over one-fourth occur before the victim is eleven years old (U.S. Department of Justice 1991b). Older women are also victims of rape, including women over the age of sixty-five. In terms of prevalence, it is estimated that one in three women in the United States will be raped in her lifetime (Quina and Carlson 1989).

Contexts

Rape occurs in various social contexts. Despite popular myths, few rapes are perpetrated by strangers in dark alleys. Women are far more likely to be sexually assaulted by someone they know, a casual acquaintance, date, husband, partner, or former partner, than by strangers, who account for less than 20 percent of all incidents (Koss 1988). Nearly nine out of ten victims in a study of 3,107 college women were raped by someone they knew — 76 percent were raped by a date and 9 percent by family members.[3]

"Marital" rape in which a woman is sexually assaulted by her husband is also common. Diana Russell's (1990) pathbreaking research found that one in seven married women had been raped by their husbands — often violently and repeatedly. Marital or date rapes, in which the woman knows the attacker, are particularly problematic for the victims, who often blame themselves for the attack and fear retaliation if they report the incidents. Further, the violation of trust that accompanies marital or date rape is often devastating for women. One victim of marital rape explains: "My whole body was being abused. I feel if I'd been raped by a stranger I could have dealt with it a whole lot better. . . . When a stranger does it, he doesn't know me, I don't know him. He's not doing it to me as a person, personally. With your husband it becomes personal. You say, 'This man knows me. He knows my feelings. He knows me intimately, and then to do this to me — it's such a personal abuse'" (quoted in Finkelhor and Yllo 1985:118). The criminal justice system is often apathetic about rape charges in cases where the attacker is known to the victim, and convictions in such cases are extremely rare (Parrot and Bechhofer 1991). Further, in a number of states it is still legal for a husband to rape his wife.

Another context in which rape occurs is "gang rape" or multiple attackers of one or more victims. College fraternities are frequently a setting for gang rape (Yancey Martin and Hummer 1989). In these organizations gang rape serves as a ritualistic means of male bonding. Fraternity brothers who participate believe that they did nothing wrong, or they blame the victim for the incident. Judge Lois Forer, who has presided over numerous gang rape trials, describes one typical case: "At trial, all the defendants admitted what they had done but insisted that they had not committed any crime. To them it was a customary form of amusement for normal males, which is how they saw themselves. And, of course, they blamed the victim. She 'asked for it'; she should not have been where she was; she should not have complained; she wasn't harmed" (quoted in Sanday 1990:xv).

Criminal Justice

Despite the large numbers of rapes each year in the United States, the criminal justice system responds slowly. Although there are laws against certain types of rape in every state, they are not uniform nor are they uniformly enforced.

Arrest and conviction rates for reported cases of rape are lower than for any other violent crime. Less than 5 percent of all reported rapes result in a conviction (U.S. Department of Justice 1991b). In cases where a complaint does result in a trial, victims are often subjected to harassment and humiliation in court. The "credibility" of the victim is often the focus of the trial, rather than the violent acts committed against her person. A statement by the presiding judge in a recent rape case in which the victim was a poor Latina prostitute who was violently raped and beaten illustrates the problem faced by marginalized women. Addressing the jury after granting his own motion for dismissal, the judge explained to the jurors: "I would like to apologize for having you spend your time doing what essentially was trying to reform or decide a breach of contract between a whore and a trick. A woman who goes out on the street and makes a whore out of herself opens herself up to anybody. She steps outside the protection of the law. That's a basic fundamental legal concept" (Bourque 1989:4). On the infrequent occasions when a rapist is convicted, prison sentences are short in comparison with such crimes as robbery and burglary.

Difference also plays a fundamental part in rape as violence against women. The rape victim's particular social position shapes her experiences of victimization and the ways in which the criminal justice system responds. Her race, class, and sexual orientation and the race and class position of the rapist intersect in ways that may be consequential. The legal system often ignores or minimizes the complaints of women of color and poor women. Furthermore, black rape victims must also face pervasive racist sexualized images of African American women (Davis 1983; hooks 1990). The discriminatory and often violent treatment of black men by the predominantly white criminal justice system may also serve as a barrier. The criminal justice system responds differently to men of color who rape: black men convicted of rape receive longer prison sentences and are more likely to get the death penalty than white men (Bourque 1989). Thus black women may feel pressure to remain quiet about the rape or to keep the incident within their communities. "Black women are less likely to report their rapes, less likely to have their cases come to trial, less likely to have their trials result in convictions, and, most disturbing, less likely to seek counseling and other support services" (Collins 1993:101).

Consequences and Help Seeking

Rape may have a number of consequences for emotional and physical health. Depression, fear, nightmares, and other sleep disturbances are common after an assault. Victims may experience these for years after the rape (Carosella 1995; Koss 1993b; Quina and Carlson 1989; Resick 1993). Rape victims are nine times more likely to commit suicide than non-victims. Rape victims often experience a number of persistent physical health problems including headaches, chronic pelvic pain, gastrointestinal disorders, and general body pain (Koss 1993b; Koss and Heslet 1992). Many women who are raped feel stigmatized and are pressured by others not to talk about the pain of their victimization, thus prolonging recovery (Carosella 1995). Sexual assault may also affect a woman's economic viability, because victims often miss work after an attack or find it difficult to concentrate.

Poor women have fewer resources to rely on and often face further mistreatment by social service agencies they may contact for help. Little or no access to health care for economically disadvantaged women may result in untreated physical and/or emotional conditions. Some victims use self-medication to cope. In particular, women who do not have access to physicians or prescription medication may use less reliable or effective substances to self-medicate such as alcohol or illicit drugs (Boyd 1993; Britton 1992). Substance abuse is itself related to a number of serious health problems for rape victims, including HIV infection (Zierler et al. 1991). One poor woman who received no medical care or other help after she was raped explains: "When I got raped that was very traumatic. And no matter how I tried to be successful at something, I would get so close to where I thought I wanted to be only to find myself going off using drugs. . . . They helped me keep my mind together, so like I didn't freak out. . . . They've kind of like blocked the scars, made them easier to live with" (Britton 1996).

Seeking help is also complicated by the victims' sexual orientation. Lesbian women may feel uncomfortable or even endangered by disclosing their sexual identity to health care providers or to the police (D'Augelli 1992).

Feminist Scholarship

Feminist research and scholarship on rape has expanded dramatically since the early 1970s, when rape emerged as a public issue. One of the first feminist theories of rape was outlined by Susan Brownmiller (1975) in her now classic *Against Our Will: Men, Women, and Rape*. Other feminist scholars (Bart and Moran 1993; Collins 1990; Davis 1978, 1989; Griffin 1977; Scully 1990; Scully and Marolla 1993) provide social, cultural, and political explanations for rape. They argue that rape is but one of many violent and coercive acts perpetrated against women that create and reinforce male dominance. Rather than an act of individual "deviance," rape is seen as an extension of other learned and accepted male behaviors, "a violent method for keeping women in their place . . . a product of a patriarchal society" (Bourque 1989:6).

Scully's study of convicted rapists showed that offenders reported that they raped women in a conscious effort to wield power over their victims and over women as a group. She develops the concept of "collective liability," which "suggests that all people in a particular category are held accountable for each of their counterparts. Thus a man's intent may not be to punish the woman he is raping but to use her because she represents a category to him" (Scully 1990:138).

Male dominance and the attendant acceptance of violence against women is magnified for women of color. The institution of slavery and the routine rape of black women by white slave owners and overseers for

pleasure and reproductive goals helped to establish the cultural acceptance of the rape of black women. Resultant cultural stereotypes have
constructed black women's sexuality as related to violent sex, lust, and
promiscuity and as undeserving of protection against rape, indeed, invit-
ing it (Collins 1990; Higginbotham 1992).

Feminist research and activism have helped to legitimate rape as a
social problem. Since the early 1970s, services for victims have been
established across the country. Hotlines provide referral and counseling to
rape victims, and antirape organizations often do medical and legal advocacy for victims (Matthews 1993, 1995).

However, rape is still a crime frequently perpetrated against women
in the United States, and recent statistics indicate that the incidence of
rape continues to rise.[4] Studies of attitudes toward rape indicate that men
continue to believe that the use of force or coercion to obtain sex from a
woman is acceptable and even desirable (Malamuth 1986; Sanday 1990).[5]
The male-dominated criminal justice system continues to respond apa-
thetically to rape victims. It appears as though the women's movement
and victims of sexual violence have embraced rape as a legitimate social
problem, whereas many social institutions and subcultures in the United
States have not.

NOTES

1. The National Crime Victimization Survey (NCVS), a federal study, is also
done annually to determine the total number of rapes occurring each year, including
both reported and unreported incidents. Although the NCVS measures more accurately, it is fraught with methodological problems that lead to underreporting on the
part of victims (Koss 1993a). These include vague and ambiguous screening questions,
interviews that impede rapport, lack of confidentiality of responses, and a survey
context that assumes that only violent rapes involving strangers are of interest to the
interviewer (Koss 1993b:1062).

2. Among developed countries, the United States has one of the highest per
capita rates of rape in the world; a woman is twenty times more likely to be raped in
the United States than in Japan and about thirteen times more likely than in England
(U.S. Department of Justice 1988).

3. In a widely publicized book, Roiphe argues that antirape activists have exaggerated the prevalence of rape on college campuses (1993). In her view, stranger rape is rare
and date rape is even less common. She argues that women's claims of rape are simply
interpretations of "bad sex." She holds that such women are too passive to refuse sex and
are then encouraged by feminists to label such experiences as rape when they feel uncomfortable or disturbed. These arguments have drawn substantial criticism from feminist

scholars and antirape activists. Pollit (1994), for instance, notes that Roiphe's arguments are based on "personal testimony" derived from limited experience in the class-specific environment of an Ivy League campus. Pollit claims that Roiphe's work is poorly researched and characterized by "misleading use of data," the very charge Roiphe levels against antirape activists.

4. In 1970 the rate of rape in the United States per 100,000 females age twelve and older was 46.3. By 1990 that had increased to 96.6 (U.S. Bureau of the Census 1994). The reasons for this are not clear. The rise may reflect increased reporting by victims or an actual elevation in the number of rapes, or both. Sociologist Diana Scully's "transitionary" theory holds that the rise is caused by backlash: men are angered by women's gains since the 1970s.

5. When the boxer Mike Tyson was released from prison after serving time for raping Deseree Washington, he was greeted with a parade. Black and white feminists vigorously protested this "hero's welcome."

REFERENCES

Bart, Pauline B., and Eileen Geil Moran, eds.
    1993   Violence against Women: The Bloody Footprints. Newbury Park, CA: Sage.

Bourque, Linda B.
    1989   Defining Rape. Durham, NC: Duke University Press.

Boyd, Carol J.
    1993   "The antecedents of women's crack cocaine abuse: family substance abuse, sexual abuse, depression, and illicit drug use." Journal of Substance Abuse Treatment 10:433-38.

Britton, Brandy M.
    1992   "Women's increased exposure to HIV: sex work, needle sharing, and condom use." Research presentation at the third annual Conference for the Reduction of Drug Related Harm, Melbourne, Australia.
    1996   "Women, violence, and AIDS: exploring the relationships between sexual and domestic violence and women's drug use and HIV risk." Research presentation, Charlestown/University of Maryland Lecture Series.

Brownmiller, Susan
    1975   Against Our Will: Men, Women, and Rape. New York: Simon and Schuster.

Carosella, Cynthia, ed.
    1995   Who's Afraid of the Dark? A Forum of Truth, Support, and Assurance for Those Affected by Rape. New York: Harper Collins.

Collins, Patricia Hill
    1990   Black Feminist Thought: Knowledge, Consciousness, and the Politics of Empowerment. New York: Routledge.
    1993   "The sexual politics of black womanhood." Pp. 85-104 in Pauline B. Bart

and Eileen Geil Moran (eds.), Violence against Women: The Bloody Footprints. Newbury Park, CA: Sage.

D'Augelli, Anthony R.
1992   "Lesbian and gay male undergraduates' experiences of harassment and fear on campus." Journal of Interpersonal Violence 7:383-95.

Davis, Angela
1978   "Rape, racism, and the capitalist setting." Black Scholar 9:24-30.
1983   Women, Race and Class. New York: Random House.

Finkelhor, David, and Kersti Yllo
1985   License to Rape: Sexual Abuse of Wives. New York: Free Press.

Griffin, Susan
1977   Rape: The Politics of Consciousness. New York: Harper and Row.

Higginbotham, Elizabeth B.
1992   "African American women's history and the metalanguage of race." Signs: Journal of Women in Culture and Society 17:251-74.

hooks, bell
1990   Yearning: Race, Gender, and Cultural Politics. Boston: South End Press.

Koss, Mary P.
1988   "Hidden rape: sexual aggression and victimization in a national sample of students in higher education." Pp. 3-25 in Anne Burgess (ed.), Rape and Sexual Assault. New York: Garland.
1993a   "Detecting the scope of rape: a review of prevalence research methods." Journal of Interpersonal Violence 8:198-222.
1993b   "Rape: scope, impact, interventions, and public policy responses." American Psychologist 48:1062-69.

Koss, Mary P., and Laura Heslet
1992   "Somatic consequences of violence against women." Archives of Family Medicine 1:53-59.

Malamuth, Neil
1986   "Predictors of naturalistic sexual aggression." Journal of Personality and Sexual Psychology 45:432-42.

Matthews, Nancy A.
1993   "Surmounting a legacy: The expansion of racial diversity in a local anti-rape movement." Pp. 177-92 in Pauline B. Bart and Eileen Geil Moran (eds.), Violence against Women: The Bloody Footprints. Newbury Park, CA: Sage.
1995   Confronting Rape: The Feminist Anti-Rape Movement and the State. New York: Routledge.

National Victims Center
1992   Rape in America: A Report to the Nation. Arlington, VA: National Victims Center.

New York Times
1992   "Survey shows number of rapes far higher than official statistics." 24 April.

Parrot, Andrea, and Laurie Bechhofer, eds.
    1991   Acquaintance Rape: The Hidden Crime. New York: John Wiley.
Pollit, Katha
    1994   Reasonable Creatures: Essays on Women and Feminism. New York: Alfred A. Knopf.
Quina, Kathryn, and Nancy L. Carlson
    1989   Rape, Incest, and Sexual Harassment: A Guide For Helping Survivors. New York: Praeger.
Resick, Patricia A.
    1993   "The psychological impact of rape." Journal of Interpersonal Violence 8:223–55.
Roiphe, Katie
    1993   The Morning After: Sex, Fear, and Feminism on Campus. Boston: Little, Brown.
Russell, Diana E.
    1990   Rape in Marriage. Bloomington: Indiana University Press.
Sanday, Peggy Reeves
    1990   Fraternity Gang Rape: Sex, Brotherhood, and Privilege on Campus. New York: New York University Press.
Schechter, Susan
    1982   Women and Male Violence. Boston: South End Press.
Scully, Diana
    1990   Understanding Sexual Violence: A Study of Convicted Rapists. Cambridge, Mass: Unwin, Hyman.
Scully, Diana, and Joseph Marolla
    1993   "'Riding the bull at Gilley's': convicted rapists describe the rewards of rape." Pp. 26–46 in Pauline B. Bart and Eileen Geil Moran (eds.), Violence against Women: The Bloody Footprints. Newbury Park, CA: Sage.
U.S. Bureau of the Census
    1994   Statistical Abstract of the United States: 1994, 112th ed. Washington: Government Printing Office.
U.S. Department of Justice
    1988   Report to the Nation on Crime and Justice, Second Edition. Washington: Bureau of Justice Statistics.
    1991a   Criminal Victimization in the United States, 1989. Washington: Bureau of Justice Statistics.
    1991b   Female Victims of Violent Crime. Washington: Bureau of Justice Statistics.
Warshaw, Robin
    1988   I Never Called It Rape. New York. Harper and Row.
Yancey Martin, Patricia and Robert A. Hummer
    1989   "Fraternities and rape on campus." Gender and Society 3:457–73.

Zierler, Sally, Lisa Feingold, Deborah Laufer, Priscilla Velentgas, Ira Kantrowitz-Gordon, and Kenneth Mayer
    1991   "Adult survivors of childhood sexual abuse and subsequent risk of HIV infection." American Journal of Public Health 81:572–75.

A Survivor Speaks about the Victim Input Program

SALLY PICKELS

A little more than twenty-one years ago, I was the victim of a brutal rape. During that crime, I was beaten with a hammer, held at knifepoint, and then robbed. As a result of that beating, I still suffer a neurological disorder and some loss of vision.

The perpetrators of the crime against me were apprehended. One was a juvenile with a record of six prior arrests, who was on probation. At the time of his arrest, he was adjudged delinquent and was sent away for stealing a car. I tried for four years to have him brought to trial for the crime against me, but the system failed me and society. He is now serving time for murder.

The other perpetrator was tried and convicted, and in 1974 he was sentenced to twenty-three-and-one-half to forty-seven years in prison. However, in 1977 he won the right to another trial on a legal technicality. Again I went through the trial, and he was again convicted and received the same sentence. I thought my dealings with the criminal justice system were over, and I could try to get on with my life.

In January 1993, I heard of the Victim Input Program operated by the Pennsylvania Board of Probation and Parole, which provides the victim of a crime the opportunity to express her or his opinion concerning the release of the defendant. This program went into effect in October 1986 with the passage of Act 134. The inmate has always had the right to participate in the legal process, but now the victim can actually participate, too.

After I heard of the Victim Input Program, I contacted the district attorney's office and the Pennsylvania Board of Probation and Parole and asked for more information about the program. I told them that I wanted

to be notified before the inmate was up for parole so that I could participate in the process.

This was a difficult decision. It meant that I had to dig up all the
feelings that I had buried for so many years, and because I needed moral
support I had to tell my sons and a few very close friends the exact nature
of the crime. My sons were fifteen, sixteen, and eighteen years old when
the crime took place, and because I was ashamed to tell them about the
rape, I only let them know about the beating and the robbery. When I
told my sons and friends and other relatives of my intention to participate
in the program, they had mixed reactions. Some were supportive, and
others couldn't handle it, so I accepted the support of those who were
willing to give it and just let the others go.

In December 1993, accompanied by supporters from Women Organized Against Rape and Northwest Victim Services, I appeared before a
hearing examiner at the parole board. I presented my testimony about the
effects of the crime, including the physical, mental, and emotional trauma
from which I still suffer. I presented letters from my sons stating the effects
of the crime on their lives, letters from a few close friends supporting our
claims, and documentation from several of my doctors. In all of these
letters, we asked that parole be denied to this inmate. Because of the
viciousness of the crime, I am permanently disabled. We feel that because
I will suffer for the rest of my life, he should be required to serve his full
sentence.

Participation in this process has its drawbacks, but it also has its
pluses. It makes you think of the entire crime and acknowledge that it
actually happened: this nightmare is real. For the first time since the
crime, I have asked for help to deal with the emotional turmoil it has
caused, and I have been attending individual and group therapy sessions
at Women Organized Against Rape. I'm no longer hiding the facts of the
crime from my children and close friends. I am just now beginning to talk
to the counselor about what actually happened to me, but it is a start! I'm
dealing with issues a little at a time, but I feel this is progress.

Another plus is that participation in this process gave me a feeling of
control. From the moment of the crime and all during the trials, I felt that
the laws were all in favor of the criminal. The only time I was allowed to
speak was in response to questions from people in the criminal justice
system. Now I feel that I have finally been able to say what I wanted to
say, without objections.

I am very happy to be able to say that in June 1994 the man who assaulted me was denied parole. He is staying in prison where he belongs. This is a personal victory for me and, I feel, for all survivors.

Anti-Lesbian Violence

BEATRICE VON SCHULTHESS

> He shot from where he was hidden in the woods eighty-five feet away, after he stalked us, hunted us, spied on us. Later his lawyer tried to assert that our sexuality provoked him. He shot us because he identified us as lesbians. He was a stranger with whom we had no connection. He shot us and left us for dead. (Brenner 1992:12)

Claudia Brenner suffered five bullet wounds, and her lover was mortally injured.

Other such violence is less tragic but also very frightening: On 10 November 1990, a male driver hit a car outside Club Q, a gay and lesbian bar in San Francisco. He got out and confronted the lesbian occupants of the struck car, shouting, "What the fuck are you looking at, you dyke bitches? There's no damage, get back in your car." The man then drove a short distance and was involved in another confrontation with patrons leaving the club. He injured seven women, two of them seriously (Conkin 1990).

Violence against lesbians is most commonly examined in terms of its interconnections with broader homophobic violence against gay men and lesbians. However, there are aspects to violence against lesbians that require distinct analysis. For lesbians, such violence intensifies the intimidation they already experience as women.

This essay explores the nature and extent of violence and harassment directed specifically against lesbians in the United States and describes the contexts within which such violence occurs.

Extent and Types of Violence

The above incidents are examples of the many acts of violence committed against lesbians in the United States (Berrill 1992).[1] Although there has been no systematic collection of information on anti-lesbian violence in the United States, the National Gay and Lesbian Task Force (NGLTF), local gay and lesbian organizations, and a few social scientists have surveyed anti-gay and anti-lesbian violence. The first national survey of anti-gay/lesbian violence in 1984 in eight cities revealed that one in ten lesbians reported having been physically assaulted because of their sexual orientation (NGLTF 1986). In addition, 16 percent reported that objects had been thrown at them, and 31 percent were chased or followed. The Philadelphia Lesbian and Gay Task Force study of violence showed that lesbians there were at least four times more likely to have been victims of violence than persons in general urban populations (1988). Twenty percent also reported they had been subjected to criminal violence during the preceding year because of their sexual orientation.

Homophobic violence falls into two major categories: verbal harassment and physical violence or its threat. A 1989 San Francisco survey that focused solely on violence against lesbians found that of the 398 respondents, 84 percent reported they had experienced anti-lesbian verbal harassment, two-thirds of these within the previous year (von Schulthess 1992). Other studies of gay men and lesbians have found similar patterns of verbal harassment against lesbians: 86 percent of lesbians in a 1986 national study (Comstock 1991) and 81 percent of lesbians in a Philadelphia study (Philadelphia Lesbian and Gay Task Force 1988). Nor are verbal assaults isolated events. Most (86 percent) of the women in the San Francisco study who had experienced some sort of verbal harassment reported more than one incident of verbal harassment within the previous year.

Fifty-seven percent of the women in the San Francisco survey reported that they had experienced physical violence or the threat of violence because of their sexual orientation. Of these women, 40 percent had been threatened with physical violence, 33 percent had been chased or followed, 27 percent had objects thrown at them, and 12 percent had been punched, hit, kicked, or beaten. Fully 16 percent suffered injuries ranging from bruises and black eyes to internal injuries and knife wounds.

Only two studies have examined types of anti-lesbian violence and the victim's race/ethnicity, and both studies found that lesbians of color experienced violence at a greater rate than white lesbians (Comstock 1991; von Schulthess 1992). In the San Francisco study, although white lesbians were more likely to have been verbally assaulted than were lesbians of color, the picture shifted when physical violence, threats, vandalism, and rape were involved. Lesbians of color consistently experienced a higher level of all types of anti-lesbian violence than did white lesbians.[2]

Reporting Violence

Data consistently indicate that the great majority of victims of anti-lesbian violence do not report these crimes to the police (NGLTF 1986; Winslow 1982). In the San Francisco study only 15 percent of the victims reported the incident to the police. One commented on the criminal justice system: "I'm not even sure I would report it [an incident of physical violence] to the police . . . because they wouldn't do anything about it. I think that when gays and lesbians are involved with violence and law enforcement and the courts . . . nothing is done" (von Schulthess 1992).

There are several possible reasons for this reluctance to report. Many lesbians fear exposure, stigmatization, and discrimination if an incident (and therefore their sexual orientation) becomes known to their employer, family, or even friends. In addition, secondary victimization is a major concern. "Like victims of rape, the victims of anti-gay hate crimes often are blamed for the incident by police, prosecutors, judges, and jurors" (Berrill and Herek 1990:404). A study funded by the National Institute of Justice found that most respondents "believed that for the most part, for various reasons, the criminal justice system has not recognized the seriousness of hate violence, or that many criminal justice personnel do not want to believe that hate motivated violence exists in their community" (Finn and McNeil 1987:4).

The Anti-Woman/Anti-Lesbian Continuum

> Violence can be rape or a sexually assaultive remark of one kind or another. Women are expected to accept that. As a lesbian, I put up with homophobia. That's institutionalized. So is sexism. The pervasiveness is alarming. I'm not sure if it's possible for women to know what safety is, because women experience violence all their lives. You can be safer but . . .
> ("Pam" in Stanko 1990:138)

Pam's statement raises three important issues concerning the nature of violence against lesbians. First, lesbians experience harassment and physical violence on the streets because of their gender. As women, they have been conditioned to cope with street harassment and violence as an inevitable part of life. One woman said, "You realize that San Francisco is just like any other place and you're going to be harassed either for being a woman or for being a lesbian" (von Schulthess 1992:70). Another lesbian explained, "Like other women, [lesbians] are so conditioned to expect violence in their lives [because of their gender], so trained to accept the threat of violence, that when they are assaulted it may not even occur to them to question why it occurred" (Tallmer 1984:14). In short, without the existence of explicit labeling language, it is difficult to distinguish anti-lesbian violence from anti-woman violence. One respondent in the San Francisco study commented: "I just get harassed so often, walking to and from the bus each day, on the bus, at work, at lunchtime, that I have a 'mask' or face I put on when I'm in public. Most of the time I don't even listen to the comments unless I feel physically threatened, and the looks . . . well, you never know what they are thinking." In addition, lesbians frequently referred to incidents where both anti-lesbian and anti-woman insults occurred.

There are, of course, incidents that are clearly focused on the woman's sexual orientation from the start. One respondent explained: "My lover and I were on the Muni. . . . We had just been to an event with lots of queers. We had just been comfortable being ourselves, holding hands. . . . This guy starts calling us names, uh, you know, like 'dyke,' 'pussy lover,' and we felt trapped and scared. He had a knife on his belt."

A second closely related issue is that attacks often began as anti-woman and then added an anti-lesbian dimension. Men expect women to act in certain ways in response to a "come on." In research on street remarks, Carol Brooks Gardner (1980:346) suggested that "retaliation is not considered feminine behavior." Women who answer back, physically respond, or do something that is construed as retaliation are seen by their assailants as nonfeminine and gender inappropriate (Gardner 1995). If the assailant is displeased by the victim's response, one way of escalating the attack and highlighting the woman's unfeminine actions is to shift the harassment from anti-woman to anti-lesbian commentary.

One lesbian illustrated this pattern in her analysis of an incident that began with a man asking to see her breast as she walked past him on the street. She ignored the comment and walked on. He continued the harassment by calling her "dyke." She concluded, "So the worst kind of woman that he can imagine, a woman that won't respond to him at all, must be a lesbian. Otherwise I would've been flattered that he wanted to see my breast" (von Schulthess 1992:71). Another woman reported similar verbal abuse from a man whose dog had attacked hers (Baum 1995:7). In several cases in the San Francisco study the women believed that their assailants did not even know they were lesbians (based, for example, on their clothing, on the locations of the assault, or on the assailants' initial remarks). Only when the women did not respond in a "properly" gendered manner did the situation escalate.

Thus it is not sufficient to frame the issue of violence against lesbians only in terms of sexual orientation. Instead, lesbianism needs to be conceptualized as an extension of gender and anti-lesbian violence as an extension of misogynist violence. The types of remarks that women experience can be seen as falling along a continuum, ranging from exclusively anti-woman at one end to exclusively anti-lesbian at the other with varied hateful combinations in between. It is important to remember, of course, that some incidents are clearly focused on the women's lesbianism.

Third, like other women, lesbians have developed habits of continually monitoring and analyzing their immediate social situations for safety. An NGLTF study found that although anti-gay/lesbian violence affected both gay men's and lesbians' behavior, lesbians were much more likely to change their behavior because of the fear of future violence (Berrill 1990). Although verbal incidents do not necessarily lead to physical violence, the threat of violence and uncertainty regarding the outcome can and does affect the day-to-day actions of lesbians. "Most gay [and lesbian] respondents to victimization surveys indicate that their public behavior is affected by their fear of physical attack. Verbal harassment and intimidation reinforce this climate of fear" (Garnets et al. 1990:373). Many women in the San Francisco study constructed what could be called a "safety map" through which they then analyzed their situations. One woman explained: "You're going to be harassed . . . and because of that you have to take precautions and that means letting go of the hand of the person you're with in certain areas or if certain groups of people are standing around looking menacing, and not going certain places late at night by yourself" (von Schulthess 1992:71). The safety map included such factors as clothing and appearance, interpersonal behavior, destination, companions, time of day, and location in the city. In her discussion of how she uses body language to negotiate the streets and put space between herself and a potential aggressor, another respondent shows the sophistication involved in constructing the safety map:

> If I hear somebody walking behind me at night on the side-
> walk, I turn to see who it is. I relax a little bit if it's a woman.
> . . . If it's a man and it's late and dark and I'm alone, I perhaps
> cross the street, depending on what he is doing. You know, if
> he's carrying two bags of groceries and walking his dog just like
> I am and he's not following me, I probably stay on the sidewalk.
> But if he was sort of, whatever, I'll walk faster or cross to the
> other side of the street or I'll stop and go in a store or pretend
> I'm going in the store. I often try to make the person pass me.
> That clears up the whole mystery of whether or not they are
> following me.

Although lesbians carefully take these factors into consideration, this does not mean that they have control over them, nor does it mean that such vigilance and behavior change can be an answer to the problem of anti-lesbian violence. At most these are management strategies to attempt to avoid violence.

I have found that lesbians not only experience both anti-lesbian violence and anti-woman violence but that some continuum, doubtless deeply rooted in cultural views of women and gender in American life, connects these two violences for many women. Anti-lesbian harassment and violence demonstrate the everyday danger in women's lives. "Anticipation of violence, manifest in the conscious or unconscious use of precaution, reflects the power and influence of racism, sexism, and homophobia today" (Stanko 1990:144). Lesbians, like others, not only react to specific situations with specific responses but also alter their ways of being because of violence in the streets. All women have limited access to the streets in our society. Lesbians have even more limited and less protected rights to be themselves and to go about their daily lives free from violence.

NOTES

Portions of this section originally appeared in von Schulthess 1992.

1. According to a report prepared for the Department of Justice, there is "plenty of documentation that criminal violence against the gay [and lesbian] community is widespread and may be increasing" (Illinois Criminal Justice Authority 1988).

2. Some lesbians in the study commented on their triple minority status (lesbian women of color). Women who are Latina and lesbians, for instance, do not experience the world as one or the other. All are part of their identities. In certain contexts these women may experience violence because of one or all of these statuses.

REFERENCES

Baum, Terry
    1995   "Unleashing homophobia." Dykespeak. January.
Berrill, Kevin T.
    1990   "Anti-gay violence and victimization in the United States." Journal of Interpersonal Violence 5(3):274–94.
    1992   "Anti-gay violence and victimization in the United States: an overview." Pp. 65–75 in Gregory M. Herek and Kevin T. Berrill (eds.), Hate Crimes: Confronting Violence against Lesbians and Gay Men. Newbury Park, CA: Sage.
Berrill, Kevin T., and Gregory M. Herek
    1990   "Primary and secondary victimization in anti-gay hate crimes: official response and public policy." Journal of Interpersonal Violence 5(3):401–13.
Brenner, Claudia
    1992   "Survivor's story: eight bullets." Pp. 11–15 in Gregory M. Herek and Kevin T. Berrill (eds.), Hate Crimes: Confronting Violence against Lesbians and Gay Men. Newbury Park, CA: Sage.
Comstock, Gary David
    1991   Violence against Lesbians and Gay Men. New York: Columbia University Press.
Conkin, David
    1990   "Felony charges filed in Club Q incident." Bay Area Reporter, 6 December, 1.
Finn, Peter, and T. McNeil
    1987   The Response of the Criminal Justice System to Bias Crime: An Exploratory Review. Washington: National Institute of Justice, Department of Justice.
Gardner, Carol Brooks
    1980   "Passing by: street remarks, address rights, and the urban female." Sociological Inquiry 3–4:328–56.
    1995   Passing By: Gender and Public Harassment. Berkeley: University of California Press.
Garnets, Linda, Gregory M. Herek, and Barrie Levy
    1990   "Violence and victimization of lesbians and gay men: mental health consequences." Journal of Interpersonal Violence 5(3):366–83.
Illinois Criminal Justice Information Authority
    1988   Chicago Community Anti-Violence Program: Office of Federal Assistance Programs.
National Gay and Lesbian Task Force
    1986   Anti-Gay Violence: Causes, Consequences, Responses. Washington: National Gay and Lesbian Task Force.
Philadelphia Lesbian and Gay Task Force
    1988   Violence and Discrimination against Lesbians and Gay People in

Philadelphia and the Commonwealth of Pennsylvania. Philadelphia: Lesbian and Gay Task Force.

Stanko, Elizabeth
1990   Everyday Violence: How Women and Men Experience Sexual and Physical Danger. London: Pandora Press.

Tallmer, Abby
1984   Anti-Lesbian Violence. Task force report 4. Washington: National Gay and Lesbian Task Force.

von Schulthess, Beatrice
1992   "Violence in the streets: anti-lesbian assault and harassment in San Francisco." Pp. 65–75 in Gregory M. Herek and Kevin T. Berrill (eds.), Hate Crimes: Confronting Violence against Lesbians and Gay Men. Newbury Park, CA: Sage.

Winslow, Cindy L.
1982   Mayor's Survey of Victims of Violence, Personal Crimes in San Francisco. Criminal Justice Council, Office of the Mayor.

Sexual Harassment

BRANDY M. BRITTON

Sexual harassment was never a major issue as long as it only threatened the careers of millions of women. It only became a major issue when it threatened the career of one man.

—*Susan Pepperdine*

In the fall of 1991 — as millions of American television viewers watched — at Senate confirmation hearings, a witness testified that a Supreme Court nominee had sexually harassed her ten years earlier.

Professor Anita Hill's testimony, Judge Clarence Thomas's refutation, and the behavior of the all-white, all-male Senate Judiciary Committee dramatically altered American awareness in ways that have transformed cultural consciousness about sexual harassment. A firestorm of discussion and argument about this topic, long recognized but almost never acknowledged, burst forth and has continued long after the contentious hearings, themselves the focus of considerable debate, ended (Chrisman and Allen 1992; Morrison 1992; Phelps and Winternitz 1992).

Sexual harassment, perpetrated primarily by men against women in all ethnic groups, social class settings, and across color and social class lines, is unwanted sexual attention of any kind. It can, though more rarely, occur when females harass males or between same-sex pairs in an interaction.

Sexual harassment can be verbal, physical, and visual or written and can range from a derogatory remark to rape. Sexual harassment includes sexist depictions, sexist or sexual jokes, propositions, touching, brushing against a person's body, physical and sexual assault, and under Title VII of the Civil Rights Act of 1994 a hostile work environment that makes it difficult for the victim to fulfill her work responsibilities (California Commission on the Status of Women 1986; Chan 1994; Pollack 1990). For instance, a woman who worked in a predominantly male shipyard in Jacksonville, Florida, sued her employer for sexual harassment when her supervisors ignored her complaints that pornographic pictures of women were prominently displayed in the workplace. These pictures depicted a woman with a meat spatula pressed against her pubic area, a nude woman holding a whip, and a dartboard designed to resemble a woman's breast—with the nipple as the bull's-eye (Fitzgerald 1993).

The Workplace

The key to sexual harassment is the power differential between the harasser and the victim who may suffer negative sanctions and retaliation if she spurns the unwanted attention (MacKinnon 1979). These power dynamics are sometimes mistaken for "sex games at work," when in fact "unwelcome sexual conduct in this context sends the victim a clear message by reminding her of the historical myth that woman's place is in the home" (Chan 1994:16).

Sexual harassment has been assumed to take place primarily in the workplace between a male and a female subordinate, because most working women hold lower-status positions than men. If he is a supervisor, the harasser may influence decisions about promotions or write letters of reference for employees to whom he is making unwanted verbal or physical advances. Harassed women fear retaliation, such as demotions or job loss, if they reject advances or report the harassment to someone else (Gruber 1989). When a woman's economic survival is threatened, her alternatives for action against the harasser are severely limited. These fears are not unfounded: one-third of women who have been harassed report suffering such consequences as being transferred, fired, or forced to resign (California Commission on the Status of Women 1986).

Unfortunately, such experiences are widespread. More than half of all working women report that they have been sexually harassed on the job at some time (Fitzgerald 1993; Shrier 1990). Conversely, less than 1 percent of employed men report that they have experienced a negative consequence as a result of sexual harassment.[1] "While men report that they frequently receive sexual overtures from women they often do not view these overtures as unwanted. Thus although men generally report a lot of sexual activity at work, they report almost no sexual harassment" (California Commission on the Status of Women 1986:24). Workplace harassment is not, however, limited to male superiors: other coworkers, customers or clients, and subordinates may advance unwanted sexual attentions. These events are more likely to occur in settings where there are few women employees relative to the number of male workers and in occupations, such as clerical work, where women are in the majority but have little status and low pay (Gruber 1989). However, it must be noted that even women in presumably high-status occupations, such as physicians and lawyers, suffer sexual harassment (see chapter 16 on caregivers) (Lenhart and Evans 1991; Rosenberg, Perlstadt, and Phillips 1993).

Educational Settings

Women also experience sexual harassment in educational settings where men disproportionately occupy positions of power relative to women. Male professors and administrators can and do use their power to coerce female students and colleagues into unwanted sexual interactions (Williams, Lam, and Shively 1992). Harassment of female students by male professors is common. Between 30 and 50 percent of all female students are verbally or physically harassed during their college years, and as many as 60 percent of women experience "everyday harassment" on campus such as sexual jokes or unwanted physical contact. Many women report dropping courses, changing majors or graduate programs, or leaving higher education altogether to avoid further harassment (Dziech and Weiner 1984; Fitzgerald 1992; Paludi et al. 1990; Schneider 1987).

Despite their formal power over male students, female professors often encounter behaviors by male students that they perceive as sexual harassment. These acts of "contrapower harassment" (Benson 1984) include sexual comments, jokes, heckling directed at female professors during lectures, poor evaluations, obscene or threatening phone calls and letters, sexual bribery, and physical and sexual assault. "That many women professors feel harassed by their male students reflects cultural differences between men and women and highlights . . . women's vulnerability to sexual harassment" (Grauerholz 1989:797-98).

Other Settings

In addition, harassment of women is also found in housing projects, in the military, and in prisons, mental hospitals, homes for the retarded, nursing homes, and therapeutic settings (Buehler and Britton 1992; California Commission on the Status of Women 1986). Landlords harass women, especially single mothers who have difficulty finding housing and often feel they cannot escape. In prisons, power differentials between male guards and female prisoners exacerbate cultural power differences between them as males and females creating optimum conditions for harassment.

Widespread harassment of women in military service came under public scrutiny in 1991 with the widely publicized Tailhook convention where more than two dozen women, some of them navy officers, were physically and sexually assaulted by a group of male officers. This led to investigations of the sexual harassment of female military personnel, en-listed and officers. The navy's survey found that 75 percent of women in the navy said that sexual harassment occurred within their work environ-ments (Rubin 1992). Moreover, these unwanted sexual attentions also occur in housing on military bases.

Even settings where women seek care are not free of sexual harass-ment. Victims of unwanted sexual attention from all types of providers commonly fear that needed services or medications will be withheld from them if they refuse or complain about the harassment (Sumrall and Taylor 1992). In one study of clients in treatment for substance abuse, women reported that their drug treatment counselors made unwanted sexual ad-vances toward them and in some instances demanded sexual favors, threatening to throw them out of treatment if they did not consent (Buehler and Britton 1992). Male physicians may also sexually harass female patients, particularly emotionally or physically vulnerable women. One woman, seeking an abortion, was physically assaulted as her doctor attempted to pressure her into unwanted sex in exchange for his services. She explains:

> [My doctor] put an arm around my shoulders. "You girls are re-ally horney, aren't you?" I pulled away. "No harm in being a little friendly," he said squeezing my thigh. I pushed his hand

off my leg. "Please . . . don't!" I moved as far from him as I could. I was feeling nauseated as I tried to discourage his passes. Did the delay mean this man was going to mess around with me and I wouldn't get the abortion I needed so desperately? . . . During the surgery as I lay on the table the two men fondled my breasts. I was repulsed but didn't try to resist. What could I do?" (Capelle 1992:43)

Consequences

Sexual harassment can have a number of deleterious economic, physical, and emotional consequences for victims. Inability to concentrate and persistent anger, fear, or helplessness often result (Koss 1990; Pollack 1990; Shrier 1990). The psychological impacts are similar to those of rape: nightmares, flashbacks, long-term depression, anxiety disorders, insomnia, and symptoms of posttraumatic stress disorder (Farley 1978; Kilpatrick 1992). Physical health consequences include frequent headaches, gastrointestinal disorders, weight loss or weight gain, nausea, and sexual dysfunction (Fitzgerald and McInnis 1989).

Race, class, and sexual orientation all affect women's experiences of harassment. "Often particular groups of women are chosen as targets of harassment because of their economic, political or social vulnerability, all of which make it more unlikely that these women will publicly resist or report the harassment. Among these groups are women of color, single mothers, working-class women, older women, disabled women, lesbians and feminists" (California Commission on the Status of Women 1986:17).

Responses and Strategies

Victims' responses range from remaining silent to quitting their jobs to filing formal complaints against their harassers (Maypole 1986). Gruber (1989) outlines four "typical" responses to victimization:

1. Avoidance strategies include ignoring the harassment and attempting to physically and structurally remove oneself such as by transferring or leaving a job.
2. Diffusion actions mask the nature of the harassment and redefine it as a superficially or temporarily legitimate inter-

action. Tactics are going along, stalling, or joking with the harasser to buy some time so that the victim may seek social support or advice about how to manage the situation.

3. Negotiation, a more direct response, includes asking or telling the harasser to cease the interaction. It is riskier for the victim, especially for women with little economic and cultural power, as the harasser may refuse to stop or retaliate against the victim as a result of her request. Because of the risk, negotiation is most often employed in situations where the power relations between the harasser and the victim are more symmetrical.

4. Confrontation focuses on use of organizational and legal power to stop the harassment. It presents a number of risks for women including retaliation and escalated harassment for reporting events, disbelief, accusations, defamation of character, and being fired.

Women often use a combination of these four strategies to cope with sexual harassment.

Although there have been several widely publicized court victories for women who have opted to sue their harassers (*Baltimore Sun* 1994; Higham 1995; Hoover and Chiang 1994; Hosler 1995), these cases are anomalies. Many women employing confrontational strategies by seeking legal assistance have great difficulty in convincing attorneys to accept their cases for several reasons. First, sexual harassment is difficult to prove because it almost always takes place in private—between the perpetrator and the victim. Second, women often lack the necessary resources to pay attorney and court fees in order to pursue a complaint. Litigation is frequently protracted, consuming the victim's and her attorney's time and resources. Third, men continue to dominate the legal profession. Some male lawyers and judges do not always take such complaints seriously, and they view women who wish to pursue legal action as hysterical, overzealous, and not worthy of the court's time. Additionally, attorney Anne Weills of Oakland, California, who specializes in representing women who have been sexually harassed, explains:

> The current conservative political climate and the attack on civil rights law have served to discourage, chill, and undermine the rights of women to pursue these legal actions. . . . Many lawyers, who would have been loath to mock these cases before, do so openly—they now feel as though they have permission

to mock women's claims of sexual harassment and to not take them seriously. . . . The retaliation women are now experiencing for filing complaints is tremendous. It really has become a new phenomenon for men who are harassers to file complaints of defamation against women who dare to complain. It is a defensive tactic that perpetrators use to try to intimidate women into not taking action. If you think that if you file a lawsuit you will be sued for defamation for filing it, that's pretty chilling and scary for a lot of women. Sexual harassment litigation has become a much meaner and tougher environment for victims than ever before.[2]

Legislation

A number of federal and state laws and guidelines address sexual harassment. Federal legislation, Title VII of the Civil Rights Act of 1964, made sexual harassment a form of gender discrimination in the workplace. It allows an employee to sue an employer for failure to create and maintain a harassment-free workplace. Additionally, employers are held legally and fiscally liable for harassment perpetrated by their employees against co-workers, regardless of whether the business owner was aware of the harassment. A second piece of federal legislation, Title IX of the Educational Amendments of 1972, made sexual harassment illegal in schools and universities. But it is limited. Only institutions receiving federal monies may be held liable, and victims may only be compensated for loss and cannot be awarded punitive damages. The Federal Equal Employment Opportunity Commission, formed in 1980, also issues guidelines and monitors reporting incidents of sexual harassment.

Like other forms of violence against women, sexual harassment sustains the gender hierarchy and power differentials between men and women. Some women are at greater risk, but every woman who experiences it undergoes corrosion of her autonomy and self-esteem. A note for the future on reducing this problem was sounded by Professor Anita Hill to the Civil Justice Foundation: "It's important that we not only understand what harassment is but that we understand how the process discourages people from coming forward. We have to empower people to come through a system that has disempowered them in the past" (quoted in Walker 1993).

NOTES

1. An important element in all sexual harassment situations and contexts is the victim's perception of the experience. Even if the harasser does not intend or mean to coerce his victim, the woman often feels threatened or intimidated by the unwanted sexual advances. Pollack (1990) found that much of the behavior that women experience and define as offensive and as sexual harassment is both defined and accepted by men as normal heterosexual behavior.

2. Personal communication from Anne Weills, attorney, Oakland, California.

REFERENCES

Baltimore Sun
    1994   "Woman who sued CIA decries agency culture: settlement pays her $410,000." 25 December.

Benson, Kathleen
    1984   "Comment on Crocker's 'An analysis of university definitions of sexual harassment.'" Signs: Journal of Women in Culture and Society 9:516–19.

Buehler, Janice, and Brandy M. Britton
    1992   "Gender issues in the treatment of heroin addicts." Progress report to the National Institute on Drug Abuse, Grant #R01DA05277. Rockville, MD.

California Commission on the Status of Women
    1986   Help Yourself: A Manual for Dealing with Sexual Harassment. Sacramento: California Commission on the Status of Women

Capelle, Eleanor
    1992   "A woman's choice." Pp. 42–45 in Amber Coverdale Sumrall and Dena Taylor (eds.), Sexual Harassment: Women Speak Out. Freedom, CA: Crossing Press.

Chan, Anja A.
    1994   Women and Sexual Harassment: A Practical Guide to the Legal Protections of Title VII and the Hostile Environment Claim. Binghamton, NY: Harrington Park Press.

Chrisman, Robert, and Robert L. Allen, eds.
    1992   Court of Appeal: The Black Community Speaks Out on the Racial and Sexual Politics of Thomas v. Hill. New York: Ballantine Books.

Dziech, Billie Wright, and Linda Weiner
    1984   The Lecherous Professor. Boston: Beacon Press.

Farley, Lin
    1978   Sexual Shakedown: The Sexual Harassment of Women on the Job. New York: McGraw-Hill.

Fitzgerald, Louise F.
1992 Sexual Harassment in Higher Education: Concepts and Issues. Washington: National Education Association.
1993 "Sexual harassment: violence against women in the workplace." American Psychologist 48:1070-76.

Fitzgerald, Louise F., and Hesson McInnis
1989 "The dimensions of sexual harassment: a structural analysis." Journal of Vocational Behavior 35:309-26.

Grauerholz, Elizabeth
1989 "Harassment of women professors by students: exploring the dynamics of power, authority, and gender in a university setting." Sex Roles 21:789-801.

Gruber, James E.
1989 "How women handle sexual harassment: a literature review." Social Science Review 74:3-7.

Higham, Scott
1995 "Police sex harassment suit settled." Baltimore Sun, 2 June.

Hoover, Ken, and Harriet Chiang
1994 "Harassment damages total $7.1 million: award against law firm, attorney may be a record." San Francisco Chronicle, 2 September.

Hosler, Karen
1995 "Senate panel to probe allegations of Packwood sexual misconduct: ethics committee details 18 incidents." Baltimore Sun, 18 May.

Kilpatrick, Douglas G.
1992 "Treatment and counseling needs of women veterans who were raped, otherwise sexually assaulted, or sexually harassed during military service." Testimony before the Senate Committee on Veterans' Affairs.

Koss, Mary P.
1990 "Changed lives: the psychological impact of sexual harassment." Pp. 73-92 in Michele A. Paludi (ed.), Ivory Power: Sex and Gender Harassment in the Academy. Albany: SUNY Press.

Lenhart, Sharyn A., and Clyde H. Evans
1991 "Sexual harassment and gender discrimination: A primer for women physicians." Journal of the American Medical Women's Association 46:77-82.

MacKinnon, Catherine A.
1979 Sexual Harassment of Working Women. New Haven, CT: Yale University Press.

Maypole, Donald E.
1986 "Sexual harassment of social workers." Social Work 31:29-34.

Morrison, Toni, ed.
1992 Race-ing Justice, En-gendering Power: Essays on Anita Hill, Clarence Thomas, and the Construction of Social Reality. New York: Pantheon.

Paludi, Michele, Marc Grossman, Carole Ann Scott, Jodi Kinderman, Susan Matula, Julie Ostwald, Judie Dovan, and Donna Mulcahy
　　1990　　"Myths and realities: sexual harassment on campus." Pp. 1–14 in Michele A. Paludi (ed.), Ivory Power: Sexual Harassment on Campus. Albany: SUNY Press.

Phelps, Timothy M., and Helen Winternitz
　　1992　　Capitol Games: Clarence Thomas, Anita Hill, and the Story of a Supreme Court Nomination. New York: Hyperion.

Pollack, Wendy
　　1990　　"Sexual harassment: women's experience vs. legal definitions." Harvard Women's Law Journal 13:149–61.

Rosenberg, Janet, Harry Perlstadt, and William R. F. Phillips
　　1993　　"Now that we are here: discrimination, disparagement, and harassment at work and the experience of women lawyers." Gender and Society 7:415–33.

Rubin, Sylvia
　　1992　　"Get sensitive—that's an order: navy's sex harassment seminar is cheered, booed." San Francisco Chronicle, 10 August.

Schneider, Beth E.
　　1987　　"Graduate women, sexual harassment, and university policy." Journal of Higher Education 58:46–65.

Shrier, Diane K.
　　1990　　"Sexual harassment and discrimination: impact on physical and mental health." New Jersey Medical Journal 87:105–7.

Sumrall, Amber Cloverdale, and Dena Taylor
　　1992　　Sexual Harassment: Women Speak Out. Freedom, CA: Crossing Press.

Walker, Thaai
　　1993　　"Anita Hill tells of stress in sex harassment cases." San Francisco Chronicle, 5 August.

Williams, Elizabeth A., Julie A. Lam, and Michael Shively
　　1992　　"The impact of university policy on the sexual harassment of female students." Journal of Higher Education 63:50–64.

[20]

The Ongoing Politics of Contraception:
Norplant and Other Emerging Technologies

CHERI A. PIES

Cheri Pies takes a public health perspective to explore how complex issues of power and control have accompanied contraceptive technology development. She carefully weighs what different groups see as advantageous or excessively hazardous, and she raises troubling questions about promoting contraceptive methods that do not prevent sexually transmitted diseases in an era of HIV infection.

From the moment it was introduced, the most remarkable thing about the birth control device Norplant has not been the medical technology involved but the rapid emergence of a popular consensus on who ought to use it.
      —Tim Rutten, Los Angeles Times, 31 May 1991

It took twenty-four years to develop, test, and approve an implantable device that can prevent pregnancy for as long as five years. It took less than two weeks for Norplant to be billed as a new method of coercion. . . .
Norplant has been most publicly and ardently taken up by those who want to cap social problems by getting a lock on the womb.
      —Ellen Goodman, Oakland Tribune, 19 February 1991

In December 1990, the U.S. Food and Drug Administration (FDA) approved the sale of Norplant, a long-acting, health care provider–dependent, reversible contraceptive device for women. The FDA's actions were greeted by widespread media response heralding Norplant as the "most effective birth control method yet" (Scott 1991). At the same time, the FDA approval generated alarm and concern among women's health advocates, ethicists, social policy analysts, public health practitioners, and consumers. These concerns were based on fears about the potential abuse and misuse of a contraceptive "whose effectiveness in preventing pregnancy does not depend on the user's behavior" (Gladwell 1990), a contraceptive that cannot be altered "short of having the implant surgically removed" (Mertus 1991). Two years later, Depo-Provera, an injectable contraceptive that lasts three months, was also approved for use in the United States.

Norplant and Depo-Provera appeared on the contraceptive market at a time when legislators, policymakers, and others were looking for a "quick fix" to a range of overwhelming and seemingly intractable social problems. The very nature of the Norplant implant—that it can be inserted and removed only by a clinician and once implanted prevents pregnancy regardless of the user's behavior—added fuel to a debate already heated by the abortion issue concerning who is and ought to be in control of women's reproductive decisions. The availability of Depo-Provera further complicates this debate, because once the injection is given, the effects cannot be reversed until the drug has worn off. Competing claims were at issue: Would Norplant and Depo-Provera enhance a woman's reproductive freedom or curtail it? Would Norplant and technologies like Depo-Provera be made available to increase the contraceptive options of all women, or would they be used to control the fertility of certain groups of women? The most vulnerable are poor women, women of color, women with emotional and mental disabilities, and HIV-infected women.

Contraceptive technologies are always introduced in social, cultural, historical, political, and economic contexts. Any number of significant factors influence the reactions to these innovations and subsequently contribute to the ways in which these technologies are embraced and utilized. To understand the controversies surrounding Norplant and Depo-Provera, it is useful to examine other controversies in the birth control movement in the United States since the late nineteenth century. This provides a framework for linking a documented need for contraception in the United States with the development of Norplant, Depo-Provera, and still other experimental contraceptive technologies. Broader issues and concerns are better understood in historical perspective than when viewed as peculiar to a particular technology.[1] Only then can we grasp the implications of distinctive attributes of the individual technologies, such as Norplant as an implant and Depo-Provera as an injectable.

Birth Control in the United States

From the earliest rumblings of the birth control movement in the United States during the mid-nineteenth century, "birth control has always been primarily an issue of politics, not of technology" (Gordon 1976:xii). The birth control movement has been concerned with who has children, who does not, and who decides—issues of power and control. Prominent players in framing this movement have had different agendas and often competing priorities. For example, "Neo-Malthusians supported birth control as a means of improving the condition of the poor by limiting population growth; feminists and socialists believed it was a fundamental women's right; eugenicists embraced it as a way of influencing genetic quality" (Hartmann 1987:92).

Feminists in the nineteenth-century birth control movement directed their efforts toward securing women's rights to reproductive self-determination, autonomy, and sexual freedom rather than toward the design and development of methods to avoid conception. Their campaign for "voluntary motherhood" was developed as part of a larger campaign for women's political equality, and it promoted abstinence as the preferred method of contraception (Gordon 1976).[2] However, this movement, led largely by middle-class women and framed from their perspective, failed to address the realities of the lives of growing numbers of immigrant and working-class women in the United States, many of whom were plagued by poverty, ill health, and poor working conditions. For these women, the goals of voluntary motherhood were seen as ones that could "only be achieved by women possessing material wealth" (Davis 1990:18). Not surprisingly, vast numbers of poor and working-class women did not identify with the early birth control movement.

Toward the end of the nineteenth century, as significant numbers of middle-class women chose to curtail their sexual activity, the birthrate among this group of white, Protestant women declined even without access to or the benefits of "modern contraception" (Brodie 1994). At the same time, births among black, immigrant, and working-class women did not decline (Gordon 1976; McCann 1994). Many leading politicians and industrialists argued that the falling birthrate among native-born whites threatened a so-called race suicide, a disappearance of their white race. This threat was greeted by such alarm and dismay that President Theodore Roosevelt insisted that steps be taken so that "race purity . . . would be maintained." To this end, and under the guise of preventing "race suicide," birth control was introduced specifically to prevent "the proliferation of the 'lower classes'" (Davis 1990:19). "Within birth control circles it was assumed that poor women, Black and immigrant alike, had a 'moral obligation' to restrict the size of their families" (Davis 1990:20).[3]

Early in the twentieth century, Margaret Sanger, well known for coin-ing the term *birth control,* worked closely with socialists to further the progressive, and frequently radical, efforts of the birth control movement.[4] The means of contraception, Sanger argued strongly, should be woman-controlled to enhance women's autonomy. Specifically, she promoted the development and distribution of diaphragms and improved spermicides through research in Britain and in the many American birth control clinics she helped to found. Later, however, Sanger enlisted the support of professionals, most notably doctors, to further the cause of birth con-trol.[5] Then, in 1919, in a statement issued in the *Birth Control Review,* Margaret Sanger embraced eugenic ideology and called for "more children from the fit and less from the unfit." "This," she said, "is the chief issue of birth control." In 1932, as the new leaders in the birth control movement continued to advocate "racial progress and sterilization," in an attempt to "prevent American people from being replaced by alien or Negro stock," Sanger reiterated her ideology and went along with eugenicists' recom-mendations for "sterilization of those suspected of producing 'unfit' off-spring" (Hartmann 1987:95).[6]

In 1942, the Birth Control Federation of America, which had been influential in limiting births among blacks in the South during the late 1930s through the "Negro Project," changed its name to Planned Parent-hood (McCann 1994). The organization then began to use the term *family planning* to describe their efforts to lower birthrates and motivate women to have fewer children, with the goal of stabilizing the family and rein-forcing women's commitment to the role of motherhood. These were not easy times, however, for an organization of this nature. The Comstock Laws, which were not fully overturned until 1965, defined all contracep-tive devices as obscene and forbade the sending of obscene matter through the U.S. mail, thus preventing Planned Parenthood and other organiza-tions like it from advertising and openly serving unmarried women. The organization was, however, instrumental in making contraceptives avail-able, accessible, and acceptable to married women and in helping women avoid unwanted pregnancies.

For most of the twentieth century, women's reproductive options have been selectively restricted. Due in large part to Sanger's strategies for birth control distribution, physicians came to control the distribution of con-traceptives. Legislators regulated the laws of that distribution, and eugen-icists promoted the "science" of improving human heredity (Duster 1990). Poor women and women of color, who were targets of birth control and eugenic rhetoric during the first half of the twentieth century, then fell victim to the population control strategies of the late 1960s and 1970s (Clarke 1997). Population control is built on the assumption that over-population is the cause of poverty, and if population growth could be controlled, poverty and other related problems would not exist. In practice, it focuses on controlling births by dictating ideal family size "without respect for cultural, social or political self-determination" (Gordon 1976:xv n). These same themes resonate in contemporary debates over the uses of new contraceptive technologies and contrast sharply with woman-controlled contraception and reproductive rights.

Population Control and Sterilization Abuse

Population control ideology is evident in the history of involuntary sterilization and subsequent sterilization abuse in the United States as well. Before 1975, significant numbers of poor and minority women were sterilized without their knowledge (Presser 1980; Reilly 1991; Rodriguez-Trias 1984; Shapiro 1985), and others were pressured to "accept" steriliza-tion as a requisite to receiving welfare payments (Hartmann 1987). In her seminal work, *Woman's Body, Woman's Right*, Linda Gordon explains that by 1974 in the United States, women of color on welfare had about one-third more sterilizations than women who did not receive welfare; in arguments later condemned as coercive, women "suffering primarily from inadequate housing, inadequate nutrition, and inadequate medical care, from poverty in short, [were] told that reducing their family size and/or unwanted pregnancies" would better their lives (Gordon 1976:400). This use of coercion, seen by many critics as a blatant attempt to reduce the nonwhite birthrate, brought renewed attention to both the racism and sexism inherent in U.S. society (Clarke 1984; Duster 1990; Hartmann 1987; Hubbard 1984; Rowland 1984; Terry 1991, 1995).

In 1974, regulations issued by the Department of Health, Education, and Welfare (HEW) required written informed consent for all women seeking sterilization via federal funding and prohibited using federal funds to sterilize women under the age of twenty-one. In 1978, HEW extended the required waiting period for federally funded sterilizations from three to thirty days, required translators as needed, and put a ban on the signing of consent forms while a woman was in labor, during childbirth, or at the time of an abortion (Gordon 1976). These regulations came about through the sustained efforts of feminist women's health activists.[7]

Scientific Contraceptive Technologies

Since the mid-1950s, introduction of new scientific reproductive and contraceptive technologies has profoundly affected the birth control and population control movements. Before the advent of birth control pills, the intrauterine device, sterilization, and legalized abortion, women and their partners typically relied on simple, low-tech methods, such as self-induced abortion, barrier methods (the diaphragm, condom, spermicides, pessary, or sponge), the rhythm method, or coitus interruptus.[8] As the ideology of population control gained popularity, reproductive researchers focused increasingly on contraceptive technologies that were long acting, highly effective, provider dependent, and easy to use (Clarke 1997). Substantial private and government funding for contraceptive research was readily available to pharmaceutical companies and agencies involved in family planning and population control efforts. Such contraceptive technologies as birth control pills, intrauterine devices, injectables, and implants made women more dependent on medical professionals for their administration and removal (Hardon and Achthoven 1990).

Women's health advocates have long criticized both the safety and the provider-dependent nature of scientific contraceptives and suggested that continued emphasis on such methods has compromised women's health and threatened women's reproductive rights (Arditti, Klein, and Minden 1984; Clarke 1984; Hardon and Achthoven 1990; Hartmann 1987; Seaman 1970/1995). To use these new methods, women need access to clinics, they have to be able to afford these services, and they often need the aid of clinicians to stop using these contraceptives. Reproductive scientists defended their interest in designing contraceptives that would be effective and "easy to use," although the question of "easy to use for whom?" was not addressed by the producers and distributors of these technologies, thus raising suspicion about the primary goal of these technologies among those concerned with women's health.[9]

Debates soon arose concerning the ethics of disseminating these science-based, provider-controlled technologies. Of particular concern was the overwhelming focus on the development of contraceptive technologies solely for use by women, with what appeared to be little consideration of the potential for abuse with provider-dependent rather than user-controlled contraceptives (i.e., coercion, lack of access to removal). Nor was there adequate attention to the adverse effects of these new technologies on women's health (infertility, no protection from sexually transmitted diseases, and increased risk of chronic, life-threatening illnesses). Furthermore, some commentators suggested that the length of time new contraceptive technologies had been under investigation was too limited, making it impossible to provide consumers with information they would need to make fully informed choices with regard to future fertility, long-term health effects, and risks to future children (Oudshoorn 1996). This is an inevitable problem with all new contraceptives as the long-term effects cannot be fully known until the technology has been used for several decades by women in diverse settings and circumstances. However, more often than not, the absence of this information is frequently downplayed, or perhaps ignored, in discussions of contraceptive "safety."

Other ethical concerns emerged as well. Some of the new contraceptive methods that were produced by U.S. pharmaceutical companies but had not been approved for use in the United States, such as Depo-Provera, were being distributed by government-funded agencies in developing countries. In addition, women being offered these new contraceptives were expected to make a commitment to long-term contraception, given the nature of intrauterine devices, injectables, and implants, raising questions as to whether these methods were enhancing or diminishing the rights of users. Moreover, many observers challenged the balance of benefits of these new technological advances over their potential harms especially in settings where primary health care is inadequate or nonexistent (Dixon-Mueller 1993a, 1993b). Given the availability of low-tech, user-controlled barrier methods, is the goal of preventing pregnancy worth exposing women to the risks of severe short- and long-term side effects?

To some observers, it appears that racism, sexism, class politics, and power relations continue to drive the current development and application of most new contraceptive technologies in the United States today (Mastroianni, Donaldson, and Kane, 1990). The themes of population control and Malthus still echo in legislatures, public policy reports, and newspaper articles. Feminist voices concerned with women's health are too often silenced. The history of the birth control movement in the United States provides an essential backdrop for understanding the current, and frequently contentious, overlap of public policies regarding women's reproductive behaviors, efforts to secure reproductive rights for all women, and directions in contraceptive research in the United States and elsewhere today. As we look more closely at how Norplant and Depo-Provera fit into this historical picture, let us first turn our attention to what are considered the contemporary needs of American women for effective contraception.

Contemporary Need for Contraception

The United States has one of the highest rates of abortion, teenage pregnancy, and unintended pregnancy in the industrialized world (Forrest 1987; Trussell and Vaughan 1989). Many reproductive researchers agree that these high rates are a result of the fact that women in America have fewer contraceptive options than women in some other countries (Kaeser 1991; Mastroianni, Donaldson, and Kane 1990). There are, however, competing explanations. Problems of access to medical care for large segments of the population, a range of cultural attitudes about sexuality and reproduction rarely considered in the development of contraceptive devices, a lack of reliable data on safety and efficacy, and the fact that many consumers are often misinformed about safety and efficacy of contraceptive methods all contribute to higher rates. Further, some women decide to use no birth control method for periods of time because they fear side effects and risks of potential health problems (Harlap, Kost, and Forrest 1991).[10]

Even among women using contraception, unintended pregnancies occur. A 1991 report issued by the Alan Guttmacher Institute indicates that 47 percent of all unintended pregnancies occur while women are using contraceptives. Each year one in nine women ages fifteen to forty-four become pregnant. Of the 6.4 million pregnancies in 1988, 56 percent were unplanned. Unintended pregnancies often occur as a result of method failure, failure to use a back-up method when necessary, incorrect or inconsistent use of a method, or discontinuance of use.

Several studies point to the effects of socioeconomic status, family stability, mother's educational level, and age at first intercourse on whether a woman uses contraception (Mosher and Bachrach 1987; Mosher and McNally 1991; Zelnick, Kanter, and Ford 1981). Moreover, contraceptive services are not readily accessible to all women. In particular, poor women, young women, women of color, and rural women may find they have limited access to these services for financial reasons, geographic distances, misinformation, lack of education, and legal barriers. For these same groups of women and others, personal barriers to contraceptive use exist as well. These may include "an inability to talk about sex, confusion or violence in the home, lack of self-esteem, and feelings of powerlessness and hopelessness" (Harlap, Kost, and Forrest 1991:9). Commenting on these barriers and the issue of access, Faye Wattleton, then president of Planned Parenthood Federation of America, wrote in a 1991 editorial in the *Los Angeles Times* that "access to birth control is woefully inadequate—so inadequate, in fact, that one can argue that poor and young women are effectively coerced to have children."

Setting the Stage for Norplant, Depo-Provera, and Other Emerging Technologies

In 1990, a National Academy of Science report on contraceptive research and development estimated that contraceptive failure alone probably led to 1.6 million to 2.0 million accidental pregnancies in the United States in 1987 (Mastroianni, Donaldson, and Kane 1990). It is not surprising, then, that reproductive scientists, contraceptive researchers, and others interested in assisting women and their partners to avoid unintended pregnancies are eager to develop a contraceptive method that will not only be highly effective in preventing pregnancies while protecting future fertility but will also be less susceptible to the possibility of contraceptive failure.

Increasing numbers of women between fifteen and forty-four years of age rely on female sterilization as a method of contraception. From 1982 to 1988, female sterilization rose from 23 to 27 percent among women of childbearing years (Kost, Forrest, and Harlap 1991; Mosher 1990). Some women and their partners have had all the children they want and prefer a method that is unobtrusive, does not interrupt sexual interludes, and is highly effective. It may be that because "currently available methods are not well suited to the religious, socioeconomic or health circumstances of many Americans," many couples choose sterilization while others wait for a "wider array of safe and effective methods" to be available (Kaeser 1991:131).

Most of the newest contraceptive technologies that offer the promise of greater protection and "convenience" of use are not yet widely available in the United States. These include long-lasting injectables (such as Noristerat), new and supposedly reversible means of sterilization (such as Filshie clips and Ovabloc silicone plugs), and new kinds of IUDs (such as Multiload, hormone-releasing and copper-bearing IUDs). All are in use in other countries, including India, Singapore, Bangladesh, Chile, and Brazil.[11]

By the 1990s, the stage was set for Norplant and then Depo-Provera. Thus when Norplant arrived on the U.S. contraceptive scene, with the promise to be long acting, reversible, safe, easy to use, and highly effective, women, policymakers, and those interested in population control all hoped it would fill needs that other methods did not. Reproductive science was moving in the direction of longer-lasting, drug-reliant birth control rather than imposed barrier and spermicide methods. According to contraceptive researchers, American women were looking for contraception that was effective, safe, and easy to use. Legislators, judges, and other policymakers were looking for ways to solve society's pressing social problems such as teen pregnancy. Norplant and Depo-Provera were about to become "part of the ongoing historical controversy," a "contested technology" where, as Clarke and Montini suggested, history would echo loudly (1993).

Development of Norplant

Research and development for a long-acting contraceptive that could be placed underneath the skin of a woman's upper arm began in 1966 at the Population Council, a private organization founded by John D. Rockefeller III in 1952.[12] (The Population Council had earlier pioneered the development of the IUD.) Ultimately, levonorgestrel, a synthetic progestin used in several types of oral contraceptives, was selected for use in an implant. The Norplant system consists of six capsules, each about the size of a matchstick, containing levonorgestrel. The capsules are inserted just under the skin of a woman's upper arm in a minor surgical procedure (Population Council 1990a). The levonorgestrel diffuses through the capsule at a slow, steady rate over five years. This dose of levonorgestrel is comparable to the daily dose in progestin-only oral contraceptives and is about one-fourth the dose found in combined estrogen-progestin oral contraceptives (*Population Reports* 1987).

It is the slow, sustained release of the drug into the bloodstream that makes Norplant different. Other new forms of contraception, such as the injectable Depo-Provera, biodegradable implants, vaginal rings, transdermal patches, transdermal wearable contraceptive accessories (e.g., bracelets, watches), and steroid-releasing IUDs, contain synthetic hormones like progestin. But only Norplant offers long-term, continuous administration of the contraceptive agent.[13]

Between 1975 and 1982, clinical trials were conducted with women volunteers in eight countries: Brazil, Chile, Denmark, the Dominican Republic, Finland, Jamaica, Sweden, and the United States. Between 1983 and 1990, Norplant was tested in over forty-six countries with more than 55,000 volunteers. In the United States, more than 1,000 women participated in clinical trials (Croxatto, Diaz, and Sivin 1991; Darney et al. 1990a, 1990b; *Population Reports* 1993, Shoupe et al. 1991; Sinofsky, Pasquale, and Gonzalez 1990). In 1983, Finland became the first country to give regulatory approval to the method.[14]

In December 1990, the United States became the seventeenth country to approve Norplant for distribution. At the time of FDA approval, more than a half-million women had used Norplant, either in countries where the method was approved for distribution or in clinical and pre-introduction trials. In addition, researchers at three international training centers—in Egypt, Indonesia, and the Dominican Republic—had conducted extensive acceptability studies with women in several countries in both rural and urban settings (Affandi et al. 1987b; Basnayake, Thapa, and Balogh 1988; Diaz et al. 1982; Population Council 1990b; Sivin 1988). These studies have provided the basis for much of what is technically known about Norplant's mechanisms of action, its effectiveness, side effects, and continuation rates. What had not been studied, however, were the social and political consequences of making this type of contraceptive available.

FDA Approval and Public Reaction to Norplant

Immediately following FDA approval of Norplant, conflicts emerged. Within one day of the FDA announcement, an editorial in the *Philadelphia Inquirer* (1990) entitled "Poverty and Norplant: Can contraception reduce the underclass?" encouraged readers to "think about" Norplant as a tool in the fight against poverty in the African American community. Shortly thereafter, David Duke, a member of the Louisiana legislature, introduced legislation that would pay "a cash bounty to any poor woman who would accept Norplant along with her welfare payments" (Yukins 1991). Taking these proposals one step further, in early January 1991, before the device became available for purchase, a judge in Tulare County, California, ordered the use of Norplant as a condition of probation for a woman convicted of child abuse. Later that month, the Kansas legislature held hearings on a bill that was hailed as a way to "save taxpayers' money," by proposing to pay five hundred dollars to women receiving AFDC who agreed to have the Norplant implant inserted. Discussion of this legislative proposal prompted syndicated columnist Ellen Goodman (1991) to observe, "The state would offer an incentive to one class of women—poor, single mothers on welfare—for one kind of birth control—Norplant."

In April 1991, California governor Pete Wilson "hoped to make Norplant available through state-financed family planning clinics and the Medi-Cal health care program for the poor." Wilson's other plans involved setting aside special funds to ensure that Norplant would be available free of charge to teenagers and women identified as "drug users." When asked if future plans included legally compelling women who used drugs during pregnancy to use Norplant, Governor Wilson stated, "Frankly, we haven't decided" (Rutten 1991).

Shortly after the announcement of Governor Wilson's proposal, a *Los Angeles Times* poll found that 60 percent of the Californians polled thought that "Norplant should be mandatory for women who abuse drugs" (*Los Angeles Times* 1991:E1). Echoing these views, in the fall of 1991, an estimated 28,000 readers of Ann Landers's nationally syndicated newspaper advice column wrote to express their opinions about Norplant and a welfare system that they believed "rewards unwed mothers with cash for each child." Letters published in the 3 September 1991 column read, "We resent paying taxes to support unwed mothers who know they'll get bigger welfare checks if they have more babies," "These irresponsible brood mares should be sterilized after the second baby," and "Forced birth control is the only solution."

During 1991–92, twenty measures were introduced in thirteen states proposing legislation that would encourage or require women on welfare or those convicted of drug use to use Norplant. None of these bills passed, though several nearly did. In response to many of these government proposals, the board of trustees of the American Medical Association (1992:1818) issued a statement recommending only voluntary use of this long-acting contraceptive, citing a "person's fundamental rights to refuse medical treatment, to be free of cruel and unusual punishment, and to procreate." Nevertheless, social policy legislation involving required or recommended use of Norplant continues to be considered.

By mid-1992, the use of Norplant was being identified by public health officials as one way to reduce teenage pregnancies among African Americans and Latinos. In December 1992, officials at the Baltimore Health Department announced their intention to make Norplant available at several

school-based clinics in the Baltimore area, beginning with a school attended by pregnant teens and teenage mothers (Beilenson, Miola, and
Farmer 1995). At the same time, in several other metropolitan areas,
Norplant was offered to adolescents at school-based clinics with high rates
of teen pregnancies (Kaplan and Johnson 1993). The responses from parents, teenagers, community leaders, religious groups, clinicians, social policy experts, and others to these actions have been mixed. Initially, the
Baltimore community was not involved in the decision to make Norplant
available at these school-based sites. Upon learning of the health
department's decision to offer Norplant to adolescents at two high schools,
many people raised concerns about the risk of unknown long-term side effects of Norplant use on young adolescents, the risk of HIV and other STDs
with a contraceptive that only prevents pregnancy, and the threat of genocide posed by the use of a long-acting contraceptive. From the Baltimore
experience with Norplant, public health professionals learned that "with
any public health initiative that might be perceived as having a disproportionate impact on minorities," it is essential that the affected communities
be involved from the beginning in the development, identification, and implementation of potential public health policies (Beilenson, Miola, and
Farmer 1995:311).

In July 1994, a class action suit was filed against Wyeth-Ayerst (the
pharmaceutical company that sells Norplant) on behalf of almost four
hundred women as a result of reported problems occurring during and after
removal of the device (Lewin 1994). The women involved in the suit
suffered severe pain during removal and experienced scarring following
removal. The lawsuit seeks damages for the women involved and furthermore requests an injunction to prevent the sale of Norplant to clinicians
who have not been trained in both insertion and removal. As media
attention to this class action suit gained prominence, requests for Norplant by clinic patients declined. At the same time, competition from the
availability of Depo-Provera is thought to have brought about a substantial drop in interest and use of Norplant (Vrazo 1994).

In addition to these public criticisms of Norplant, several major public
policy controversies have emerged. These include (1) the potential for
coercive use of the device, particularly with vulnerable populations of
women, (2) the court-ordered use of Norplant in cases involving women
convicted of child abuse or drug use, (3) Norplant as a social policy option
in addressing the problem of teenage pregnancy, and (4) the question of
balancing the need for pregnancy prevention with an equally demanding

need for disease prevention. Simultaneously, the high cost of Norplant (approximately $365 for the device, and an additional $450 to $750 for insertion and removal) presented additional concerns over who would have access to it. Because most women's insurance will not pay for Norplant, this technology is likely to become a contraceptive option only for the very poor (through Medicaid or MediCal) or for the affluent.

Without a doubt, the availability of Norplant threatened to resurrect real problems of coercive misuse and abuse, as well as targeting certain populations for fertility control. These are problems reminiscent of the early years of the birth control movement in the United States, as well as more recent times. Women might choose Norplant for its effectiveness and long-acting nature; however, once the device is inserted, they may find that control of their future fertility rests with health care providers' willingness to remove it.[15] An inevitable tension has evolved, a tension between the potential for coercive use of this long-acting contraceptive and the failure to provide adequate access to Norplant for a broad cross-section of women. As a result, contradictory critiques of contraceptives such as Norplant and Depo-Provera have emerged among women's health advocacy groups. This contradiction focuses on the needs of all women for equal access to a wide array of contraceptive options and the potential for misuse, abuse, and coercion in the service delivery setting of certain contraceptives, especially with particular populations of women.

Different Values, Multiple Viewpoints about Norplant

In a 1991–92 study I conducted in California, reproductive health care consumers, reproductive health care providers, and policymakers participated in focused group interviews designed to identify their values and viewpoints with regard to the complex ethical, social, and political issues raised by the debate over Norplant. In this work, the different sociopolitical contexts that affect ethical decision making became clearer. Policymakers placed a great deal of emphasis on their obligation to the public, an obligation that requires them to support actions that appear to preserve and support the social good. This obligation, however, was not without conflicts. As one policymaker explained, "People are desperate for some sort of solution to the problem of pregnancy among substance-using women. They want to find a way of preventing the ongoing problem and the perpetuation of it. When something like Norplant comes around and it looks like a possible solution, well—there you have it" (Pies 1993:146). On the other hand, concerns about the potential for mandatory or recommended use of Norplant for certain groups of women prompted policymakers to ask about the implications of such actions: "If we agree to compromise one groups' rights, whose are next?" and "Once you mandate something for one group, where do you draw the line?"

In contrast, health care providers focused on the needs of their clients for effective, safe contraceptives, while repeatedly drawing attention to the risks of exposure to HIV and other STDs with Norplant, the unknown effects of long-term use, and the potential for women to fail to return for routine gynecologic care with a long-acting contraceptive in place. At the same time, health care providers were conflicted about how to address some of the recurring problems they saw among their patients—teen pregnancies, repeat abortions, HIV-infected women bearing children, etc.—without infringing on a woman's right to choose when, whether, and with whom to be pregnant. As one health care provider explained, "Years of exposure to certain problems often makes something like Norplant look good" (Pies 1993:149). Although many of the health care providers agreed with that statement, most believed that Norplant was "only a Band-Aid," not an adequate solution to the recurrent social problems they were seeing.

Finally, consumers (who were teenage mothers, women at risk for HIV infection, women on welfare, and homeless pregnant women) spoke to similar concerns about the problems of teenage pregnancy, drug-exposed newborns, and women having more children than they can comfortably care for. However, they were adamant that controlling or restricting women's reproduction was not the solution. They pointed to social and political factors to explain why people act in ways that others deem "irresponsible," "immoral," or "wrong," including racism, discrimination, unemployment, lack of education, and poverty. From their perspectives, individuals do not have much control over their own lives. Instead, their lives are controlled by the actions of others, largely legislators, policymakers, judges, welfare workers, and other government officials. These consumers expressed skepticism that other people, or society in general, would have their own best interests at heart. As one consumer commented, "If they are going to let people on welfare have Norplant for free, something's got to be wrong with it" (Pies 1993:91). Furthermore, in each and every consumer focus group, participants raised concerns about the history of sterilization abuse, particularly in communities of color, and the potential for the subtler, if shorter term, form of sterilization abuse that Norplant presented.

This glimpse at different perspectives suggests the depth of real conflicts (and some of the major actors such as reproductive scientists and international population controllers were not studied). Such conflicts will not be easily resolved through appeals to a single standard of rationality—a standard frequently based on a worldview generated by those who believe that they are free of economic and social constraints. Norplant represents a significant shift in the balance of control over fertility—a shift of control away from the woman and into the hands of others—health care providers, legislators, judges, and agencies (Kaufert 1990).

Norplant, Depo-Provera, and Emerging Technologies

The introduction and development of other contraceptive technologies in the 1990s further intensifies this shift in control. For example, Depo-Provera, a long-acting injectable contraceptive for women, must be administered by a clinician every three months.[16] And, although it is effective for approximately three months, "many users do not ovulate for five or more months after an injection of the usual dose." Furthermore, many critics of the method fear that because it is "easy to use" by those interested in controlling the reproductive behavior of others such as poor women, mentally disabled and institutionalized women, and women of color, this could lead to the adoption of coercive, nonvoluntary contraceptive programs targeting these women (Klitsch 1993:37).

Development of immunological contraceptives has stirred similar fears. Research on immunological contraceptives began in the 1970s and was aimed at developing a contraceptive method given in a single injection to prevent pregnancy for one to two years. Judith Richter, author of a 1993 report on immunological contraception, explains the mechanism of action in this way: "These new methods work in a totally new way, tricking the body into attacking part of reproduction (hormones, or part of the egg, sperm or early embryo) as if it were a germ." Still in the testing stage, the potential availability of this so-called contraceptive vaccine is troubling. According to a contraceptive policy report issued by HAI-Europe, "immunological contraceptive cause the immune system to attack a body function which would otherwise be protected" (1994:1). Furthermore, once administered, immunological contraceptives are irreversible. Critics also point to the fact that this type of contraceptive could be easily administered without a woman's informed consent. Moreover, referring to immunological contraceptives as a "vaccine" may lead women to assume a false impression of safety and potential health benefits.

Several women's health advocacy groups, such as the National Women's Health Network, the National Black Women's Health Project, the National Latina Health Organization, and the National Women's Survival Summit, have argued that in the age of HIV/AIDS, more priority must be given to improving existing user-controlled barrier and natural methods. Women need greater control over their fertility, and they need to be able to protect themselves from HIV/AIDS and other STDs. Although the availability of the female condom promised such protection and control, the reality of its use has proved otherwise. Studies completed for the FDA suggested that the female condom was comparable to other female barrier methods, such as the diaphragm and cervical cap. However, once women began using this method, effectiveness seemed to be lower than initially predicted. And although women were considered to be in control of the female condom, its use still requires male participation and cooperation.

Conclusion

The controversies sparked by the development and use of long-acting, provider-dependent, reversible contraceptive technologies are complicated by issues of power and control, the complex cultural contexts of people's lives, and control over women's reproduction for social benefits. Certainly, there are any number of factors that contribute to explanations of why a technology is embraced at a particular point in time. A quick glance at any leading newspaper in the United States today provides an all-too-graphic picture of the compelling social, political, and economic problems this country is facing. Articles on growing unemployment, a failing economy, and blatant, indiscriminate violence have become more and more common. Stories citing the increase in births of drug-affected newborns, the global incidence of HIV infection, the persistent problems of homelessness, the rise in gang violence among adolescents, boarder babies with no hope of foster placement, and growing numbers of people living in poverty chart a bleak trend of the health and welfare of

America's men, women, and children. In an attempt to "put a cap" on this proliferation of controversial social issues, more social control over women's reproduction has been offered as a solution. It is no wonder then that Norplant has been proclaimed "as perfect a method as you can have" (Painter 1990) and Depo-Provera has taken its place among other contraceptive options despite lingering concern about its long-term safety and potential for misuse. Not surprisingly, the debates prompted by Norplant, Depo-Provera, and the emerging technologies echo the controversies of the past.

Since 1991, more than 900,000 American women have chosen to have Norplant inserted (Vrazo 1994). One early study of Norplant users in Texas suggests that users are young (under twenty-five), unmarried, and poor (60 percent with a household income of $10,000 or less) (Frank et al. 1992). In a 1992 study comparing women choosing Norplant over oral contraceptives, the authors note that "Medicaid reimbursement for Norplant appears to be a powerful incentive for . . . inner city clinic patients to adopt Norplant rather than oral contraceptives" (Weisman et al. 1993).

Before its approval in the United States, Depo-Provera was used extensively outside the United States and was approved for use in thirty countries. Because of complicated side effects, results of animal studies, and potential for abuse, women's health movement activists worked vigorously in the 1980s against its approval. Since receiving FDA approval in 1992, Depo-Provera has proved to be a very popular method among consumers and providers alike. Some commentators suggest that the interest of U.S. women in Depo-Provera may in fact drive Norplant off the contraceptive market. Questions still abound about the long-term safety of Depo-Provera, and certainly the questions of potential misuse remain.

Given that the politics of race and class surrounding emerging contraceptive technologies are bound to persist and that the long-term effects of Norplant and Depo-Provera use are not yet evident, it is likely that these long-acting, provider-dependent contraceptives will continue to be controversial. Historically, women have demonstrated a strong desire to control their own fertility. Not surprisingly, social, economic, and political forces have converged in an attempt to control the reproductive behaviors of certain groups of women. The tensions between these desires on the part of women for reproductive freedom and the pressures on the part of others to shape women's reproductive choices speak volumes about the politics of contraception. These complications and contradictions are not likely to abate.

NOTES

1. "Certain technologies almost inevitably become part of ongoing historical controversies and cannot be meaningfully abstracted from them. Nuclear power, genetic testing, and new abortion technologies . . . are examples of such contested technologies, sites where history echoes loudly. These technologies are constructed within as well as disseminated through extant, contentious arenas composed of heterogeneous actors committed to action on the core issue" (Clarke and Montini 1993:42).

2. It was a campaign based on "the notion that women could refuse to submit to their husbands' sexual demands" (Davis 1990:18), and it advanced the idea that they had a right to choose when to become pregnant. "Voluntary motherhood" reflected values and aspirations of the white Protestant middle class. It encouraged women to break out of traditional gender roles by pursuing education, careers, and self-advancement through avenues other than having children (Gordon 1976).

3. Thus "what was demanded as a 'right' for the privileged came to be interpreted as a 'duty' for the poor." And what began as a movement committed to advancing the rights of women rapidly became a movement linked to dominant eugenic thinking. Eugenics is the "science" of improving human heredity by applying agricultural principles of "breeding good stock" to humans. It offers a philosophy that "the rich and powerful were genetically superior to the poor, and that whites were in general superior to other races" (Hartmann 1987:96). This ideology led to calls for compulsory sterilization of "inferior" races and classes and inaugurated more concerted efforts to supplant women's rights, particularly the rights of certain groups of women.

4. Margaret Sanger was a leading figure in the drive to challenge traditional views of sexual morality and to advance a morality that separated sex from reproduction. Along with Emma Goldman, Sanger was influential in bringing about a fundamental reorientation of sexual values. Between 1916 and 1921, however, her alliances with the more radical factions of this movement weakened, and she turned her attention to establishing credibility of the birth control movement among political conservatives, physicians, and the wealthy (Chesler 1992; Gordon 1976; Hartmann 1987).

5. With them she advocated legislation that would allow only physicians to prescribe contraceptives. Such legislation was opposed by a number of groups who believed that contraceptive services would become inaccessible to women who did not have access to clinics or regular medical care. Others believed that one did not have to be a physician to know how to fit a woman for a diaphragm, the primary technology of contraception along with spermicides at that time (Rothman 1984).

6. In a recent Sanger biography, *Woman of Valor*, Ellen Chesler attempts to clarify Sanger's apparently eugenicist leanings by explaining that Sanger "deliberately courted the power of eugenically inclined academics and scientists to blunt the attacks of religious conservatives against her" (1992:216). Chesler argues that Sanger embraced eugenic viewpoints and built alliances with particular individuals at the time in an attempt to engage secular support for her cause. McCann (1994) has demonstrated how Sanger also used academic eugenicists and biologists to control and limit the power of medical doctors in the birth control movement. Questions remain, however,

as to Sanger's motivation for this shift in her views. Was this the only avenue—one that strongly suggested an intention to limit the "proliferation" of the lower classes—that she saw as viable in her efforts to champion the availability of contraception, ensure women's liberation, and guarantee genuine social reform?

7. Groups of physicians and representatives of population agencies sought to relax federal regulation of sterilization practices, however, arguing that "protection against involuntary pregnancy is as much an individual right as is protection against involuntary sterilization" (Hartmann 1987:242). Birth control advocates, women's health activists, and representatives of various women's groups countered that there were other ways to avoid pregnancy and, above all, that each woman should have the right to choose, without threats, pressure, or incentives and with full knowledge and informed consent, in what ways she wants to control her fertility. The State of California and the City of New York are the only places in the United States where there are regulations requiring informed consent for private-pay sterilizations.

8. For a detailed description of each of these methods, see *Our Bodies, Ourselves* by the Boston Women's Health Book Collective (1992).

9. Barbara and Gideon Seaman's 1970 groundbreaking book, *Women and the Crisis in Sex Hormones,* exposed the dangers of oral contraceptives and offered an incisive critique of the development, testing, and distribution of this contraceptive and the social, psychological, and physical effects of hormones on women. However, despite growing questions and fears about the long-term safety and benefits of many new methods, the menu of contraceptive methods available to consumers grew.

10. According to the 1988 National Survey of Family Growth, of the 58 million U.S. women between the ages of fifteen and forty-four who have ever had intercourse, about 67 percent are at risk of unintended pregnancy at any given time (Kost, Forrest, and Harlap 1991). That is, they are fertile and sexually active, not pregnant, and not seeking to have a child in the near future. Included in this group are the 39 million women, ages fifteen to forty-four, who practice a reversible method of birth control or rely on contraceptive sterilization, and the 3.9 million who do not use any method of contraception at all. Results from several studies confirm that approximately 40 percent of all U.S. births in 1988 were unintended—28 percent were mistimed and 12 percent were unwanted (Forrest and Fordyce 1988; Mosher 1990).

11. From this list, only the copper-bearing IUD and Depo-Provera are currently available in the United States. Before the FDA approved Depo-Provera as a contraceptive in 1992, the injectable was being used in some locales because it had received FDA approval for other health-related uses.

12. Early laboratory research involved testing the feasibility of subdermal steroid-filled Silastic capsules for the prevention of pregnancy. The silicone rubber used to make the Silastic capsules has been used in surgical applications (e.g., heart valves) and medical prostheses (e.g., IUDs, clips for female sterilization) for decades (Roy, Mishell, and Robertson 1984; Segal 1987; Zeidenstein 1990). In the initial experimental stages, these capsules were filled with different steroid compounds to determine which compound would be released most uniformly and would result in "desirable measures of safety and effectiveness" (Segal 1983).

13. It is believed that Norplant prevents pregnancy by (1) inhibiting ovulation, (2) causing a thickening of the cervical mucus, making it less penetrable by sperm, and (3) changing the lining of the uterus, making it less able to accept a fertilized egg.

14. Leiras, a Finnish pharmaceutical company, began manufacturing and distributing the implant. Before this, the U.S.-based pharmaceutical company Wyeth-Ayerst had been the sole manufacturer of the device for the Population Council.

15. Morsy (1994) has documented refusal to remove Norplant in tests in southern Egypt. In desperation, some women have attempted to cut Norplant out of their arms themselves.

16. FDA approval of Depo-Provera came after many years of contentious debate about the safety of this method. Depo-Provera was manufactured by Upjohn during the late 1950s and was approved for use to treat renal and kidney cancer in 1960. Beginning in 1963, Upjohn sought approval of Depo-Provera for contraceptive purposes. The FDA repeatedly denied Upjohn permission for this use based largely on the results of a series of animal studies conducted between 1968 and 1975. Data from these studies indicated that Depo-Provera caused cancer in test animals.

In 1978, it was determined that Depo-Provera did not meet the FDA's safety standards. Further studies were conducted over a period of ten years, and in June 1992, Upjohn presented additional information to secure approval for use of Depo-Provera as a contraceptive. In October 1992, despite protests from women's health advocates, medical and public health practitioners, and others, the FDA approved Depo-Provera for use in the United States. Some observers suggest that at this time, it is important to "separate medical safety aspects from problems in service delivery, where abuses regarding information and choice of methods remain" (Reproductive Health Matters 1993:101).

REFERENCES

Affandi, B., J. Prihartono, F. Lubis, H. Sutedi, and R. S. Samil
    1987a   "Insertion and removal of Norplant contraceptive implants by physicians and nonphysicians in an Indonesian clinic." Studies in Family Planning 18(5):302–6.
Affandi, B., S. S. I. Santoso, W. Hadisaputra, F. A. Moeloek, J. Priahartono, F. Lubis, and R. S. Samil
    1987b   "Five-year experience with Norplant (in Indonesia)." Contraception 36:417–28.
American Medical Association Board of Trustees
    1992   "Requirements or incentives by government for the use of long-acting contraceptives." Journal of the American Medical Association 267(13):1818–21.
Arditti, Rita, Renate Duelli Klein, and Shelley Minden (eds.)
    1984   Test-Tube Women: What Future for Motherhood? London: Pandora Press.

Basnayake, S., S. Thapa, and S. Balogh
    1988   "Evaluation of safety, efficacy, and acceptability of Norplant implants in
            Sri Lanka." Studies in Family Planning 19(1):39-47.
Beilenson, P. L., E. S. Miola, and M. Farmer
    1995   "Politics and practice: introducing Norplant into a school-based health
            center in Baltimore." American Journal of Public Health 85(3):309-11.
Boston Women's Health Book Collective
    1992   The New Our Bodies, Ourselves. New York: Simon and Schuster.
Brodie, Janet Farrell
    1994   Contraception and Abortion in Nineteenth-Century America. Ithaca,
            NY: Cornell University Press.
Chesler, Ellen
    1992   Woman of Valor: Margaret Sanger and the Birth Control Movement in
            America. New York: Simon and Schuster.
Clarke, Adele
    1984   "Subtle forms of sterilization abuse: a reproductive rights analysis." Pp.
            188-212 in Rita Arditti, Renate Duelli Klein, and Shelley Minden (eds.),
            Test-Tube Women: What Future for Motherhood? London: Pandora Press.
    1997   Disciplining Reproduction: Modernity, American Life Sciences, and the
            Problem of Sex. Berkeley: University of California Press.
Clarke, Adele, and Teresa Montini
    1993   "The many faces of RU 486: tales of situated knowledges and technologi-
            cal contestations." Science, Technology, and Human Values 18(1):42-78.
Croxatto, H. B., S. Diaz, and I. Sivin
    1991   "Contraceptive implants." Pp. 22-29 in M. Seppala and L. Hamberger
            (eds.), Frontiers in Human Reproduction. New York: New York Academy
            of Sciences.
Darney, P. D., E. Atkinson, S. Tanner, S. MacPherson, S. Hellerstein, and A. Alvarado
    1990a   "Acceptance and perceptions of Norplant among users in San Francisco,
            USA." Studies in Family Planning 21(3):152-60.
Darney, P. D., C. M. Klaisle, S. Tanner, and A. Alvarado
    1990b   "Sustained-release contraceptives." Current Problems in Obstetrics, Gy-
            necology, and Fertility 13:90-125.
Davis, Angela
    1990   "Racism, birth control, and reproductive rights." Pp. 15-26 in Marlene
            Gerber Fried (ed.), From Abortion to Reproductive Freedom: Transform-
            ing a Movement. Boston: South End Press.
Diaz, S., M. Pavez, P. Miranda, D. M. Robertson, I. Sivin, and H. B. Croxatto
    1982   "A five-year clinical trial of levonorgestrel Silastic implants (Norplant)."
            Contraception 25(5):447-56.
Dixon-Mueller, Ruth
    1993a   "The sexuality connection in reproductive health." Studies in Family
            Planning 24(5):269-82.

1993b   Population Policy and Women's Rights: Transforming Reproductive Choice. New York: Praeger.

Duster, Troy
1990   Eugenics through the Back Door. Berkeley: University of California Press.

Forrest, Jacqueline D.
1987   "Unintended pregnancy among American women." Family Planning Perspectives 19(2):76–77.

Forrest, Jacqueline D., and R. R. Fordyce
1988   "U.S. women's contraceptive attitudes and practice: how have they changed in the 1980s?" Family Planning Perspectives 20(3):112–18.

Frank, M. L., A. N. Poindexter, M. L. Johnson, and L. Bateman
1992   "Characteristics and attitudes of early contraceptive implant acceptors in Texas." Family Planning Perspectives 24(5):208–13.

Gladwell, Malcolm
1990   "Science confronts ethics in contraceptive implant." Washington Post, 31 October, A1.

Goodman, Ellen
1991   "Contraceptive and threat of coercion." New York Times, 19 February, B7.

Gordon, Linda
1976   Woman's Body, Woman's Right: A Social History of Birth Control in America. New York: Grossman.

HAI-Europe (Health Action International)
1994   "Immunological contraceptives." Contraceptive Policy Report. May. Amsterdam.

Hardon, A., and L. Achthoven
1990   "Norplant: a critical review." Women and Pharmaceuticals Bulletin (November):14–17.

Harlap, S., Kathryn Kost, and Jacqueline D. Forrest
1991   Preventing Pregnancy, Protecting Health: A New Look at Birth Control Choices in the United States. New York and Washington: Alan Guttmacher Institute.

Hartmann, Betsy
1987   Reproductive Rights and Wrongs: The Global Politics of Population Control and Contraceptive Choice. New York: Harper and Row.

Hubbard, Ruth
1984   "Personal courage is not enough: some hazards of childbearing in the 1980s." Pp. 331–35 in Rita Arditti, Renate Duelli Klein, and Shelley Minden (eds.), Test-Tube Women: What Future for Motherhood? London: Pandora Press.

Kaeser, Lisa
1991   "Contraceptive development: why the snail's pace?" Family Planning Perspectives 22(3):131–33.

Kaplan, T., and J. Johnson
   1993   "Birth control implants at valley school defended." Los Angeles Times,
           26 March, A20.
Kaufert, Patricia A.
   1990   "Ethics, politics, and contraception: Canada and the licensing of Depo-
           Provera." Pp. 121-44 in George Weisz (ed.), Social Science Perspectives
           on Medical Ethics. Dordrecht, The Netherlands: Kluwer Academic.
Klitsch, Michael
   1993   "Injectable hormones and regulatory controversy: an end to the long-run-
           ning story?" Family Planning Perspectives 25(1):37-40.
Kost, Kathryn, Jacqueline D. Forrest, and S. Harlap
   1991   "Comparing the health risks and benefits of contraceptive choices." Fam-
           ily Planning Perspectives 23(2):54-61.
Landers, Ann
   1991   "Resentment reigns." Oakland Tribune, 3 September, B5.
Lewin, Tamar
   1994   "'Dream' contraceptive's nightmare." New York Times, 8 July, A7.
Mastroianni, Luigi, Jr., Peter J. Donaldson, and Thomas Kane, eds.
   1990   Developing New Contraceptives: Obstacles and Opportunities. Washing-
           ton: National Academy Press.
McCann, Carole R.
   1994   Birth Control Politics in the United States, 1916-1945. Ithaca, NY:
           Cornell University Press.
Mertus, Julie
   1991   "The politics of forced contraception." California Advocates for Pregnant
           Women 14(Spring):1-3.
Morsy, Soheir
   1991   "Safeguarding women's bodies: the white man's burden medicalized."
           Medical Anthropology Quarterly 5(1):19-24.
   1994   "Deadly reproduction among Egyptian women: maternal mortality and the
           medicalization of population control." Pp. 162-76 in Faye D. Ginsberg and
           Rayna Rapp (eds.), Conceiving the New World Order: The Global
           Stratification of Reproduction. Berkeley: University of California Press.
Mosher, William
   1990   "Contraceptive practice in the United States, 1982-1988." Family Plan-
           ning Perspectives 22(5):198-205.
Mosher, William, and C. Bachrach
   1987   "First premarital contraceptive use: United States, 1960-82." Studies in
           Family Planning 18(2):83-95.
Mosher, William, and James W. McNally
   1991   "Contraceptive use at first premarital intercourse: United States, 1965-
           1988." Family Planning Perspectives 23(2):108-16.

Oudshoorn, Nelly
    1996   "For better or worse: scientists strive for universal reproductive technologies." Social Studies of Science, forthcoming.

Painter, K.
    1990   "As perfect a method as you can have." USA Today, 6 December, 1A.

Philadelphia Inquirer
    1990   "Poverty and Norplant: can contraception reduce the underclass?" Editorial, 12 December.

Pies, Cheri
    1993   Controversies in Context: Ethics, Values and Policies Concerning Norplant. Ann Arbor: University Microfilms.

Population Council
    1990a   "NORPLANT implants are approved for use in the United States," press release, 10 December.
    1990b   "Norplant levonorgestrel implants: a summary of scientific data." Prepared by the Population Council in collaboration with the INTERCARE Consulting Network.

Population Reports
    1987   "Injectables and implants—hormonal contraception: new long-acting methods." Population Reports, ser. K, no. 3 (Mar.-Apr.):K57-87.
    1993   "Injectables and implants—decisions for Norplant programs." Population Reports, ser. K, no. 4, (November).

Presser, H. B.
    1980   "Puerto Rico: recent trends in fertility and sterilization." Family Planning Perspectives 12(2):102-5.

Reilly, Peter R.
    1991   The Surgical Solution: A History of Involuntary Sterilization in the United States. Baltimore: Johns Hopkins University Press.

Reproductive Health Matters
    1993   "Research round-up: safety of Depo-Provera." Reproductive Health Matters 1 (May):101-2.

Richter, Judith
    1993   Vaccination against Pregnancy: Miracle or Menace? BUKD and HAI.

Rodriguez-Trias, Helen
    1984   "The women's health movement: women take power." Pp. 107-26 in Victor W. Sidel and Ruth Sidel (eds.), Reforming Medicine: Lessons of the Last Quarter Century. New York: Pantheon Books.

Rothman, Barbara Katz
    1984   "The meanings of choice in reproductive technology." Pp. 23-34 in Rita Arditti, Renate Duelli Klein, and Shelley Minden (eds.), Test-Tube Women: What Future for Motherhood? London: Pandora Press.

Rowland, R.
    1984   "Reproductive technologies: the final solution to the woman question?" Pp. 356-70 in Rita Arditti, Renate Duelli Klein, and Shelley Minden

(eds.), Test-Tube Women: What Future for Motherhood? London: Pandora Press.

Roy, S., D. R. Mishell, and D. N. Robertson
1984   "Long-term reversible contraception with levonorgestrel-releasing Silastic rods." American Journal of Obstetrics and Gynecology 148:1006–13.

Rutten, Tim
1991   "Norplanting or supplanting private rights." Los Angeles Times, 31 May, E1.

Scott, Julia
1991   Legislative Alert, "Norplant." National Black Women's Health Project, public policy report, July.

Seaman, Barbara, and Gideon Seaman
1995   Women and the Crisis in Sex Hormones. 25th anniversary ed. New York: Hunter House.

Segal, Sheldon
1983   "The development of NORPLANT implants." Studies in Family Planning 14(6/7):159–63.
1987   "A new delivery system for contraceptive steroids." American Journal of Obstetrics and Gynecology 157:1090–92.

Shapiro, Thomas M.
1985   Population Control Politics: Women, Sterilization, and Reproductive Choice. Philadelphia: Temple University Press.

Shoupe, D., D. R. Mishell Jr., B. L. Boop, and M. Fielding
1991   "The significance of bleeding patterns in Norplant implant users." American Journal of Obstetrics and Gynecology 77(2):256–60.

Sinofsky, F. E., S. A. Pasquale, and S. J. Gonzalez
1990   "Long-acting contraceptive implants—acceptance by U.S. women." San Francisco: American College of Obstetrics and Gynecology. Abstract.

Sivin, Irving
1988   "International experience with Norplant and Norplant-2 contraception." Studies in Family Planning 19(2):81–94.

Terry, Jennifer
1991   "Body politics in the 1990s: a feminist agenda for theory and action." Unpublished.
1995   Deviant Bodies: Critical Perspectives on Difference in Science and Popular Culture. Bloomington: Indiana University Press.

Trussell, James, and B. Vaughan
1989   "Aggregate and lifetime contraceptive failure in the United States." Family Planning Perspectives 21(5):224–26.

Vrazo, Fawn
1994   "Difficulties surfacing for Norplant." Philadelphia Inquirer, 7 July, A1.

Weisman, C. S., S. B. Plichta, D. E. Tirado, and K. H. Dana
1993   "Comparison of contraceptive implant adopters and pill users in a family

planning clinic in Baltimore." Family Planning Perspectives 25(5):224–26.

Yukins, Elizabeth
1991   "New birth control drug receives mixed reaction." Gay Community News, 4–10 March.

Zeidenstein, George
1990   Statement at news conference following FDA approval of Norplant. 11 December.

Zelnick, M., J. Kanter, and K. Ford
1981   Sex and Pregnancy in Adolescence. Beverly Hills, CA: Sage.

[PART VII]

Challenges and Choices for
the Twenty-first Century

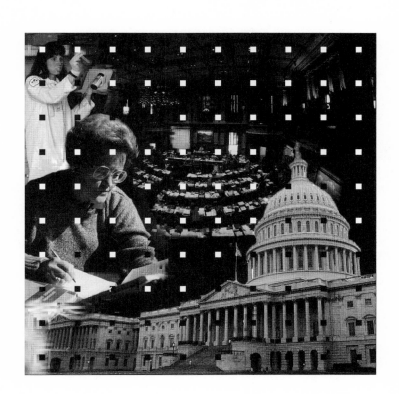

The health consequences of the complexities and differences in women's life circumstances are not well researched. To gain a fuller understanding of what actually produces health and what women in different situations need to sustain or restore their health, we need research that builds on but goes beyond current thinking. For feminist health researchers and policymakers who believe that it is time to broaden our perspectives on women's health, what will help us transcend narrow and incomplete bio-medical models? What will help policymakers and health professionals recognize important aspects of health and healing for women whose situations are poorly understood? What shapes or directions might research agendas take?

Part 7 opens with an agenda, formulated by the National Women's Health Network, to achieve equity for women by expanding ongoing biomedical research to address issues that women find particularly pressing (see chapter 21). Although there are serious gaps in biomedical knowledge about women's health, Olesen, Taylor, Ruzek, and Clarke emphasize in chapter 22 that a substantial research literature already includes women. Rather than posit that women's health has not been studied, these contributors argue that much of the extensive literature on sociocultural aspects of women's health and healing has simply been overlooked. In their view, research agendas could include assessing and integrating this knowledge as part of the groundwork for moving into new areas that hold great promise for improving women's health.

Realistically, there are finite resources available for research, just as there are for health care services. In looking across the array of research agendas on women's health, which, one might ask, seem most promising? How are judgments to be made about what warrants funding by whom? On the basis of what criteria are research agendas adopted or rejected, and how do research interest groups influence these decisions? What are some of the effects that adoption of research agendas have on what we know about women's health, and how might different agendas contribute to sustaining and promoting health for all, not just some, women?

These are questions that need to be answered as we press forward with research agendas around which claims are made about improving women's health. In chapter 23, we (Ruzek, Olesen, and Clarke) present an overview of research that we see as potentially promising in five areas: (1) women's actual experiences of health and illness, (2) a broader epidemiology of women's health, (3) culturally and sociodemographically specific studies of clinical efficacy, (4) access to and actual use of a broad array of traditional and alternative or complementary health services as well as conventional medical services, and (5) recruitment, training, and practice patterns of both conventional and alternative health care providers. We challenge readers to consider how they would allocate resources to pursue these agendas and the biomedical research agendas proposed by Narrigan and her colleagues in chapter 21. What values and principles might particular groups of women prefer to use to make decisions about how to allocate national research resources as well as deliver medical care services?

[21]

Research to Improve Women's Health:
An Agenda for Equity

DEBORAH NARRIGAN, JANE SPRAGUE ZONES,
NANCY WORCESTER, AND MAXINE JO GRAD

Since its inception in 1975, the National Women's
Health Network has worked vigorously to improve national health policy and practice affecting women's
health. The network is the only national, membership-
based advocacy organization devoted exclusively to
women's health issues. Its original goals were to develop a
strong women's voice in the national political arena and
to provide women a source of balanced information on
health issues (National Women's Health Network 1986).
These goals rested firmly on prevailing assumptions of the
women's health movement of the 1970s. Those assumptions proposed first that health concerns are a fundamental, common ground for women and consequently that
these commonly held concerns could unite women into
an effective voice for change. Even as we identify common concerns, however, we must acknowledge the vast
differences in women's experiences and health needs that
arise from those experiences.

The National Women's Health Network has evolved over the last twenty
years and is now self-consciously and explicitly building the organization's
membership, board, and staff into a body of diverse women. The organization brings together women representing a wide range of constituencies
and viewpoints who respect each other's differences and who are committed to finding areas of consensus. The following essay is an example of a
position paper that the network's board of directors periodically writes to
inform network members and the public of the educational and advocacy
work of the organization. These papers represent one of the ways we
actively work for consensus. The papers develop through board discussion
of the issue, a small group of the board members writing a draft, circulation
of several drafts for comments, and finally board discussion and agreement

on the paper's final version. Such an attempt at compromise and consensus is sometimes halting, often time-consuming, but always rewarding.

We originally wrote this paper in 1991 as our response to heightened public awareness of the glaring inequity in biomedical research on women's health. We have recently updated it. The paper begins with a brief overview of roots of this inequity, continues with a chronology of recent public policy and action that recognize and begin to remedy the inequities, and closes with the National Women's Health Network agenda for continued improvement in the conduct of woman-centered biomedical research.

Improving Women's Health: An Agenda for Equity

At first glance, scientific inquiry can appear quite neutral, but looking more closely, its processes, progress, and theories are intimately tied to the values of the larger society, which are essentially male dominated and profit focused (Birke 1986; Brighton Women and Science Group 1980; Hubbard 1990). These values affect which problems are studied, how they are studied, how the results are communicated and applied, and how future research priorities are developed.

Research into women's health serves as a case in point. Gender inequities in this arena periodically come into view. Recently two issues have caught the attention of the American public. First, although women make up more than half the population and receive more than half the health care in this country, most illnesses specific to diverse groups of women have not been given adequate research attention or funding. Second, diseases that affect all types of people often have been studied in only one type of population, such as middle-aged men or college students. Information from studying only very specific groups must then be extrapolated to the widely differing populations of our country. Generalizing findings so far beyond study populations violates one of science's own rules.

Roots of Gender Inequity in U.S. Biomedical Research

Within the hierarchical discipline of science, efforts devoted to health rank well below science for power and profit in the United States and elsewhere. For example, relatively little of the national budget in most western industrialized nations goes to health research. Much more goes for defense research and development. Feminist critics point out that science has been conceptualized and constructed almost exclusively by upper-middle-class and upper-class men, and it consequently represents a particular male political and cultural experience (Hubbard 1990; Schiebinger 1987). The scientific questions that are asked, and the answers that are sought, depend more on who has the power to do the asking than on which biologic or behavioral questions need answers. Thus, it retains an androcentric bias in choice of problems, methods, and interpretation of results (Keller 1982). Science done from this androcentric position thus easily perpetuates and undergirds the status quo. The inherent danger here is that scientific rationales such as biological determinism will find their way into value-laden explanations for differences in rates of illness in different groups of people.

The very concept of illness is also gender based. Critics of the U.S. system of biomedical research have noted that "an insidious tendency to see disease as either a women's or men's disease grips the scientific community" (Pettiti 1990:2). These characterizations are often incorrect. For example, both lung cancer and coronary artery disease have been characterized as men's diseases, even though they affect women as severely as men. Given the masculine dominance in scientific research, and in our social and political systems at large, it is not surprising that the study of "men's diseases" predominates.[1] Diseases affecting significant numbers of diverse groups of American women have not been investigated with the same rigor and intensity.

The categoric exclusion of one gender from clinical studies violates the principle of distributive justice. In the context of clinical research, distributive justice is characterized by fairness. Fairness "requires that no one group—gender, racial ethnic, or socioeconomic group—receive disproportionate benefits or bear disproportionate burdens of research." Thus, denying women access to participation in studies also denies women as a class the benefits of the research, and this denial is plainly "presumptively unjust" (Mastroianni, Faden, and Federman 1994a:76, 78).

Another factor has to do with scientific method. Characteristically in the natural sciences, a researcher "objectively" analyzes one or more variables that are systematically changed, while other variables are experimentally or statistically held constant (Birke 1986). This method works well to explain phenomena that are measurable or repetitive, but it cannot deal with unique occurrences or with systems that are gradual, that change slowly, or that cannot be broken into measurable parts (Hubbard 1990). The scientific method usually offers specific but very limited answers to a research question. This entire enterprise is inescapably shaped by the worldview of a particular society, time, and person carrying out the research project (Kuhn 1970; Rosser 1992).

How Women Are Excluded from Biomedical Research

Excluding women from biomedical research occurs in three important ways. First, a research study may intentionally exclude women. Second, the number of women participants may be insufficient to allow analysis of findings by gender. Third, if women subjects are included, investigators may choose not to analyze or report outcome differences (or similarities) by gender (Mastroianni et al. 1994a). The reason the first type of exclusion is standard procedure is that one of the variables easiest to control is the kind of subjects taking part in an investigation. The more homogeneous the subjects are, the easier it is to see if the experimental variable itself—and not differences among people—explains the experimental effect. Clinical research done this way is easier, less expensive, and relatively certain to yield statistically significant results. This dominant approach accounts in part for the preponderance of work done exclusively with white male subjects.

Critics of this approach point out that a precise answer could be seen as a deficit, because the specificity denies the complexity of most natural or biological events (Birke 1986). Designing a study "which maximizes the likelihood of clear results and also acquires information that can be reliably generalized to the health care needs of the more heterogeneous population" (U.S. Department of Health and Human Services 1985:IV-58) would be much more complicated, as well as more costly and time-consuming—but absolutely necessary. Just how much heterogeneity in any given study population would capture real differences among groups of people in, for example, effects of a treatment remains unclear. Establishing what constitutes "adequate" inclusion of women in clinical trials has been debated (Bennett 1993). The National Institutes of Health published a set of guidelines (U.S. Department of Health and Human Services 1994) that ironically could be used to justify exclusion of women subjects (Merton 1994). Regardless of what guidelines are applied, any guideline assumes women (and men) are a set of uniform, biologically interchangeable bodies. If, as most scientists assume, there are actually few gender differences in responses to treatments or medications, this assumption "reinforces rather than reduces the justification for a principle of inclusion" (Mastroianni et al. 1994a:6). One of the difficult questions that remains is this: To what extent are we biologically interchangeable?[2]

Exclusion by Virtue of Hormones

One might ask why, in the name of homogeneity, women-only studies might not be useful as well as easy to design. One rationale given for not doing this has been the hormonal changes of the menstrual cycle, pregnancy, or lactation. Although seldom explicitly stated, researchers reason that hormonal variation is a factor that cannot easily be controlled, creating problems in designing a study that will yield clear answers. In a governmental report on women's health, for example, the comment is made that "if the menstrual cycle were not expected to contribute to variability in other measurements, then women might be included more often in research studies, along with men" (DHHS 1985:IV–59). Thus, women's normal hormonal cycles are viewed as methodological problems, or biological deviations from the male norm, rather than as pertinent factors that might reveal important sources of variation in findings.

Further, potential pregnancy itself is a biological rationale that has caused categorical exclusion of women from clinical trials, particularly those examining medications or interventions. The possibility of adverse effects on the embryo or fetus, or "teratogenic liability," is the most common reason given for excluding women from study samples (Cotton 1990). Although this exclusion affects women, its intent demonstrates concern not for the woman but for the health of the future child. In 1977, the Federal Food and Drug Administration issued formal rules banning women with childbearing potential from participating in the two early phases of drug trials. A woman of childbearing potential was defined as a "premenopausal female capable of becoming pregnant." This included women who were using contraception or whose partner had had a vasectomy (U.S. Food and Drug Administration 1977). Prohibiting such a large group of women from being subjects in clinical studies leaves scientists as well as women in the dark about a drug's impact and allows "the understudied group to receive no medical treatment, ineffective treatment or even harmful treatment" (Mastroianni et al. 1994a:79).

This is ironic and dangerous as drugs certainly are used widely by women with the confounding factors of menstrual cycles and pregnancies (Cotton 1990). This prohibition was recently lifted and is discussed below.

Issues of Women's Participation as Subjects in Biomedical Research

Ironically, some women, particularly poor women, have been overly represented in clinical research. This has occurred because poor women often receive care at inner-city hospitals staffed by physicians affiliated with medical schools who are eager to do research. Patients at such institutions would be likely candidates for recruitment into clinical studies, and in turn, this recruitment might be experienced as a form of exploitation. On the other hand, little effort has been made to successfully recruit and retain women from diverse backgrounds into clinical studies. For example, caregiving for dependent relatives, for which women are primarily responsible, may interfere with keeping clinical study appointments. Or, women enrolled in heart disease studies who might be ten to twenty years older than male counterparts may be less mobile and thus less able to carry out a study exercise regimen (Stoy 1994). If women are subjects in clinical studies, one commentator has suggested that, given women's socialization, they may feel "less empowered" than men to assert their right to withdraw from a study (Levine 1994). In addition, unless special needs of some women and men (non-English speakers, for example) are met, they would not be able to enroll or comply with many research design requirements and may drop out of the study. Thus, the research project would not yield satisfactory results (Kolata 1991).

The lack of biomedical research on needs of women of color has been recognized as a glaring deficit for more than a decade. As a Public Health Service report (DHHS 1985:II-47) indicates, "The nearly 21.4 million women in the United States who are members of minority groups have more than their share of illness. . . . Ethnic minority women . . . experience higher infant and maternal mortality rates, greater prevalence of chronic diseases, and a lower life expectancy." Several contradictory circumstances account for this deficit. First, women of color might decline to participate in clinical research trials given the historic exploitation of persons of color in high-risk clinical trials.[3] Second, historically, many communities of color have relied on spirituality and alternative treatments as their first choice for healing (Mitchell 1994). An individual who seeks health and healing by placing her faith in a spiritual healer may see little benefit in volunteering for a biomedical research project. In short, women of color may have different—and equally sound—reasons to participate or not participate in clinical trials from Euro-American women (Stoy 1994).

Developing creative methods that bring diverse women into research trials is about to become a newly valued venture for biomedical researchers. Federal funding will be based on evidence that the project is designed to enroll and retain women and men from diverse backgrounds. Recent suggestions for ensuring women's participation include scheduling flexibly, providing transportation, and designing recruitment materials that are sensitive to women (Stoy 1994). On the other hand, in the quest to rectify the long history of exclusion, the scientific community will need to be vigilant in seeing that recruitment means voluntary participation, not undue inducement (Mastroianni et al. 1994a). Until a substantial amount of this new, inclusive, biomedical research is completed, research reports should include broad descriptions of study population characteristics beyond age and gender to include race, ethnicity, region, and economic status.

Even when women do participate in large clinical studies, findings are seldom analyzed to yield answers that consider diversity in a meaningful way. Inequities that low-income women, adolescent, older, disabled, rural, urban, or women of color and lesbian women experience in access to and in quality of health care are reflected in the lack of research on conditions significantly affecting these groups. In addition, scientific investigators schooled in conventional biomedical methods may be skeptical about treatment outcomes that differ among demographic subgroups unless a biological rationale for the differences is evident (Mastroianni et al. 1994a).

Recent Advances in Drug Research

Recently, some drug research has begun to consider variation in therapeutic effects based on ethnicity, age, and gender of subjects, utilizing well-known information on these differences. For example, on average, women are smaller than men in weight, height, surface area, and metabolic rate—all characteristics that could theoretically influence the concentration of a drug or the body's responses to a drug (Merkatz et al. 1993).[4] Ethnicity may also influence responses to drugs.[5] Investigations of biologically founded gender and ethnic differences are imperative in order to understand the effectiveness and safety of drugs.

Biomedical research has systematically ignored the complex relationships of race, ethnicity, and health, failing to distinguish whether these characteristics are thought of as biological or social attributes and failing to study the intersection of these characteristics and their relationship to health. Even if attempts are made to be inclusive, they tend to be an afterthought. Biomedical researchers will need to carefully conceptualize, define, and measure race and ethnicity, and they would profit from using social science methodologies designed specifically for these purposes. The need for research that seriously examines diverse responses to widely used therapies is urgently needed to prevent unanticipated harm (Mastroianni et al. 1994a; Woods 1994).

Doing Biomedical Research: Where Are the Women?

The business of doing scientific research contributes to the paucity of investigation of women's health for several reasons. First, individual scientists do not usually work on problems entirely of their own choosing; instead, they carry out research to produce marketable results, which means publications, promotion, and peer recognition (Hubbard 1990). Second, most research endeavors are financed by private industry or government to address problems geared specifically to meet the needs of private profit or the military-industrial complex (Brighton Women and Science Group 1980). Thus, even if a scientist wants to investigate a question in women's health, these realities might act as deterrents. Recent widespread attempts to control spending within the health care system and the political goal to decrease the national deficit have depleted health research funding. One result of these pressures is a proposal in Congress to decrease the National Institutes of Health budget by 10 percent for 1996 (Rosenthal 1995).

Furthermore, women constitute a small proportion of scientists and research physicians in the United States despite notable increases in the last fifteen years. In 1989, although women constituted 45 percent of the total workforce, only 16 percent of scientists and engineers were women. Among all doctorally prepared employed women scientists and engineers, only 3 percent were African American, 7 percent were Asian, and 0.2

percent were Native American in 1989. Although these percentages are very small, the actual number of African American and Asian women with doctorates in science or engineering more than doubled between 1979 and 1989 from 785 to 2,236 and from 2,028 to 5,328, respectively. The proportion of women of color scientists, however, did not change in that decade: in 1979, 9 percent of all women with doctoral preparation in sciences were women of color, and in 1989 the total was 10 percent (National Science Foundation 1992).

Women have made larger inroads in medicine with many of the most prestigious medical schools enrolling as many women as men (see chapter 16). In academic health centers, however, where the vast majority of biomedical research is based, women made up only 18 percent of all faculty members. According to a 1994 American Medical Association report, of those physicians identifying themselves as researchers, 16 percent are women, or 2,396 of the total of 14,716 physician researchers (Roback et al. 1994).

NIH and the Process of Doing Research

Funding for large-scale biomedical research comes primarily from the U.S. Department of Health and Human Services (DHHS), specifically the National Institutes of Health (NIH). The total 1994 budget for all sixteen institutes and three centers that make up the NIH was $10.9 billion, up from $10.3 billion in 1993 (NIH 1994). Competition for dollars within each institute, and among them, is fierce.

The NIH research project review and approval process reflects and adds to the inequities in women's research in a number of ways. First, NIH administrators and scientific advisors are rarely women. In fact, only 18 percent of the tenured scientists at NIH are women; few are in high-level positions, and women are paid from 2 to 9 percent less than men in each employment category (Watson 1993). In the scientific review process, it is these NIH scientific advisors who first review the scientific merits of proposals and then assign priority scores to allocate funding. Thus, advisors and staff have immense discretionary control not just over dollars but over which problems are chosen for study, by whom, and in what manner. In addition, NIH staff annually set priorities for research topics based on their assessment of political concerns and pressure and scientific fashion. In the end, only a small number of all research proposals approved after scientific review are funded (Nadel 1990), and the proportion funded appears to be declining: in 1993, only 25 percent of all proposals were funded, whereas nearly one-third were funded in 1989 (Rosenthal 1995).

NIH receives comparatively few applications from women scientists including doctorally prepared nurses and physicians, although the proportion has been growing.[6] The NIH process to select and fund research projects is weighted in favor of investigators with a track record. In general, the more recognized research the applicant has done, the higher the priority for funding. The hierarchy so familiar to women thus persists here: older, experienced men control the academic research system, and to progress, women must position themselves with a powerful mentor, hoping for advancement in the research market through association as well as merit and longevity. Furthermore, because of the recent increases in women entering scientific professions, women are more prevalent among researchers at the lower rungs of the hierarchy and have not accumulated the extensive research record generally expected for funding (Pettiti 1990). One positive note in research funding is that women who sought awards as new investigators received funding on par with men, with both genders achieving 18 percent success. However, 18 percent funding is a decrease in success rate for all investigators over the decade. In 1984, 25 percent of new investigators were funded (Division of Research Grants 1994). In times of budgetary pressures, funding new ideas may be constrained by commitments to fund mainstream work (Woods 1994).

To ameliorate inequities in research grant funding will require multiple strategies. Suggestions for increasing the number of women in higher echelons of academic science include postponing the standard tenure decision to allow for childbearing and formal part-time appointments for women faculty (Koshland 1988). For women of color, barriers to careers in science or biomedical research are intensified. For many, even contemplating such a career choice reportedly "appear[s] unrealistic and out of reach" (Office of Research on Women's Health 1992c).

Traditionally, feminists have posited that the practice of science will not change until women secure education that puts them in the "pipeline" to a career in science and until more feminists become scientists and move into powerful positions (Birke 1986; Rosser 1992) such as principal investigators in their own research specialty. Additionally, however, some feminists are calling for a more socially responsible science. Some also argue that science itself should change to "accommodate the qualitative methods of inquiry at which women are alleged to excel" (Koertge 1994). They point out the dilemma inherent in trying to advance knowledge for and about women through the use of mainstream scientific methods (Woods 1994). The question remains: How can science truly pursue information that will benefit women rather than merely be about women, and how can women conduct science?

Funding for Research in Women's Health

Women's health has not fared well in the competition for research dollars until recently. With political pressure to pay attention to selected women's diseases, a new willingness to spend federal research dollars for women's health has emerged. A review of the National Cancer Institute's budget emphasizes willingness to spend on breast cancer. Although the dollar amount is vastly increased, still it is proportionately small. In 1986, for example, $51 million was allocated for all breast cancer research and in 1994, the allocation totaled $306 million. The increase is undeniable, but the total spent on cancers unique to women (breast, uterine, cervical, ovarian, and vaginal) constituted only about 15 percent of NCI's total budget in 1993 (National Cancer Institute 1993).

Of the total NIH budget for research of $10.9 billion for 1994, $833 million, or less than 10 percent, was allocated to health issues unique to women. The allocation for HIV/AIDS and women is an additional $706 million—nearly equal to the total spending on all other women's health research (NIH 1994). The large AIDS appropriation may start to redress a decade of relative inactivity in the federal research enterprise on women and AIDS (Mastroianni et al. 1994a).

Ironically, the rapid expansion in funding for women's health research may not be entirely beneficial. The dramatic rise in dollars for breast cancer research, for example, has spawned studies that focus on "novel technologies" (National Cancer Institute 1993:112) rather than on environmental or behavior factors that may reduce risk of disease. The Tamoxifen Breast Cancer Prevention Trial is a case in point.

Tamoxifen is a medication with unusual dual properties. It resembles estrogen, but it also can block estrogen's natural activity. It has been used widely as treatment after surgery for early breast cancer because it appears to reduce recurrence of breast cancer in the other breast for about one-third of postmenopausal women who receive it. Half the 16,000 subjects who are pre- and postmenopausal women with some increased risk of developing breast cancer will receive a daily dose of Tamoxifen for five years; the other half will receive a placebo. Like many chemotherapeutics for cancers, Tamoxifen has both side effects and major adverse effects. It is associated with the development of endometrial and liver cancer, as well as thromboembolic phenomena (blood clots) and ocular toxicity (National Cancer Institute 1993:110, 112, 228). The increased risk of endometrial cancer is fivefold; the rate of increase for liver cancer is unknown; thromboembolism occurs seven times more for women taking Tamoxifen, whereas eye damage is rare (Fugh-Berman and Epstein 1992).

Critics have argued that participants will stand to lose more than they gain from being in this trial. It is difficult to justify exposing healthy women to an agent with such significant risks in the name of primary disease prevention. Further, the study has been beset by charges of fraud and incomplete, inaccurate informed consent procedures regarding the increased risks (Raloff 1992). This controversial example shows that with an infusion of money targeted for research on women's illness and health, pharmaceutical manufacturers and research entrepreneurs—not women themselves—may be the winners.

Summary

The following factors contribute to gender inequity in biomedical research:

1. Scientific research has been largely a white, upper-class male endeavor and culture.
2. The predominant scientific method—testing of hypotheses about the relationships among several variables—frequently excludes women from research samples. Instead, clinical trials have relied on homogeneous samples, most often white, middle-class men.
3. Research that preferentially would benefit diverse populations has not been viewed as a research priority.
4. Funds for health care research are scarce, creating intense competition among researchers, although allocations have increased recently for study of specific diseases, namely, breast cancer.
5. The dearth of women, particularly women of color, in upper echelons of public and academic research institutions has meant very few women are deciding what or how diseases in women should be studied and what national women's health priorities should be.

Public Policy's Turnabout on Gender Inequity in Biomedical Research

Over a decade ago the U.S. Public Health Service (PHS), a major division of the DHHS, quietly created a task force to investigate inequities in women's health research. In 1985 this task force published a key document, *Women's Health: Report of the Public Health Service Task Force on Women's Health Issues*, which identified five criteria to categorize a health condition or disease as a woman's issue. The disease or condition must be unique, more prevalent, more serious, have different risk factors, or require interventions that are different for women or a subgroup of women (DHHS 1985). These criteria are based solely on a biomedical definition of disease. This narrow definition has remained central in public policy descriptions of women's health issues, although more socially inclusive definitions of health have been proposed—but not adopted. Instead of focusing on diseases, a social model of health places women's core needs at the center and pays attention to the diversity of women's health over their life span while also critically examining the concepts of risk and risk reduction (Ruzek 1993).

The task force pleaded for improved research: "The need for data that are relevant to health and are sex- and age-specific by race and ethnicity is crucial" (DHHS 1985:9). The report also called for expanded biomedical and behavioral research emphasizing conditions and diseases in women in all age groups and systematic efforts to address gender bias in research that leads to inadequate attention to the needs of women. These recommendations were largely ignored by the Public Health Service agencies. NIH did, however, follow a PHS directive to set up the Women's Health Advisory Committee, which remains in place today. In 1986, and again in 1987, the NIH Women's Health Advisory Committee urged applicants for clinical research grants to include women and minorities in study populations, requested applicants excluding them to justify the exclusion, and asked researchers to evaluate gender differences in their findings (Nadel 1990). This policy, however, did not lead to any substantial changes.

This committee also concluded that in 1987, only 13.5 percent of the total NIH budget had been spent on women's health issues, but cautioned that "this does not mean that the remainder . . . of the budget is spent on diseases of men. . . . The majority of funds . . . are expended for studies of diseases which affect both men and women" (Kirschstein 1990:3).

In summary, although the PHS formally recognized inequity in women's biomedical research a decade ago, its recommendations for improvement lay dormant until 1990, when political inquiry and public criticism propelled NIH to change. (For a chronology of policy actions influencing biomedical research, see appendix A.)

Congressional Action and Influence on Women's Biomedical Research

In 1989, the Congressional Caucus for Women's Issues pointed out that because women pay substantial tax dollars for health research, "they deserve to derive greater benefit from that research" (Southwick 1990). The House of Representatives Subcommittee on Health and the Environment of the Committee on Energy and Commerce joined the Congressional Caucus for Women's Issues in requesting a General Accounting Office (GAO) investigation of NIH's lack of implementation of its own policies to increase women's health research. The landmark GAO report of 1990 concluded that the NIH had made "little progress in implementing its policy to encourage inclusion of women in research populations" (Nadel 1990) and recommended research grant policy revisions to require that applicants include women or justify exclusion.

The Congressional Caucus for Women's Issues also drafted an omnibus bill in 1989, the Women's Health Equity Act. It called for establishing a permanent office for women and health under the assistant secretary of health, codifying the NIH policy of required inclusion of women in research studies, and allocating large sums for research into several diseases specific to women, such as breast cancer. The bill was reintroduced in each session of Congress from 1989 to 1994 and portions of it have become law. After the 1994 Republican sweep of Congress, the Office of the Congressional Caucus for Women's Issues was abolished, and the original Health Equity Act was replaced by a bill introduced in 1995 in the House of Representatives by Constance Morella of Maryland. H.R. 1736 includes requests for increased funding directed to governmental efforts for improved health care services for women. At time of publication, the bill was pending and had no Senate sponsor (personal communication, Representative Morella's staff).

The other significant legislation that structurally altered health care research is Public Law 103-43, the NIH Reauthorization Act of 1993, which revised and extended NIH programs. Its provisions included permanently establishing the Office of Research on Women's Health (ORWH) as well as an Office for Minority Health. It also required "blanket" inclusion of women and other subgroups in clinical studies. The regulatory language accompanying this law was published in March 1994. It begins to grapple with many of the issues discussed here. For example, NIH-supported studies will be required to include women and minorities and their subpopulations "such that valid analyses of differences in intervention effects can be accomplished." The term *valid analysis* is defined as "unbiased assessment" yielding, on average, the correct estimate of difference in outcomes between two groups of subjects, which is clinically significant but not necessarily statistically significant (DHHS 1994:14511).

This law and its regulations compel biomedical research to be systematically conducted with a new goal: to discover generalizable answers to questions posed by the widely varying health needs of the people of this nation. This mandate, however, has been criticized on several fronts. First, to meet the inclusion guidelines, clinical study design will be more complex and costly, and sample sizes will have to be much larger than in the past, potentially decreasing the number of research projects that NIH will fund (Hamilton 1994). Second, concern has been raised that these "global rules" could be interpreted as "quotas" or that mandated inclusion of women and other groups "might be applied so uncritically as to hamper rather than enhance the advancement of scientific information about these groups" (Bennett 1993:289, 291). Or, investigators might seek exemptions rather than attempt to comply (Hamilton 1994). As one critic has noted, simply adding a cohort of women to a study designed from the "male as norm" perspective cannot add to our understanding of women and their health (Woods 1994).

On the other hand, the new rules suggest trying models other than clinical trials for some questions in health research. In some situations observational, epidemiologic techniques may be useful, as well as meta-analysis, a statistical method that combines data from several studies for analysis and stronger conclusions than could be provided by any single study (Mastroianni et al. 1994a).

Recent Steps Forward by National Institutes of Health

Three months after receiving the GAO report, NIH unveiled the Office of Research on Women's Health within the Office of the Director of the NIH, complete with funding and authority. This was a victory. The

ORWH has been charged with three broad mandates: to strengthen research related to diseases that affect women and ensure NIH-supported research adequately addresses issues of women's health; to see that women are adequately represented in biomedical and behavioral studies supported by NIH; and to support recruitment, retention, and reentry of women in biomedical careers (ORWH 1992a). Dr. Vivian Pinn, formerly chief of pathology at Howard University College of Medicine, has been ORWH director since 1991. The budget for the first year was $1.5 million and rose to $10.2 million in 1994.

Since its founding in 1990, the ORWH has taken several impressive steps to respond to the three mandates noted above. To formulate a long-range women's health research agenda, the ORWH solicited public comment and held an invitational conference in 1991. The conference has been criticized, however, because it did not include representatives of women's health advocacy groups. A published conference report proposed "a comprehensive research agenda . . . with a multidisciplinary approach" (ORWH 1992b:12). Despite the agenda's comprehensiveness, it focuses primarily on clinical dimensions of health, reflecting the agenda first articulated by the 1985 Public Health Service Report. Feminists question whether this agenda will "provide explanations about women's health that are liberating, that have the capacity to be used by women for women's good" (Woods 1994:475).

As short-term goals, the ORWH has selected four research priority topics for 1995 that have been "understudied": occupational health, autoimmune diseases, reproductive health, and women's urological health. Demonstrating fiscal support for women's health, the ORWH allocates discretionary funds to augment ongoing NIH-supported studies that implement the ORWH research agenda. A total of 270 projects have received this funding supplement on topics ranging from gestational diabetes in Hispanics to the genetic basis of osteoporosis (ORWH 1995).

To address the second mandate, ensuring women are included in clinical studies, the ORWH has held a workshop and public hearing and in 1994 published a resulting report, "Recruitment and Retention of Women in Clinical Studies." This report is designed for use by researchers "and advocates in the appropriate and sensitive recruitment and retention of women, particularly minority women, in clinical studies" (ORWH 1995:3). The ORWH has also implemented a systematic, centralized tracking system on enrollment of women and minorities in NIH-supported clinical research, but results are not yet available (Mastroianni et al. 1994a).

Acting on the third mandate, to increase opportunities for women scientists, the ORWH convened a task force to gather information and held a public hearing and workshop in 1992. The conference report, "Women in Biomedical Careers: Dynamics of Change, Strategies for the Twenty-first Century" (1994), outlines issues in education, career advancement patterns, and social barriers along with strategies for improvement (ORWH 1992c, 1995). At the direction of Congress, the ORWH has also begun a survey of medical schools on the current content of women's health and to design a model curriculum. In summary, in its first five years, the ORWH has proven to be intent on unraveling some of the long-standing NIH institutional neglect of scientific work on behalf of women.

The Food and Drug Administration has also begun to promote inclusion of women in clinical drug trials. In 1988 the FDA urged researchers to examine safety and efficacy in specific population groups. However, according to a 1992 GAO investigation, only about 50 percent of the pharmaceutical studies done between 1989 and 1992 included analyses of drug effects in women.

In 1993 the FDA examined its restrictions on women in early phases of drug trials. An FDA statement declared that the 1977 "restriction on women with childbearing potential implies a lack of respect for their autonomy and decision-making capacity" (Merkatz et al. 1993:295). New guidelines encourage the inclusion of women of all age groups in all phases of most drug trials. The agency noted that study design could reduce the risk of accidental fetal exposure, for example, by administering a study drug immediately after menstruation or by taking advantage of highly sensitive pregnancy testing to avoid this risk. The most important method for safety, however, remains meticulous informed consent procedures.

The Women's Health Initiative's Potential for Answers

Women's health research received wide publicity when NIH launched the Women's Health Initiative in early 1991. This project is "the largest of its kind, clearly transcending the categorical structure of the NIH. . . . It will have an ecumenical approach . . . that allows all of the Institutes to contribute" (Healy 1991:1). The WHI seeks to understand causes, treatment, and particularly prevention of the three diseases that are the leading killers of women: cancer, cardiovascular disease, and osteoporosis (Women's Health Initiative 1994).

The study has three components: a randomized controlled trial of promising but unproven approaches to prevention, an observational study of predictors of these diseases, and a study of "community approaches to developing healthful behaviors" that have not been widely adopted (Women's Health Initiative 1994:1). The clinical trial component is under way and will enroll a total of 64,500 menopausal women for nine years in one of two intervention studies: a low-fat diet to see its effect on breast or colon cancer and cardiovascular disease, and hormone replacement therapy to evaluate its effect on preventing osteoporosis and coronary heart disease. Women enrolled in either of the trials will be recruited to a study of calcium/vitamin D supplementation to examine its effect on preventing colon cancer and osteoporotic fractures. The observational study will enroll an additional 100,000 women for nine years who either decline to participate or do not meet requirements to participate in the randomized intervention trials. The three-part clinical trial and the observational study will take place in forty clinical centers across the United States to ensure broad geographic distribution of subjects. The entire WHI is estimated to require fifteen years to complete with an end date of 2007 (Women's Health Initiative 1995, personal communication). The total cost is estimated to be $628 million. Funding, however, will be allocated annually out of the congressional appropriation to NIH, which introduces the uncertainty that accompanies political funding decisions. In 1994, $59 million was allocated.

Several features of the WHI's organization are unique and may in themselves advance women's health. The WHI directors have successfully recruited women scientists to head at least fifteen of forty clinical centers that began carrying out the prevention trial in early 1995. Also, recruitment efforts are targeting medically undeserved women and women of color so that the study sample is a "representative cross section of the U.S. population" (Women's Health Initiative 1994). Nine of the forty centers have enrollments averaging 60 percent minority participants (Brody 1996).

The WHI is breaking new ground and holds enormous promise for finally providing answers to many of the most pressing health problems for older American women, because of the size of the study populations as well as its rigorous design. Early criticism voiced by women's health advocates and the Institute of Medicine concerning the consent form for the clinical trials has led to an improved consent form. The study also responded promptly to a 1995 research report that demonstrated serious problems with one of the interventions in the hormone replacement clinical study (administering estrogen alone to healthy postmenopausal women). Within three months of reviewing this report, WHI changed part of the hormone replacement clinical study design to reflect the findings. This demonstration of the WHI's ability to "act swiftly to incorporate new information to the study plan" (Finnegan, Rossouw, and Harlan 1995:2) is reassuring.

Some scientists have expressed concern about having NIH personnel decide the research questions. However, given the magnitude of the study's costs, health activists consider the locus of power to be appropriately in the hands of public servants. In a broader sense, despite the promise of the WHI, the population and the questions being studied still leave many pressing health problems (such as mental health) for the future.

Thus, since the 1990 GAO report, governmental actions have begun to rectify some of the glaring inequities in biomedical research on women's health: the 1993 NIH Reauthorization Act requires inclusion of women and minorities in research studies funded by NIH, and it institutionalized the Office of Research on Women's Health; Congress has passed portions of the Women's Health Equity Act; FDA has liberalized its guidelines for women's participation in drug trials; and the Women's Health Initiative is funded and under way. It is tempting to think that these changes herald a major shift in the way biomedical research is done, but such onerous examples as the Tamoxifen prevention study must not be ignored. Women's health activists will need to hold the biomedical research community accountable for "formulating scientifically meaningful questions and then testing them in rigorous studies" (Bennett 1993:291). In fact, an Institute of Medicine Committee convened in 1992 to study ethical and legal issues in including women in clinical studies goes further, suggesting "guiding principles" for just conduct of clinical research: "Where it is established that specific health interests of women, men or other groups have not received a fair allocation of research attention or resources, justice may require a policy of preferential treatment toward these specific areas in order to remedy a past injustice and to avoid perpetuating that injustice" (Mastroianni et al. 1994a:83).

National Women's Health Network Position and Action Plan

We recognize the deeply embedded social and political influences on the conduct of science and the serious need to rectify the inequities in biomedical research in the United States which have recently garnered positive governmental responses. In light of these circumstances and events, the National Women's Health Network (NWHN) has delineated the following seven-point position and action plan. (Appendix B contains a list of specific priority women's health problems.)

1. We hold NIH accountable for consistent application of policies to rectify the underrepresentation of women in clinical research studies.
2. We urge the Office of Research on Women's Health (ORWH) to insist that health research endorsed by NIH meaningfully examines the wide range of health needs arising from the diverse lives women lead.
3. We support ORWH efforts to increase recruitment and retention of women from diverse backgrounds and ethnicities to careers in health research.
4. We strongly endorse the Office of Research on Women's Health's discretionary funding of high-quality research on risk reduction and disease prevention "that might not have been designated for funding" (Schneider 1990).
5. We support the development of methods to enroll childbearing-aged women in clinical research projects that examine drug or therapeutic interventions with appropriate, complete, and closely monitored informed consent.
6. The NWHN will make our positions known to, and will collaborate with, the Office of Research on Women's Health.
7. The NWHN encourages women to influence the national research agenda by seeking opportunities to actively participate in design, recruitment, and conduct of health research.

Conclusion

Improving biomedical research is a component of improving the health of American women. Such research has been flawed by gender bias imbedded in our culture and compounded by lack of respect for the diversity of health needs among us. Research has also been hindered by scarce research funds. The predominant androcentric scientific method has severely limited women from participating in biomedical research, and it provides findings that are not generalizable to our diverse population. Women, particularly women of color, constitute a shockingly small proportion of scientists, a fact that further limits progress in seeking mean-ingful answers about women. Governmental policy has been weakly ap-plied to these inequities, although recent legislative and regulatory changes should lead to improvements. The Women's Health Initiative offers some promise of change in the manner that clinical research is conceived and carried out. In a broader sense, the task ahead is to forge a more socially responsible and just science of health for us all.

APPENDIX A
Chronology of Policy Actions
Influencing Biomedical Research on Women's Health

1985   Public Health Service publishes Women's Health Report of the Public Health Service Task Force on Women's Health.

1986   NIH establishes Advisory Committee on Women's Health Issues, which recommends increasing women's participation in biomedical research funded by NIH.

1987   NIH policy of 1986 is reissued with emphasis on inclusion of minorities.

1989   Congressional Caucus for Women's Issues introduces the Women's Health Equity Act Omnibus bill.
        Caucus and House of Representatives Subcommittee on Health and Envi-ronment call for General Accounting Office investigation of NIH im-plementation of 1986 policy.

1990   GAO reports serious gender inequities in NIH and recommends major pol-icy changes.

1990   NIH mandates inclusion of women for all research grants; establishes and funds Office of Research on Women's Health.

1991   Bernadette Healy appointed NIH director. She proposes Women's Health Initiative, an "ecumenical" NIH study of the three leading causes of death in American women.
        Vivian Pinn appointed first director of the Office of Research on Women's Health (ORWH).
        ORWH convenes Hunt Valley Conference "Opportunities for Research on Women's Health."

1992   ORWH holds hearing and conference on recruitment and retention of women in biomedical careers.

1993   Women's Health Initiative subject recruitment is begun for prevention trials.
        ORWH holds hearing on recruitment and retention of women in clinical studies.
        1993 NIH Revitalization Act passed; includes permanent ORWH and mandates inclusive policy for NIH-supported studies.

FDA publishes new guidelines for study of gender differences in clinical evaluation of drugs, including participation of women of childbearing age.

1994   ORWH publishes two reports from 1992 conferences: *Women in Biomedical Careers: Dynamics of Change, Strategies for the Twenty-first Century* and *Recruitment and Retention of Women in Clinical Studies.*

1995   Women's Health Initiative completes selection of all forty clinical centers for the intervention clinical trials, and subject recruitment continues; the community study is pending.

ORWH begins survey of medical schools on current curricula on women's health and begins developing a model curriculum.

H.R. 1736 replaces the Women's Health Equity Act in Congress; the Office of the Congressional Caucus for Women's Issues is abolished.

1996   Women's Health Initiative subject recruitment lags; 109,500 more participants needed.

APPENDIX B
*National Women's Health Network Current Priority
Women's Health Conditions Needing Significant Research*

Each topic meets one or more of the PHS criteria for a condition or disease that affects women significantly and is not included in the Women's Health Initiative. Study of prevention of each of these problems for diverse groups of women is of highest priority.

1. Cardiovascular disease
    a. coronary artery disease—gender differences in treatment effects
    b. stroke
2. Cancer
    a. lung
    b. breast—prevention
    c. endometrial—relationship to hormone replacement therapy
    d. ovarian
    e. cervical—particularly new screening modalities
3. AIDS/HIV
    a. gender differences in diagnostic criteria and access to care
    b. gender differences in experimental drug response
    c. policy development specific to women with AIDS
4. Violence against women—health consequences and outcomes
5. Reproductive tract function and dysfunction
    a. menstrual cycle in relation to pharmacologic effects of widely used agents, such as antihypertensive and antidepressant medications
    b. menopause
    c. endometriosis
    d. uterine fibroids

6. Childbearing health
    a. causes of maternal mortality and morbidity
    b. premature labor
    c. contraceptive methods—development
    d. medical induction of therapeutic abortion
    e. prevention of infertility
7. Chemical Dependency
    a. gender-based smoking and alcohol cessation program development and evaluation
    b. illicit substance abuse—evaluation of treatment programs specific to women
    c. metabolic or other biological gender differences in response to the agents
8. Systemic collagen diseases
    a. systemic lupus erythematosus
    b. arthritis
    c. chronic fatigue syndrome
9. Mental health, particularly depression
    a. diagnosis—developing gender-neutral criteria
    b. treatment and outcomes specific to women
10. Environmental and occupational health
    a. investigation of toxic compounds in foods, water, and air as risk factors for major diseases
    b. evaluation of health effects of specific working conditions such as food service and hospitals
11. Thyroid diseases
    a. hyperthyroidism (five times more frequent in women)
    b. hypothyroidism (four times more frequent in women)
12. Cosmetic and reconstructive surgery
13. Urinary tract
    a. infections
    b. incontinence
14. Eating disorders/obesity
15. Gallbladder disease (women under fifty develop stones four times as often as men)
16. Health behaviors
    a. evaluation of differences in medical decisions by provider gender
    b. consequences of gender differences in patients' use of health care services

NOTES

1. A noteworthy example of research carried out in this framework is the study of low-dose aspirin as a heart disease preventative, which used 22,000 subjects—all of

whom were male physicians (Steering Committee of the Physicians' Health Study Research Group 1989). Despite a report on aspirin's benefit for women (Manson et al. 1991), the evidence of low-dose aspirin as a primary means of preventing myocardial infarction in women remains "promising but incompletely evaluated" (Appel and Bush 1991:566; Manson et al. 1992).

2. A related issue in health care research that has contributed to limited information for women is that for some major illnesses (e.g., coronary heart disease), women tend to develop the disease later in life than men. To understand the progression of coronary heart disease in women, female subjects in prospective studies would need to be studied longer than male subjects to observe the same number of new cases of heart disease. Generally, the longer a study continues, the more costly it will be.

3. The most infamous example is the Tuskegee Institute experiments from 1932 to 1972, in which syphilis was deliberately left untreated in black men (Cotton 1990). Oral contraceptive pills, developed during the 1950s, were tested on thousands of Puerto Rican women. "The ethical and scientific standards of the early pill studies in Puerto Rico in fact left much to be desired" (Katz 1972:745). More recent examples of the risk of exploitation arise from reports of Norplant and Depo-Provera being potential aids in controlling fertility of the "underclass" (*Philadelphia Inquirer* 1992). A report on use of these methods by Native American women receiving health care from the U.S. Indian Health Service noted inconsistency and inaccuracy in the information they received before accepting these methods (Krust and Asetoyer 1993). Such accounts of abuse might well be a factor in deep-seated mistrust of clinical research among people of color.

4. For example, in a study of theophylline, a drug commonly prescribed for asthma, the drug's effect lasted half as long for women as for men, apparently because of differences in liver metabolism (Nafzinger and Bertino 1989). Natural hormonal variations of the menstrual cycle also appear to alter drug responses. The effectiveness of insulin has been found to decrease during the second half of the menstrual cycle (Widom, Diamond, and Simonson 1992).

5. In a study comparing Caucasian and Chinese subjects taking propranolol, a drug widely used to control high blood pressure, Chinese subjects required less than half as much medication as their Caucasian counterparts to achieve a therapeutic effect. An explanation for the difference is that for the Chinese patients, more of the drug remains unbound, thus more potent, in their blood than in the Caucasian subjects' blood (Cotton 1990).

6. A report on women in NIH grant programs from 1984 to 1993 notes that 16.5 percent of applications to NIH in 1989 for competing research grants were from women, and 16.4 percent of the grants actually awarded were for female investigators. In 1993, the latest year for which data are available, 21 percent of competing grant applications were from women, and 25 percent of projects funded were led by female investigators (Division of Research Grants 1994). As might be expected, the National Institute of Nursing Research was the only institute that reviewed more applications from women than men—332 women and 41 men. Of the 43 applicants who received funding, 36 were women (personal communication, National Institute of Nursing Research 1995). Interestingly, the average dollar amount of awards also differs by

gender, with women receiving about 7 percent less than their male counterparts each year from 1984 to 1993. The difference in 1993 was $16,000, with a male recipient garnering on average $240,000 whereas a female recipient received $214,000 (Division of Research Grants 1994).

REFERENCES

Appel, Lawrence, and Trudy Bush
  1991   "Preventing heart disease in women another role for aspirin?" (editorial). Journal of the American Medical Association 266:565-66.
Bennett, J. Claude; Board on Health Sciences Policy of the Institute of Medicine
  1993   "Inclusion of women in clinical trials—policies for population subgroups." New England Journal of Medicine 329:288-91.
Birke, Lynda
  1986   Women, Feminism, and Biology: The Feminist Challenge. New York: Methuen.
Brighton Women and Science Group
  1980   Alice through the Microscope: The Power of Science over Women's Lives. London: Virago.
Brody, Jane
  1996   "Personal health: a 15 year study focuses on guiding women toward a healthier old age." New York Times, 8 May, B9.
Cotton, Paul
  1990   "Is there still too much extrapolation from data on middle-aged white men?" Journal of the American Medical Association 263:1050.
Division of Research Grants
  1994   Women in NIH Extramural Grant Programs Fiscal Years 1984-1993. Bethesda, MD: National Institutes of Health.
Finnegan, Loretta, Jacques Rossouw, and William Harlan
  1995   "A peppy response to PEPI results." NIH News-2B25/31, 1-2.
Fugh-Berman, Adriane, and Samuel Epstein
  1992   "Tamoxifen: disease prevention or disease substitution?" Lancet 340:1143-45.
Hamilton, Jean
  1994   "Going to extremes." Women's Review of Books 11:15-16.
Healy, Bernadette
  1991   Overview statement on the new initiative to study women's health. Bethesda, MD: National Institutes of Health.
Hubbard, Ruth
  1990   The Politics of Women's Biology. New Brunswick, NJ: Rutgers University Press.
Katz, Jay
  1972   Experimentation with Human Beings. New York: Russell Sage Foundation.

Keller, Evelyn
    1982   "Feminism and science." Signs: Journal of Women in Culture and Society 7:589-602.

Kirschstein, Ruth
    1990   "Statement at the National Institutes of Health meeting on women's health research issues." National Institutes of Health.

Koertge, Noretta
    1994   "Are feminists alienating women from the sciences?" Chronicle of Higher Education, 14 September, A80.

Kolata, Gina
    1991   "In medical research equal opportunity doesn't always apply." New York Times, 10 March, E16.

Koshland, Daniel
    1988   "Women in science" (editorial). Science 239:1473.

Krust, Lin, and Charon Asetoyer
    1993   A Study of the Use of Depo-Provera and Norplant by the Indian Health Services. Lake Andes, SD: Native American Women's Health Education Resource Center.

Kuhn, Thomas
    1970   The Structure of Scientific Revolutions, 2d ed. Chicago: University of Chicago Press.

Levine, Robert
    1994   "Recruitment and retention of women in clinical studies." Vol. 2, pp. 58-64 in Anna C. Mastroianni, Ruth Faden, and Daniel Federman (eds.), Women and Health Research: Ethical and Legal Issues of Including Women in Clinical Studies. Washington: National Academy Press.

Manson, Joann, Meir Stampfer, Graham Colditz, Walker Willett, Bernard Rosner, Frank Seizer, and Charles Hennekens
    1991   "A prospective study of aspirin use and primary prevention of cardiovascular disease in women." Journal of the American Medical Association 266:521-27.

Manson, Joann, Heather Tosteson, Paul Ridker, Suzanne Satterfield, Gerald O'Conner, Julie Buring, and Charles Hennekens.
    1992   "The primary prevention of myocardial infarction." New England Journal of Medicine 326:1406-20.

Mastroianni, Anna C., Ruth Faden, and Daniel Federman, eds.
    1994a   Women and Health Research: Ethical and Legal Issues of Including Women in Clinical Studies. Vol 1. Washington: National Academy Press.
    1994b   Women and Health Research: Ethical and Legal Issues of Including Women in Clinical Studies. Vol. 2, Workshop and Commissioned Papers. Washington: National Academy Press.

Merkatz, Ruth, Robert Temple, Solomon Sobel, Karyn Feiden, David Kessler, and the Working Group on Women in Clinical Trials
    1993   "Women in clinical trials of new drugs." New England Journal of Medicine 329:292-96.

Merton, Vanessa
 1994 "Impact of current federal regulations on the inclusion of female subjects in clinical studies." Vol. 2, pp. 65–83 in Anna C. Mastroianni, Ruth Faden, and Daniel Federman (eds.), Women and Health Research: Ethical and Legal Issues of Including Women in Clinical Studies. Washington: National Academy Press.

Mitchell, Janet
 1994 "Recruitment and retention of women of color in clinical studies." Vol. 2, pp. 52–56 in Anna C. Mastroianni, Ruth Faden, and Daniel Federman (eds.), Women and Health Research: Ethical and Legal Issues of Including Women in Clinical Studies. Washington: National Academy Press.

Nadel, Mark
 1990 National Institutes of Health: Problems in Implementing Policy on Women in Study Populations. Statement before the Subcommittee on Health and the Environment Committee of Energy and Commerce, U.S. House of Representatives. GAO/HRD-90-38. Washington: General Accounting Office.

Nafzinger, A., and J. Bertino
 1989 "Sex-related differences in theophylline pharmacokinetics." European Journal of Clinical Pharmacology 37:97–100.

National Cancer Institute
 1993 1995 Budget Estimate. Washington: National Cancer Institute.

National Institutes of Health (NIH)
 1994 Women's Health Research. Bethesda, MD: Budget Office, National Institutes of Health.

National Science Foundation
 1992 Women and Minorities in Science and Engineering: An Update. Washington: Government Printing Office.

National Women's Health Network
 1986 Ten Years of Leadership, 1976–1986. Washington: National Women's Health Network.

Office of Research on Women's Health (ORWH)
 1992a Overview. Bethesda, MD: National Institutes of Health.
 1992b "Report of the National Institutes of Health: opportunities for research on women's health, 4–6 September 1991, Hunt Valley, Maryland." NIH Pub. No. 92-3457.
 1992c Public hearing on recruitment, retention, re-entry, and advancement of women in biomedical careers. Bethesda, MD: National Institutes of Health.
 1995 Overview. Bethesda, MD: National Institutes of Health.

Pettiti, Diane
 1990 Testimony before the House Select Committee on Aging Subcommittee on Housing and Consumer Interests (unpublished).

Philadelphia Inquirer
 1992 "Poverty and Norplant: can contraception reduce the underclass?" (editorial). 12 December.

Raloff, Janet
    1992   "Tamoxifen and informed consent." Science News 142:378-80.
Roback, Gene, Lillian Randolph, Bradley Seidman, and Thomas Pasko
    1994   Physician Characteristics and Distribution in the United States. Chicago: American Medical Association.
Rosenthal, Elizabeth
    1995   "Hospital research falling victim to lean budgets." New York Times, 30 May, A1, A12.
Rosser, Sue
    1992   Biology and Feminism: A Dynamic Interaction. New York: Macmillan.
Ruzek, Sheryl Burt
    1993   "Towards a more inclusive model of women's health." American Journal of Public Health 83:6-8.
Schiebinger, Linda
    1987   "The history and philosophy of women in science review essay." Pp. 32-40 in Sandra Harding and Jean O'Barr (eds.), Sex and Scientific Inquiry. Chicago: University of Chicago Press.
Schneider, Iris
    1990   Personal communication to Beverly Baker, executive director, National Women's Health Network.
Southwick, Karen
    1990   "Women excluded from tests on new drugs, critics contend." Healthweek, 26 March, 48.
Steering Committee of the Physicians' Health Study Research Group
    1989   "Final report on the aspirin component of the ongoing physicians' health study." New England Journal of Medicine 321:129-35.
Stoy, Diane
    1994   "Recruitment and retention of women in clinical studies: theoretical perspectives and methodological considerations." Vol. 2, pp. 45-51 in Anna C. Mastroianni, Ruth Faden, and Daniel Federman (eds.), Women and Health Research: Ethical and Legal Issues of Including Women in Clinical Studies. Washington: National Academy Press.
U.S. Department of Health and Human Services (DHHS)
    1985   Women's Health: Report of the Public Health Service Task Force on Women's Health Issues. DHHS Pub. No. (PHS) 85-50206. May. Washington: Government Printing Office.
    1994   "NIH guidelines for the inclusion of women and minorities as subjects in clinical research; notice." Federal Register, 28 March:14508-13.
U.S. Food and Drug Administration (FDA)
    1977   General Considerations for the Clinical Evaluation of Drugs. Rockville, MD: FDA.
U.S. General Accounting Office
    1992   FDA Needs to Ensure More Study of Gender Differences in Prescription Drug Testing. HRD-93-17. Washington: Government Printing Office.

Watson, Traci
    1993   "Task force: level the playing field." Science 260:888–89.
Widom, Barbara, Michael Diamond, and Donald Simonson
    1992   "Alterations in glucose metabolism during menstrual cycle in women with IDDM." Diabetes Care 15:213–20.
Women's Health Initiative
    1994   Overview. Bethesda, MD: National Institutes of Health.
Woods, Nancy
    1994   "The United States women's health research agenda analysis and critique." Western Journal of Nursing Research 16:467–79.

[22]

Strengths and Strongholds in Women's Health Research

VIRGINIA L. OLESEN, DIANA TAYLOR,
SHERYL BURT RUZEK, AND ADELE E. CLARKE

Reviewing the extensive bodies of research in nursing, sociology, and anthropology, this multidisciplinary group of scholars points out that there is a rich, empirically based literature on sociocultural differences in health and healing that includes women. This literature includes case studies and other qualitative research as well as quantitative studies. These contributions should not be ignored but used as a background for shaping specific research agendas for the future.

Growing recognition of the issues surrounding multiple axes of diversity has characterized the twenty-year history of research on women's health. In spite of slow acknowledgment of the needs, interests, and concerns of diverse women, scattered research in a variety of fields has started to open awareness of cultural diversities. This chapter reviews various sociocultural, public health, and nursing inquiries, none of them perfect, which have probed some fundamental issues about or described diverse women's participation in health care systems.[1] These serve as leads to crucial questions for future research, which will be discussed in chapter 23.

Brief History of Women's Health Research

Social and Behavioral Sciences

Stimulated by health activism in the growing feminist movement, research interest in the social and behavioral aspects of women's health grew dramatically in the academic branches of the women's health movement during the 1970s and 1980s. Scholars whose work already encompassed women's health issues found themselves taken seriously, and their work quickly coalesced into an emerging research agenda which recognized that mere anger with inadequate health care for women would not suffice and that serious research in numerous areas was required if aspects of the problem were to be understood and eventually embedded in policy (Olesen 1976:1–2).

The question of minority women's health issues as grounded in race- and class-specific conditions was raised but for some years largely ignored. Even in the emergent history of women's health, which had acknowledged historical issues of particular salience especially for African American women (e.g., Davis 1981), early analyses did not center on such fundamental forms of stratification as race and gender (Apple 1990; Leavitt 1984).

In the social sciences, both race and class remained largely invisible as attention focused on sex differences in health status, women's conceptualizations and experiences of health and medical events, utilization of health services, the roles of women as health providers, and social and psychological dimensions of conditions that were of particular concern to women—for example, breast cancer, reproduction, rape, and domestic violence. These early studies contributed four important elements to the history of women's health research:

- First, perspectives on women's health were at least being generated by women rather than by (mostly male) physicians.
- Second, women and their health/illness experiences and needs were lodged in sociocultural-historical contexts rather than exclusively biomedical frameworks.[2]
- Third, misleading stereotypes were overturned or destabilized, thus problematizing aspects of medical care where women had been taken for granted: for example, invidious, sexually stereotyped diagnoses (Lennane and Lennane 1973), doctor-patient relationships that demonstrated differential and negative attitudes toward women (Armitage, Schneiderman, and Bass 1979), women's knowledge of their own bodies (Jordan 1977), and the very categories of diagnoses (Boskin-Ludehl 1976).[3]
- Fourth, the sociocultural findings about women qua women moved away from making inferences about women's health based on male experiences, a substantial problem in biomedical research and epidemiological research, as chapter 21 makes clear.[4]

These studies started to break open ossified views of women in health care. They varied, however, in the extent to which they acknowledged race and class. Thus, what should have been a wedge into larger considerations of diversity was obscured in continued universalizing rhetoric. Much work still reflected a generic conceptualization of "women's health issues."

Margaret Nelson's (1983) classic study of what women in different social classes want in birth interventions broke with the prevailing tendency to characterize "what women wanted" homogeneously. She found that middle-class women were then seeking "natural birth" whereas working-class and poor women were delighted with the idea of drugs to provide a pain-free birth experience. In an earlier but less widely circulated study, Manzanado, Walters, and Lorig (1980) had reported their findings of Chicanas' preferences for female versus male health providers. This analysis linked provider preference to language and place of birth and clearly articulated the task ahead.

The 1980s were marked by an acknowledgment, but not necessarily an analysis, of diversities in women's health needs and experiences, though some work was beginning.[5] During this period, diverse health needs were conceptualized largely as "special needs."[6]

Recognition slowly grew that in studies of health and healing neither members of different social classes nor members of minority groups could be lumped together and studied without reference to their own multiple statuses and life experiences and that there were significant variations *within* groups once thought to be homogeneous (Schur, Bernstein, and Berk 1987).[7] In this same era women's health research conferences flourished. Some focused specifically on health of minority women, and almost all included sessions on women in diverse situations and commitments, thus emphasizing the long overdue recognition of the topic and providing outlets for dissemination and discussion of diversity-relevant research.[8]

Nursing Research

Whereas most scientific disciplines have typically adopted a unidimensional view of health and illness, nursing research proposes a biopsychosocial model built upon a core of "holism" where multiple levels of inquiry (individual, group, community) can be considered and applied to visualize the diversity of factors that may be involved in women's health or illness.[9] However, although a central strength of nursing is the attempt to maintain a holistic perspective, gender and its relations to health and illness have not yet been investigated in the same way or with the same intensity as other social factors.

Further, as is true of social and behavioral research in women's health, nurse researchers' explorations of diverse women's situations have been slow to develop. Few studies have assessed the impacts of interventions on complex person-environment relationships. However, two theoretical models do speak to the interaction of individual women with the environment (Shaver 1985) and the necessity to think beyond the individual and health promotion in a context of environmental modification and personal change (Pender 1987). These provide important frameworks for women's health research that would allow greater exploration of diversity. Moreover, a feminist critique of American health promotion rejects the emphasis on individual behavior as the most important factor in health and reiterates the critical matter of social location (e.g., Williams 1989).

An important theme related to diversity has been the relatively recent recognition that women's health is distinct from maternal-child health. A 1981 review of women's health research in nursing showed continued focus on women's reproductive function and biomedical disease phenomena (Dunbar et al. 1981). The reviewers found twice as much research on women in childbearing and child-rearing roles than on women's other health problems. Further, there was a strong focus in the area of diagnosis and treatment of disease, rather than in health promotion and disease prevention. In short, there was little growth in women's health nursing research in the 1970s during the rise of the women's movement.

By 1988, however, another review found that nursing research had begun to address all aspects of women's health with a variety of methods (Woods 1988) and sounded a wide-ranging call for future nursing research on women's health that would emphasize diverse women, their lived experiences, and the necessity for recognition and integration of biological, psychological, social, and cultural contexts.[10] Although culturally oriented research was scarce in the 1980s, by the late 1980s, very much as in social and behavioral science investigations of women's health, nurse researchers had begun to explore diversity, looking at AIDS and African American and Hispanic women's beliefs (Flaskerud and Nyamathi 1989; Flaskerud and Rush 1989), and at depression, stress, and mastery of coping skills in immigrants from four cultures (Franks and Faux 1990).[11] Research on older women, which had lagged in the early 1980s (Woods 1988), also picked up considerably.

Since 1990, nursing research about women's health has expanded, both methodologically and substantively, to generate new knowledge particularly attuned to issues of diversity.[12] In 1993, twelve data-based studies specifically related to gender, race, or class could be identified in the nursing research literature, a number that increased to twenty-five in 1994 and early 1995, numbers which clearly signaled a departure from the previous orientation to women's health as part of reproductive and child health and a new move to focus on diversity.[13] These studies have yielded knowledge about how clinicians themselves contribute to the social construction of gender, race, class, health, and illness (Caroline and Bernhard 1994). Continuing to incorporate a holistic and bio-psychosocial framework, using a wide variety of qualitative and quantitative research designs, nursing research has focused on multiple factors related to women's health and illness, in addition to women's lived experience, though critics have commented on how much more can and must be done (Jackson 1993), a point also made about social science research.

Some of nursing research plus work in the social and behavioral sciences that has explored diversity will be reviewed below. Before doing so, however, it is important to discuss the difficulties that researchers face in moving the complexities of diversity from "margin to center," to use bell hooks's apt phrase (1984).[14]

How Methodologies Make Studying Diversity Difficult

Both quantitative and qualitative research methodologies contain problems that make it difficult to learn what we need to learn. Because concepts and methods shape our knowledge, they bear on the issues of diversity and commonality in women's health.[15] (See Reinharz 1992 for an in-depth exploration of feminist research methods.)

Quantitative Research

Those who have studied statistics know how researchers opt for very homogeneous samples in order to identify causal factors. People who are "different" might introduce unwanted intervening variables ("noise") and/or contribute data that might dilute or mask the "dominant pattern" that scientists seek to identify. Such researchers therefore narrow subjects' eligibility criteria in hopes of focusing more clearly on their topic of study. They justify this on grounds that by reducing variation they can achieve statistical significance more readily, and this is indeed true. However, they also sacrifice the generalizability of their findings to diverse populations, although this is rarely acknowledged. If we later replicated such studies on samples from different populations, populations composed of women in a variety of life circumstances, we could *eventually* come to understand what factors are involved in health and disease processes in the human population. But this is not what happens.

Instead, scientists and the media quietly ignore the core dictum that every student learns in basic quantitative research methods: you cannot generalize beyond the population from which a sample has been drawn. In health research and practice, this is violated wantonly and without attention to the institutionalized race, gender, and class biases that are literally built into the enactment of most research methodologies. People ignore the question of who has been intentionally excluded from samples and assume or proceed to declare that research findings are widely generalizable.[16]

Methodological and conceptual issues that have impeded and obscured explanations of the relationship between socioeconomic status and health have been described in the nursing literature. Researchers have forgotten the problems with reciprocal effects (poverty leads to poor health, which may lead to diminished earning capacity); confounding factors (smoking, obesity, and high blood pressure are linked to low income), and measurement issues (education, occupation, and income have unique strengths/weaknesses as indicators of socioeconomic status) in understanding and explaining the relationship between economic impoverishment and women's health and illness (Nelson 1994). This raises the second core dictum of quantitative research: correlation does not signify *causation*.

Qualitative Research

In qualitative research, lowest on the hierarchy of scientific research, not only the results but the method must be marketed. Naturalistic inquiries into existing social groups and their practices *in situ* have always been questioned regarding generalizability. Qualitative research selectively studies individuals with particular characteristics but sometimes wrongly assumes that the findings apply to others. For example, Margaret Nelson's (1983) work on birth preferences may be interpreted to suggest that middle-class women "want" natural birth and working-class women "want" drugs in labor—whether or not this is true in a setting outside the one Nelson studied. Uncritical generalizations of this kind easily lead to stereotyping or glossing over group or individual differences.

Because of the difficulty of doing qualitative research with people very different from the researcher with whom there are incongruences of status, and particularly race and linguistic differences (Edwards 1990; Riessman 1987), the scarcity of women of color in social science research has hampered increasing the qualitative knowledge base. A three-year ethnographic study of a senior citizen center in a poor, inner-city African American community by a nurse researcher described issues of ethnicity, age, and class between the outsider researcher and the insider study group, analyzed the outsider/insider dilemma, and suggested strategies to help researchers study groups different from themselves (Kauffman 1994).

Defining experiences of minorities as deviant behavior has also impeded knowledge acquisition. More qualitative research has been done on illicit activities (drug use, prostitution) than on the normal course of health and health-seeking behavior among women of color. Fortunately, qualitative work by female researchers of color on topics such as Latino family life and health (Baca Zinn 1989; Zambrana 1982; Zambrana and Aguirre-Molina 1987); African American family relations (Dill 1988), sickle cell and stress (Hill 1993), and HIV/AIDS (Fullilove et al. 1990; Mays 1987, 1988; Nyamathi and Vasquez 1989; Romero, Arguelles, and Rivero 1993) promises to shift the focus of scholarship on the health of women of color.

Because qualitative or interpretive research can be particularly powerful in grasping women's lived health experiences, researchers have posed critical questions that go beyond data gathering such as how women's experiences are conceptualized and presented and whose voices are heard (Olesen 1994:167-68). (Such questions are rarely, if ever, raised in quantitative work.) Although the voices of women of color, disabled women, lesbian and bisexual women, and women who hold stigmatized status (e.g., imprisoned women) are increasingly heard, they are sometimes individual voices, individual stories (Browne, Connors, and Stern 1985; White 1990). This must be followed by systematic research to avoid overgeneralizing from individual experience.

Regardless of the difficulties inherent in both qualitative and quantitative research methods for investigation of differences originating from women's diverse contexts, new and developing methods can advance our understanding. In quantitative research, when little is known about the intra-individual variability of any particular phenomena, such as pain, fatigue, or perimenstrual symptom experience in different ethnic groups, a time-series methodology can answer questions of individual experience yet approximate the internal validity of experimental designs (Taylor 1990). In addition, structural equation modeling strategies (using LISREL, EQS, etc.) that better reflect the complexity of the dimensions compared with simple linear analytic models can analyze multiple indicators of diversity (ethnicity, race, occupation, income, class, education, etc.) as well as build and test complex theoretical models using multidimensional data that represent both the individual woman and her environment (social, political, cultural) (Taylor 1991). Further, some researchers are moving to hybrid or triangulated designs (Mitchell 1990) where both quantitative and qualitative methods are used in the investigation of women's experiences.

In qualitative research, advances in narrative and phenomenological analysis can facilitate deeper exploration of the meaning of women's diverse experiences (Bell 1988; Benner 1994; Paget 1988; Riessman 1990; Stevens, Hall, and Meleis 1992b).

Selected Reports on Research in Diversity

Bearing in mind these difficulties, we now turn to reviews of selected research[17] on differences from several strongholds of recent research on diversity in women's health: the social and cultural sciences, public health, and nursing.[18] (Chapters in this volume contain other examples.) Although limited in their scope in terms of what is critical for realization of more efficacious knowledge of difference, a topic discussed in chapter 23, these selections nevertheless suggest that a research agenda more fully attuned to diversity is possible. Our review summarizes work on women's experiences of health and illness, their health behaviors, services, providers, interpretations, or knowledge production and research that involves diverse women.

These reports vary both with regard to methodological approaches (qualitative and quantitative) and the degree to which differences are explored and analyzed. Some are sheerly descriptive of one group of diverse women's health in contexts of which we know little; others are comparative. Some explore two elements, for instance, rural living and ethnicity, ethnicity and employment status. Few take up race and gender along with the neglected category of social class, yet the intertwining of these is apparent in many realms of women's health experience and care, such as AIDS (Krieger and Fee 1994:274–76).

Experiences of Health and Illness

A number of studies depict health and illness experiences among diverse women in a variety of circumstances. These studies indicate that broad generalizations cannot hold up either across groups or within groups. An oral history study of ten elderly black women in North Carolina showed that, among other factors, declining traditional rural resources generate health and other problems for elderly black farm women (Carlton-LaNey 1992), whereas a quantitative survey of 3,237 blacks and whites age sixty-five or over documented that older black women reported the highest levels of functional morbidity and the most negative assessments of their own health (Ferraro 1993). Hmong women's health was positively related to the degree to which they were acculturated, a nursing study discovered (Faller 1992).

Nurse researchers have also focused on ethnic diversities and health/illness experiences: Haitian immigrant women's preventive care for their children (DeSantis and Thomas 1990), Native American women and biculturalism in health (Hobus 1990), childbearing practices (Phillips and Lobar 1990), management of illnesses (Goforth-Parker 1994; Wuest 1991), use of culturally specific care (Huttlinger and Tanner 1994), health care needs among five ethnic/racial groups of low-income clerical workers (Stevens, Hall, and Meleis 1992a, 1992b), African American women (Griffin 1994), health problems of low-income pregnant Hispanic women who have been battered (Torres 1993), and depression among African American women (Barbee 1992; Oakley 1986; Tomes et al. 1990). Nurse researchers have also used sociocultural and political theories to understand women's mental illness (Steen 1991) and eating disorders (White 1991).

Several studies demonstrate the importance of *within-group* differences: Utilizing a variety of variables, a survey study of 245 employed and unemployed black women found that the unemployed women were significantly more depressed than employed women, irrespective of age, household income, level of education, marital status, and presence of children (Brown and Gary 1988). Level of education, not regional residence, was the important factor in African American women's use of family planning, according to a survey of 1,074 African American women in Philadelphia and North Carolina (Turner and Darity 1987–88). An interview study of thirty-two Afghan refugee women by nurse researchers found age diversity within cultural diversity (Lipson and Miller 1994).

A rare study of race, class, and multiple role strains included 229 black and white female social workers and licensed practical nurses. Investigators found strains particularly intense for both black and white working-class women, particularly around the "double day." They also found that African American women, facing the twofold problem of race and class, had fewer rewards and greater concerns (Marshall and Barnett 1991), indicating again that race, ethnicity, and social class affect women's life chances and, consequently, their health (Nickens 1993).

Nurse researchers' descriptive study of 94 African American, white, Mexican American, and Puerto Rican American women found that the women experienced general stress, but ethnic minority women were exposed to stress unique to their ethnicity (Walcott-McQuigg 1994). Other nursing research demonstrated unique factors related to depression among African American women (Warren 1994). Different explanatory models for self-esteem and depressed mood among young adult Asian, African American, and white women were found by nurse researchers using a feminist theoretical framework (Woods et al. 1994).

Knowledge of homeless women's health and illness experiences has to this date been framed around the important issues of whether the women are single or have children. Homeless women are racially diverse. A national study of 1,704 homeless users of soup kitchens and shelters in cities over 100,000 in 1987, found that more than half of the single women and four-fifths of homeless women with children were African American, Latina, or other nonwhites (Burt and Cohen 1989:512-13). More precise knowledge of racial and ethnic differences in diverse homeless women's health and illness experiences is needed such as one nurse researcher's description of health needs of pregnant homeless women (O'Connell 1993).

Health Behaviors

Several studies illustrate the utility of the comparative approach. A quantitative investigation of 333 black and 468 white mothers in Detroit showed the link between unemployment and smoking among young black mothers, highlighting the importance of understanding "the social contexts in which mothers in different populations take up smoking and continue to smoke" (Andreski and Breslau 1995:232). A survey of 107 low-income pregnant African Americans, recent Mexican immigrants, and Mexican Americans in Los Angeles depicted important differences in substance use patterns (Zambrana et al. 1991). Two studies departed from the tendency to study health promotion behaviors in white, middle-income and upper-middle-income groups: a survey of 102 black and 141 Latina low-income females found differences in eating habits, sleep, and visits to the doctor that have implications for health promotion programs (Sanders-Phillips 1994); a nursing inquiry described health-promoting behaviors of African American women (Ahijevych and Bernhard 1994). A nurse researcher examined differences between African American and Caucasian women in seeking care for breast cancer symptoms (Lauver 1994). All these studies demonstrate the importance of not generalizing across groups.

A nursing study that draws attention to health practices of low-income working women of color, a group relatively invisible in the literature on health promotion and protection, investigated nursing assistants in long-term care facilities, almost all women of color. Using both qualitative and quantitative approaches, the researcher was able to identify their health practices and concerns (job-related injuries and financial worries) (Nelson 1995).

Access to Services

Barriers to diverse women's access to services include economic, social, and psychological issues that vary for different groups and for different women within groups. A quantitative study of 586 white, 277 black, and 150 Latina women discovered that obtaining a mammogram depended on socioeconomic status. In all three groups, women with upper socioeconomic status had similar rates. Within the generally lower rates in women of lower economic status, Latina women's rates were much lower. This group lacked resources and language because they were less acculturated (Stein, Fox, and Murata 1991:109), an important *within*-group difference.

A nursing study of 450 Mexican American women over age forty found that strong traditional attitudes toward family was the best predictor of getting a Pap smear and mammography (Suarez 1994). Age was a factor for African American women seeking cancer detection, according to other nurse researchers (Brown and Williams 1994). Barriers to prenatal care among 177 black women in three high-risk communities in Chicago, such as job demands, travel time to providers and child care, were significant factors for those who used affiliated providers as against those who turned to alternative sources of care (Kelley et al. 1992). Nursing research has described lesbians' problems with receiving culturally appropriate health care (Stevens and Hall 1991; Trippet and Bain 1992) and the Southeast Asian refugees' search for healers in the American health system (Muecke 1983).

Several nursing research studies departed from merely investigating women's situations and looked at women and their providers: One nursing investigator looked at cultural sensitivity among women's health care providers concerning breast-feeding (Abramson 1992); another looked at the efficacy of AIDs counseling programs for black and Latina women (Nyamathi 1993). A third study examined differential views of pain by Mexican American and white women and their nurses (Calvillo and Flaskerud 1993).

Interpretation and Knowledge Production

Because of the emphasis on subjectivity, qualitative research can reveal diversities in how women interpret, construct and use knowledge about illness and health. Among fifteen Native American women, all reported using both Indian and "white" medicine, depending on what was accessible. Older women used Indian medicine more frequently, whereas many of the younger women believed in preventive western practices (Drevdahl 1993). Religious belief and scientific understandings were intertwined in forty low-income black women's explanatory models for cancer (Gregg and Curry 1994), whereas twenty-six rural black women in North Carolina drew on several sources of knowledge (popular, indigenous, medical) in coming to terms with the diagnosis of breast cancer (Mathews, Lannin, and Mitchell 1994).

One nurse researcher detailed the importance of healing beliefs and values to Navajo women (Bell 1994). Explanatory models for depression varied among Chinese American immigrant women: women who thought their problem was physical sought professional help, but those who held a psychological explanation sought help from family and friends (Ying 1990). Variations between Chicanas and Mexicanas around the constructions of such important concepts as motherhood point to the necessity of not placing all Latina women into one analytic category (Segura 1991). Differential processes of health decision making and experiences of family violence among Cambodian refugee women have been detailed in nursing research (Frye 1991; Frye and D'Avanzo 1994). Young African American and European American women construct their bodies differently, as one nurse researcher discovered (Harris 1994).

Quantitative research, though limited with regard to the capacity to understand how women construct meanings, nevertheless can disclose how distribution of interpretations varies: in a study of 409 Latina women over age fifty on beliefs about breast cancer, older women, less educated women and less acculturated women expressed more denial and less hope (Saint-Germain and Longman 1993), another indication of the importance of within-group differences. A quantitative nursing study described beliefs about health in various ethnic groups (Woods et al. 1988).

Involved Research

The Women's Health Advisory Committee of the San Francisco Department of Public Health (Taylor and Dower 1995; WHAC 1994) combined concern with improvement of women's health care services with active involvement of diverse women in a focus group research project. The committee, itself a composite of diverse women from professional backgrounds, convened nineteen groups that reflected diversity in San Francisco (African American, Asian American, Native American, Latinas, Middle Eastern women, sex workers, Vietnamese immigrants, seniors, teen mothers, young women, lesbians, and women who are deaf, homeless, incarcerated, bisexual, disabled, HIV positive, cancer patients, and cancer survivors). The women had differing degrees of insurance—private, public, or none.[19]

Common themes came up in almost every discussion.[20] The women spoke of both health care providers and staff and the system (structures of delivery such as insurance, hospitals, regulations, etc.) as areas ripe for improvement. Regarding providers, women spoke of providers' attitudes (superiority, insensitivity, discrimination, rudeness, lack of compassion) and quality of care (mistakes, low-quality care, inappropriate touching or requests, lack of information about complaint processes and accountability).

The participants' concerns also spoke to the health care system as a source of inadequate care.[21] Worries about access and narrow views within health care professions dominated their statements. Access related to lack of provider diversity was reflected in one woman's statement, which others echoed: "When I go for health care, I never see any providers that look like me." African American women said they found providers' insensitivity and inability to interact effectively with speech patterns, established cultural practices of health care and darker skin colors disrespectful. Many women were frustrated by narrow views in the current system, specialized treatment of one body part to the exclusion of the total person, a focus on disease and drugs without looking at health promotion and wellness, exclusive reliance on western medicine while ignoring alternative or complementary therapies. Women of color, those with chronic illnesses, and immigrant women expressed particular concerns about mental health, violence, growing dependency in illnesses, and restrictive regulations. All of these themes are being used to plan women-centered relevant health care delivery.[22]

Paths Just Taken—Work to Come

Although awareness of the necessity to avoid generalizations in women's health and to take greater cognizance of diversity has developed too slowly, a body of work in nursing, the social sciences, and public health has begun to emerge. Some of this work has analyzed important differences among and between groups, whereas other sectors of it have outlined the critical differences within groups that reflect age; rural versus urban residence; being or not being employed and type of job, if employed; education; socioeconomic status; degree of acculturation; religious beliefs, etc. In spite of this and in spite of methodological issues in both quantitative and qualitative research that make investigating diversity difficult, though not impossible, much remains to be done in research on women's health if we are to recognize, as Krieger and Fee put it, that "in reality, we are a mixed lot, our gender roles and options shaped by history, cultural and deep divisions across class and color lines" (1994:272). Chapter 23 takes up this challenge.

NOTES

1. A review of the extensive biomedical research related to women's health is beyond the scope of this chapter and, from the biopsychosocial perspective of this book, too limited. Chapter 21 provides a critical review of that type of research, particularly the federal Women's Health Initiative, as well as discussion of women scientists (those who hold science degrees, as well as female physicians and nurses with doctoral preparation in basic sciences).

2. That early criticism (women seen exclusively in a biomedical frame) continues to be heard about NIH's 1991 Women's Health Initiative, as the authors from the National Women's Health Network make clear in chapter 21.

3. Destabilizing taken-for-granted views of women continues with studies of patient-provider communication and the importance of nurse practitioners in the "politics of location" (Fisher 1995:221); diagnosis and concepts of illness (Hunt, Jordan, and Irwin 1989); the invidiousness and misogynist use of the medical-psychological term *compliance* (Hunt, Jordan, and Browner 1989); delegitimizing women's complaints, for example, chronic fatigue syndrome (Ware 1992); and women's knowledge of illness (Arksey 1994).

4. Social science research has not been completely free of the problem of assuming knowledge about women's health from male experiences, as evidenced in two areas, homelessness and AIDS. Although an early study (Garrett and Bahr 1976) detailed differences between homeless men and women, for some time the assumption remained that homeless men and women were similar. One study found that homeless single women, homeless women with children, and single men differ significantly on a number of variables, including histories of mental illness and going without food (Burt and Cohen 1989). Other research has documented gender differences and health symptoms among the homeless (Gove et al. 1993; Ritchey, LaGory, and Mullis 1991), the needs of single homeless mothers (Bassuk 1993a, 1993b), and mental health issues among homeless women (Buckner, Bassuk, and Zima 1993). Nursing research has also begun to address these differences (Nyamathi 1991; Nyamathi and Flaskerud 1992). An AIDS outreach program oriented to poor women of color at risk for HIV infection utilized participant observation and ethnography to recognize complex differences between men and women in exposure to AIDS and to assess women's culture for more effective outreach (Romero 1993).

5. At the level of government, a series of national task forces (Moore 1980; U.S. Public Health Service 1985, 1987, 1991) directed attention to women's health issues. Parallel efforts were also occurring internationally. Here, the agenda was to get women's health issues into the health policy arena where the emphasis on generality clearly overshadowed specificity.

6. The first Public Health Task Force on Women's Health noted that care should be taken to consider the needs of minorities, the handicapped, and other disadvantaged groups (Moore 1980), and the first text on women and the health care system (Marieskind 1980) highlighted attention to the health needs of minority groups. In 1986, Dr. Jane S. Lin-Fu specifically addressed the special health concerns of ethnic minority women, noting both shared and specific disadvantages and problems.

7. When the editors of this book conducted three summer international faculty development institutes (1984–86) on women, health, and healing, research findings on diverse women's health had advanced enough (although not far enough, as this volume makes clear) that it was possible for the institute's curriculum to cover a wide spectrum of groups. Working in the era before computer-assisted searches were as easy as they are now (for some people), the institutes generated a much-needed bibliography on the health of minority women in the United States (Ruzek et al. 1986). The

Center for Research on Black and Southern Women at the University of Memphis has also published bibliographies on black women's health.

8. Notable in this regard were the 1992 and 1994 conferences at the University of Illinois at Chicago on reframing women's health (1994), the 1983 Spelman conference on black women's health (Christmas 1984), ongoing conferences at the University of Washington's Center for Women's Health Research, and policy-oriented meetings at the Institute for Women's Policy Research in Washington. This tradition carried forward with the 1995 colloquium at the University of California, San Francisco, "Re/Visioning Women, Health, and Healing," which brought together feminist, cultural, and technosciences studies perspectives (Clarke and Olesen 1997).

9. The clinical application of nursing research pays special attention to everyday concerns. Instead of labeling women with a negative diagnosis (e.g., hypochondriacal), nurses seriously explore the meaning of complaints and symptoms. In the nursing process, the woman's thoughts, feelings, symptom experiences, and sociocultural environment provide the basis for diagnosis, therapy, and clinical outcomes. The nurse places the woman (a whole human being) in her lived environment rather than viewing the woman as a collection of component parts who is isolated from the social and cultural environment (McBride 1986).

10. Most studies during this seven-year review (1980–86) were correlational in design, with five experimental or quasi-experimental study designs. Studies related to women, health, and nursing practice during the 1980s addressed attitudinal correlates of health promotion or risk screening behaviors (such as performance of breast self-examination, weight management behaviors, correlates of exercise performance, images of health, health beliefs, roles, coping, and social support), which was a distinct shift in emphasis from earlier research focused on maternal roles.

11. Also important in the developing research on diversity was the establishment in 1989 of the *Journal of Transcultural Nursing*, which has provided a forum for reports on cultural diversity in human health and illness. Transcultural nursing research began in the 1950s, but it accelerated in scope in the 1970s to become a major theme in nursing research on diversity.

12. One of the unrecognized yet valuable types of nursing research is the report found in the clinical literature. Though not reported as case studies, which are in the style of medical journals, clinical reports nevertheless contain rich details about health care for diverse women.

13. Of the 1993 studies on diversity, one-third were descriptive or exploratory, one used case study, three were epidemiological or correlational, one relied on phenomenological analysis, one incorporated structural equation analysis, and one used experimental design to test therapeutic treatments. Of the 1994–95 studies, seven used epidemiological, phenomenological, experimental, or causal modeling designs; the remainder were descriptive.

14. Though a full discussion of the problematics of science is beyond the scope of this chapter, it is nevertheless useful to note briefly that human sciences, both qualitative and quantitative, which emphasize what people say about their health or illness, rank far below physics or biochemistry, which rely on "objective" instrumentation, in the scientific status hierarchy that influences funding. Whether in the social

sciences, public health, or nursing, social science researchers thus enter a problematic research situation. Feminists critical of this situation fault traditional sciences for excluding modes of conceptualization important to people in their own words.

15. As Narrigan and her colleagues argue in chapter 21, current epidemiological research certainly does not reflect what it ought to reflect in our understanding of general disease processes, particularly social aspects of disease, because much of the existing literature gives us a very gender-distorted view of disease processes. Phenomena studied in men are generalized to women without any empirical evidence. Differences among men or among women are still largely ignored unless these differences were created as part of an experiment. For example, a research report might state those women taking hormone A had this outcome, but those who did not had another outcome. The range of variation within groups typically goes unreported, too.

16. Aronson (1984) sees some parts of this as making political claims—part of the marketing that needs to be done to secure funding, an important issue as science must be sold to be done (Nelkin 1987). Politically, scientists of various sorts compose different interest groups in competition for funding. Similar structural conditions prevail in qualitative research. (For other gender issues in quantitative research see especially Rosser 1988; Oakley 1990.)

17. This review is based on extensive searches of various bibliographic resources (Socio-File, Index to Nursing Literature, Med-Line) and the authors' own knowledge of research trends. Reports were selected to illustrate some attention to diversity. It is not possible to say whether or not these inquiries are "representative" of work done in the 1980s and 1990s, because the decisions made by creators of bibliographies may not include all work on women's health in journals not included in the index, and certain vagaries of indexing sometimes obscure relevant references. However, it was clear that what is discussed here is but a small portion of research on women's health, thus underscoring the core point of this volume that much more attention to diversity in women's health research is necessary.

18. Two major research centers on women's health issues are the Institute for Women's Health at the University of Illinois at Chicago, founded by Alice Dan, which offers postgraduate research training, and the Center for Women's Health Research, the first such NIH-funded center, at the University of Washington School of Nursing. The Washington center was started by Nancy Woods, Joan Shaver, Margaret Heitkemper, Ellen Mitchell, and Martha Lentz. At the University of California, San Francisco, two doctoral programs, one in sociology and the other in nursing, offer graduate research training with emphases on women, health, and healing.

19. Both cultural and feminist principles shaped the methods. After they were unable to contact women by mail, organizations personally contacted women they knew. Women wanted to be invited and to be assured they would be taken seriously. Recognizing many women's responsibilities that limit participation, the committee offered stipends, transportation reimbursement, child care, meals, and language translation. Committee members were paired with culturally similar cofacilitators (and/or interpreters). For example, a cancer survivor led the women living with cancer group. Participants later said this combination made for informed, sensitive, and supportive leadership.

20. A subgroup of the Women's Health Advisory Committee read, cheered, and

cried over all tape transcripts. Data synthesis categorized participants' voices and visions. Two-thirds of the committee members were able to contact participants to discuss participants' responses to the conceptual themes summarized from the text analysis, thus marking a convergence of methodology, cultural awareness, and community participation. The whole committee heard the combined voices of all 250 women from the nineteen focus groups, yielding a mechanism for discussion of barriers to women's health and to the committee's own functioning.

21. This nebulous concept of system included the training, education, and regulation of health care providers; insurance and the legal system; hospitals and health clinics; and traditional versus emergent thoughts regarding disease, health, and specialization.

22. To begin this project, another focus group project with diverse women's health providers and health advocates is planned. In an interesting example of how diversity-oriented research can change the researchers, the Women's Health Advisory Committee has tried to integrate focus group recommendations into the committee's internal functioning. New processes for working together provide a forum for considering and resolving conflicts within the committee related to diversities of race, class, and age.

REFERENCES

Abramson, Rachel
    1992   "Cultural sensitivity in the promotion of breast-feeding." NAACOG Clinical Issues in Perinatal and Women's Health Nursing 3:717–22.
Ahijevych, Karen, and Linda Bernhard
    1994   "Health-promoting behaviors of African American women." Nursing Research 43:86–89.
Andreski, Patricia, and Naomi Breslau
    1995   "Maternal smoking among blacks and whites." Social Science and Medicine 41:227–34.
Apple, Rima, ed.
    1990   Women and Health in America: Historical Essays. Columbus: Ohio State University Press.
Arksey, Hillary
    1994   "Expert and lay participation in the construction of medical knowledge." Sociology of Health and Illness 16:448–68.
Armitage, K. J., S. Schneiderman, and R. Bass
    1979   "Response of physicians to medical complaints in men and women." Journal of the American Medical Association 241:2186–87.
Aronson, Naomi
    1984   "Science as a claims-making activity: implications for social problems research." Pp. 1–30 in Joseph W. Schneider and John I. Kitsuse (eds.), Studies in the Sociology of Social Problems. Norwood, NJ: Ablex.
Baca Zinn, Maxine
    1989   "Family, race, and poverty in the eighties." Signs 14:35–50.

Bair, Barbara, and Susan E. Cayleff, eds.
 1993   Wings of Gauze: Women of Color and the Experience of Health and Illness. Detroit: Wayne State University Press.

Barbee, Evelyn
 1992   "Dimensions of depression in African American women." Paper presented at the Midwest Nursing Research Society meeting, Chicago.

Bassuk, Ellen L.
 1993a   "Homeless women—economic and social issues: introduction." American Journal of Orthopsychiatry 63:337-39.
 1993b   "Social and economic hardships of homeless and other poor women." American Journal of Orthopsychiatry 63:340-47.

Bell, Roxanne
 1994   "Prominency of women in Navajo healing beliefs and values." Nursing and Health Care 15:232-40.

Bell, Susan E.
 1988   "Becoming a political woman: The reconstruction and interpretation of experience through stories." Pp. 97-123 in A. D. Todd and S. Fisher (eds.), Gender and Discourse: The Power of Talk. Norwood, NJ: Ablex.

Benner, Patricia
 1994   "The tradition and skill of interpretive phenomenology in studying health, illness, and caring practices." Pp. 99-128 in Patricia Benner (ed.), Interpretive Phenomenology: Embodiment, Caring, and Ethics. Thousand Oaks, CA: Sage.

Boskin-Ludehl, Marlene
 1976   "Cinderella's step-sisters: a feminist perspective on anorexia nervosa and bulimia." Signs 2:342-56.

Brown, Diane Robinson, and Lawrence E. Gary
 1988   "Unemployment and psychological distress among black American women." Sociological Focus 21:209-21.

Brown, Linda W., and Roma Williams
 1994   "Culturally sensitive breast cancer screening programs for older black women." Nurse Practitioner 19:21-31.

Browne, Susan E., Debra Connors, and Nanci Stern, eds.
 1985   With the Power of Each Breath: A Disabled Women's Anthology. San Francisco: Cleis Press.

Buckner, John C., Ellen Bassuk, and Bonnie T. Zima
 1993   "Mental health issues affecting homeless women: implications for intervention." American Journal of Orthopsychiatry 63:385-99.

Burt, Martha R., and Barbara E. Cohen
 1989   "Differences among homeless single women, women with children, and single men." Social Problems 36:508-24.

Calvillo, Evelyn R., and Jacquelyn H. Flaskerud.
 1993   "Evaluation of the pain response by Mexican American and Anglo-American women and their nurses." Journal of Advanced Nursing 18:451-549.

Carlton-LaNey, Iris
    1992   "Elderly black farm women: a population at risk." Social Work 37:517-23.
Caroline, Harlene A., and Linda A. Bernhard
    1994   "Health care dilemmas for women with serious mental illness." Advances
            in Nursing Science 16:78-88.
Christmas, June J.
    1984   "Black women and health care in the '80s." Spelman Messenger 100:8-11.
Clarke, Adele E., and Virginia L. Olesen, eds.
    1997   Revisioning Women, Health, and Healing. New York: Routledge.
Dan, Alice J., ed.
    1994   Reframing Women's Health: Multidisciplinary Research and Practice.
            Newbury Park, CA: Sage.
Davis, Angela Y.
    1981   Women, Race, and Class. New York: Random House.
DeSantis, Lydia, and Janice Thomas
    1990   "The immigrant Haitian mother: a transcultural nursing perspective on
            preventive health care for children." Journal of Transcultural Nursing
            2:2-15.
Dill, Bonnie Thornton
    1988   "Our mothers' grief: racial ethnic women and the maintenance of fami-
            lies." Journal of Family History 13:415-31.
Drevdahl, Denise
    1993   "Images of health: perceptions of urban American-Indian women." Pp.
            122-29 in Barbara Bair and Susan E. Cayleff (eds.), Wings of Gauze.
            Detroit: Wayne State University Press.
Dunbar, Doris, E. Patterson, C. Burton, and G. Stuckert
    1981   "Women's health and nursing research." Advances in Nursing Science
            3:1-10.
Edwards, Rosalind
    1990   "Connecting method and epistemology: a white woman interviewing
            black women." Women's Studies International Forum 13:477-90.
Faller, Helen S.
    1992   "Hmong women: characteristics and birth outcomes." Birth 19:144-48.
Ferraro, Kenneth F.
    1993   "Are older black adults health-pessimistic?" Journal of Health and Social
            Behavior 34:201-14.
Fisher, Sue
    1995   Nursing Wounds: Nurse Practitioners/Doctors/Women Patients and the
            Negotiation of Meaning. New Brunswick, NJ: Rutgers University Press.
Flaskerud, Jacqueline H., and Adeline Nyamathi
    1989   "Black and Latina women's AIDS-related knowledge, attitudes, and prac-
            tices." Research in Nursing and Health 12:339-46.
Flaskerud, Jacqueline H., and C. E. Rush
    1989   "AIDS and traditional health beliefs and practices of black women."
            Nursing Research 38:210-15.

Franks, Ferne, and Sandra A. Faux
  1990   "Depression, stress, mastery, and social resources in four ethnocultural women's groups." Research in Nursing and Health 13:283-92.
Frye, Barbara A.
  1991   "Cultural themes in health care decision making among Cambodian refugee women." Journal of Community Health Nursing 8:33-44.
Frye, Barbara A., and Carolyn D. D'Avanzo
  1994   "Cultural themes in family stress and violence among Cambodian refugee women in the inner city." Advances in Nursing Science 16:64-77.
Fullilove, Mindy T., Robert E. Fullilove, Katherine Haynes, and Shirley Gross
  1990   "Black women and AIDS prevention: a view towards understanding the gender rules." Journal of Sex Research 27:47-64.
Garrett, Gerald R., and Howard M. Bahr
  1976   "The family backgrounds of Skid Row women." Signs 2:369-81.
Goforth-Parker, Judy
  1994   "The lived experience of Native Americans with diabetes with a transcultural nursing perspective." Journal of Transcultural Nursing 6:5-11.
Gove, Walter R., Ferris J. Ritchey, Mark LaGory, and Jeffrey Mullis
  1993   "Higher rates of physical symptoms among homeless women do not appear to be due to reporting bias: a comment on Ritchey et al. (1991)." Journal of Health and Social Behavior 34:178-81.
Gregg, Jessica, and Robert H. Curry
  1994   "Explanatory models for cancer among African American women at two Atlanta neighborhood health centers: the implications for a cancer screening program." Social Science and Medicine 39:519-26.
Griffin, F. N.
  1994   "The health care system: factoring in the ethnicity, cultural, and health care needs of women and children of color." Association for Black Nursing Faculty Journal 5:130-33.
Harris, Sharrette M.
  1994   "Racial differences in predictors of college women's body image attitudes." Women and Health 21:89-104.
Hill, Shirley
  1993   "Cognitive coping strategies among the mothers of children with sickle cell disease." Pp. 79-88 in Barbara Bair and Susan E. Cayleff (eds.), Wings of Gauze. Detroit: Wayne State University Press.
Hobus, Ruth
  1990   "Living in two worlds: a Lakota transcultural nursing experience." Journal of Transcultural Nursing 2:33-36.
hooks, bell
  1984   From Margin to Center. Boston: South End Press.
Hunt, Linda M., Brigitte Jordan, and Carole Browner
  1989   "Compliance and the patient's perspective: controlling symptoms in everyday life." Culture, Medicine, and Psychiatry 13:315-34.

Hunt, Linda M., Brigitte Jordan, and Susan Irwin
   1989   "Views of what's wrong: diagnosis and patients' concepts of illness." So-
           cial Science and Medicine 28:945-56.
Huttlinger, Kathleen W., and Dennis Tanner
   1994   "The peyote way: implications for culture care theory." Journal of Trans-
           cultural Nursing 5:5-11.
Jackson, Eileen M.
   1993   "Whiting out the difference: why U.S. nursing research fails black fami-
           lies." Medical Anthropology Quarterly (n.s.) 7:363-85.
Jordan, Brigitte
   1977   "Self-diagnosis of early pregnancy: an analysis of lay competence." Med-
           ical Anthropology 2:14-30.
Kauffman, Karen S.
   1994   "The insider/outsider dilemma: field experience of a white researcher
           'getting in' a poor black community." Nursing Research 43:179-83.
Kelley, Michele A., Janet D. Perloff, Naomi M. Morris, and Wang-yue Liu
   1992   "The role of perceived barriers in the use of a comprehensive prenatal
           care program." Journal of Health and Social Policy 3:81-89.
Krieger, Nancy, and Elizabeth Fee
   1994   "Man-made medicine and women's health: the biopolitics of sex/gender
           and race/ethnicity." International Journal of Health Services 24:265-83.
Lauver, Diane
   1994   "Care-seeking behavior with breast cancer symptoms in Caucasian and
           African American women." Research in Nursing and Health 17:421-31.
Leavitt, Judith Walzer, ed.
   1984   Women and Health in America. Madison: University of Wisconsin Press.
Lennane, K. J., and Lennane, R. J.
   1973   "Alleged psychogenic disorders in women—a possible manifestation of
           sexual prejudice." New England Journal of Medicine 288:288-92.
Lipson, Juliene, and Sue Ellen Miller
   1994   "Changing roles of Afghan refugee women in the United States." Health
           Care for Women International 15:171-80.
Manzanado, Hector Garcia, Esperanza Garcia Walters, and Kate Lorig
   1980   "Health and illness perceptions of the Chicana." Pp. 191-207 in Marga-
           rita Melville (ed.), Twice a Minority: Mexican American Women. St.
           Louis: Mosby.
Marieskind, Helen
   1980   Women and the Health Care System. St. Louis: Mosby.
Marshall, Nancy L., and Rosalind C. Barnett
   1991   "Race, class, and multiple role strains and gains among women employed
           in the service sector." Women and Health 17:1-19.
Mathews, Holly F., Donald R. Lannin, and James P. Mitchell
   1994   "Coming to terms with advanced breast cancer: black women's narratives
           from eastern North Carolina." Social Science and Medicine 38:789-800.

Mays, Vickie M.
:   1987   "Acquired immune deficiency and black Americans: special considerations." Public Health Reports 10:224-31.
:   1988   "The interpretation of AIDS risk and AIDS risk reduction by black and
Hispanic women." American Psychologist 43:11.

McBride, Angela B.
:   1986   "Women's health: where nursing and feminism converge." Pp. 3-10 in J.
Griffith-Kenney (ed.), Contemporary Women's Health: A Nursing Advocacy Approach. Menlo Park, CA: Addison-Wesley.

Mitchell, Ellen S.
:   1990   "Multiple triangulation: a method for nursing science." Advances in
Nursing Science 8:18-26.

Moore, Emily, ed.
:   1980   Women and Health, United States, 1980. Supplement to Public Health
Reports, Sept.-Oct. Washington: Public Health Service.

Muecke, Marjorie
:   1983   "In search of healers: Southeast Asian refugees in the American health
care system." Western Journal of Medicine, special issue: Cross-cultural
Medicine 139:31-36.

Nelkin, Dorothy
:   1987   Selling Science: How the Press Covers Science and Technology. New
York: Freeman.

Nelson, Margaret K.
:   1983   "Birth and social class." Social Problems 30:284-97.

Nelson, Martha A.
:   1994   "Economic impoverishment as a health risk: methodological and conceptual issues." Advances in Nursing Science 16:1-12.
:   1995   "Health practices and risk-related behaviors among low-income working
women: nursing assistants employed in long-term care agencies." Ph.D.
diss., School of Nursing, University of California, San Francisco.

Nickens, Herbert W.
:   1993   "Minority health research issues." Science, Technology, and Human Values 189:506-10.

Nyamathi, Adeline M.
:   1991   "Relationship of resources to emotional distress, somatic complaints and
high-risk behaviors in drug recovering and homeless minority women."
Research in Nursing and Health 14:269-77.
:   1993   "Outcomes of specialized and traditional AIDS counseling programs for
impoverished women of color." Research in Nursing and Health 16:11-21.

Nyamathi, Adeline M., and Jacqueline H. Flaskerud.
:   1992   "A community-based inventory of current concerns of impoverished
homeless and drug addicted minority women." Research in Nursing and
Health 15:121-29.

Nyamathi, Adeline M., and Rose Vasquez
:   1989   "Impact of poverty, homelessness, and drugs on Hispanic women at risk
for HIV infection." Hispanic Journal of Behavioral Sciences 11:299-314.

Oakley, Ann
    1990   "Who's afraid of the randomized controlled trial? Some dilemmas of the
            scientific method and 'good' research practice." Pp. 167-94 in Helen
            Roberts (ed.), Women's Health Counts. London: Routledge.
Oakley, L. D.
    1986   "Marital status, gender role attitude, and black women's report of depres-
            sion." Journal of the National Black Nurses Association 1:41-51.
O'Connell, Mary Lee
    1993   "Childbirth education classes in homeless shelters." AWHONN Clinical
            Issues in Perinatal and Women's Health Nursing 4:102-11.
Olesen, Virginia
    1976   "Rage is not enough: scholarly feminism and research in women's health."
            Pp. 1-2 in Virginia Olesen (ed.), Women and Their Health: Research
            Implications for a New Era. Washington: National Center for Health Ser-
            vices Research, Research Proceedings Series, U.S. Department of Health,
            Education, and Welfare.
    1994   "Feminisms and models of qualitative research." Pp. 158-74 in Norman
            K. Denzin and Yvonna S. Lincoln (eds.), Handbook of Qualitative Re-
            search. Newbury Park, CA: Sage.
Paget, Marianne
    1988   The Unity of Mistakes: A Phenomenological Interpretation of Medical
            Work. Philadelphia: Temple University Press.
Pender, Nola J.
    1987   Health Promotion in Nursing Practice. Norwalk, CT: Appleton, Century,
            Crofts.
Phillips, Suzanne, and Sandra Lobar
    1990   "Literature summary of some Navajo child health beliefs and rearing
            practices within a transcultural nursing framework." Journal of Trans-
            cultural Nursing 1:13-20.
Reinharz, Shulamit
    1992   Feminist Methods in Social Research. Oxford: Oxford University Press.
Riessman, Catherine K.
    1987   "When gender is not enough: women interviewing women." Gender and
            Society 1:172-207.
    1990   "Strategic uses of narrative in the presentation of self and illness." Social
            Science and Medicine 30:1195-1200.
Ritchey, Ferris J., Mark LaGory, and Jeffrey Mullis
    1991   "Gender differences in health risks and physical symptoms among the
            homeless." Journal of Health and Social Behavior 32:33-48.
Romero, Gloria J., Lourdes Arguelles, and Anne M. Rivero
    1993   "Latinas and HIV infection/AIDS: reflection on impacts, dilemmas, and
            struggles." Pp. 340-52 in Barbara Bair and Susan E. Cayleff (eds.), Wings
            of Gauze. Detroit: Wayne State University Press.
Romero, Mary
    1993   "Women's culture in AIDs outreach." Pp. 353-63 in Barbara Bair and
            Susan E. Cayleff (eds.), Wings of Gauze. Detroit: Wayne State Univer-
            sity Press.

Rosser, Sue, ed.
   1988   Feminism within the Science and Health Care Professions: Overcoming Resistance. New York: Pergamon Press.
Ruzek, Sheryl, Patricia Anderson, Adele Clarke, Virginia Olesen, and Kristin Hill
   1986   Minority Women, Health, and Healing in the United States: Selected Bibliography and Resources. San Francisco: Women, Health, and Healing Program, Department of Social and Behavioral Sciences, School of Nursing, University of California.
Saint-Germain, Michelle, and Alice Longman
   1993   "Resignation and resourcefulness: older Hispanic women's responses to breast cancer." Pp. 257–72 in Barbara Bair and Susan E. Cayleff (eds.), Wings of Gauze: Women of Color and the Experience of Health and Illness. Detroit: Wayne State University Press.
Sanders-Phillips, Kathy
   1994   "Health promotion behavior in low-income black and Latino women." Women and Health 21:71–84.
Schur, Claudia L., Amy B. Bernstein, and Marc L. Berk
   1987   "The importance of distinguishing Hispanic subpopulations in the issue of medical care." Medical Care 25:627–41.
Segura, Denise
   1991   "Ambivalence or continuity? Motherhood and employment among Chicanas and Mexican immigrant women workers." Azatlan 20:119–50.
Shaver, Joan
   1985   "A biopsychosocial view of health." Nursing Outlook 33:186–91.
Steen, Melva
   1991   "Historical perspectives on women and mental illness and prevention of depression in women, using a feminist framework." Issues in Mental Health Nursing 12:359–74.
Stein, Judith A., Sarah A. Fox, and Paul J. Murata
   1991   "The influence of ethnicity, socioeconomic status, and psychological barriers on use of mammography." Journal of Health and Social Behavior 32:101–13.
Stevens, Patricia E., and Joanne H. Hall
   1991   "A critical historical analysis of the medical construction of lesbianism." International Journal of Health Services 21:271–307.
Stevens, Patricia E., Joanne Hall, and Afaf I. Meleis
   1992a   "Examining vulnerability of women clerical workers from five ethnic/racial groups." Western Journal of Nursing Research 14:754–74.
   1992b   "Narratives as a basis for culturally relevant holistic care: ethnicity and everyday experiences of women clerical workers." Holistic Nursing Practice 6:49–58.
Suarez, Lucina
   1994   "Pap smear and mammogram screening in Mexican American women: the effects of acculturation." American Journal of Public Health 84:742–46.

Taylor, Diana
  1990   "Time-series analysis: use of autocorrelation as an analytic strategy for describing pattern and change." Western Journal of Nursing Research 12:254–61.
  1991   "Perimenstrual symptoms: an explanatory model." Pp. 103–18 in Diana Taylor and Nancy Woods (eds.), Menstruation, Health, and Illness: Neuroendocrine, Sociocultural, and Clinical Perspectives. Washington: Hemisphere.

Taylor, Diana, and Katherine Dower
  1995   "Toward a women-centered health care system: women's experiences, women's voices, women's needs." Health Care for Women International, in press.

Tomes, E. K., A. Brown, K. Semenya, and J. Simpson
  1990   "Depression in black women of low socioeconomic status: psychological factors and nursing diagnosis." Journal of the National Black Nurses Association 5:37–46.

Torres, Sara
  1993   "Nursing care of low-income battered Hispanic pregnant women." AWHONN Clinical Issues in Perinatal and Women's Health Nursing 4:416–23.

Trippet, S. E., and J. Bain
  1992   "Reasons American lesbians fail to seek traditional health care." Health Care for Women International 13:145–53.

Turner, Castellano B., and William A. Darity
  1987   "Education and family planning among black American women." Inter-
  –88   national Quarterly of Community Health Education 8:117–27.

U.S. Public Health Service
  1985   Women's Health: Report of the Public Health Service Task Force on Women's Health Issues. DHHS Pub. No. (PHS) 85-50206. May. Washington: Government Printing Office.
  1987   Women's Health. Proceedings of the National Conference on Women's Health, 17–18 June 1986, sponsored by Food and Drug Administration and Public Health Service Coordinate Committee on Women's Health Issues. Public Health Reports to the July–August issue.
  1991   Action Plan for Women's Health. Office of Women's Health. DHHS Pub. No. (PHS) 91-50214 (Sept.).

Walcott-McQuigg, Janet A.
  1994   "Worksite stress: gender and cultural diversity issues." American Association of Occupational Health Nursing Journal 42:528–33.

Ware, Norma C.
  1992   "Suffering and the social construction of illness: the delegitimation of illness experience with chronic fatigue syndrome." Medical Anthropology Quarterly (new series) 6:347–61.

Warren, Barbara Jones
  1994   "Depression in African American women." Journal of Psychosocial Nursing 32:29–33.
White, Evelyn
  1990   The Black Women's Health Book: Speaking for Ourselves. Seattle: Seal Press.
White, J. H.
  1991   "Feminism, eating, and mental health." Advances in Nursing Science 13:68–80.
Williams, D. M.
  1989   "Political theory and individualistic health promotion." Advances in Nursing Science 12:14–25.
Women's Health Advisory Committee
  1994   "Restructuring health care delivery: woman-centered health services." San Francisco: San Francisco Department of Public Health.
Woods, Nancy F.
  1988   "Women's health." Vol. 6, pp. 210–36 in J. J. Fitzpatrick, R. L. Taunton, and J. Q. Benoliel (eds.), Annual Review of Nursing Research. New York: Springer.
Woods, Nancy F., Martha Lentz, Ellen Mitchell, and L. D. Oakley
  1994   "Depressed mood and self-esteem in young Asian, black, and white women in America." Health Care for Women International 15:243–62
Woods, Nancy F., Shirley Laffrey, Mary Duffy, Martha Lentz, Ellen Mitchell, Diana Taylor, and Kathy Cowan
  1988   "Being healthy: women's images." Advances in Nursing Science 11:36–46.
Wuest, Judith
  1991   "Harmonizing: a North American Indian approach to managing middle ear disease with transcultural nursing implications." Journal of Transcultural Nursing 3:5–14.
Ying, Yu-Wen
  1990   "Explanatory models of major depression and implications for help-seeking among immigrant Chinese-American women." Culture, Medicine, and Psychiatry 14:393–408.
Zambrana, Ruth E., ed.
  1982   Work, Family, and Health: Latina Women in Transition. Monograph No. 7. Bronx, NY: Fordham University Hispanic Research Center.
Zambrana, Ruth E., and Marilyn Aguirre-Molina
  1987   "Alcohol abuse prevention among Latino adolescents: a strategy for intervention." Journal of Youth and Adolescence 16(2):97–113.
Zambrana, Ruth E., Marta Hernandez, Christine Dunkel-Schetter, and Susan C. M. Scrimshaw
  1991   "Ethnic differences in the substance use patterns of low-income pregnant women." Family and Community Health 13:1–11.

[23]

Conversing with Diversity:
Implications for Social Research

SHERYL BURT RUZEK, VIRGINIA L. OLESEN,
AND ADELE E. CLARKE

Moving toward the future, both commonalities and diversities in women's health must be addressed. The idea of commonalities as fixed, bounded life experiences may need to be reconceptualized as similarities or resemblances to break out of unproductive ways of thinking that overlook important differences among women. Taking this perspective, the authors sketch out five broad research agendas that might provide valuable knowledge that could enhance women's health.

Widening Visions of Women's Health:
Complexities and Contradictions

The critical space that women's health now occupies in national arenas is not the same space that absorbed the three of us and many others when many women's health movements emerged twenty years ago. It is infinitely more complex, peopled with many more players, and characterized by often contradictory concerns that buffet and shift players and issues. As we consider the future of women's health, what are some of the research implications for the social and behavioral sciences that emerge out of our growing awareness of women's diversities? The themes and issues raised by contributors to this volume and others are multifaceted, and we make no attempt here to summarize them. Rather, our intent is to identify what appear to us, as feminist social scientists, to be some of the urgent research questions that arise from focusing on diversities. Replacing narrow, reductionist models of both mental and physical health with more complex ones entails altering current research agendas, favored methodologies, and perceptions of what is important to know about women's health. These research agendas have implications for clinical practice and policy.

In this volume, we and others have shown how both health and illness are socially and economically produced and experienced in very different ways by very different women. The ways in which women make a living in the paid or unpaid labor force, their racial or ethnic identity, age, sexual orientation, living conditions, and social and cultural heritages and involvements all interact. These intersections of social and economic statuses, culture, and roles critically influence health, including the experience of health and illness, in myriad ways.

In terms of future research, we need more intensive focus on the social processes involved in the production of health, not just the avoidance of diseases. That is, producing health must be not only valued but studied. We need more complex models to understand women's illnesses and diseases, how differences are played out in the experience of and response to serious disease. We now know how inaccurate generalizations about broad racial/ethnic groups' health behavior are likely to be, and we know that cultures and subcultures change, especially in and through immigration. Static models of culture can be insidious to women, especially in groups where women are directly attempting to change and improve their situations. Clinicians need training that prepares them to practice in ways that truly address the social and psychological needs of diverse patients.

The essays in this volume also emphasize the importance of people of color, women with particular health needs, and women who live in different cultural and geographic locations defining their own health agendas. They also raise questions about how to shape clinical services to fit particular sociocultural needs. Involving women of color organizations, disability rights groups, older women's health advocacy groups, and others in setting national research and service priorities will alter the directions in women's health. More diverse health providers, researchers, and policymakers will need to interact in new ways to address both the particular and common needs of all women.

New questions emerge around the social desirability of race/ethnic, age, and gender-specific services. Ann Metcalf's (chapter 11) analysis of "culture cultivating" interventions for Native American women raises an important policy issue: If genuinely culturally relevant and effective care will more likely emerge from ethnically distinct service providers than "mainstream" institutions or dominant group providers, what provisions can be made to foster the continued existence of community-based services that are targeted to specific racial/ethnic groups? Do some forms of ethnically/culturally targeted services offer advantages that benefit women? What are the opportunities for fostering culturally appropriate services for other groups? Can such models of care, developed by and for specific populations, be "mainstreamed" successfully? Finding ways to support innovative models of culturally relevant and sensitive care in larger institutions seems particularly pressing and different from current trends — promoting uniform practice guidelines and large, bureaucratic medical systems to deliver a "standardized level of care." Variations in the sociocultural conditions and subjective experiences of health care are becoming both politically and socially invisible. How can we meet diverse needs and widen access to care?

Larger transformations in the global economy affect the socioeconomic and cultural conditions of all women. At this time, no one can fully comprehend what effects these transformations will have on women's health in the United States and in other industrialized or less developed nations. Work becomes exceptionally unstable for most people, especially women. Single mothers are becoming more common globally, not just in the United States. Massive shifts in education and employment are inevitable. Linking medical care benefits to employment is risky indeed for women in such a labile economic situation. This specter of economic displacement also renews concern about what we see as an excessive focus on biomedical, rather than social, determinants of health. Unless women have jobs and homes, the existence of advanced medical technologies is hardly relevant to our health.

Other social transformations in the United States not addressed in this volume will have their own impact on women's health, including growing controversy over immigration, the visibility of lesbian and gay communities, emergent bisexual and transgender communities, the actions of the radical right to restrict access to abortion and sex education, and a growing split between "haves" and "have-nots." The wide range of issues linked to health makes it abundantly clear that generalizing about women is highly problematic. Indeed, assuming that all women have similar needs and interests in health and medical care confuses profound issues. Recognizing how diversities lead to different perceptions of what is important, a point we made in chapters 1 and 3, seems an understatement. When we actually grasp the concept of diversity, we realize the urgency of conceptualizing women's health in new ways "beyond diversity."

Yet we are facing contradictions. Although absolutely requisite, emphasizing diversities alone can lead to fragmented visions of women's health. Perceiving the issues as too complex or contradictory could discourage some from taking any social action on women's health or be used to justify the status quo. As feminist scholar Nancy Tuana (1993:281) asks, how "can we recognize the importance of the differences between women without losing sight of what we have in common?"

Searching for the Contours of Our Commonalities

To provide access to medical care for all women requires coming to some degree of social consensus about what "all women need," agreeing on some medically necessary services. The need to define what constitute medically necessary services will inevitably lead to policymakers adopting what they view as manageable definitions of women's common health and medical care needs. Depending on how medically necessary services are conceptualized and by whom, this development could be positive or negative. Given the history of a priori judgments about women's "common needs," the task ahead will be arduous. Women from all walks of life must define medically necessary needs and make accommodations. Developing the ability to see diversity without losing sight of common ground is a pressing issue for women's health activists and policymakers. If we don't undertake these efforts, others will make policy "for our own good." This has not turned out well in the past (Ehrenreich and English 1979)!

National efforts to restructure the American health care system have already set in motion changes that affect women's health at the federal, state, and local levels. Asking what women have in common is urgent because new research agendas, service policies, and financing mechanisms will affect women in various life circumstances differently. Will an agenda for equity emerge to improve all women's health?

Analyzing health statistics for women within and between specific racial/ethnic groups and socioeconomic groups reveals widely divergent patterns of health and ill health. Such data can provide useful information for social planners who need to know how particular health conditions are distributed if they are to target preventive and therapeutic efforts. For scholars, these data raise new research questions about links between race/ethnicity, socioeconomic status, the cultural context of health practices, and the availability of health services (Krieger et al. 1993). However, it is not enough to describe patterns of morbidity and mortality or the misery of poor women seeking attention for their health; the conditions which brought them to that point must also be examined (Scott 1991). The common threads of what thrusts women into poor health, when identified along with differences, may be of paramount importance in preventing or treating health problems. In short, both the common and more particular pathways to health and illness need elucidation.

One approach that might facilitate identifying women's commonalities without losing sight of differences would be to carefully examine women's health experiences in specific realms to clarify the general and particular features of such experiences. Examples here could include health problems of office workers who use computers or women with chronic illnesses such as arthritis and lupus. In this endeavor, understanding how experiences or health conditions came about by virtue of social, economic, and historic factors seems particularly important. A growing body of scholarship on women's health makes such an enterprise feasible. Thus definitions of commonalities and clarifications of differences could be identified inductively from empirical observations of women's diverse, specific experiences. To do this, however, will require involving a broad range of scholars, policymakers, and clinicians in a search for new ways of conceptualizing "women's health." Such an approach seems more productive than relying on a deductive model that starts with the assumption that "since we are all women, we *must* share common concerns."

Inductive approaches require suspending expectations about the very nature of commonalities, including abstract theorizing about commonalities. In searching for what women share in common, Nancy Tuana (1993:283) suggests: "It is more realistic to expect pluralities of experiences that are related through various intersections or resemblances of some of the experiences of some women to some of the experiences of others. In other words, we are less likely to find a common core of shared experiences that are immune to economic conditions, cultural imperatives, etc., than a family of resemblances within a continuum of similarities, which allows for significant differences between the experiences." If our commonalities can be defined more accurately as similarities or resemblances than as fixed, fully bounded shared life experiences, health problems, or health needs, how will this conceptualization be used productively in policymaking arenas? What lobbying strategies will facilitate public policymaking that recognizes group *and* individual differences?

We ourselves, along with many others in women's health, are struggling with how to conceptualize commonalities and common needs. It is far easier to declare that all women need health services that are affordable and accessible than to define what this actually means or to agree on priorities for spending resources. The recent health care reform debates demonstrated how easily the fragile consensus on the need to make medical care universally available can give way to particularistic priorities. What is seen as essential by some women is seen as trivial, excessive, or unimportant by others. Dziech (1993) argues that debates over the nature of commonalities or common differences indicate the success of feminists in recognizing and bringing issues of difference to the fore and allowing various groups to explore and explain them in their own ways. But explaining and exploring does not make social policy, though it is a requisite first step.

Coming to terms with "what's important" at the national level necessarily entails making choices. It requires setting priorities for investing finite resources in improving social factors that promote health (such as education, housing, and economic development), and/or investing in research and biomedical services that more often focus on curing than preventing health problems. If women do not step forward and attempt to define at least the contours of our commonalities, their broad resemblances and similarities of social as well as biomedical health needs, who will do it for us? How will women's health be constructed and represented by decision makers in Congress and by the medical insurance, biotechnology, and medical industries? Whose voices will define what constitutes women's health?

Increased awareness of diversity is likely to make decision making and social action more, not less, difficult. We must accept that in many situations, particularly in policy arenas, more time and resources must be allocated to consider carefully the interests and needs of potential users of services. Moreover, even with good intentions to meet the needs of all, some degrees of dissatisfaction are inevitable. It is not possible to act in ways that please everyone all the time. That is, in seeking to improve women's health, it is essential to recognize that there are indeed dilemmas, conflicts, and contradictions. In all likelihood there will be conflicts of *interest* among women. Sisterhood is powerful, but so are race, class, age, sexual orientation, physical and mental (dis)abilities, religious affiliation, and regional attachments. These and other social characteristics and alliances will inevitably come into play, pitting some women against others in profound ways. What values will guide how women wield power in these conflicts?

Given the inevitability of compromise, how will women forge compromises that reflect both their understandings of the diversity of women's health needs and the pragmatic politics of social action? How can dilemmas be resolved in new ways that move beyond the impasses generated by conventional interest group politics? Can women transcend some interest group allegiances under some circumstances, and if so, under what conditions and for what reasons? How can health be transformed into something more than a commodity to be designed, marketed, and sold to the highest bidder? Are there moral and ethical principles that could assist in crafting strategies that would allow women to pursue shared, but more inclusive, goals?

A few examples of emerging conflicts portend the future. Health advocates who successfully lobbied for a broad array of maternity benefits for Medicaid recipients must confront the fact that most working women do not have medical benefit packages that are nearly so generous. In establishing a national comprehensive medical benefits package, women who are uninsured or poorly insured would certainly have improved access to medical care, but Medicaid clients might face reduced benefits. How can health advocates support wider access to medical care when it might require reductions in service to groups they have traditionally supported in policy arenas? Will they/we be willing to accept limitations on our own coverage in exchange for wider access for more vulnerable women?

Faced with overwhelming public demands and strong resistance from powerful interest groups, policymakers may find inaction easier and "safer" than action. If we allow a vacuum of leadership, powerful interest groups will define services that they want to provide as necessary—whether such services are beneficial to most or even some women. A challenge of this decade will be crafting definitions of what is "medically necessary" out of emerging concepts of effectiveness, cost-effectiveness, futility, and equity. This endeavor cannot be turned into a technocratic exercise. Moral and ethical precepts such as social justice and social good are sorely needed to move discussions of widening access to medical care in new directions.

Diverse Research Agendas for Women's Health

Biomedical agendas for improving women's health dominate national research funding arenas. Although biomedical interventions are often valued and valuable, biomedical research agendas focus primarily on basic science, treatment-oriented questions. Prevention is framed largely in terms of screening or early intervention. To us, these are *not adequate prevention* activities. Because secondary prevention is widely promoted as preventive health care, it is easy to lose sight of the need for "primary prevention," preventing disease from occurring at all. Some of us would argue that we are distracted from primary prevention because of the levels of social change necessary to genuinely promote health.

Broader social definitions of women's health need clearer articulation. To prevent disease, far more research is needed on the actual social conditions that promote or inhibit disease processes—ranging from individual behaviors to social and environmental conditions. This mandate to study the social production of health and of illness is not easy to realize either methodologically or fiscally. Despite widely shared criticisms of both quantitative and qualitative work, well-entrenched research modalities impede the development of new research questions and agendas. Scientific focus on women's biology must be understood in the social context of women's actual working and living conditions. Women's biology, not women's social experience, is widely viewed as the basis for women's commonality. We urge the extensive and innovative exploration of the domain of women's health in all its diversity precisely to foreclose the narrowing consequences of such research modalities (Olesen and Lewin 1985:19). As part of that endeavor we challenge critical aspects of that domain, namely, the structure, organization, and funding of science and technology development both nationally and internationally. We also challenge the propriety of allocating vast financial resources to developing treatments and technologies that will be available only to the few, especially when these developments are funded by public monies. There needs to be much broader participation—democratization—in the setting of research agendas of all kinds.

This book has provided an overview of diverse women's knowledge and perspectives on health issues that are situated within their particular life circumstances. Much of this knowledge is still embryonic. For example, we need more fully articulated framing of the varied situations and understandings of health of women of color and rural women, of their families and communities in the United States, of different classes, ethnic traditions, ages, and life situations. Such research needs to move beyond the view that morbidity and mortality rates per se tell us what we need to know about women's health. More complete understanding of the realities of health-promoting and health-damaging life conditions, not just health statistics, are needed to make better decisions about how and where health resources need to be spent to improve the health of all women. In short, we need to rethink what we define as important to research about women and women's health. Persons whom health policies are intended to "help" must have a central voice in articulating what directions research should take. New strategies for policymaking and priority setting need to emerge to ensure that health systems do not silence voices only now being heard or misconstrue their perspectives.

Defining what is worthy of scientific investigation is a social and political act, not a neutral value-free position. The Women's Health Initiative, initiated in 1991 in the NIH, reflects a biomedical conceptualization of health that is widely promoted simply as *the* national women's health agenda. In our view, far more attention needs to be directed at understanding the politics and social construction of women's health research agendas. Biomedical research always runs the risk of further medicalizing women and women's bodies, which can constrain us unnecessarily (Riessman 1983).

Women's health research agendas are being promoted by groups with diverse interests. Advocacy groups increasingly seek to influence research agendas through priority-setting mechanisms and public pressure campaigns. For example, the National Breast Cancer Coalition has emerged as a powerful lobby for cancer research. Other agendas focus on particular populations. The Older Women's League has long sought to increase spending on health services research that affects older women. Zambrana (1987) has proposed a research agenda on issues that are particularly salient for poor and minority women. Black women, who constitute the largest and most organizationally networked group among women of color in the United States, seek to establish their own research agendas and priorities (Rodgers-Rose 1994). Lesbians are actively seeking to address the focus and direction of research on their health (Stevens 1992). The feminist disability rights community has sought to influence the amount and content of research particularly salient to women with disabilities. Gill's (1994) articulation of disabled women's research needs at the NIH reflects the centrality of research priority setting for previously silent groups.

These developments suggest that wider publics perceive what feminist scholars have argued, that science reflects gender, race, and class bias and has too many consequences for women to be left to scientists alone (Bleier 1984; Harding 1986; Hubbard 1990; Rosser 1988). Additionally and painfully, no single research agenda is likely to address the multiplicity of interests women have in research enterprises. As feminist social scientists, we see the need for creative approaches to research of various kinds that utilize the best of varying styles and methods in the social and behavioral sciences and the humanities (Olesen 1994; Reinharz 1992).

To elaborate, we believe that certain issues raised recently by feminist scholars are fundamental to emerging social and cultural research agendas in the applied as well as traditional social and behavioral health sciences. Donna Haraway's provocative formulation (1991) of all knowledge as situated, context-dependent, historical, and cultural provides a strong starting point. We do not yet have an adequate array of what Haraway terms "situated knowledges" about diverse women's health experiences and beliefs. Many groups we can merely name (e.g., multiracial or transgendered women) have not yet articulated their health experiences and thus cannot be represented even at a token level. We simply do not know what additional "groups" might emerge if the concept of "situated knowledges" is legitimated, encouraged, and supported—if research on them is even funded.

Directions for Social Research

In our view, the narrow biomedical focus that is widely viewed as the singular women's health research agenda is both limited and limiting. Understanding the breadth and varieties of other emerging women's health research agendas puts biomedical research agendas into a larger social context. Social research agendas themselves are varied, reflecting both disciplinary and cross-disciplinary efforts. As feminist social scientists we would hope to see future research that includes the perspectives and situations of diverse women in the following areas:

1. women's actual experiences of health and illness, including what women want and don't want;
2. new epidemiologies of women's health;
3. culturally and sociodemographically specific studies of clinical efficacy of all major treatment interventions used on women;
4. women's experiences of access to and actual use of a broad array of health services; and
5. recruitment, training, certification, and practice patterns of women as health care providers.

Each of these types of research, discussed below, require the skills and training of scholars from many different disciplines who grasp the intersections of sex/gender, race/ethnicity and class, and other salient characteristics and identities of differently situated women.

1. *Women's experiences of health and illness* might include historically and economically grounded sociocultural and sociobehavioral research on diverse women's health understandings, situations, and self-perceived needs. The focus of this research might include investigation of how women in different life situations socially construct health, disease, and health-related issues in their own terms, drawing out culturally relevant concepts. It would also entail study of the lived experiences and immediate social and economic contexts of women's lives—the frames in which women can and do or cannot and do not seek extant health care services.

This in turn requires investigation of women's own constructions of their health care needs and goals that are grounded in their actual contexts of care. Shirley Hill's (1994) work on how African American mothers cope with their children's sickle cell disease and make reproductive decisions for themselves is a good example of this kind of qualitative research. In short, to answer the question "What do women want?" we must begin by asking women—in the full diversities of their lived situations. For it is only through understanding women's own perceptions of their health and health caring experiences that socially and culturally acceptable and effective interventions can be developed.

To learn what women want necessarily requires also studying what women in specific life situations do *not* want. That is, researchers need to discover what experiences with health care are perceived as poor, bad, or demeaning and what actions are experienced as coercive. Cheri Pies's study of Norplant is a good example of user-focused research that allows women to articulate their own perspectives on issues that affect them profoundly. Too often, research on controversial or socially contested issues such as Norplant remains at the biomedical level or focuses only on easily quantifiable measures such as "discontinuation rates." Although such indicators of dissatisfaction with medical technologies are easily produced, they tell us little about women's actual experiences or feelings about their health or medical care.

We need more research on how women perceive themselves as being blocked from participation in health care decision making, both formal and informal. Research that evokes women's own full and rich stories— their narrative accounts—would be especially helpful here. Hurst and Zambrana's (1980) exploratory study of low-income Puerto Rican women details the women's voices as they discussed their health care needs and the barriers to their use of the health care system. At times, narrating experiences can help women formulate more clearly what they do want and why they want it. Stevens's (1992) work on marginalized women's access to medical care is a useful model for narrative analysis. Narrative accounts and case studies provide distinctive insights into the actual conditions of women's lives that may offer clues for more effective preventive or treatment efforts. For example, Lewis's (1993) sensitive case accounts of black IV drug users' perceptions of risk of AIDS uncovered beliefs about the risks of drug treatment programs (such as loss of custody of children) that deter women from enrolling. Behar's (1990, 1994) moving accounts of unwanted hysterectomies move the reader beyond seeing wombs as "unnecessary organs."

In short, better research on women's actual experiences in clinical situations and informal care contexts (rather than mythic "physician/patient" interactions which today form only a small part of health care) are sorely needed. How are women actually treated? How do they feel when medical technicians process them through mammography screening, draw blood for laboratory tests, or carry out the myriad common medical procedures today? How is the experience different for women with disabilities? for women who do not speak the language of providers? for women whose cultural background differs? What is the actual experience of being an experimental subject to test a new drug or treatment? How does social class shape this and other health care experiences?

Given the documented use of alternative therapies, studies might also profitably judge how patients are treated in such settings compared with mainstream medical institutions (More and Milligan 1994; O'Connor 1995). Eisenberg and his colleagues (1993) stunned the medical community with their national survey, which showed that adults may actually consult unconventional practitioners such as chiropractors, acupuncturists, and massage therapists as or more often than conventional primary care providers. Anecdotal evidence suggests that alternative practitioners often interact with patients in ways that are experienced as supportive and healing—and rarely found in impersonal conventional medical institutions. The appeal of lay and nurse-midwives may similarly lie in their interpersonal skills and their ability to respect the diversity of women's desires for positive birthing experiences. Taken together, the popularity of midwives and alternative practitioners strongly suggests the need for research into how diverse groups of women feel about their health and their bodies when they utilize various types of health practitioners.

In the field of mental health, where the cultural fit between patients and practitioners may be especially important, case studies of traditional healers may reveal conceptualizations of mental health and illness that are much more congruent with people's lived experience than the diagnostic categories currently used. For example, Fontenot's (1993) study of ethno-psychiatry among African Americans in rural Louisiana reveals important links between spirituality and healing that secular practitioners might attempt to grasp. For women of color and ethnic women, the constructs of psychotherapy need to be enlarged and revised to address ethnic and cultural issues that bridge the gap between the usually white middle-class world of feminist (and other) therapists and their clients who are women of color and ethnic women (Boyd 1994).

2. *The epidemiology of women's health* includes research on the distribution and causes of health and diseases among and between social, economic, and cultural groups. Epidemiologists must find new ways to study social and environmental as well as biological and behavioral risk factors in diverse groups. Socioeconomic status and race simply cannot be treated as "control" variables but must be reconstructed as important independent causes of poor health status. O'Campo and her colleagues (1995) have proposed a promising contextual analytic approach. The focus of epidemiological research needs to shift in other ways as well, to better elucidate the relations of race, sex/gender, class, and so on, which are now being reconceptualized (e.g., Krieger et al. 1993).

Ruzek and Hill (1986) have argued that new definitions of significant health problems, especially problems related to chronic illness and mental health, need to emerge in epidemiological research. The distribution of women's experience of violence (rape, assault, sexual harassment, domestic violence, war) and economic insecurity (low wages, high unemployment, threat of loss of income through divorce, widowhood, spousal disability) need to be investigated as major sources of mental and physical illness for women. A broader range of conditions than the "leading causes of death" also need to be studied in an epidemiological framework to counterbalance the dominant view that the so-called killer diseases, such as cancer and heart disease, are more "important" to control than the living and working conditions that reduce well-being over the entire life cycle.

Despite growing attention to violence prevention, an adequate epidemiology of violence for women must include the social and psychological effects of violence and perceptions of risk of violence, not just homicide rates. Although it is often argued that homicide is the "tip of the iceberg," women should ask why the whole iceberg is not being mapped. The

question is particularly pertinent given the resources being spent on map-
ping the human genome and probing for ways to motivate people to
improve personal health habits. Although genetic information and individual lifestyle choices may, but do not necessarily, lead to improved
health, changing social, psychological, and environmental conditions to
prevent or reduce occupational stress, sexual harassment, rape, domestic
violence, and economic insecurity through sociopolitical changes that
improved the status of women would surely have large payoffs in terms of
women's health and well-being (Ruzek and Hill 1986). And, as O'Campo
and her colleagues (1995) point out, a clearer understanding of which
elements of social environments are most predictive of violence against
women could lead to better targeting of resources.

There are significant policy implications of collecting a wider range
of more precise epidemiological data. Better data clarify where the burden
of ill health falls in society. Under pressure from advocacy groups, better
national data on many forms of violence are emerging. These data have
legitimated concerns and helped the American Medical Association and
the American Public Health Association redefine violence beyond being
only a criminal justice or "mental health" concern.

As prestigious groups have redefined violence as a national health
issue, public and private funding is more available to stem or ameliorate
violence. However, in some of the new programs, violence against women
is ignored or given short shrift. Richie and Kanuha (1993) point out that
racism and sexism in public health care systems themselves create barriers
to helping battered women of color. Others are concerned, for example,
that new laws which mandate that health providers report domestic violence to police, whether or not the woman involved wants it and even
without her knowledge, will make battered women less likely to seek
necessary health care and may even endanger them further. Understanding the diversity of forms of violence against women, including those
embedded in institutions ostensibly designed to help women, is essential.

Epidemiological research on the distribution and causes of disease
among and between groups of women merits further development. This is
especially true in terms of social groupings that might make sense to
women themselves. The finding that black women and their families
experience greater infant mortality and morbidity than Native American
women and families came as a surprise to some people, even in health
fields. Similarly, differences in infant mortality and morbidity *among*
Hispanic groups were unexpected by some scientists and raise important

questions about the meaningfulness and usefulness of health statistics that aggregate such diverse populations. The favorable health status of Asian American women should raise questions about how some groups generate such good health.

Potentially, more complete information on the distribution of health problems could help guide where to target health interventions to maximize health outcomes, something that is increasingly important because of cost-containment concerns. Nonetheless, "health facts" do not ensure action, nor do they in and of themselves alter negative conditions. Women need to ask hard questions about the relative benefits of investing national resources in finer and finer health statistics compared with other types of research, direct services, or social investments that might improve women's working and living conditions. Although surveillance plays an important role in public health, questions do need to be asked about the costs of improved biostatistical reporting compared with other health investments.

3. Culturally and sociodemographically specific studies of how diverse groups respond clinically to specific treatment modalities including medications, medical procedures, and devices are needed. These should include studies of "alternative therapies" provided outside of conventional medical settings. We also need to know how much clinical research is funded for addressing specific diseases or syndromes and the extent to which women with different characteristics respond to studied treatment modalities. That is, we cannot now easily determine how research that is currently funded attends to differences among women.

As Rosser (1994) points out, gender bias in clinical research currently neglects relevant research questions based on women's personal experiences. Thus research on conditions such as interstitial cystitis, a chronic bladder inflammation disorder that afflicts ten times more women than men, has been largely ignored (Webster 1994). Such oversight has, in Webster's clinical experience, resulted in women's complaints being ignored or misinterpreted. What other conditions do women suffer in silence?

Because of the historical exclusion of women from participation in clinical trials, the health sciences have failed to address many pressing issues for women. Recent changes in requirements for federally funded clinical research to include women in clinical trials came only under political pressure (Mastroianni et al. 1994a, 1994b; Oberman 1994). Some clarifications must also be added. Krieger and Fee (1994:16) challenge the popular assertion that lack of research on white women and on nonwhite racial/ethnic men and women resulted from the perception of white men as the "norm": "In fact, by the time that researchers began to standardize methods for clinical and epidemiologic research, notions of difference were so firmly embedded that whites and nonwhites, women and men, were rarely studied together. . . . For the most part, the health of women and men of color and the nonreproductive health of white women were simply ignored. It is critical to read these omissions as evidence of a logic of difference rather than as an assumption of similarity." As Narrigan and her colleagues pointed out in chapter 21, new questions must also be raised about how culture and class, region, race/ethnicity, and other characteristics of research subjects affect the efficacy of treatments. So little is known now about differential effects of treatment for different groups that it is impossible to assess how the inclusion of diverse research subjects will affect findings. In addition, differential access to medical services (because of geographic isolation or financial status) may affect the safety and efficacy of drug treatments such as RU-486 and Norplant, issues that are lost by taking evidence of risk and effectiveness established in major medical centers to represent what women will actually experience in their own communities.

With the push for standardized practice guidelines and limits on hospitalization for people being treated for specific illnesses, it is imperative that practitioners and insurers understand *variations* in effects and recovery rates to provide adequate care. In short, women need to lobby the NIH, Congress, related interest groups, and researchers themselves on the need for more diversity in studies of clinical treatments. An issue that will have to be addressed eventually is how much diversity is feasible to achieve in research given multiple demands for research resources. Questions about who benefits from research investments need to be raised by diverse groups.

The interest of the Agency for Health Care Policy Research in comparing the effectiveness of different treatment modalities and analyzing outcomes by type of medical insurance is a positive sign. It suggests that the social, not just the biological, dimensions of patient populations are finally being recognized. We suspect that one of the changes to be brought about by the restructuring of health care services and coverage will be that effectiveness of treatment will be studied more often, more appropriately, and with more adequate attention to the social factors that shape medical outcomes. At the very least, investigators are likely to report more fully on the sociodemographic characteristics of their subjects when reporting their "outcomes."

4. Access to and use of conventional and alternative health services for diverse groups of women require ongoing examination. Research on the availability and actual use of all kinds of health services to women in all life circumstances and age groups is needed. We include here what are often termed *alternative approaches* to healing as well as conventional medicine. Eisenberg and his colleagues (1993) reported considerable variation in use of unconventional practitioners by sociodemographic groups. In this study, nonblack persons (ages 25-49) who had more education and income were the major users of unconventional therapies. It should be noted that racial and ethnic minority groups, including new immigrants, native peoples, and rural African Americans have all historically used traditional healers and healing practices not likely to have been asked about by Eisenberg and his colleagues (Galanti 1991; O'Connor 1995; Snow 1993). More research on alternative practitioners used by women in all ethnic groups in both rural and urban settings would alter dominant views of what constitutes *the* American health care system. Serious study of utilization of traditional healers, as well as other less conventional therapies, would tell us how women protect and improve their health.

Also in need of study is differential access to both high- and low-technology care. Although access to maternity care has been well researched, women's access to higher technology nonreproductive services ranging from transplantation to angioplasty and cancer treatments are rarely reported by race, region, or socioeconomic status. We do not mean to assert here that such care is unproblematic or necessarily "better" in the long run than other options. We simply note that little is known about who gets what types of treatments, although there is widespread belief that wealthier people have better access to all kinds of care. Because gaps in service vary so, meaningful health reform can emerge only with a clearer view of what various women actually have.

5. Research on who is recruited and trained to provide health care is needed. We need to know how practice patterns of health providers enable female practitioners to make use of their skills and training as nurses, physicians, curanderas, spiritual healers, dentists, physical therapists, lay and licensed midwives, and pharmacists. Historians of medicine and nursing widely recognize how central gender and race are to recruitment into the health professions (Fee 1983; Hine 1985, 1989; Litoff 1990; Melosh 1982; Morantz-Sanchez 1990; Reverby 1987). But the proliferation of ancillary and allied health professions raises new questions about women's roles as health providers. Butter and her colleagues (1987) have described in detail the patterns of sex segregation in the health workforce and the structural conditions that limit women's mobility.

Additional research is needed on the actual interactions between gender, race, class, and different provider occupational groups. For example, it is important to understand how certified nurse-midwives and nurse-practitioners face practice limitations imposed by largely male medical groups who see women practitioners as unwanted competition, even in some geographical areas in which they themselves do not intend to practice. Research is needed that addresses questions about the relative effectiveness of different types of generalist and specialist practitioners, from varying backgrounds, given emerging debates over who will provide primary care to women.

There are important research questions about women physicians and obstetrician-gynecologists' roles in women's medical care. National efforts to increase the supply of primary care providers will likely result in economic incentives for professions that lay claim to this designation. In an analysis of the actual functions of primary care providers, Harrison (1994:83) argues that although physicians are assumed to be the best providers of medical care, "most primary care does not require a physician, other than for consultation and referral." Thus debates over developing a medical specialty devoted to women's health come at a time when the most cost-effective way to ensure that women have access to female primary care providers is to turn most primary care over to nurse-practitioners or perhaps multidisciplinary health practitioners. Harrison believes such primary practitioners need grounding in the social and behavioral sciences more than they need specialized biomedical skills. Such strategies would also dramatically increase the number of women of color engaged in primary care. Research on many aspects of the training, practice, and utilization of different types of primary care providers will be critical for policymaking that actually leads to improvements in women's health care.

Methods for Women's Health Research

Some of the research questions posed here can be addressed using existing methods whereas others will require innovative approaches. We are not arguing that social science researchers (who self-identify as feminist or not) need to invent all new wheels. Rather, researchers need to invent some new wheels and carefully retread some old ones to handle the complexity of women's diverse health situations. How can this be done? Multiple leads exist. For over two decades feminists have wrestled with many methodological and theoretical issues, such as the practices and ethics of interviewing (DeVault 1990; Finch and Mason 1984), the problematics of objectivity and validity (Acker, Barry, and Esseveld 1991; Lather 1988, 1995), the position of the researcher (Collins 1986), handling respondents' voices (Fine 1992; Riessman 1987), the nature of the everyday world and women's silencing (Smith 1987), hidden oppressive ideologies within method (Gorelick 1991), and the challenges of including race and class diversity in small qualitative studies (Denzin and Lincoln 1994; Weber Cannon, Higginbotham, and Leung 1991).

Some important issues in research methodologies/paths to situated knowledges in terms of women's health include starting with a conceptual understanding of how women have been universalized in health research so that future scholars do not replicate past mistakes. This history will require studies of the ways in which women and women's bodies have been universalized, totalized, homogenized to delete differences and erase the range of variations that are in fact important to understand.

Extant research categories, when deconstructed, can be replaced with categories of women's own construction. For example, Oudshoorn (1994) recently analyzed the construction of generic woman in terms of the history of contraceptive development, especially the Pill. Here one can see how women were used as research objects to construct a composite menstrual cycle that varied considerably from the experiences of individual women. Women's experiences were obscured through the concept of "woman cycles." Similarly, Rothman (1983) has shown how medical concepts such as "normal labor" have been constructed out of observations of highly medicalized, in-hospital birth experiences that bear little resemblance to the "stages of labor" observed in planned home births.

In epidemiological and survey research it will be critical to involve women scientists from widely varied backgrounds. Issues about how to classify groups and subgroups and select meaningful health indicators will only be resolved with the inclusion of a much wider array of scholars. Zambrana (1992) notes that instrument development is an area in which reconceptualizing how to study sociocultural diversity is particularly needed.

Simply translating existing instruments or using bilingual interviewers is inadequate for seriously including more diverse groups in health research. Many of the conceptualizations of health and illness or strategies for seeking health care are culturally inappropriate and fail to tap dimensions of health that are meaningful to many women outside of mainstream cultures.

To have more participatory research means involving more diverse researchers and more diverse respondents. There is an urgent need to recruit and train a wider range of women as social and behavioral scientists to facilitate the emergence of women's own frames and categories of sense making. Greater diversity of scholars will be needed to move beyond relying on a priori categories constructed by others—men or women who have not, do not, and cannot share in certain experiential realms. At the same time researchers need to be open to developing research formats where participation takes on new forms and incorporates new voices. Such research has been done occasionally (e.g., Craddock and Reid 1993; Lather 1988, 1995; Light and Kleiber 1981). These new forms challenge feminist health researchers in several ways. Genuinely participatory research leads to complicated and sometimes difficult research relationships, particularly when views of participants differ from most feminist outlooks (Hess 1990). Other scholars working in this mode note the need for careful attention to unwitting appropriation of participant-generated data for the researcher's own personal interests (Opie 1992).

More diverse perspectives and persons are needed particularly in policy-oriented research where unintended consequences of proposed policy changes are most likely to be anticipated by scholars who share common background characteristics with those populations who will be affected by the policies. Though feminist research on policy has produced insights on how policies are framed (Estes and Edmonds 1981; Petchesky 1985), the part that feminist organizations have played (Gelb and Palley 1987), women's "needs" (Fraser 1989), the state's control of women (Brown 1992), multiple issues in women's health policy—at every level from local and nongovernmental through federal—await scrutiny from feminists and other scholars who self-identify with other perspectives.

Stacey (1988) cautions that feminist research approaches should be neither romanticized nor demonized. The mandate, however, is for multiple women's voices, muted or excluded from health discourses, to be heard not only through the media of other researchers but through their own work. Critical questions abound that can be answered only through research grounded in particular women's experiences and circumstances with recognition of how the experiences came about (Scott 1991).

One of our agendas in writing and editing this volume has been to open doors to the field of women's health to a diversity of readers many of whom, we sincerely hope, will become the next generation of researchers whose work will lead to the improvement of the lives of women all over the world. The creation of new knowledge that is situated in the specific conditions of women's lives is fundamental. As feminist scholars of all methodological preferences have come to recognize, to do this necessitates the involvement of diverse women as full participants and critical interpreters of particularized contexts, not merely as inhabitors of those contexts. Just being a woman is not necessarily enough; the capacity to be aware of and to sensitively interpret differences is fundamental (Riessman 1987). The needs for more diverse respondents as well as researchers are closely linked. Weber Cannon, Higginbotham, and Leung (1991), for example, discuss how researchers must seriously extend themselves and their efforts far beyond the usual in order to recruit women of color at all for many studies. Efforts to increase diversity become even more arduous for those who do rural research, research on stigmatized women, or work that requires particularly good rapport between researchers and subjects.

Broadening the pool of researchers in terms of background experience, linguistic skills, identities, and status characteristics is critical. At times, a "one-to-one match" may be the only or best way to gain certain kinds of information—particularly subjective meanings and understandings. But it is important to recognize that in the process of broadening the pool of researchers, and thus the range of research questions likely to be addressed, heretofore "hidden" diversities will emerge and be salient, as Segura and Pesquera (1993) found in their study of labile Chicana identities. The work of Ito and her colleagues in chapter 12 underscores the range of ethnic diversity among Asian/Pacific women scholars themselves and the magnitude of difficulty of "matching" researchers with subjects in terms of particular characteristics. Sometimes emergent diversities themselves will be barriers to the research process (e.g., social class or regional ethnic differences).

As social scientists, however, at least some of us would argue that careful training and awareness of nuances of sociocultural differences can increase scholars' ability to conduct meaningful research with persons who are in fact different from themselves in significant ways. Evaluation researchers Loevy and O'Brien (1994:103), who argue that community-based focus group research can serve as "the voice of the community," argue that simplistic views on the need to match researchers and participants in all circumstances need to be rethought. They preface their methodological discussion of the conduct of focus groups by stating: "We no longer ascribe to the myth that, to conduct a successful focus group or to do an interview, the researcher must be of the same sex and race/ethnicity as the participants. The success of the focus group depends on the circumstances, the topic, the style and the approach of the researcher."

As scholars, we believe that more attention must be directed to these issues. To assume that understanding of others is unattainable beyond one's own group may underestimate the ability of some to transcend their own particularistic and ethnocentric worldviews, at least for the purpose of knowing and understanding others at a level that facilitates more adequate research, public policy, and clinical practice. At the same time, the politics of research and the needs of diverse groups to define their own research agendas and their own social realities pose a different set of issues. The long held view of feminists and others that persons who are marginal to a group may be able to see things that insiders fail to see is a theoretical and methodological concept that warrants discussion in light of current controversies over the ability of insiders and outsiders to comprehend and report on diverse women's health issues.

Whose Voices Will Define Women's Health?

All three of us, authors of this chapter and editors of this volume, are qualitative researchers, deeply embedded in interpretive symbolic interactionist and grounded theory research traditions. All of us have done (and/or still do) quantitative research. Thus when we raise the issue of enhancing the capacities of research to allow diverse women's own conceptual categories to emerge, we fully recognize how challenging—and how partial—this is likely to be.

If American society in the 1990s is highly labile, so are American feminisms where shifts and alterations reflect, as this volume has shown through the topic of women's health, emergent voices, different perspectives, and conflicts of interest and of commitment. Despite differences, in some instances very sharp differences between certain views and methodological approaches, the multiple feminisms of this era all have something to offer to those who aspire to understand women's health. The magnitude and complexity posed by issues of diversity seen in this volume, issues that are bound to increase, require multiple feminisms and multiple methodological and policy approaches if feminist and other women's health agendas are to be realized. Indeed, coming to terms with diversity and finding ways to make space for diverse women's health agendas will be a challenge for all pluralistic societies.

It is our hope that this book will open intellectual space to yet more players and more ideas. We expect that this volume itself will be surpassed by the work of others as they locate and analyze emergent issues for specific women in diverse situations. Sorting out dilemmas and contradictions in women's health and opening up dialogue on the contours of women's commonalities are sorely needed. We hope that the essays in this volume will contribute to this endeavor. We also hope that these essays, taken as a whole, provide convincing evidence that coming to understand commonalities is an enterprise that must be grounded in the experience and insights of women from widely divergent backgrounds. Embracing and elaborating differences are necessary steps toward genuinely addressing our differences, something that we must do to find real common grounds.

NOTE

Susan Reverby and Mira Katz made particularly helpful comments on an earlier draft of this chapter.

REFERENCES

Acker, J., K. Barry, and J. Esseveld
    1991   "Objectivity and truth: problems in doing feminist research." Pp. 119-32 in M. M. Fonow and J. A. Cook (eds.), Beyond Methodology: Feminist Scholarship as Lived Research. Bloomington: Indiana University Press.

Bair, Barbara, and Susan E. Cayleff, eds.
    1993   Wings of Gauze: Women of Color and the Experience of Health and Illness. Detroit: Wayne State University Press.

Behar, Ruth
    1990   "The body in the woman, the story in the woman: a book review and personal essay." Michigan Quarterly Review 29(4):694-738.

1994 "My Mexican friend Marta, who lost her womb on this side of the border." Pp. 129-38 in Alice J. Dan (ed.), Reframing Women's Health: Multidisciplinary Research and Practice. Thousand Oaks, CA: Sage.

Bleier, Ruth
1984 Science and Gender: A Critique of Biology and Its Theories on Women. New York: Pergamon.

Boyd, Julia A.
1994 "Ethnic and cultural diversity in feminist therapy: keys to power." Pp. 226-34 in Evelyn C. White (ed.), The Black Women's Health Book, rev. ed. Seattle: Seal Press.

Brown, Wendy
1992 "Finding the man in the state." Feminist Studies 18:7-34.

Butter, Irene H., Eugenia S. Carpenter, Bonnie J. Kay, and Ruth Simmons
1987 "Gender hierarchies in the health labor force." International Journal of Health Services 17(1):133-49. Reprinted in Elizabeth Fee and Nancy Krieger (eds.), Women's Health, Politics, and Power: Essays on Sex/Gender, Medicine, and Public Health. Amityville, NY: Baywood, 1994.

Collins, Patricia Hill
1986 "Learning from the outsider within: the sociological significance of black feminist thought." Social Problems 33:14-32.

Craddock, E., and Margaret Reid
1993 "Structure and struggle: implementing a social model of a well woman clinic in Glasgow." Social Science and Medicine 19:35-45.

Denzin, Norman K., and Yvonna S. Lincoln
1994 Handbook of Qualitative Research. Newbury Park, CA: Sage.

DeVault, Marjorie
1990 "Talking and listening from women's standpoint: feminist strategies for interviewing and analysis." Social Problems 37:96-116.

Dziech, Billie Wright
1993 "The bedeviling issue of sexual harassment." Chronicle of Higher Education, 8 December, A48.

Ehrenreich, Barbara, and Deirdre English
1979 For Her Own Good: 150 Years of the Experts' Advice to Women. Garden City, NY: Anchor Press/Doubleday.

Eisenberg, David M., Ronald C. Kessler, Cindy Foster et al.
1993 "Unconventional medicine in the United States: prevalence, costs, and patterns of use." New England Journal of Medicine 328(4):246-52.

Estes, Carroll, and Beverly Edmonds
1981 "Symbolic interaction and social policy analysis." Symbolic Interaction 4:75-86.

Fee, Elizabeth, ed.
1983 Women and Health: The Politics of Sex in Medicine. Amityville, NY: Baywood.

Finch, Janet, and Jennifer Mason
    1984   "It's great to have someone to talk to." Pp. 7–87 in Colin Bell and Helen
            Roberts (eds.), Social Researching: Politics, Problems, Practice. London:
            Routledge and Kegan Paul.
Fine, Michelle
    1992   "Passions, politics and power: feminist research possibilities." Pp. 205–32
            in Michelle Fine (ed.), Disruptive Voices. Ann Arbor: University of
            Michigan Press.
Fontenot, Wonda Lee
    1993   "Madame Neau: the practice of ethno-psychiatry in rural Louisiana." Pp.
            41–52 in Barbara Bair and Susan E. Cayleff (eds.), Wings of Gauze.
            Detroit: Wayne State University Press.
Fraser, Nancy
    1989   "Struggle over needs: outline of a socialist-feminist critical theory of late
            capitalist political culture." Pp. 161–87 in her Unruly Practices: Power,
            Discourse, and Gender in Contemporary Social Theory. Minneapolis:
            University of Minnesota Press.
Galanti, Geri Ann
    1991   Caring for Patients from Different Cultures: Case Studies from American
            Hospitals. Philadelphia: University of Pennsylvania Press.
Gelb, Janet, and Marion Lief Palley
    1987   Women and Public Policies. Princeton, NJ: Princeton University Press.
Gill, Carol J.
    1994   "Becoming visible: personal health experience of women with disabili-
            ties." Paper presented to the National Institutes of Mental Health. May.
            A revised version of this paper will appear in Danuta Krotoski, Margaret
            Nosek, and Margaret Turk (eds.), The Health of Women with Physical
            Disabilities: Setting a Research Agenda for the Nineties. Baltimore:
            Brookes (in press).
Gorelick, S.
    1991   "Contradictions of feminist methodology." Gender and Society 5:459–77
Haraway, Donna
    1991   "Reading Buchi Emecheta: contests for 'women's experience' in women's
            studies." Pp. 109–26 in her Simians, Cyborgs, and Women: The Rein-
            vention of Nature." London: Routledge.
Harding, Sandra
    1986   The Science Question in Feminism. Ithaca, NY: Cornell University Press.
Harrison, Michelle
    1994   "Women's health: new models of care and a new academic discipline."
            Pp. 79–92 in Alice J. Dan (ed.), Reframing Women's Health: Multidis-
            ciplinary Research and Practice. Thousand Oaks, CA: Sage.
Hess, Beth
    1990   "Beyond dichotomy: drawing distinctions and embracing differences."
            Sociological Forum 5:75–94.

Hill, Shirley A.
    1994   Managing Sickle Cell Disease in Low-Income Families. Philadelphia: Temple University Press.
Hine, Darlene Clark
    1985   Black Women in the Nursing Profession. New York: Garland.
    1989   Black Women in White: Racial Conflict and Cooperation in the Nursing Profession, 1890-1950. Bloomington: Indiana University Press.
Hubbard, Ruth
    1990   The Politics of Women's Biology. New Brunswick, NJ: Rutgers University Press.
Hurst, Marsha, and Ruth E. Zambrana
    1980   "The health careers of urban women: a study in East Harlem." Signs 5:3 (suppl.):S112-S126.
Krieger, Nancy, and Elizabeth Fee
    1994   "Man-made medicine and women's health: the biopolitics of sex/gender and race/ethnicity." Pp. 11-29 in Elizabeth Fee and Nancy Krieger (eds.), Women's Health, Politics, and Power: Essays on Sex/Gender, Medicine, and Public Health. Amityville, NY: Baywood.
Krieger, Nancy, D. Rowley, A. Herman, B. Avery, and M. Phillips
    1993   "Racism, sexism, and social class: implications for studies of health, disease, and well-being." American Journal of Preventive Medicine 9(6 suppl.):82-122.
Lather, Patti
    1988   "Feminist perspectives on empowering research methodologies." Women's Studies International Forum 11:569-81.
    1995   "The validity of angels: interpretive and textual strategies in researching the lives of women with HIV/AIDS." Qualitative Inquiry 1(1):41-68.
Lewis, Diane K.
    1993   "Living with the threat of AIDS: perceptions of health and risk among African American women IV drug users." Pp. 312-27 in Barbara Bair and Susan E. Cayleff (eds.), Wings of Gauze. Detroit: Wayne State University Press.
Light, Linda, and Nancy Kleiber
    1981   "Interactive research in a feminist setting." Pp. 167-84 in Donald A. Messerschmidt (ed.), Anthropologists at Home in North America: Methods and Issues in the Study of One's Own Society. Cambridge: Cambridge University Press.
Litoff, Judy Barrett
    1990   "Midwives and history." Pp. 435-50 in Rima Apple (ed.), Women, Health, and Medicine in America: A Historical Handbook. New Brunswick, NJ: Rutgers University Press.
Loevy, Sara Segal, and Mary Utne O'Brien
    1994   "Community-based research: the case for focus groups." Pp. 102-10 in Alice J. Dan (ed.), Reframing Women's Health: Multidisciplinary Research and Practice. Thousand Oaks, CA: Sage.

Mastroianni, Anna C., Ruth Faden, and Daniel Federman, eds.
   1994a   Women and Health Research: Ethical and Legal Issues of Including
            Women in Clinical Studies. Vol. 1. Institute of Medicine. Washington:
            National Academy Press.
   1994b   Women and Health Research: Ethical and Legal Issues of Including
            Women in Clinical Studies. Vol. 2, Workshop and Commissioned Pa-
            pers. Institute of Medicine. Washington: National Academy Press.
Melosh, Barbara
   1982   The Physician's Hand. Philadelphia: Temple University Press.
More, Ellen Singer, and Maureen A. Milligan, eds.
   1994   The Empathic Practitioner: Empathy, Gender, and Medicine. New Bruns-
            wick, NJ: Rutgers University Press.
Morantz-Sanchez, Regina
   1990   "Physicians." Pp. 469–88 in Rima Apple (ed.), Women, Health, and
            Medicine in America: A Historical Handbook. New Brunswick, NJ:
            Rutgers University Press.
Oberman, Michelle
   1994   "Real and perceived legal barriers to the inclusion of women in clinical
            trials." Pp. 266–76 in Alice J. Dan (ed.), Reframing Women's Health:
            Multidisciplinary Research and Practice. Thousand Oaks, CA: Sage.
O'Campo, Patricia, et al.
   1995   "Violence by male partners against women during the childbearing years:
            a contextual analysis." American Journal of Public Health 85:1092–97.
O'Connor, Bonnie Blair
   1995   Healing Traditions: Alternative Medicine and the Health Professions.
            Philadelphia: University of Pennsylvania Press.
Olesen, Virginia
   1994   "Feminisms and models of qualitative research." Pp. 158–74 in Norman
            K. Denzin and Yvonne S. Lincoln (eds.), Handbook of Qualitative Re-
            search. Newbury Park, CA: Sage.
Olesen, Virginia, and Ellen Lewin
   1985   "Women, health, and healing: a theoretical introduction." Pp. 1–24 in
            Ellen Lewin and Virginia Olesen (eds.), Women, Health, and Healing:
            Toward a New Perspective. London: Tavistock-Methuen.
Opie, Ann
   1992   "Qualitative research, appropriation of the 'other' and empowerment."
            Feminist Review 40:52–69.
Oudshoorn, Nelly
   1994   Beyond the Natural Body: An Archaeology of Sex Hormones. New York:
            Routledge.
Petchesky, Rosalind
   1985   "Abortion in the 1980s: feminist morality and women's health." Pp.
            139–73 in Ellen Lewin and Virginia Olesen (eds.), Women, Health, and
            Healing: Toward a New Perspective. London: Tavistock-Methuen.

Reinharz, Shulamit
    1992   Feminist Methods in Social Research. Oxford: Oxford University Press.
Reverby, Susan
    1987   Ordered to Care: The Dilemma of American Nursing, 1850-1945. Cambridge: Cambridge University Press.
Richie, Beth E., and Valli Kanuha
    1993   "Battered women of color in public health care systems: racism, sexism, and violence." Pp. 288-99 in Barbara Bair and Susan E. Cayleff (eds.), Wings of Gauze. Detroit: Wayne State University Press.
Riessman, Catherine Kohler
    1983   "Medicalization of women's health." Social Policy 14:3-18.
    1987   "When gender is not enough: women interviewing women." Gender and Society 2:172-207.
Rodgers-Rose, La Frances
    1994   Health Research Priority Setting Conference, 23-24 September 1994, Newark, NJ. International Black Women's Congress.
Rosser, Sue V.
    1988   "Women in science and health care: a gender at risk." In S. V. Rosser (ed.), Feminism within the Science and Health Care Professions: Overcoming Resistance. Elmsford, NY: Pergamon.
    1994   "Gender bias in clinical research." Pp. 253-65 in Alice J. Dan (ed.), Reframing Women's Health: Multidisciplinary Research and Practice. Thousand Oaks, CA: Sage.
Rothman, Barbara Katz
    1983   "Midwives in transition: the structure of a clinical revolution." Social Problems 30:262-71.
Ruzek, Sheryl, and Jessica Hill
    1986   "Positive approaches to promoting women's health: redefining the knowledge base and strategies for change." Health Promotion 1(3):301-9.
Scott, Joan
    1991   "The evidence of experience." Critical Inquiry 17:773-79.
Segura, Denise, and Beatriz Pesquera
    1993   "Chicana political consciousness: cultural good girls, white, middle-class wannabees and soldaderas." Paper presented at the University of California Women's Studies Conference on the Feminist Future, Lake Arrowhead. November.
Smith, Dorothy
    1987   The Everyday World as Problematic. Boston: Northeastern University Press.
Snow, Loudell F.
    1993   Walkin' over Medicine. Boulder, CO: Westview Press.
Stacey, Judith
    1988   "Can there be a feminist ethnography?" Women's Studies International Forum 11:21-27.

Stevens, P. E.
  1992   "Lesbian health care research: a review of the literature from 1970 to
          1990." Health Care for Women International 13(2):91-120.
Tuana, Nancy
  1993   "With many voices: feminism and theoretical pluralism." Pp. 281-89 in
          Paula England (ed.), Theory on Gender, Feminism on Theory. New York:
          Aldine de Gruyter.
Weber Cannon, Lynn, Elizabeth Higginbotham, and M. L. A. Leung
  1991   "Race and class in qualitative research on women." Pp. 107-18 in M. M.
          Fonow and J. A. Cook (eds.), Beyond Methodology: Feminist Scholarship
          as Lived Research on Women. Bloomington: Indiana University Press.
Webster, Denise C.
  1994   "Tension and paradox in framing interstitial cystitis." Pp. 377-85 in Alice
          J. Dan (ed.), Reframing Women's Health: Multidisciplinary Research and
          Practice. Thousand Oaks, CA: Sage.
Zambrana, Ruth E.
  1987   "A research agenda on issues affecting poor and minority women: a model
          for understanding their health needs." Women and Health 12(3-4):137-
          60.
  1992   "The relationship between use of health care services and health status:
          dilemmas in measuring medical outcome in low-income racial/ethnic
          populations." Pp. 103-14 in Mary L. Grady and Harvey A. Schwartz
          (eds.), Medical Effectiveness Research Data Methods. AHCPR Pub. No.
          92-0056. Rockville, MD: Agency for Health Care Policy Research.

Contributors

Brandy M. Britton, Ph.D., is assistant professor of sociology at the University of Maryland, Baltimore County. Her research has focused on violence against women, the battered women's movement, women's political activism, women's drug use, and HIV/AIDS among women. Currently, she is working with other faculty in her department to develop a specialty track for graduate students in women's health. She is also principal investigator for a grant sponsored by the University of Maryland that examines the roles of incest, rape, and partner violence in the onset of drug and alcohol problems and risky HIV practices among women.

Rita Chi-Ying Chung, Ph.D., received her Ph.D. in psychology in New Zealand and was awarded the Medical Research Council (MRC) Fellowship for postdoctoral work abroad. She was the former project director for the National Research Center on Asian American Mental Health at the University of California, Los Angeles, and was recently a visiting professor in the psychology and psychiatry departments at the Federal University of Rio Grande Do Sul in Brazil. She has written extensively on Asian and refugee mental health and has worked in the Pacific Rim, Asia, and Latin America. Currently, she is an adjunct professor at the Johns Hopkins University.

Adele E. Clarke, Ph.D., is associate professor of sociology and of the history of health sciences at the University of California, San Francisco. Her work centers on cultural studies of science, technology, and medicine with special emphasis on common medical technologies that affect most women's health such as contraception. Published works include *The Right Tools for the Job: At Work in Twentieth-Century Life Sciences,* coedited with Joan Fujimura, (Princeton, 1992, and Synthelabo Press, Paris, 1996). Her book *Disciplining Reproduction: American Life Scientists and the "Problem of Sex"* is forthcoming (University of California, 1997); she is also coediting, with Virginia Olesen, *Revisioning Women, Health and Healing: Cultural, Feminist and Technoscience Perspectives* (Routledge, 1997). Her current project is a book on qualitative research methods, "New Directions in Grounded Theory," emphasizing cartographic and positional approaches, including social worlds analysis.

Christine Dunkel-Schetter, Ph.D., received her Ph.D. in social psychology from Northwestern University and with a National Science Foundation fellowship conducted postdoctoral research at the University of California, Berkeley. She is currently professor of psychology and director of the Health Psychology Program at the University of California, Los Angeles. She oversees a program of research on psychological and social risk factors in pregnancy and effects on birth outcomes. She has published extensively on stress, coping, and social support. Her publications also include a coedited book on infertility, research on coping with breast cancer, and papers on stress and social support processes in pregnancy and birth.

Carroll L. Estes, Ph.D., is director of the Institute for Health and Aging, and professor of sociology in the Department of Social and Behavioral Sciences, School of Nursing, University of California, San Francisco. She is president elect of the Gerontological Society of America (1995-96), vice president for the National Older Women's League, and past president of the American Society on Aging and the Association for Gerontology in Higher Education. Her many honors and awards include the Distinguished Scholarship Award, Pacific Sociological Association; the American Society on Aging Award; the Helen Nahm Research Award; the Faculty Research Lecturer Award at the University of California, San Francisco; the Donald P. Kent Award, Gerontological Society of America; and the Beverly Award, Association for Gerontology in Higher Education. Two recent coedited books are *The Nation's Health* (4th ed., Jones and Barlett, 1994) and *Health Policy and Nursing: Crisis Reform in the U.S. Health Care Delivery System* (Jones and Bartlett, 1994), and one pending is "The Political Economy of Health and Aging."

Julia Faucett, Ph.D., R.N., is an academic faculty member in the Department of Community Health Systems, School of Nursing, University of California, San Francisco. She is director of the Occupational Health Nursing Program of the Center for Occupational and Environmental Health, a multidisciplinary and multicampus graduate education and research program. Her research focuses on musculoskeletal disorders in the workplace, which she is studying in newspaper, public service, manufacturing, and agricultural settings.

Nikki V. Franke, Ed.D., is an associate professor at Temple University. She received M.Ed. and Ed.D. in health education from Temple University. She is coordinator of the community health field placement program for the Department of Health Education. She is on the board of directors of the Health Promotion Council and the Black Women in Sport Foundation. Her primary areas of research are health issues in the black community and sports nutrition.

Carol J. Gill, Ph.D., is a clinical and research psychologist specializing in health and disability. Her professional positions have included director of rehabilitation psychology at Glendale Adventist Medical Center and commissioner on mental health for the Los Angeles County Commission on Disabilities. She is currently president of the Chicago Institute of Disability Research, adjunct assistant professor of Physical Medicine and Rehabilitation at Northwestern University Medical School, and research chair of the Health Resource Center for Women with Disabilities in Chicago. She teaches, conducts research, publishes widely in professional journals and books as well as the disability press, and identifies proudly as a woman with a disability.

Maxine Jo Grad is an attorney, women's health activist, and mediator. She is a director of the National Women's Health Network, a Washington, D.C., based consumer organization. Her areas of concentration are breast cancer and reproductive health. She is also a governor's appointee to the Vermont Governor's Commission on Women and served a three-year term on the Vermont Victim's Compensation Board. She teaches at Woodbury College in Montpelier, Vermont. She advocates that women will be provided with current and accurate information upon which they can make their own health care choices. Maxine lives in Vermont with her husband and their two daughters.

Tina Hancock is associate professor in the School of Social Work, University of South Florida, Tampa. She holds a doctoral degree in clinical social work from the University of Alabama and an M.S.W. from the University of North Carolina, Chapel Hill. She teaches human behavior and the social environment and clinical practice to graduate social work students and has published articles on single-parent families.

Elizabeth Higginbotham, Ph.D., is associate director of the Center for Research on Women and professor of sociology and social work at the University of Memphis. Her publications have appeared in *Gender and Society, Women's Studies Quarterly,* and in many edited collections. The chapter here is one of many selections from the project, "Social Mobility, Race, and Women's Mental Health." This study, a collaboration with Lynn Weber, is a broad investigation of the role of upward mobility in the educational experiences, work life, family life, well-being, and mental health of two hundred black and white professional and managerial women in the Memphis area.

Karen L. Ito, Ph.D., is assistant research anthropologist at the Neuropsychiatric Institute, Division of Social Psychiatry, University of California, Los Angeles, and senior research associate for LTG Associates, Inc. She has conducted research on health care alternatives of Asian American women in southern California, cultural behavior and concepts of pregnancy among Mexico-born mothers in San Diego, cultural barriers and tuberculosis among Vietnamese Americans in Orange County, reproductive decision making in the highlands of Papua, New Guinea, and cultural constructions of illness and self among native Hawai'ians in Hawai'i. Her book *The Ties that Define: Metaphor, Morality, and Aloha among Urban Hawai'ians* (Cornell) is forthcoming.

Vida Yvonne Jones, Ph.D., is principal administrative analyst for the Institute for Health and Aging and lecturer for the Department of Social and Behavioral Sciences, School of Nursing, University of California, San Francisco. She directs the education and training activities of the institute and is responsible for the coordination of key institute administrative activities. She has done research on the management of systemic lupus erythematosus, a complex chronic illness affecting mainly women. Her research interests include issues related to chronicity, women, and the informal support and housing of the minority elderly. She received her Ph.D. from the University of California, San Francisco.

Marjorie Kagawa-Singer, Ph.D., R.N., M.N., is a nurse-anthropologist and assistant professor in the School of Public Health and the Asian American Studies Center at the University of California, Los Angeles. At UCLA she earned her master's degree in nursing and her master's and doctorate in anthropology. She has published on issues in cross-cultural health care and has lectured extensively on the influence of culture on patient and family responses to chronic diseases as well as on the dynamics involved in multicultural staff interactions.

Lora Bex Lempert, Ph.D., is assistant professor of sociology at the University of Michigan, Dearborn. Her published works include "The Line in the Sand: Definitional Dialogues in Abusive Relationships" in *Studies in Symbolic Interaction* and "A Narrative Analysis of Abuse" in the *Journal of Contemporary Ethnography*. Her current research focuses on African American grandparents raising adolescent grandchildren.

Ann Metcalf, Ph.D., is associate professor of anthropology at Mills College in Oakland, California. She received her Ph.D. from Stanford University and for the last two decades has worked with American Indian programs in the San Francisco Bay area. Most recently, she has done needs assessment and evaluation research at a Native American substance abuse treatment center for Indian women and their children.

Deborah Narrigan is a certified nurse-midwife and educator in women's health and midwifery. She was a member of the board of directors of the National Women's Health Network from 1988–94. While on the board, she collaborated on the position paper that is the basis for the coauthored chapter in this book.

Virginia L. Olesen, Ph.D., is professor of sociology (emerita) in the Department of Social and Behavioral Sciences, School of Nursing, at the University of California, San Francisco, where she continues to teach and do research in women's health issues and qualitative methods. Publications include *Culture, Society, and Menstruation*, edited with Nancy Fugate Woods (Hemisphere, 1986), *Women, Health, and Healing: Toward A New Perspective*, edited with Ellen Lewin (Tavistock, 1985), and essays on estrogen replacement therapy, toxic shock, women's occupational health, aging and professional women, definitions of success among professional women, sociology of emotions, and issues in fieldwork methods.

Judy M. Perry, R.N., M.S.N., is assistant professor of community health nursing at Berea College. She is presently a doctoral student in sociology at the University of Kentucky, where her research area is women's health and Appalachian studies. She is currently focusing on a sociohistorical analysis of fertility patterns and the birth control movement in Kentucky. Since 1988 she has been involved in program development and training of indigenous lay health workers in rural Appalachia, working with Appalachian Communities for Children, the Kentucky Homeplace Project, and the Central Highlands Appalachian Leadership Initiative on Cancer.

Cheri A. Pies, Dr.P.H., M.S.W., is associate director of the Maternal and Child Health Program at the School of Public Health, University of California, Berkeley. Her writing, teaching, and advocacy are focused on ethical, social, and political issues in reproductive health and contraceptive technologies. Her publications include articles on lesbian parenting, Norplant and other long-acting contraceptives, and ethical issues related to women, HIV, and pregnancy, and the book *Considering Parenthood* (Aunt Lute, 1988). She also coedits *Face to Face: A Guide to AIDS Counseling.*

Sally Pickels. Upon learning about the Victim Input Program, I realized that I had the power to possibly influence the decision of the parole board regarding the fate of the perpetrator of the crime against me. I didn't feel very confident about the legal system because of my past experiences, but in my heart I knew that I had to do something. I could no longer allow my fears of the system and the perpetrators to control me—I had to act! I made up my mind that I was going to participate in the Victim Input Program. No matter what the outcome of the legal procedures, I could not fail: if parole was denied, I would be victorious; if granted, it would be because the system had failed. After making my decisions, I finally admitted that my life had been a charade for twenty-one years. I needed professional help to deal with this turmoil, so I contacted Women Organized Against Rape and started therapy. I wrote the piece included here to share with other victims/survivors that we do have power to influence the system. We do have the right to survive. We can take back control. Although the crime has changed our lives, we can learn to incorporate it into our lives and start to live again. We have that right!

Helen Rodriguez-Trias, M.D., F.A.A.P., is a pediatrician, a consultant on health programming, and a longtime activist for health rights, particularly for women and children. After seven years in academic medicine at her alma mater, the University of Puerto Rico's School of Medicine, she directed pediatric programs in several major hospitals in New York and New Jersey, while teaching at the pediatric departments of the Albert Einstein College of Medicine, Columbia University's College of Physicians and Surgeons, the University of Medicine and Dentistry of New Jersey, and the Department of Social Medicine at Montefiore. She was also medical director at the AIDS Institute in New York, a division of the New York State Department of Health. During the past three years she has served on the executive board of the American Public Health Association and been its president elect, president, and immediate past president. She is a member of several boards of national organizations addressing health inequities, most notably, the National Women's Health Network.

Sheryl Burt Ruzek, Ph.D., M.P.H., is professor of health education and affiliated professor of women's studies at Temple University, Philadelphia. She has written and edited numerous books and articles on women's health issues. An updated version of her 1978 study, *The Women's Health Movement: Feminist Alternatives to Medical Control,* is in preparation. She is also currently working on issues related to women, health advocacy, and national health reform. She has been an advisor and consultant to many local, state, and national organizations, including the U.S. FDA Obstetrics and Gynecology Devices Panel. She chairs the ECRI/WHO Collaborating Center on Technology Transfer Committee on Women's Health Medical Technologies and lectures widely on women's health.

Susan C. M. Scrimshaw, Ph.D., is currently dean of the School of Public Health and professor of community health sciences and anthropology at the University of Illinois, Chicago. She was raised in Guatemala and has worked extensively in Latin

America. She has conducted a series of ten research projects focusing on family planning and fertility decision making, improving pregnancy outcomes, child survival programs, and on culturally appropriate delivery of health care. She was president of the National Society for Medical Anthropology in 1985, is a member of the Institute of Medicine, and is a fellow of the American Association for the Advancement of Science. The 1985 Margaret Mead Award is one of many honors she has received. Recently, she was appointed to the Chicago Board of Health by Mayor Richard Daley.

Nancy E. Stoller, Ph.D., is professor of community studies and sociology at the University of California, Santa Cruz. She has published widely in the area of women's health, with special emphasis on the health of women in prison, lesbians, and the AIDS epidemic, including *Women Resisting AIDS: Feminist Strategies of Empowerment,* coedited with Beth Schneider (Temple, 1995). She is currently completing a new book on AIDS community organizing, "Lessons from the Damned: Queers, Whores, and Junkies Respond to AIDS."

Diana L. Taylor, Ph.D., R.N., N.P., F.A.A.N., is associate professor of nursing in the Department of Family Health Care Nursing, School of Nursing, University of California, San Francisco. She has focused much of her clinical and research work on understanding the biopsychosocial and lifespan factors that affect the health and illness of women within the context of cyclic changes across the menstrual cycle. With Nancy Fugate Woods she is the coeditor of *Menstruation, Health and Illness: Neuroendocrine, Sociocultural and Clinical Perspectives* (Hemisphere, 1991), and she is the principal investigator of an NIH-funded study of the effectiveness of nonpharmacological treatments for women's symptom experience. As part of an interdisciplinary collaborative effort, she is developing a new model of women's health that will both guide research efforts and provide a curriculum for educating women's health providers.

Beatrice von Schulthess, Ph.D., M.P.H., received her doctoral degree from the Department of Social and Behavioral Sciences at the University of California, San Francisco. She received her M.P.H. degree in health education from the School of Public Health at the University of North Carolina, Chapel Hill. Her research and activist interests include violence against women, hate crimes, lesbian health, and women's health policy.

Lynn Weber, Ph.D., director of the Center for Research on Women at the University of Memphis, was on leave for the 1995–96 academic year as visiting distinguished professor of gender studies in the Department of Sociology at the University of Delaware. She is coauthor of *The American Perception of Class* (Temple, 1987). Her recent work focuses on race, class, and gender in the social mobility process. She and Elizabeth Higginbotham codirect a research project, "Social Mobility, Race, and Women's Mental Health," which is a broad investigation of the role of upward mobility in the educational experiences, work life, family life, well-being, and mental health of two hundred black and white professional managerial women in the Memphis area.

Deborah L. Wingard, Ph.D., received her doctoral degree in epidemiology from the School of Public Health at the University of California, Berkeley. She has achieved national and international recognition for her research and educational efforts in the areas of women's health (particularly, gender differences in morbidity, mortality, and lifestyle), diabetes, and the long-term effects of exposure to DES. She is currently professor of epidemiology in the Department of Family and Preventive Medicine at the University of California, San Diego, where she is a mentor for medical students, doctoral students, and junior faculty (especially women).

Nancy Worcester, University of Wisconsin-Madison's women's studies outreach specialist, regularly teaches women's health courses (to four hundred students a semester!), coordinates and teaches a wide range of community-based women's studies courses throughout Wisconsin, and coordinates the Wisconsin Domestic Violence Training Project for School and Health Professionals. She was a founding member of the Women's Health Information Center in Britain and has served eight years on the National Women's Health Network Board. Worcester is the coeditor, with Mariamne H. Whatley, of two editions of *Women's Health: Readings on Social, Economic, and Political Issues* (Kendall/Hunt).

Ruth E. Zambrana, Ph.D., is Encochs Professor and director of the Center for Child Welfare of the Human Services Program at George Mason University in Fairfax, Virginia. She has conducted research for the past fifteen years on the health of low-income Latino/Hispanic women, children, and families, with a special focus on maternal and child health. She has published extensively on issues related to health education, employment, and research methodology among low-income women of color. Her most recent edited book is *Understanding Latino Families: Scholarship, Policy and Practice* (Sage, 1995).

Jane Sprague Zones, Ph.D., is a medical sociologist in the Department of Social and Behavioral Sciences, School of Nursing, University of California, San Francisco. She has been a member of the board of directors of the National Women's Health Network since 1988, and chair of the board from 1993 to 1996. A women's health policy advocate, she is and has been a consumer representative on various Food and Drug Administration scientific advisory panels, including, currently, the Fertility and Maternal Health Drugs Advisory Committee.

Index

ableism, 97, 98
Ablon, Joan, 293
abortion: access versus quality control in, 59–61; Campaign for Abortion and Reproductive Equity, 75; defective fetuses issue, 78; differential access to, 61–62; Hyde Amendment, 61–62; supercoil procedure, 60; terrorism against providers of, 82
abuse: of African American women, 372–73; drugs and risk of child abuse, 363; of women with disabilities, 103–4. *See also* domestic violence; sexual abuse
access to service, 183–230; achieving, 207–10; to behavioral assistance, 139; to birth control, 54; to contraceptives, 527–28; differential access, 61–62; diminishment of, 183–84; for marginalized people, 452, 618; MY-PAP controversy, 64–66; versus quality control, 59–61; rationing health resources, 206–7; research on required, 623; for rural women, 79; social diversity and, 590–91; universal access, 206, 207; wider access requiring reductions elsewhere, 613
accidents, motor vehicle. *See* motor vehicle accidents

accreditation of prison health care, 462–63
activism. *See* health activism; political activism
Adams, Diane L., 248
administrative control in occupational health, 165–66
advocacy organizations, 4, 608, 615, 620
aerosols, 268
African American women, 353–79; abortion access for, 61; abuse of, 372–73; Afrocentric definition of personal health behavior, 126, 143n. 15; in agriculture, 178; AIDS in, 360, 373–74, 464; Alpha Kappa Alpha sorority health projects, 71; alternative treatments used by, 623; "Black Is Beautiful," 258; breast cancer in, 195, 323n. 9, 591; cancer incidence and survival rates for, 34; cancer mortality rates for, 32, 323n. 9, 359–60; career and marriage as goals of, 388; cervical cancer screening, 214n. 41; child-rearing stress in, 373; and children's sickle cell disease, 617; classism affecting health status of, 353, 375; color prejudice in, 254–55, 261; commitment to community of, 388; coping strategies for

Sanger, Margaret, 85n. 16, 523,
538nn. 4, 6
San Jose Indian Alcoholics Anonymous, 293
Schaefer, James M., 288
Scherr, Racquel L., 257
science: feminists on, 560-61; gender and class bias in, 553, 562,
615; women in academic, 560,
562. See also research; social and
behavioral sciences
screening, 193-97; Appalachian
women questioning, 236; for
breast cancer, 195-96; for cervical
cancer, 194, 195, 214n. 41; clinical breast examinations, 194, 195;
controversies surrounding, for
breast cancer, 193-97; errors in,
193, 214n. 35; guidelines that
treat all women alike, 193-94; as
marketing tool, 194-95; overuse
of, 183, 193; underuse of, 183;
varying by race and ethnicity,
194. See also mammography; Pap
smear
Scully, Diana, 496, 498n. 4
Seaman, Barbara, 138, 145n. 38,
211n. 5, 216n. 62, 539n. 9
Seaman, Gideon, 539n. 9
secondary prevention, 613
Segura, Denise, 627
Self-Determination policies for Native Americans, 290, 291-92
self-worth (self-esteem): beauty and,
253-55; in mental health, 384-85;
power and, 390; psychiatry for
maintaining, 263
servants, domestic, 414n. 3, 430
service, access to. See access to service
services, health. See health services
Seventh Day Adventists, 129
sewing machine operators, ergonomic
hazards for, 155, 157, 158, 161

sex: life expectancy and, 35; mortality and, 35. See also gender
sexism: African American women's
health affected by, 353, 375; competition between women in, 254;
and contraceptives, 526; personal
health behavior in context of,
126; in public health system, 620;
and sterilization, 524; in the workplace, 391
sexual abuse: culturally appropriate
programs for, 321; of Southeast
Asian refugees, 317-18, 319
sexual assault. See rape
sexual harassment, 510-19; consequences of, 514; contrapower harassment, 512; coping strategies for,
515; by drug treatment counselors,
513; in educational institutions,
512-13; Anita Hill, 390, 510-11,
517; hostile work environment as,
511; by landlords, 513; legislation
addressing, 516; in medical
schools, 410, 415n. 12; of men,
512; by physicians, 513-14; power
as key to, 511; responses to, 514-
15; retaliation against women who
file complaints, 516; retaliation
feared by women who protest, 511;
suing the harasser, 515-16; Tailhook incident, 513; Clarence
Thomas, 390, 510-11; types of,
511; victim's perception of, 517n.
1; of women in prison, 513; of
women in the military, 513; in the
workplace, 511-12
sexuality: efforts to impose conservative values on, 129; regulation of
female, 128; study of adolescent,
131. See also sexual orientation
sexual orientation: bisexual women's
health issues, 78-79; and experience of harassment, 514; as factor

Women and Health Series

RIMA D. APPLE AND JANET GOLDEN, EDITORS

The series examines the social and cultural construction of health practices and policies, focusing on women as subjects and objects of medical theory, health services, and policy formulation.

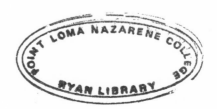

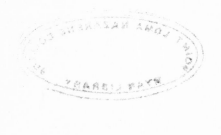